Operative Dentistry

Modern Theory and Practice

Operative Dentistry
Modern Theory and Practice

M. A. Marzouk D.D.S., M.S.D.
Professor and Head, Operative Dentistry,
Director, Graduate Program of Restorative Dentistry,
Washington University, School of Dental Medicine

A.L. Simonton D.D.S.
R.D. Gross D.D.S.
Clinical Assistant Professors, Operative Dentistry
Washington University, School of Dental Medicine

FIRST EDITION

Illustrated

Ishiyaku EuroAmerica, Inc.
St. Louis · Tokyo · 1985

Ishiyaku EuroAmerica, Inc./Dental Series

Series editor: Monika E. Strong, D.D.S.
Book editor: Harry James Cargas, Ph.D.
Illustrations: Dr. Al Chu & Marcie Hartstein
Index: Charles M. Kodner

FIRST EDITION

Ishiyaku EuroAmerica, Inc.
11559 Rock Island Court, St. Louis, Missouri 63043

Library of Congress Catalog Card Number

84-062369

ISBN: 0-912791-15-2

Composition and design: Graphic World, St. Louis, Missouri
Printed by: CBP Press, St. Louis, Missouri

Dedicated to our wives and children
for their patience and support,
and to all our former students,
without whose encouragement and class participation
as we started putting our original notes together
this book would not have been possible.

Acknowledgement

Our deepest gratitude is owed to our dear friend, Mrs. Svetlana Schuster, secretary in the Department of Operative Dentistry. Her untiring efforts on behalf of this text are in large measure responsible for the project's fruition. Her secretarial skill and intelligent advice, as well as her constant encouragement, will never be forgotten.

A special debt of gratitude also goes out to our publisher, Manuel L. Ponte. His sincere and enthusiastic belief in our manuscript was an inspiration to us from the very beginning.

Appreciation is also to be expressed to Dr. Al Chu and to Miss Marcie Hartstein. Dr. Chu's early technical drawings served to inspire Miss Hartstein's artistic talents, bringing to life the hundreds of illustrations that are an integral part of this text.

We are indebted to Dr. A. H. El-Kafrawy, Professor, Department of Oral Diagnosis and Medicine, Indiana University School of Dentistry, for his masterful contributions to chapter one. He is, indeed, an esteemed academician.

Finally, a heartfelt ''thank-you'' goes to our beloved and much-respected colleagues in the Department of Operative Dentistry, Washington University School of Dental Medicine. Without their dedication to the department's goals and their untiring efforts in maintaining the challenges of its enormous day-to day activities, we would never have been able to even consider, let alone complete, this work.

Preface

The stimulus to write this book originated from the students with whom I have been associated during 25 years of teaching in six dental schools. In the innumerable continuing education courses that I have given over the span of those years, I have been able to see many of my former students, and, invariably, these practitioners have encouraged me to formalize my teachings into a written text. If, indeed, my educational efforts have contributed to the success of my former students, then it is my sincere hope that this textbook will serve to help many others with whom I hereby share whatever knowledge I possess.

Even though Operative Dentistry is the oldest of the dental sciences, advances and developments within the last ten years have drastically changed the scope of this subject. Breakthroughs in the science of dental materials, biology of the pulp and the periodontium, preventive dentistry, occlusion and the technology which correlates these fields, have revolutionized the process of formulating a biologically, cariogenically, and mechanically sound single-tooth restoration. This book capitalizes on these breakthroughs, and tries to utilize them in every detail. Despite all the advances, however, the original work of G. V. Black, in 1898, remains unchallenged as the baseline upon which further information in the field has been built. I hope this will be obvious throughout this text.

Chapter one is an introductory chapter, detailing the definitions, objectives, nomenclature, and principles of modern Operative Dentistry. Considerable explanation is given for the mechanical, cariogenic, and biologic basis for the single tooth restoration. The contribution by Dr. A. H. El-Kafrawy in this chapter is commendable. A real effort is made to emphasize details in the text through graphic and clinical illustrations.

Chapter two details the classification, nomenclature, use and care of operative instrumentation. Hopefully, the accompanying illustrations will simplify this information for both the student and the clinician. Rather than single-out individual functions for each instrument, several modes of use were described so that practitioners will be able to assemble their tray set-ups according to their preference.

Chapter three brings to light the complexities of the oral environment, and attempts to elucidate general solutions to those problems which interfere with control of the operating field. It is hoped that the information contained herein will enable the reader to formulate a personalized procedure to achieve that control.

Chapter four is a necessary prerequisite to chapters five through seven, as it details the latest advances in amalgam technology. Hopefully, the mass of new information contained here will assist the practitioner, as well as the student, in making intelligent choices of amalgam materials to suit their individual needs.

Although chapters five, six and seven are entitled "Tooth Preparations for Amalgam," the basic preparation designs described in these chapters may be modified as necessary to suit other restorative materials. The mechanical problems (especially occlusal loading and its effect) are explained in great detail in these three chapters. Their cause and effect explanations are not confined to amalgam restorations only, but rather can be applied to all other restorative modalities. Because of newer generations of amalgam and preparation instrumentation, new designs of tooth preparation have been made possible; these are thoroughly explored in these chapters. The basic facts concerning the designing of tooth preparations enumerated in these chapters are a necessary prerequisite to more advanced application of this data in Chapters Nine, Eighteen and Twenty-six.

Chapters eight, nine and ten are devoted to Direct Tooth-Colored Restorations, with great emphasis given to the composite resins. During the process of writing the manuscript for this book (1978-1984), these were the chapters that required the most frequent alterations, due to the rapidly advancing science of these materials. It is hoped that the procedures and designs of tooth preparation described in these chapters can accommodate the expected future developments in this subject.

Chapter eleven deals in great detail with pins and posts as retaining means for restorations. Special emphasis is given to possible misuses of these modalities, and a comprehensive effort is made to present atraumatic technics in tooth preparations, and restorative designs for pins and posts.

Chapter twelve is devoted entirely to an extremely important, and often overlooked, aspect of restorative dentistry, namely contacts and contours. The subject was presented from anatomic, physiologic, and pathologic points of view. Any available technology aimed at fulfilling the objectives of this subject is thoroughly explored.

Chapters thirteen and fourteen complement one another, especially when approached in sequence. Chapter thirteen deals with the material science, biology and pathology of Intermediary Basing Materials and Procedures, with special emphasis on preservation of the physiologic integrity of the pulp-dentin organ. Chapter fourteen deals with deep carious lesions, both from a diagnostic and a therapeutic point of view. It is hoped that the reader, after thoroughly digesting these two chapters, will be able to make an intelligent choice of an intermediary base material for any situation that may arise.

Chapter fifteen emphasizes the compatibility of operative procedures and materials with the investing periodontium. It is hoped that the physical, mechanical and histological details presented in this chapter will enable the operator to gain a newer respect for periodontal tissues and for the interrelationship between these tissues and operative procedures.

Chapter sixteen culminates the previous three chapters and deals with the compatibility of operative procedures with the entire stomatognathic system.

Chapters seventeen through twenty-five are devoted to cast restorations, from "indications," to "construction," to "cementation." The text is not confined here to discussing only traditional gold alloy restorations. Rather, four additional materials, including cast-mouldable ceramics are thoroughly detailed. Considerable effort was made to describing tooth preparation designs to accommodate newer developments in this constantly changing field. These chapters also include a section on full veneer crowns because of the popularity of this procedure as a single tooth restoration.

Chapter twenty-six is devoted to direct gold restorations. Despite the traditional nature of this restorative modality, a real effort was made here to simplify procedures in the technique in order to enable more general practitioners to undertake these restorations. It is my belief that the time-proven quality and durability of this therapy will bring direct gold back into the mainstream of operative procedures.

Chapter twenty-seven is devoted to a newly expanding area in operative dentistry, namely the restoration of non-carious lesions in teeth. With increasing awareness of control measures for dental caries decreasing its incidence, there has been a corresponding increase in the diagnosis of non-carious destructive processes. This chapter discusses classification, diagnosis, and chemical and mechanical therapy for these lesions. The chapter concludes with a discussion of trauma, its classification and therapeutic solutions.

Chapter twenty-eight ties together information from all previous chapters in the discussion of restoration of badly broken down teeth. There are complex correlations in this chapter which will enable the student and practitioner to develop the proper "designing mentality" to incorporate previously presented knowledge in successfully handling complicated restorative situations.

This text, then, may be likened to a ladder which ascends from the simple to the complex. With a solid foundation in basic operative principles, this ladder will carry the reader to new horizons in knowledge of operative dentistry. This, indeed, has been my goal, both as an educator and as an author. I feel the ladder is steady but steep; yet, with determined steps from rung to rung, the reader should arrive first with an appreciation that operative dentistry is a complex and demanding science, and second, with the knowledge and skill commensurate with its demands.

M. A. Marzouk

Contents

CHAPTER 1

Principles of operative dentistry

Definition of Operative Dentistry

At one time, the term "operative dentistry" included *all* dental services for patients. This is not difficult to understand, since most dental treatment can be considered as "operations" that are delivered in a dental operating room or "operatory". However, since the appearance and recognition of dental specialties, the scope of operative dentistry has been reduced to the restoration of natural teeth. Thanks to refined techniques, sophisticated instruments and expanded knowledge, the term "operative dentistry" can now be defined as the diagnosis, prevention and treatment of defects of natural teeth. These defects may be dental decay, erosion, abrasion, attrition, hypoplasia, hypocalcification, discoloration and trauma. It is estimated that today's general dental practitioner spends 60-80% of his time dealing with such defects and utilizing the techniques of modern operative dentistry.

The functions and purposes of operative dentistry are actually derived from the definition itself:

I. Diagnosis

Proper diagnosis of lesions, including their locations and extent, is vital for planning the method of treatment, including the design of the tooth preparation and the selection of restorative materials and procedures.

II. Prevention

The ultimate goal of any dental practitioner should be disease prevention; therefore every step of an operative procedure must emphasize this. For example, the location of the margins of a tooth preparation and the shape (contour) of the final restoration are designed to prevent any recurrence of the causative diseases and their defects.

III. Interception

This procedure in operative dentistry refers to preventing further loss of tooth structure by stabilizing an active disease process.

IV. Preservation

Preservation of the vitality and important anatomy in remaining sound tooth structure are of utmost importance and this principle should prevail in every procedure in operative dentistry.

V. Restoration

The ultimate goal of operative dentistry treatment should be the restoration of health. This will include restoring form, function, phonetics, esthetics, and occlusal stability to not only the teeth themselves, but also to their surrounding tissues and to the entire stomatognathic system. Restorative treatments should be systematically compatible with and conducive to the welfare of the whole patient. Such techniques necessitate scientific and artistic knowledge, as well as manual skills, if this ultimate goal is to be achieved.

Dental Caries

This is the disease that dentists deal with more than 90% of the time in operative dentistry. A brief discussion of the dynamics, predisposing factors, theories of cariology, the signs and symptoms, and classification of decay is in order.

According to the *acidogenic* theory, dental decay is caused by acids produced by microbial enzymatic action on ingested carbohydrates. These acids will decalcify the inorganic portion

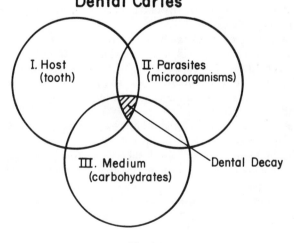

The General Mechanism of Dental Caries

Fig. 1-1

of the teeth; then the organic portion is disintegrated, creating cavities. The *proteolysis* theory, on the other hand, claims that the organic portion of the tooth is attacked first with certain lytic enzymes. This leaves the inorganic portion without a matrix support, causing it to be washed away, creating cavities. In a third theory, *microbiotic secretions*, or metabolic products of microorganisms, have the ability to chelate calcium from tooth substances, leaving the organic matrix to be disintegrated. Each of these theories fails to explain all ramifications of the disease, but all three agree on the following.

For the decay process to be established there must be (Fig. 1):

    I. Host (tooth)
   II. Parasites (plaque microorganisms)
  III. Medium, (carbohydrates in the diet)

I. The Host

In discussing the caries triad, the host is an essential element; it encompasses the tooth, salivary factors, muscular activity, habits, group susceptibility, age, and environment. The tooth, itself, is the primary host factor, but its composition, morphological characteristics, and locations influence the caries process. In terms of composition, it has been proven that the caries susceptibility of a tooth is inversely proportional to its fluorine, calcium and tin contents (Fig. 2). With regard to morphological characteristics, one must recall one of G.V. Black's contributions to dentistry, namely the definition of the relative self-cleansability of certain tooth surfaces. Imagining a bolus of food on the occlusal or incisal surface of a tooth, the areas on the tooth surface where the food can stagnate are considered non-self-cleansable; conversely, the areas on the tooth surface where the food is moving continuously are considered self-cleansable.

The bolus of food on the occlusal surface of a molar or premolar (Fig. 3) can move in three possible directions. The first direction (Fig. 4) is toward the pits and fissures where stagnation can occur. The second direction (Fig. 5) is toward the contact areas and gingival embrasures, via the occlusal, buccal and lingual embrasures, with the possibility of stagnating in the contact area, the area of near approach, and/or the gingival embrasure. The third direction (Fig. 6) is toward the facial or lingual sulcus with the possibility of stagnating there, and on the tooth surface apical to the height of contour (point of maximum convexity or the cervical ridge) of the facial or lingual surfaces.

In anterior teeth there can be similar directions of movement as in posterior teeth, with the exception that food boli will move onto the incisal surfaces (Fig. 7A). However, food boli will move both to the gingival embrasures (Fig. 7B) as well as to stagnating areas on the facial and lingual surfaces (Figs. 8 and 9).

Pits and fissures on the tooth surfaces are frequently devoid of enamel protection. Food and plaque stagnation at the pulpal extent of these defects, as a result of the first direction of movement could start a caries process that directly invades the underlying dentin.

Therefore, G. V. Black concluded that the following areas on the tooth surface are relatively non-self-cleansable:

    a. Pits and fissures (Fig. 10)

    b. Contact areas (Fig. 11, A and B)
    c. Area of near approach (Fig. 11, A and B)
    d. Gingival embrasures (Fig. 12)
    e. Facial or lingual surfaces apical to the cervical ridge (Figs. 13 and 14)

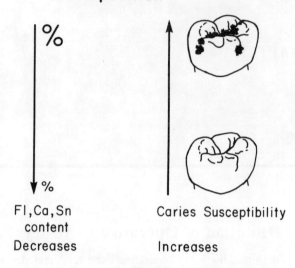

I. Composition

%

%

Fl, Ca, Sn content Decreases

Caries Susceptibility Increases

Fig. 1-2

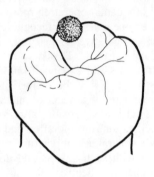

Fig. 1-3

1st direction of movement

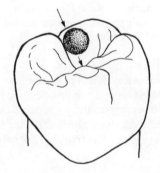

Fig. 1-4

2nd direction of movement

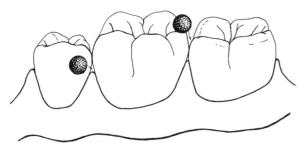

Fig. 1-5

3rd direction of movement

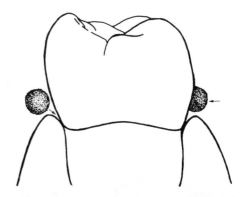

Fig. 1-6

1st direction of movement

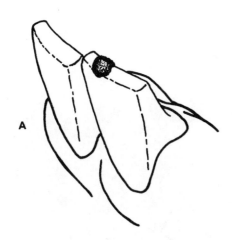

2nd direction of movement

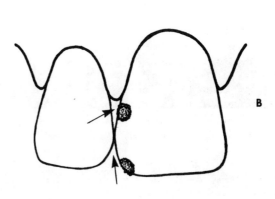

Fig. 1-7

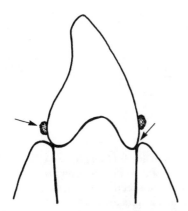

3rd direction of movement
(mandibular)

Fig. 1-8

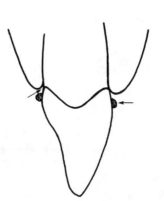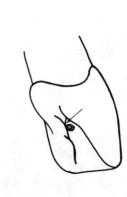

3rd direction of movement
(maxillary)

Fig. 1-9

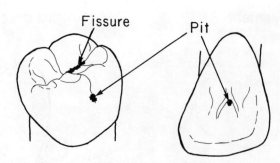

Fig. 1-10

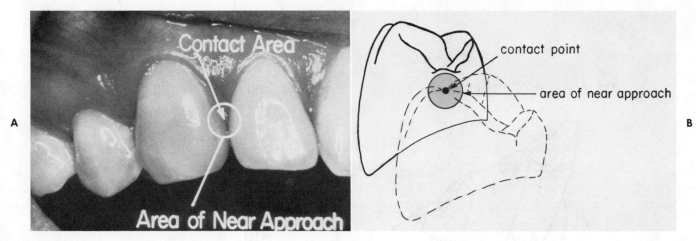

Fig. 1-11

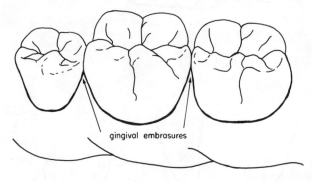

Fig. 1-12

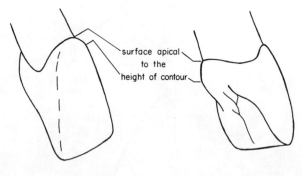

Fig. 1-13

In contrast, the following areas on the tooth are relatively self-cleansable:

a. Tips of cusps (Fig. 15)

b. Crests of marginal and crossing ridges (Fig. 15)

c. All inclined planes of cusps and ridges (Fig. 15)

d. Occlusal, incisal, facial and lingual embrasures (Figs. 16 and 17)

e. Facial or lingual surfaces incisal or occlusal to the height of contour with the exception of pits, if present (Figs. 18 and 19)

f. Axial angles of teeth (Figs. 18 and 19)

Finally, with regard to the location and alignment of teeth, the closer the posterior teeth are to the ramus (vertical portion of the mandible), the greater is the probability of food accumulation there, with a concomittant greater difficulty in cleansing them. Therefore, they will be more susceptible to decay (Fig. 20).

Malalignment of teeth, causing improper contacts and occlusal relationships, will render some (otherwise self-cleansable) areas non-self-cleansable.

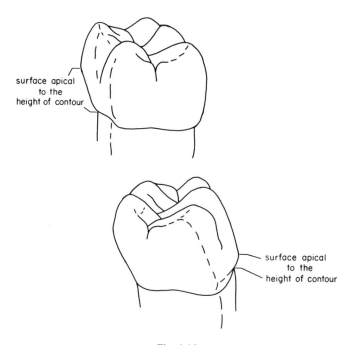

surface apical
to the
height of contour

surface apical
to the
height of contour

Fig. 1-14

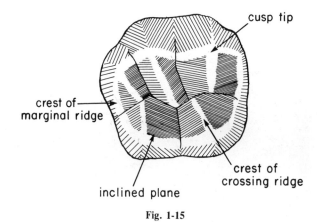

cusp tip

crest of
marginal ridge

crest of
crossing ridge

inclined plane

Fig. 1-15

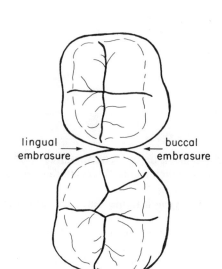

lingual
embrasure

buccal
embrasure

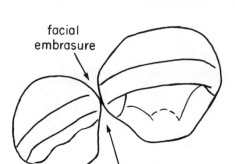

facial
embrasure

lingual embrasure

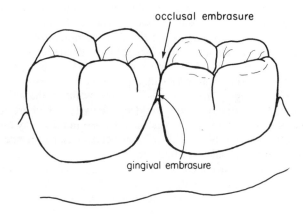

occlusal embrasure

gingival embrasure

Fig. 1-16

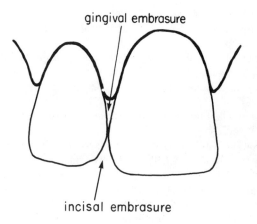

gingival embrasure

incisal embrasure

Fig. 1-17

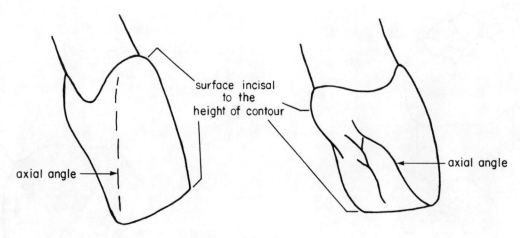

Fig. 1-18

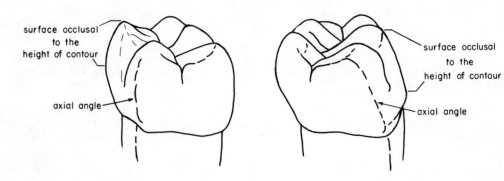

Fig. 1-19

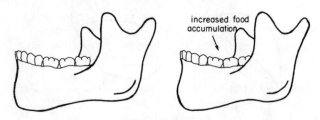

Fig. 1-20

Saliva is the second major item in the host portion of the caries formula. The following are the salivary factors involved:

1. Composition

Caries susceptibility is usually inversely proportional to salivary phosphate content. Also, higher organic content in the saliva generally indicates more stable plaque formulation.

2. pH

Higher alkaline saliva predisposes to less decay activity.

3. Viscosity

Serous saliva (low viscosity) predisposes to more self-cleansability than mucinous (high viscosity) saliva.

4. Flow

Higher quantities of saliva flowing in the oral cavity predisposes to less decay activity.

5. Antibacterial elements

Although these are usually found in saliva, their anticariogenecity depends on their nature, concentration, and amounts.

6. Antibody elements

Certain immunological activities have recently been identified in the saliva.

Host musculature (Fig. 21) i.e., activities of the tongue, cheeks, lips, and muscles of the face will create and guide the self-cleansing activities within the oral cavity. Likewise, certain host habits will enhance caries activity (e.g., poor eating habits, such as desserts and snacks, bruxism, etc.); others will discourage caries activity (e.g., disciplined oral hygiene and good eating, i.e., no snacks between meals).

With regard to group susceptibility of the host, it has been shown that females are more susceptible to decay than males (teeth erupt earlier). Also, more civilized societies incur a greater susceptibility to caries than primitive societies.

The age (Fig. 22) of the host, is significant in the caries process. Generally speaking, the decay activity is highest between the ages of 14 and 20 years. A decline in the decay rate after age 20 may be due to an enhanced conscientiousness about proper diet and oral hygiene.

The host's environment is the final influencing factor. The phosphate content of food and water, and especially the fluoride content of water, will definitely diminish the caries activity.

up to here is most emphasized in manual.

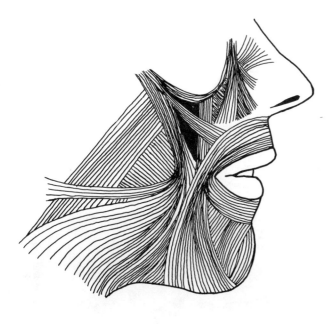

Musculature

Fig. 1-21

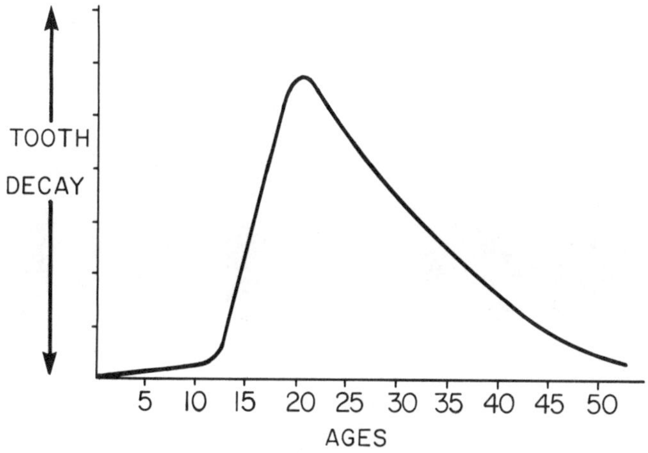

TOOTH
DECAY

5 10 15 20 25 30 35 40 45 50
AGES

Fig. 1-22

II. Parasite

The second part of the caries triad consists of the microorganisms brought into contact with the tooth surface via a bacterial plaque, thereby creating a classic parasitic relationship. The plaque is formed primarily of microorganisms, but other components are salivary glyco-proteins and inorganic salts. The plaque adheres to the tooth surface with a sticky polysaccharide carbohydrate called Dextrane. The parasite portion of the caries formula is not clearly understood, but the streptococcus mutant is thought to play a major role in the adhesion (production of Dextrane) and production of certain chemicals necessary for tooth cavitation.

III. Medium

It is well established that decay is the disease of higher civilization, and that modern diet is the third major factor in the initiation and progress of the decay process. There have been three detrimental changes in modern diets as compared to primitive diets. First, protective factors are deleted from food materials during harvesting, processing, storage and/or preparation, e.g., phytates (an organic phosphate). Second, cariogenic factors are added to food materials, e.g., refined carbohydrates such as sucrose, fructose, lactose, and glucose. Third, the frequency of meals, usually three, with between meal snacks, is a routine not experienced by primitive man.

Physical as well as chemical characteristics of a diet determine its relative cariogenecity. As an example of the influence of physical characteristics, harder and more fibrous food material necessitates increased masticatory activity and, consequently, greater ability for cleaning the teeth surfaces of any stagnating debris.

With regard to the influence of chemical characteristics, carbohydrates are known to be the most cariogenic of all food materials. Sucrose is the most detrimental, followed by fructose, lactose, galactose, and glucose. Increasing the fluoride content of a diet will decrease caries activity by decreasing the solubility of tooth structure, decreasing the surface energy of tooth surfaces, thereby discouraging plaque adhesion, and by interfering in the metabolism of carbohydrates by the microorganisms. Increasing the phosphate content in a diet will decrease the solubility product of the tooth substance in the surrounding electrolytes, thereby discouraging inorganic tooth substance solubility. Finally, vitamins may improve the uptake of fluoride, some improving calcification of tooth structure, and others being anticariogenics (e.g., vitamin K).

Classification of Decay

There are nine schemes for the classification of carious lesions. The use of these classification schemes is based upon the clinical, radiographic, and histologic appearance of the carious process, and in some instances, the involvement of a particular type of a tooth, group of teeth or a tooth surface.

The classification schemes vary in their popularity and complexity, i.e., some are more specific and detailed than others. It is certainly possible (and perhaps desirable) to utilize elements of several schemes in describing a particular carious lesion.

1. An *incipient* (Fig. 23, A and B), *initial*, or *primary carious lesion* is one that describes the first attack on a tooth surface. A *recurrent* (Fig. 24, A and B) or *secondary lesion* is one observed under or around the margins or surrounding

Incipient Caries

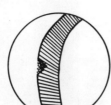

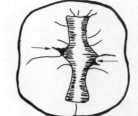

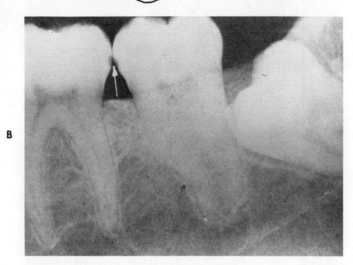

Fig. 1-23

Recurrent Caries

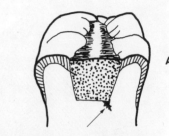

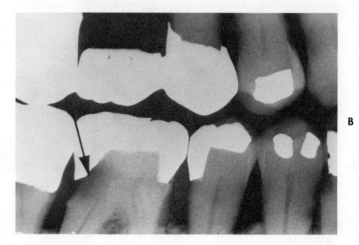

Fig. 1-24

walls of an existing restoration. Interproximal margins of a proximal restoration not involving all of the contact area, incompletely involved pits and fissures, and areas near fractured surfaces are common sites of recurrent decay.

2. *acute* or *rampant* caries (Fig. 25) is a rapidly invading process that usually involves several teeth. The lesions are soft and light-colored and are frequently accompanied by severe pulp reactions. *Chronic carious lesions* (Fig. 26) are of variable depth, longer standing, and tend to be fewer in number. The dentin in the latter lesions is hard in consistency and dark in color. Usually, the color, consistency, odor, age, duration, and pulp reaction are used to differentiate between acute and chronic decay.

3. *Pit and fissure* carious *lesions* (Fig. 27) are those originating in the pits and fissures found on the lingual surfaces of maxillary anterior teeth and on the buccal, lingual, and occlusal surfaces of posterior teeth. *Smooth-surface* carious *lesions* (Fig. 28) are those originating in all surfaces without pits, fissures, or grooves.

4. The "forward-backward" classification of decay can be considered as a graphical representation of the pathway of dental caries. The first component of the enamel to be involved in the carious process is the interprismatic substance. The disintegrating chemicals will proceed via this substance, causing the enamel prisms to be undermined (Fig. 29). The resultant caries involvement in enamel will have a cone shape. In concave surfaces (pits and fissures) the base of this cone will be toward the DEJ (Fig. 30), while in convex surfaces (smooth

surfaces) the base of this cone will be away from the DEJ (Fig. 30). The first component to be involved in the dentin is the protoplasmic extension within the dentinal tubules. These protoplasmic extensions have their maximum spacing at the DEJ, but as they approach the pulp chamber and the root canal walls, the tubules become more densely arranged with fewer interconnections. One can, therefore, imagine that caries cones in dentin will have a cone shape with the base of the cone toward the DEJ (Fig. 30).

Decay starts in enamel, and then it involves the dentin. Wherever the caries cone in enamel is larger or at least the same size as that in dentin, it is called *forward decay* (pit decay in Fig. 30). However, the carious process in dentin progresses much faster than it does in enamel, so the cone in dentin tends to spread laterally, depriving the enamel of its dentin support, i.e., creating undermined enamel. In addition, the decay can attack the enamel from its dentinal side. At this stage, therefore, it becomes *backward decay* (smooth surface lesion in Fig. 30 and lesions in Fig. 31).

5. The so called "*senile carious lesions*" (Fig. 32, A and B) are those associated with the aging process. They are located almost exclusively on the root surfaces of the teeth, but sometimes they are associated with partial denture clasps. In all situations they follow advanced gingival recession.

6. *Residual caries* is that which is not removed during a restorative procedure, either by accident (Fig. 33, A and B), neglect or intention. Sometimes a small amount of acutely carious dentin close to the pulp is covered with a specific

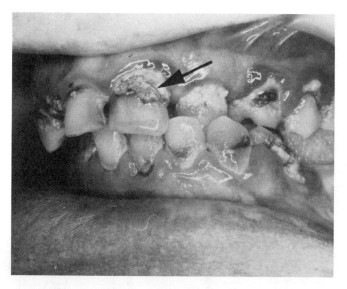

Fig. 1-25

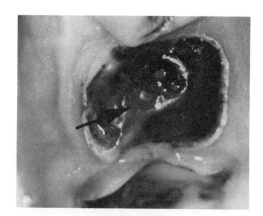

Fig. 1-26

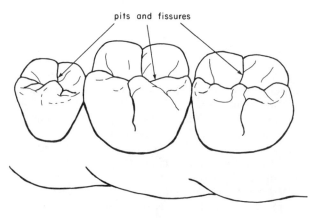

Fig. 1-27

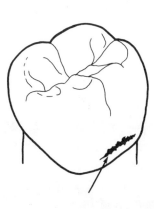

Smooth Surface

Fig. 1-28

Fissural Undercuts

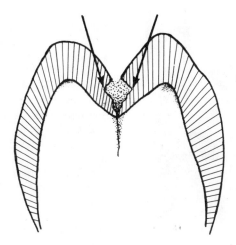

Fig. 1-29

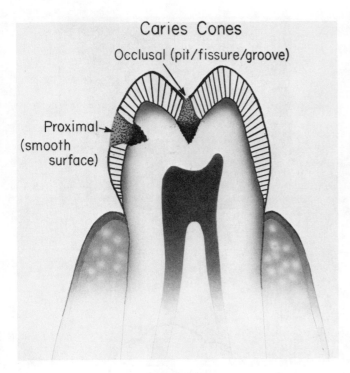

Fig. 1-30

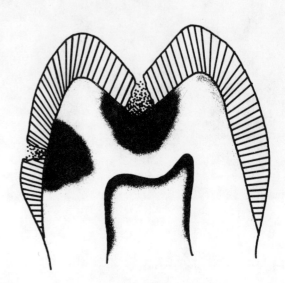

Fig. 1-31

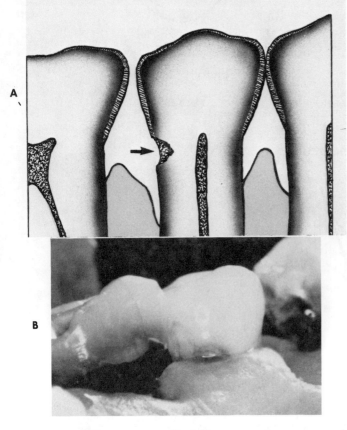

Fig. 1-32

capping material to stimulate reparative dentin deposition, isolating caries from the pulp. The carious dentin can be removed at a later time (Fig. 33A).

7. *A simple carious lesion* (Figs. 34 and 35A) is one that involves only one surface of the tooth. *A compound carious lesion* involves two surfaces of a tooth (Figs. 34B and 35B) and a *complex carious lesion* (Figs. 34C and 35C) involves three or more tooth surfaces.

8. G.V. Black's classification of caries is based on treatment and restoration design, i.e., it is a therapeutic classification.

Class I lesions (Fig. 36, A and B) begin in structural defects of teeth, such as pits, fissures, and sometimes defective grooves. They usually have three locations: the occlusal surfaces of molars and premolars, the occlusal two-thirds of the buccal and lingual surfaces of molars, and the lingual surfaces of anterior teeth.

Class II lesions (Figure 37, A and B) are found on proximal surfaces of bicuspids and molars.

Class III lesions (Fig. 38, and B) are found on proximal surfaces of anterior teeth that do not involve or necessitate removal of the incisal angle.

Class IV lesions (Fig. 39, A and B) are found on the proximal surfaces of anterior teeth and involve or require the removal and restoration of the incisal angle(s).

Class V lesions (Fig. 40, A and B) are found at the gingival third of the facial and lingual surfaces of anterior and posterior teeth.

Class VI lesions (Fig. 41) were not originally included in Black's classification. They are found on incisal edges and cuspid tips. They are also found on molar and premolar cusp tips, axial angles of teeth, or any highly self-cleansable areas. They usually start in a traumatic or a formative defect.

9. The classification scheme enjoying the most wide spread clinical utilization employs the initials of the surfaces to be

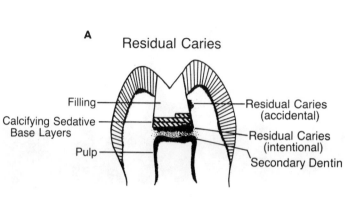

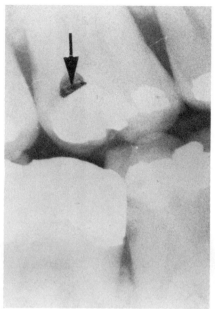

Fig. 1-33

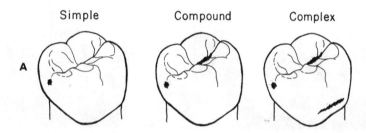

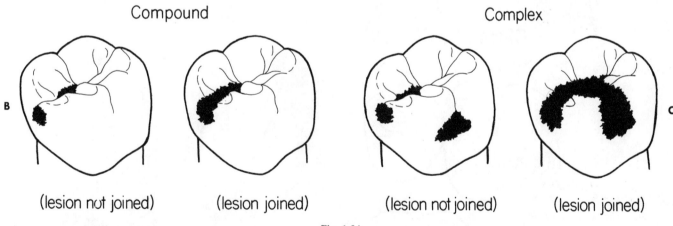

Fig. 1-34

treated, in order to describe the surfaces to be restored (Fig. 42).

O—for occlusal surfaces
M—for mesial surfaces
D—for distal surfaces

F—for facial surfaces
B—for buccal surfaces
L—for lingual surfaces

Various combinations are also possible, such as MOD—for mesio-occluso-distal surfaces.

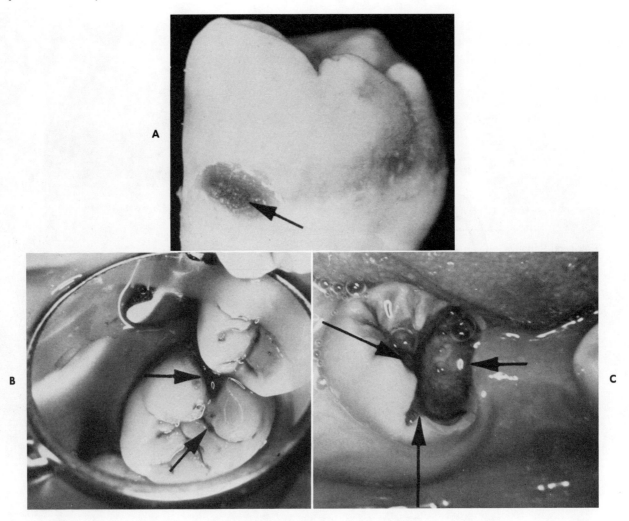

Fig. 1-35

Class I (G.V.Black)

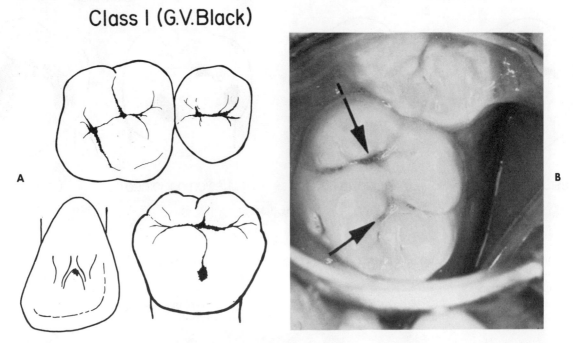

Fig. 1-36

Class 2 (G.V.Black)

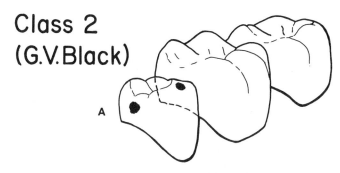

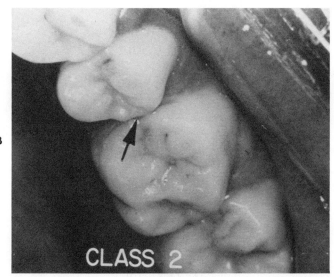

Fig. 1-37

Class 3 (G.V.Black)

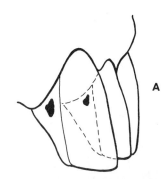

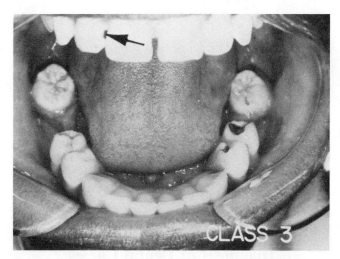

Fig. 1-38

Class 4 (G.V.Black)

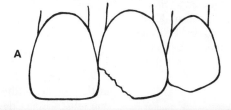

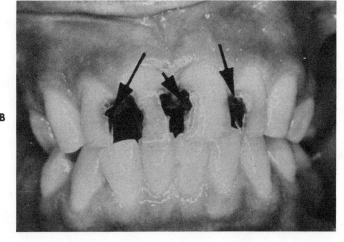

Fig. 1-39

Class 5 (G.V.Black)

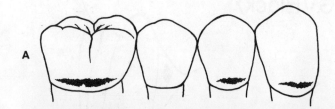

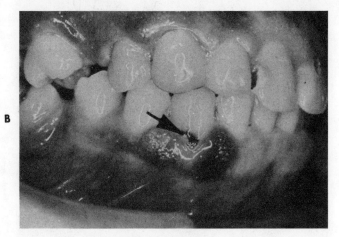

Fig. 1-40

Class 6 (G.V.Black)

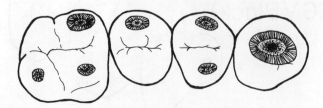

Fig. 1-41

Tooth Surfaces

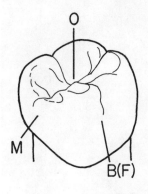
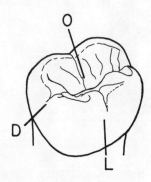

O - Occlusal
M - Mesial
B(F) - Buccal (Facial)
D - Distal
L - Lingual

Fig. 1-42

Diagnosis of Dental Caries

I. Explorers

A sharp new explorer will have a diameter of 200 microns at its tip. Pressing this tip into pits and fissures with forces parallel to the blade will cause it to penetrate the enamel and/or dentinal caries cone, making a definitive diagnosis of decay. A blunt explorer will not do this. Some interproximal carious lesions can be similarly detected by interproximal explorers. Facial and lingual lesions can be easily penetrated by an explorer, affirming diagnosis based on direct vision.

II. Radiographs (Fig. 43)

Bitewing-type radiographs are especially diagnostic for proximal decay, in which the caries cones appear radiolucent. However, the extent of the caries cone cannot be definitely defined by the radiographs. In fact, the extent that is apparent in the film is usually less than the actual decay. Radiographs are not reliable to detect occlusal, facial, or lingual decay, although the lateral spread of the dentinal caries in occlusal lesion cases can be observed at the DEJ in a radiograph.

III. Discoloration

When observed in pits and fissures, discoloration should make one suspicious of decay. However, this is not true in every case, for in older persons most of the surface enamel defects are filled with leathery brown (dark brown) organic material. Frequently, the investing enamel is quite sound. On the other hand, observing a grey hue in a marginal ridge should create a suspicion of a proximal cavity under that ridge.

IV. Patient Complaints

Whenever sweets, hot, cold, or any item that changes osmatic pressure within the dentin causes subjective complaints, one must suspect dentinal involvement of a carious lesion.

V. Dental Floss or Tape (Fig. 44)

If floss is inserted through a contact area and then dragged occlusally in a sawing action against one proximal surface causing it to fray and shread, we must suspect a cavity on this proximal surface, provided that there is no proximal calculus or overhanging restoration margin present.

VI. Separation of Teeth (Fig. 45)

Using a wood or plastic wedge or a mechanical separator, or simply the operator's thumb nail, one might visualize whether or not a contacting tooth proximal surface does have a cavity.

VII. Translumination (Fig. 46)

When a light source is located lingually while the teeth are viewed from a facial direction, one may see the shadow of the caries cone through the enamel.

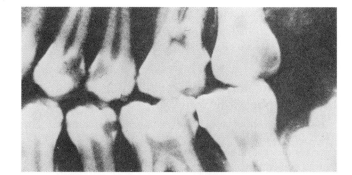

Fig. 1-43

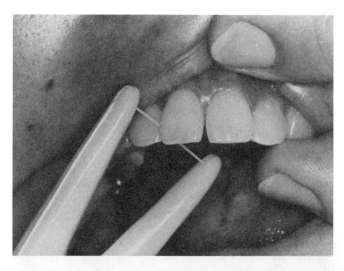

Fig. 1-44

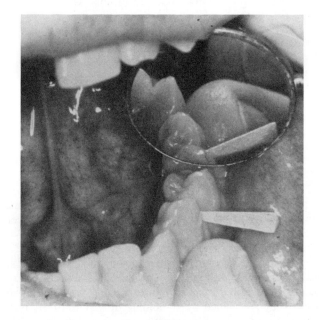

Fig. 1-45

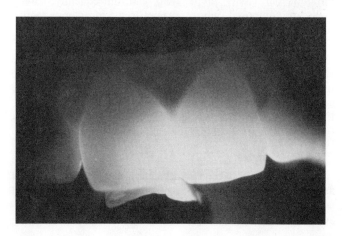

Fig. 1-46

Role of Oral Hygiene in Controlling the Carious Process

Removal of the bacterial plaque from a tooth surface will eliminate one major item from the caries triad, virtually stopping the process completely. So plaque removal is definitely an effective method of caries prevention and control.

Unfortunately, the only presently acceptable way to remove this plaque is a mechanical way, i.e., toothbrushing the more accessible areas, and dental flossing the less accessible areas. Brushing should be performed after each meal before the initiation of any bacterial activity. Toothbrushes are available in many forms, dimensions, hand-angulations, bristle consistencies, bristle diameters, bristle numbers per unit area, etc., to suit every patient's need. Floss or dental tape are the most effective aids in removing the plaque interproximally. Pulsating water under pressure, interdental stimulators, interproximal brushes, and pipe cleaners are also effective tools in specific circumstances.

Detergent foods and the "swish and swallow" technique do help to remove gross plaque and food debris, but these should not be regarded as primary methods of plaque control.

Disclosing dye tables or wafers aid in revealing those areas on tooth surfaces which are covered with the food debris and plaque that are potential causes of decay. They allow the patient to improve his technique of mechanically removing these substances.

The disciplined, frequent measures of eliminating plaque are essential before and after any operative treatment. Without them, the restorative treatment will undoubtedly fail due to recurrence of decay, necessitating more extensive treatment.

Tooth Preparation

There is no surface regeneration of enamel and dentin. To replace such lost tooth structure, it is necessary to prepare the remaining portion of the tooth to receive a restorative material. Thus, a tooth preparation can be defined as "the mechanical preparation and/or the chemical treatment of the remaining tooth structure, which enables it to accommodate a restorative material without incurring mechanical or biological failure.''

Generally, this can be attained in one of four ways:

I. Intracoronal and Intraradicular Tooth Preparation

These are cavity preparations that penetrate into the enamel and dentin substance of the crown or root portions of the tooth. Such preparations have definite surrounding walls, floors and junctions with adjacent unprepared tooth surfaces. This type of cavity preparation may have different shapes, dimensions, and relationships with the remaining tooth structures, according to variables to be discussed later. Furthermore such cavity preparations possess certain named features (Fig. 47):

A. Walls

These are named according to adjacent surfaces, and they are usually composed of enamel and dentin, with an intervening DEJ. Sometimes walls are composed of dentin only (e.g., an intraradicular cavity preparation) and, infrequently, cavity walls are composed only of enamel (e.g., in anterior teeth).

B. Floors

This refers to those portions of the preparation which are almost at right angles to the surrounding walls. Floors are usually composed of dentin only (e.g., pulpal floor), but they can be formed of enamel and dentin (e.g., gingival floor). Cavity preparation floors are named according to adjacent anatomy, e.g., gingival, pulpal, apical, subpulpal, etc.

C. Line angles

The junctions between two adjacent walls, or between a wall and a floor are referred to as line angles. They are named according to the combining walls or wall and floor (e.g., buccopulpal).

D. Point angles

The junctions between three walls or between two walls and a floor are called point angles. They are named according to the combining walls and/or floors (e.g., mesio-bucco-pulpal).

E. The cavosurface margin

The surface periphery of the cavity preparation, which is the junction between the cavity wall (floor) and the adjacent tooth surface is the cavosurface margin. It takes the name of the adjacent surface.

F. Cavosurface angle

This refers to the angle between a wall (floor) and the adjacent tooth surface. It takes the name of the wall (floor) and the adjacent surface.

II. Extracoronal or Extraradicular Tooth Preparations (Fig. 48)

Such preparations are usually for cast restorations. They involve reducing the tooth dimensions surfacewise to create a space for the restoration. Such reduction could include enamel, dentin, cementum, or a combination of these, providing the external termination of the preparation is placed on enamel or dentin only. There is also a certain nomenclature for tooth preparation features produced by this type of a preparation.

1. Preparation surface

This is simply the preparation surface resulting from the tooth reduction, and it is named according to the tooth surface it replaces, e.g., buccal, lingual, etc.

2. Finishing lines

The definite termination of the surface preparation is the ''finish line''. This could be on enamel or dentin, depending on whether the preparation ends on the anatomical crown or root. Finishing lines can be formed in different ways that will be described later.

3. The cavosurface margins and angles

These are similar to their counterparts in intracoronal-intraradicular cavity preparations, i.e., they describe the junctions and angles between the finishing lines and the adjacent tooth surfaces.

4. External angles

Extracoronal and extraradicular preparations have also line and point angles, designating the junctions between two adjacent preparation surfaces or three joining preparation surfaces. They are named by combining the names of the preparation surfaces. To differentiate them from intracoronal-intraradicular line and point angles, their names should be accompanied by the term ''external angle'', e.g., MB or OL external angles.

III. Roughened Tooth Surfaces (Fig. 49)

This procedure is performed mechanically and/or chemically and it is used for certain materials that can adequately wet these surfaces (to be described in detail with direct tooth-colored materials).

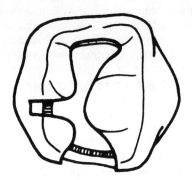

Fig. 1-47

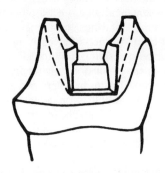

Fig. 1-48

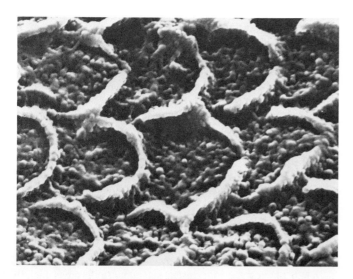

Fig. 1-49

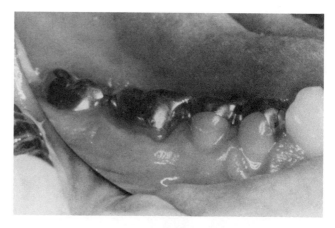

Fig. 1-50

IV. Conditioned Tooth Surface.

This involves the use of surface-active agents (usually chemical acts) to improve the adhesiveness of certain wetting restorative materials (to be described later).

Tooth Restoration (Fig. 50)

A restoration is the artifical replacement of lost tooth structure. It should be fabricated so that it is compatible both mechanically and biologically not only with the tooth, but also with the investing tissues (periodontium, musculature, etc.). As mentioned previously a restoration should impart form, function, health, proper phonetics, occlusal stability, proper axial loading and good esthetics to the tooth. It should also allow maximum freedom for mandibular movement within the physiological limits of the stomatognathic system.

Steps in Tooth Preparation

A systemized approach for a tooth preparation was originally recommended by G.V. Black. After some modifications, this approach entails the following steps:

I. Obtaining the outline form
II. Obtaining the resistance form
III. Obtaining the retention form
V. Removal of carious dentin
V. Obtaining the convenience form
VI. Establishing the configuration and correlations of enamel walls
VII. Debridement of the preparation
VIII. Observing and practicing the biologic form
These steps can seldom be done in the sequence mentioned here, e.g., step 4 may be done second, step 5 may be performed first, etc., depending on individual circumstances.

I. Obtaining the Outline Form

The outline form is defined as "the locations that the peripheries of the completed tooth preparation will occupy on tooth surfaces." In other words, it is the perimeter of tooth preparation in width, length, and depth dimensions.

The principles governing outline form were originally stated by G.V. Black and they emphasize the ideal for which one should strive. However, new materials and techniques, as well as advancements in preventive dentistry, require certain modifications from Black's original principles. These modifications and the reasons for making them will be described in detail as each restorative modality is discussed throughout this text.

The tooth preparation outline form in most of the time should:

A. Include all surface involvement of the enamel from the stage of decalcification to the stage of enamel penetration.

B. Include all enamel that has been undermined by the lateral spread of caries in the dentin and by backward decay. *Usually*, there is no place for undermined enamel in a cavity wall.

C. Extend far enough on the tooth surface so that the margins of the preparation will be located on finishable, self-cleansable areas. This is necessitated by the shortcomings of existing restorative materials, for none can completely chemically bond or adhere to the surrounding tooth. Therefore, any restoration will be surrounded by a microleakage space between itself and the adjacent tooth structure. This space will range between 20-120 microns in width, even in clinically successful restorations. Obviously, such a space can accommodate microorganisms and food substances predisposing to recurrent decay. Because this interphase is considered the weakest link against decay recurrence, it should be placed in areas that are easily cleansable by natural and/or artificial means. This may necessitate the sacrifice of some sound tooth structure. This principle is called "extension for prevention, or cutting for immunity" (Fig. 51).

D. For *most* intracoronal preparations, extend far enough pulpally and/or axially to include the dentino-enamel junction and penetrate to an average depth of 0.5 mm into the dentin. The three reasons to do this are to avoid seating the restoration on the very sensitive DEJ where maximum interconnection of the dentinal tubules exist, to give bulk for the restorative material, and to allow the restoration to take advantage of the dentin's elasticity during insertion and function.

For usual dimension extracoronal and limited dimension intracoronal preparations in anatomical crowns, it is acceptable

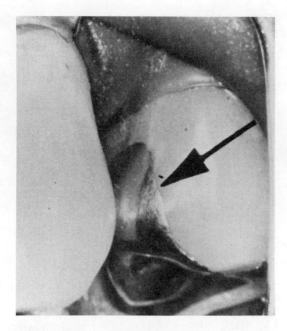

Fig. 1-51

to end the preparation surface, walls, or floor in enamel, as long as the reduction does not end at the DEJ. If the latter situation occurs, there must be further reduction to assure that preparation surfaces (walls) are in dentin.

Application of the Principal Factors

1. Pits and fissure lesions
The outline form will include:

a. All enamel directly attacked by decay (Fig. 52).

b. All undermined enamel (Fig. 53).

c. Sufficient enamel and dentin to locate the pulpal and axial walls (Fig. 54) or preparation surfaces within 0.5 mm from the DEJ as previously described.

d. All pits and fissures (Fig. 52) ending on adjacent inclined planes (of cusps, crossing or marginal ridges) or smooth surfaces, thus fulfilling the principles of the extension for prevention.

2. Proximal smooth surface cavities
The outline form will include a, b, and c as in pit and fissure cavities (in most cases) (Figs. 52, 55, 56, 57);

In order to fulfill the objectives of extension for prevention, ideally the following procedure should be undertaken. In the gingival direction, locate the gingival margin (finishing line) on the proximal tooth surface 0.5-1 mm apical to the crest of the healthy free gingiva within the gingival crevice. The apical extent of the restoration should not exceed the bottom of the crevice, because (1) the alkalinity of the crevicular fluid can neutralize, to some extent, acids produced from plaque activity (this fluid is alkaline only when the gingiva is healthy) and (2) the knife-edge relationship of the healthy free gingiva to the adjacent tooth surface will discourage food accumulation on adjacent restored surfaces occlusal to the sulcus for considerable periods during and after food ingestion.

Because of these two factors, the tooth surface forming one of the perimeters of the gingival crevice and sometimes the

area parallel with the crest of the free gingiva is considered a relatively immune area to decay recurrence (if the gingiva is healthy). If the gingiva is diseased, the dentist should estimate the future location of the crest of the free gingiva after healing occurs, and he should place the gingival margin of the preparation 0.5-1 mm apical to this estimated position. There are numerous modifications to these basic rules which will be described in the chapter on single tooth restorations and the periodontium.

In situations of severe gingival recession, with the carious lesion occlusal to the free gingiva and with no possibility of gingival regeneration, it is not necessary to extend the gingival margin of the preparation to the crevice. Here, the apical extent of the caries will define the gingival extent of the preparation. Fortunately, the gingival embrasure is also widened by the gingival recession, and this will allow artificial cleansing mechanisms to be effective there.

When placing the margins in self-cleansable areas facially and lingually, include all contact areas and the areas of near approach, ending the margins in embrasure areas (Fig. 59). The following factors will determine the extent into those embrasures:

a. The flare and mesio-distal width of the embrasures
The wider (mesio-distally) and more flared the facial and lingual embrasures are, the lower is the chance of food and plaque accumulation there. Such embrasures require less extension of the preparation facio-lingually (Fig. 60). In addition, flaring and increases in the mesio-distal width of these embrasures is at the expense of the dimensions of the contact areas. So the facio-lingual extension of the preparation would be less, as a result of the tooth anatomy itself.

b. Occlusion and masticatory forces (Fig. 61)
The more ideal the interrelationship between the adjacent and opposing teeth is, the better is the cleansability of the facial and lingual embrasures. This also requires less extension of the preparation facio-lingually. Likewise, the more ideal the masticatory loading is, the more effective will be the cleansing streams at the embrasures, and the required extension facio-lingually for the preparation will be less.

c. Caries index and oral hygiene (Fig. 62)
Understandably, the facio-lingual extension of a cavity into the corresponding embrasures is directly proportional to the caries index. In a patient with a high caries index, it would behoove the operator to place proximal margins farther into the embrasures, to improve cleansability.

d. Age
Three factors are involved here. First is the maturity of the tooth structure. An older tooth has a higher fluoride content and is more decay resistant, requiring less tooth involvement.

Second is the maturity of the patient. From the oral hygiene standpoint, greater maturity should theoretically imply a greater conscientiousness about proper oral health, necessitating less extension for prevention.

Third is the attrition on contact areas that will create wider facets at the expense of the embrasure space. In this situation, trying to bring the facial and lingual margins to the corresponding embrasures can lead to the unnecessary involvement of sound tooth structure. Taken together, these age factors will dictate that, in older patients, especially after age thirty, the facio-lingual extensions should be decreased.

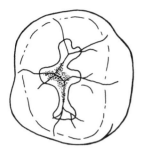
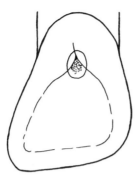

Decayed Enamel &
Inclusion of Pits and Fissures

Fig. 1-52

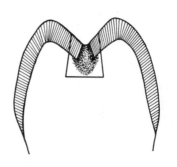
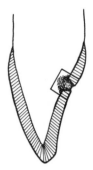

Undermined Enamel

Fig. 1-53

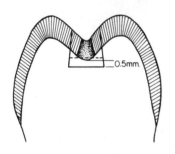
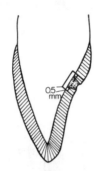

0.5mm.

0.5 mm

Depth of Preparation

Fig. 1-54

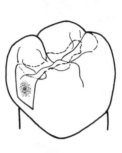
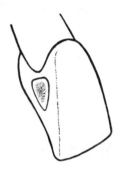

Decayed Enamel

Fig. 1-55

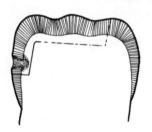
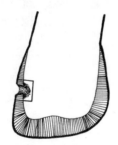

Undermined Enamel

Fig. 1-56

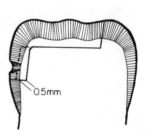
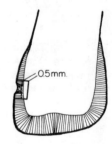

0.5mm.

0.5mm.

Depth of Preparation

Fig. 1-57

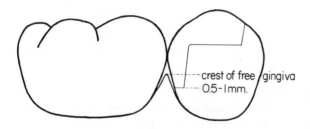
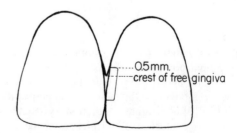

crest of free gingiva
0.5-1mm.

0.5mm.
crest of free gingiva

Relationship of Gingival Margin of Preparation
To Gingival Crest

Fig. 1-58

Extension for Prevention

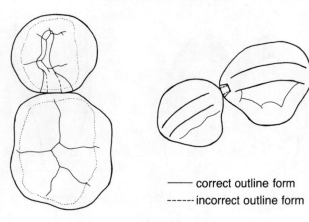

— correct outline form

------ incorrect outline form

Fig. 1-59

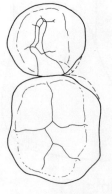

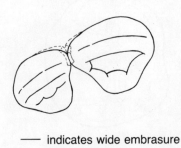

— indicates wide embrasure

----- indicates small embrasure

Wider Embrasures Reduces Facio-Lingual Extension of Cavity Preparation

Fig. 1-60

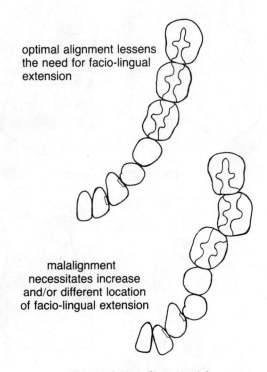

optimal alignment lessens the need for facio-lingual extension

malalignment necessitates increase and/or different location of facio-lingual extension

Extension Influenced by Masticating Forces

Fig. 1-61

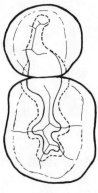

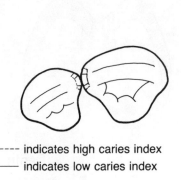

---- indicates high caries index

— indicates low caries index

Extension Influenced by Caries Index and Oral Hygiene

Fig. 1-62

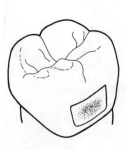

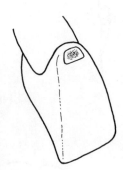

Decayed Enamel

Fig. 1-63

e. Creation of a more convex restoration proximally than that of the original proximal surface

If it is desirable, and if the periodontal and occlusion conditions allow, an increase in the facio-lingual convexity of the proximal surface of the future restoration by decreasing the dimensions of the contact area and increasing the width and flare of the embrasure, can substantially decrease the facio-lingual extension of the cavity preparation (see chapter on Class II amalgam restorations).

3. Facial and lingual gingival one-third smooth surface lesions

The outline form will include:

a. All enamel directly attached by decay (Fig. 63).

b. All undermined enamel (Fig. 64).

c. Sufficient enamel and dentin to locate the pulpal and axial walls or preparation surfaces within 0.5 mm of the DEJ (Fig. 65).

d. The principles of extension for prevention. In the gingival direction, this will be accomplished exactly as in proximal smooth surface lesions (Fig. 66). In the mesio-distal direction,

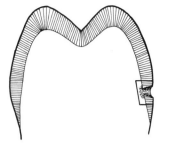 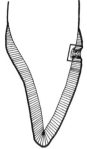

Undermined Enamel

Fig. 1-64

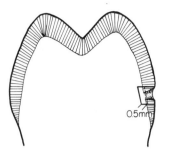 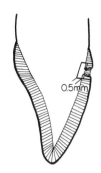

Depth of Preparation

Fig. 1-65

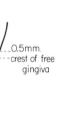

Relation of Gingival Margin of Preparation
To Gingival Crest

Fig. 1-66

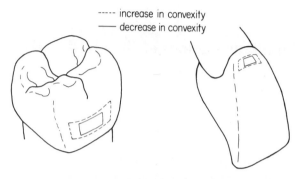

Occluso-Gingival Convexity Influencing
Mesio-Distal Extension of Preparation

Fig. 1-67

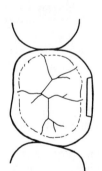 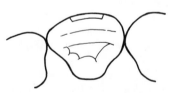

Masticatory Forces Influencing Mesio-distal Extension

Fig. 1-68

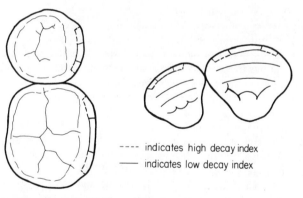

Decay Index Influencing Mesio-Distal Extension

Fig. 1-69

bear in mind that the whole facial or lingual surface apical to the height of contour is relatively non self-cleansable. Also, the mesio-distal extent should not include the axial angles. Four factors decrease the mesial-distal extension of these preparations:

i. A decreased occluso-gingival convexity, which improves the self-cleansability of these surfaces (Fig. 67).

ii. Proper occlusion and masticatory forces contributing to self-cleansability of the embrasures and axial angles (Fig. 68).

iii. Caries index and oral hygiene incapabilities of the pa-

tient, which are directly proportional to the amount of extension of these preparations (Fig. 69).

iv. Increased age of the tooth and maturity of the patient (as described in proximal, smooth surface lesions) will contribute to substantial reductions in the mesio-distal extensions, even to the point of including *only* that enamel directly attached or undermined by decay (Fig. 70).

e. Occlusally, the margins of these preparations should extend to, but should not include, the height of contour of the facial and lingual surfaces (Fig. 71).

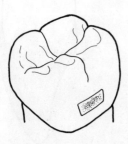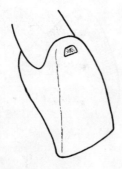

Maturity of Tooth Structure Influencing
Mesio-Distal Extension

Fig. 1-70

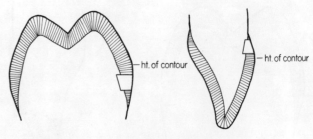

Occlusal Extension of Cavity Preparation

Fig. 1-71

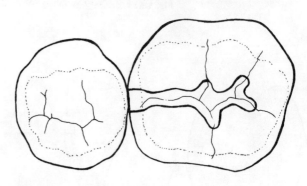

Fig. 1-72

Auxillary Factors of the Outline Form

A. Conservation (Fig. 72)

Lost tooth structures are irreplaceable. The theme in modern operative dentistry is *conservation* of as much tooth structure as possible, to the extent that it is sometimes necessary to violate some of Black's principles. Modern instruments and techniques have been invented to fulfill the objectives of conservation. However, even though the modern operator may strive for conservation of tooth structure, he must also be completely assured that decay recurrence and other complications will not occur.

B. Adjacent enamel cracks (crazing) or decalcifications could be involved in the preparation (Fig. 73A). In a sense, this is extension for prevention (see chapter on restorations of badly broken down teeth).

c. Type of the restorative material

Certain restorations that can be fabricated inside the mouth (amalgam, gold foil) need a smaller size preparation than cast restorations that are fabricated outside the mouth. Certain other restorations, such as bonded restorations, do not require removal of sound tooth structures prior to their insertion.

D. Extension for access

The obvious example of this modification is the occlusal involvement of a posterior tooth in a cavity preparation to gain access for a proximal lesion, even when the occlusal surface is intact and caries free (Figs. 73B and 74).

E. Unusual anatomy, malalignment, and steep cusps will change the locations and extent of cleansable and non-self-cleansable areas, subtantially modifying the outline form (Fig. 73B).

F. Outline form should be modified so that, if possible, no margins will be in occlusion with opposing teeth, as this will create marginal failure of the future restoration through opening and closing of the potential marginal space during masticatory loading, and through occluding with thin peripheries of the restoration or tooth structure inviting possible structural failure (Fig. 74).

G. Esthetics

Considerations of esthetics may substantially modify the outline form, e.g, labial extension of preparations in anterior teeth are limited. Margins are put into the contact areas, in an effort to make them less conspicuous. In fact, there is no other aux-illary factor that can modify the outline form more than esthetics.

Since esthetics as a modifying factor to the basic ideal outline form is of great importance, it deserves elaboration. The esthetic concern in operative dentistry is to try to convince a viewer that there is no restoration in the tooth. This can be accomplished through use of one or more of the following procedures:

1. Use tooth-colored restorative materials, which entail proper choice of shade that matches that of the surrounding tooth structure.

2. Place preparation margins, which are potentially conspicuous, into hidden locations, e.g., subgingivally, contact areas, etc. Sometimes this will locate them in non-self-cleansable areas.

3. Design the preparation outline so that the potentially conspicuous margins will be parallel to the adjacent periphery of the tooth or to the obvious anatomy there (compare a cast alloy restoration on tooth #19 and tooth #20 in Fig. 75 and that on tooth #29 and tooth #30 in Fig. 74). This can partially mask the most conspicuous portion of any restoration, i.e., the differentiating line between the restoration and tooth structure.

4. Design the preparation outline so that the conspicuous margins or surfaces of the restoration will not directly reflect light back to the viewer, but will instead reflect light first to adjacent tooth surfaces (tooth #29, Fig. 74). This will entail less facial extension of the preparation outline.

5. Execute the preparation outline in definite lines, with no irregularity or abrupt changes in the marginal outline.

6. Create as biologically smooth a surface as possible on the restoration surface in order to minimize plaque accumulation and stainability of the material.

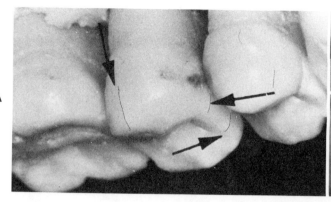
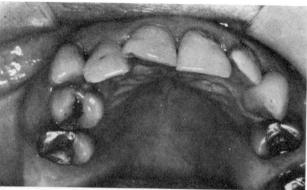

Fig. 1-73. **A**, Enamel crazings stained with tincture of iodine.

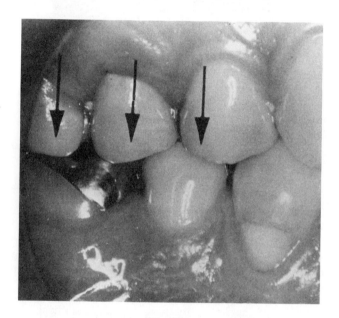

Fig. 1-74

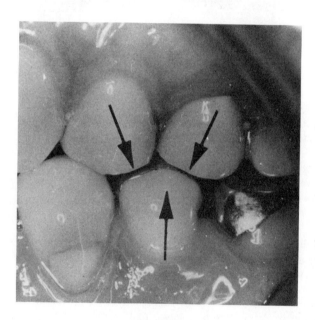

Fig. 1-75

7. Imitate the normal esthetically acceptable contour of the restored tooth in three dimensions. This may involve less extensions for the preparation in order to maintain a guiding tooth-surface contour. On the other hand, this may involve over-extension, if the original tooth contour is not esthetic and the restoration will change it completely.

8. Place surface landmarks in the restorations similar to those on adjacent natural teeth, even if they are in the form of surface defects.

H. Protect important and critical anatomy. Sometimes it is necessary to modify outline form to avoid involving a portion of the tooth that would be mechanically or biologically endangered by the regular outline form.

I. Abnormal cleansing capability, e.g., abnormal saliva, mental retardation or physical handicaps, will necessitate modifying the outline form to include new uncleansable areas (Fig. 76, A and B).

J. Use the processes of enameloplasty and enameloectomy for multiple supplementary grooves, e.g., on the occlusal surface of a molar, although not pitted or fissured, they can be hard to clean, and it is therefore not feasible to locate margins there. Since it is unrealstic to involve all of these grooves in a cavity preparation, they can be modified by making several of them into a large, saucer-shaped, shallow and easily cleansable one. This substantially improves the cleansability of the area, while sacrificing the minimal amount of enamel. The process is called enameloplasty (Fig. 77). It can be accomplished using a ball-shaped diamond stone or large round bur, to be followed by the appropriate finishing burs. If the involvement includes large deep grooves, complete penetration or badly thinned enamel will occur. In this case, include these grooves in the preparation but at shallower depths than the rest of the preparation. This is referred to as enamelectomy (Fig. 78).

K. Use the principle of extension for retention (Fig. 47).

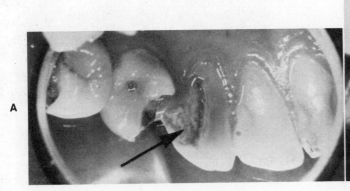

Fig. 1-76

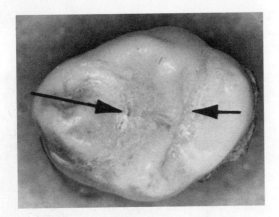

Fig. 1-77

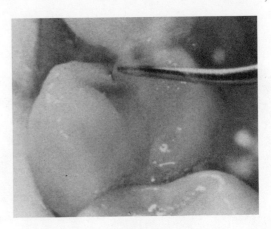

Fig. 1-78

Sometimes it is necessary to involve additional surfaces or areas of a surface to facilitate increased retention form in order to prevent the restoration from being dislodged.

L. Use the principle of extension for resistance (Fig. 48). After fulfilling all the principal objectives for the outline form, some weakened tooth structure may remain, which must be covered or supported with a restorative material. This will necessitate further extension of the preparation in order to mechanically engage these weakened areas.

II. Obtaining the Resistance Form

Resistance form is defined as the architectural form given to a tooth preparation which enables both the restoration and the remaining tooth to resist structural failure from occlusal loading stresses. Building a restoration is similar to building any mechanical structure, in that the stress patterns of the available foundation and the contemplated structure must be predetermined. Accordingly, the following items should be considered.

A. Stress patterns of teeth

Every tooth has its own stress pattern, and every location on a tooth has special stress patterns. Recognizing them is vital prior to designing a restoration without failure potential.

1. Stress bearing and stress concentration areas in anterior teeth

a. The junction between the clinical crown and clinical root bears shear components of stress (Fig. 79), together with tension on the loading side and compression at the non-loading side, during excursive mandibular movements.

b. The incisal angles (Fig. 80), especially if they are square, are subject to tensile and shear stresses in normal occlusion. Massive compressive stresses will be present in edge-to-edge occlusion, and if the incisal angles are involved in a disclusive mechanisms, these stresses are substantially increased.

c. The axial angles and lingual marginal ridges will bear concentrated shear stresses (Fig. 81, A and B). In addition, on the loading side tensile stresses are present, and on the non-loading side compressive stresses are found.

d. The slopes of the cuspid will bear concentrated stresses (three types), especially if the cuspid is a protector for the occlusion or part of a group function during mandibular excursions (Fig. 82).

e. The distal surface of a cuspid exhibits a unique stress pattern (Fig. 83, A and B) as a result of the anterior components of force concentrating compressive loading at the junction of the anterior and posterior segments of the dental arch and microlateral displacement of the cuspid during excursive movements. Both of these factors will lead to tremendous stress concentration with resultant abrasive activity there (see chapter on distal of cuspid restorations).

f. The lingual concavity in upper anterior teeth (Fig. 81B)

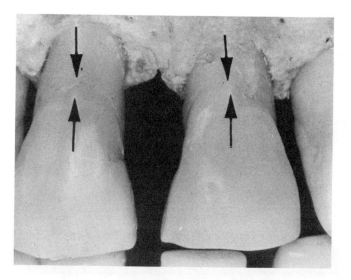

Fig. 1-79

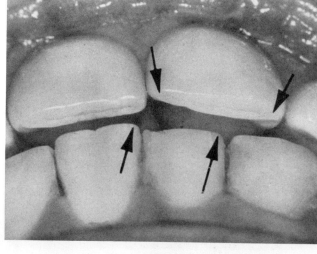

Fig. 1-80

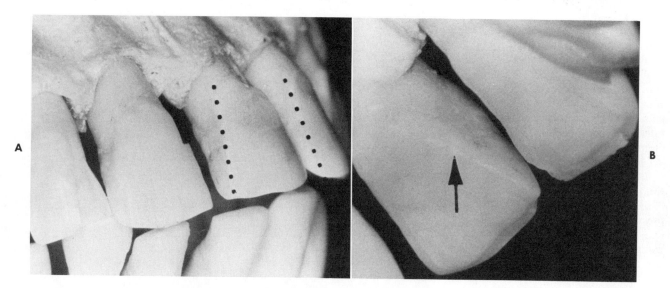

A

B

Fig. 1-81

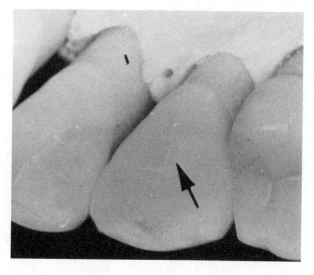

Fig. 1-82

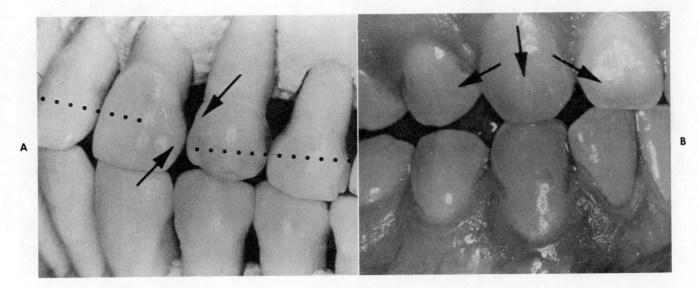

Fig. 1-83

bears substantial compressive stresses during centric occlusion, in addition to tensile and shear stresses during protrusive mandibular movements.

g. The incisal edges of lower anterior teeth are subjected to compressive stresses. In addition, tensile and shear stresses are present during protrusive mandibular movement. The incisal ridges of upper anterior teeth will have these same stresses during the mid-protrusive and sometimes at the protrusive border location of the mandible (Fig. 83B).

2. Stress bearing and stress concentration areas of posterior teeth

a. Cusp tips, especially on the functional side, bear compressive stresses (Fig. 84).

b. Marginal and crossing ridges bear tremendous tensile and compressive stresses (Fig. 85).

c. Axial angles bear tensile and shear stresses on the nonfunctional side (Fig. 86A), and compressive and shear stresses on the functional side (Fig. 86B).

d. The junction between the clinical root and the clinical crown during function (especially lateral excursion) bears tremendous shear stresses, in addition to compression on the occluding contacting side and tension on the non-contacting side (Fig. 87).

e. Any occlusal, facial, or lingual concavity will exhibit compressive stress concentration, especially if it has an opposing cuspal element in static or functional occlusal contact with it.

3. Weak areas in the tooth should be identified and recognized before any restorative attempt, in order to avoid destructive loading. They are:

a. Bi- and trifurcations (Fig. 88, A and B).

b. Cementum should be eliminated as a component of a cavity wall. The junction between the cementum and the dentin is always irregular, so the dentin surface should be smoothed flat after cementum removal.

c. Thin dentin bridges in deep cavity preparations (Fig. 89).

d. Subpulpal floors in root canal treated teeth. Any stress concentration there may split the tooth interceptally (Fig. 90).

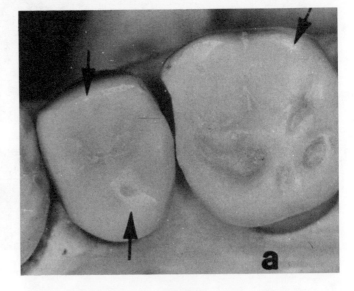

Fig. 1-84

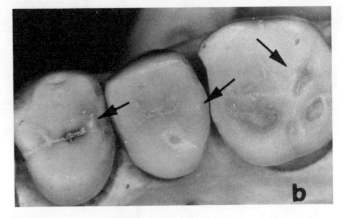

Fig. 1-85

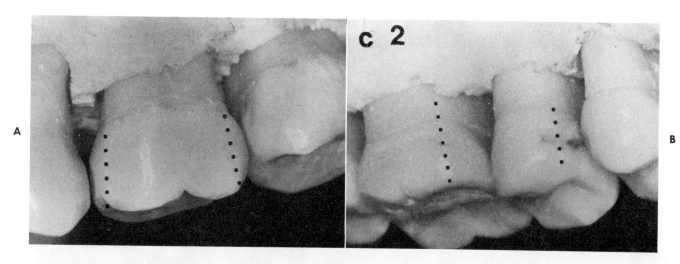

Fig. 1-86

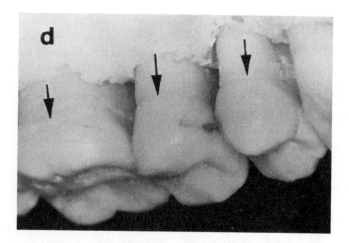

Fig. 1-87

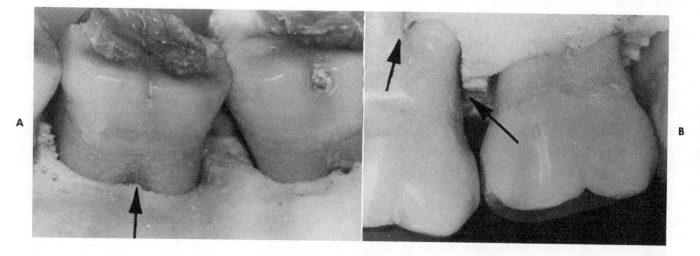

Fig. 1-88

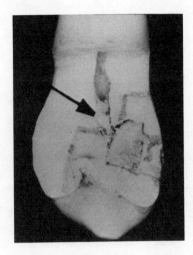

Fig. 1-89

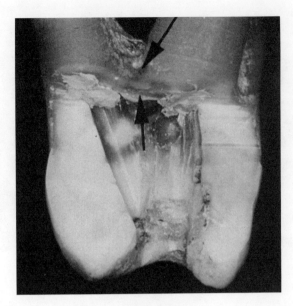

Fig. 1-90

e. Cracks or crazing in enamel (Fig. 73A), and/or dentin. Both should be treated passively in any restoration design. They may act as shear lines leading to further spread.

B. Some applied mechanical properties of teeth

1. Although the following figures are averages, they provide an idea about the principal mechanical properties of tooth structure. It must be understood that these figures can differ from one location on a tooth to another, and from one tooth to another:

a. Compressive strength of enamel supported by vital dentin is usually 36-42,000 PSI.

b. Compressive strength of vital dentin is 40-50,000 PSI.

c. Modulus of resilience of enamel supported by vital dentin is 60-80 inch-lbs/cubic inch.

d. Modulus of resilience of vital dentin is 100-140 inch-lbs/inch^3.

e. Modulus of elasticity of enamel supported by vital dentin under compression is 7,000,000 PSI.

f. Modulus of elasticity of vital dentin is 1,900,000 PSI.

2. In general, when enamel loses its support of dentin, it loses more than 85% of its strength properties.

3. Tensile strength of dentin is about 10% less than its compressive strength.

4. Tensile strength and compressive strength of enamel are similar, as long as the enamel is supported by vital dentin.

5. Shear strength of dentin is almost 60% less than its compressive strength, and this is very critical in restorative design.

6. There is minimal shear strength for enamel when it loses its dentin support.

7. When the dentin loses its vitality, there is a drop of almost 40-60% in its strength properties.

C. Vale experiment

The original experiment involved preparation of occlusoproximal cavities with different crossing dimensions at the marginal and crossing ridges with a standard depth. The teeth were then subjected to measured occlusal loads. The load that split the tooth was recorded and compared to the control, which was the load that split a sound tooth. Later, the same experiment was repeated by several investigators using more sophisticated equipment than that used by Vale. The results were consistent. A summary of their findings brought to the closest round figures is as follows:

1. By crossing one marginal ridge at ¼ the intercuspal distance, there is almost 10% loss of a tooth's resistance to splitting.

2. By crossing two marginal ridges at ¼ the intercuspal distance, there is almost 15% loss of a tooth's resistance to splitting.

3. By crossing one marginal ridge at ⅓ the intercuspal distance, there is almost 30% loss of a tooth's resistance to splitting.

4. By crossing two marginal ridges by ⅓ the intercuspal distance, there is almost 35% loss of a tooth's resistance to splitting.

5. By crossing one marginal ridge at ½ the intercuspal distance, there is almost 40% loss of a tooth's resistance to splitting.

6. By crossing two marginal ridges at ½ the intercuspal distance, there is almost 45% loss of a tooth's resistance to splitting.

7. By crossing a crossing ridge at ¼ the intercuspal distance, there is almost 20% loss of a tooth's resistance to splitting.

8. By crossing a crossing ridge at ⅓ the intercuspal distance, there is almost 35% loss of a tooth's resistance to splitting.

9. By crossing a crossing ridge at ½ the intercuspal distance, there is almost 45% loss of a tooth's resistance to splitting.

D. To best resist masticatory forces, use floors or planes at right angles to the direction of loading (Figure 91A) to avoid shearing stresses (Figure 91B).

E. If possible, walls of preparations should be parallel to the direction of the loading forces (Fig. 92A), in order to minimize or avoid shearing stresses (Fig. 92B).

F. Intracoronal and intraradicular cavity preparations can be done in box (Fig. 93A), cone (Fig. 93B) or inverted truncated cone shapes (Fig. 93C).

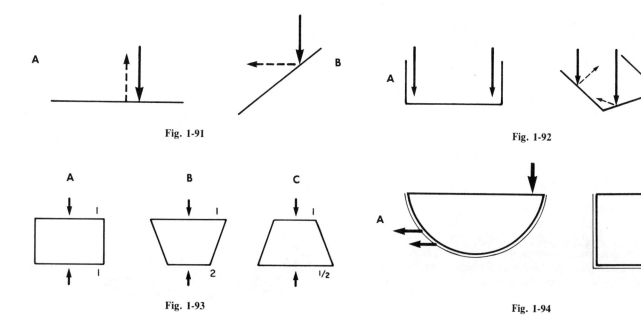

Fig. 1-91

Fig. 1-92

Fig. 1-93

Fig. 1-94

From the drawings it is possible to deduce that the inverted truncated cone shapes will have a higher resistance to loading than the box shapes, and the box shapes will have a higher resistance than the cone shapes. Therefore, if conditions and requirements allow, cavity preparations should be prepared in an inverted truncated cone shape.

G. Definite floors, walls and surfaces with line and point angles (Fig. 94B) are essential to prevent micromovements of restorations, with concomitant shear stresses on remaining tooth structures (Fig. 94A).

H. Increasing the bulk of a restorative material or leaving sufficient bulk of tooth structure in critical areas is one of the most practical ways of decreasing stresses per unit volume (compare A and B, Fig. 95).

I. Designing the outline form with minimal exposure of the restoration surface to occlusal loading will definitely minimize stresses and the possibility of mechanical failure in the restoration (Fig. 96).

J. A comparative evaluation of the mechanical properties of the restorative material relative to that of the tooth structure will dictate the preparation and restorative design, i.e., if the restorative material is stronger than the tooth structure, the design should be such that the restorative material will support the tooth structure and vice versa if the restorative material is weaker than tooth structure (compare cavity preparations in Fig. 47 to that in Fig. 48).

K. Junctions between different parts of the preparation, especially those acting as fulcra, should be rounded in order to minimize stress concentration in both tooth structure and restorations and to prevent any such sharp components from acting as shear lines for fracture failure.

L. Retentive features must leave sufficient bulk of tooth structure to resist stresses resulting from displacing forces (see chapter on pin and post-retained restorations).

III. Obtaining the Retention Form

Retention form is defined as that form given to the tooth preparation, especially its detailed anatomy and general shape,

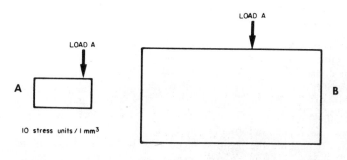

Fig. 1-95

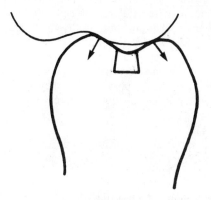

Fig. 1-96

which enables the restoration, that it will accommodate, to avoid being dislodged by masticatory loading. Retention means are divided into principal and auxillary types according to their efficiency in retaining the restoration. Any design of a tooth preparation should have at least one principal means of retention form.

According to their locations, retention means can be classified as *intracoronal* (inside a cavity preparation within the tooth) and *extracoronal* (on the preparation surface, replacing reduced external tooth surfaces).

A. Principal means of retention

1. Frictional retention (Fig. 97) depends on 4 factors:

a. The surface area of contact between tooth structure and restorative material

Greater surface area produces a greater frictional component of retention. It is directly proportional to the length, width, and depth of the walls and surfaces involved in the preparation.

b. Opposing walls or surfaces involved

More opposing walls and/or surfaces in a tooth preparation produce greater frictional components of retention and, consequently, a more stable restoration within the preparation.

c. Parallelism and non-parallelism

A higher degree of parallelism between opposing walls produces greater frictional components of retention. Higher convergence of the walls in the intracoronal preparation and higher divergence of the walls in the extracoronal preparation produce greater locking ability of the tooth preparation to restorative material, irrespective of frictional retention.

d. Proximity

Bringing the restorative material closer to tooth structure during insertion will substantially increase the frictional retention. This requires smoothing the preparation details, inserting the restorative material into the preparation with a wetting consistency compatible with its strength, forcing the proximity of restorative material to tooth by means of mechanical energy, and using the dimensional changes of both tooth and restorative material to increase their proximity to each other, etc.

2. Elastic deformation of dentin

Changing the position of dentinal walls and floors microscopically by using condensation energy within the dentin's proportional limit (From position 1 to position 2 Fig. 98), can add more gripping action by the tooth on the restorative material. This occurs when the dentin regains its original position while the restorative material remains rigid, thereby completely obliterating any remaining space in the cavity preparation.

3. Inverted truncated cones or undercuts (Fig. 99)

Undercuts can be introduced in every component of a tooth preparation. These can be in any direction, and can tremendously improve retention, provided that they are filled with the restorative material and do not interfere with the restoration fabrication.

4. Dove-tail

This is a purposeful modification in the outline form in some cases, but usually extension for prevention will create a dove-tail outline (Fig. 99).

Auxillary means of retention

Although we will mention and illustrate some examples of auxillary means of retention, they will be explained in complete detail with different designs of a cavity preparation.

A. Grooves (Fig. 100) are cut in dentin whenever bulk allows, without undermining the adjacent enamel.

B. Internal boxes (Fig. 101) have definite walls and floors.

C. Posts (Fig. 102) are made from wrought or cast metal and placed in the root canals.

D. Pins (Fig. 103) are made from cast or wrought metal.

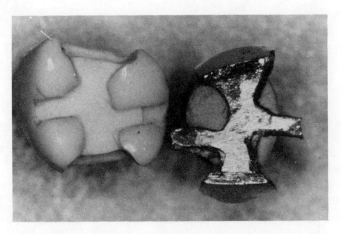

Fig. 1-97

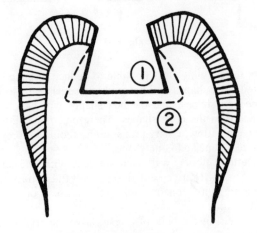

Fig. 1-98

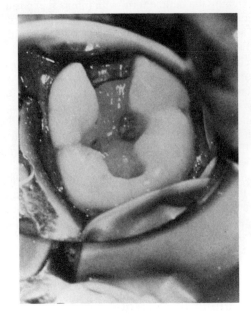

Fig. 1-99

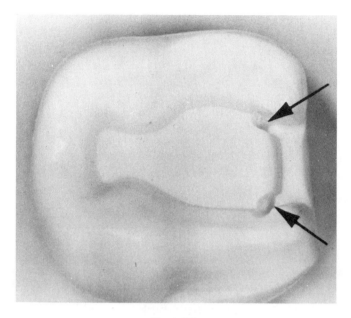

Fig. 1-100

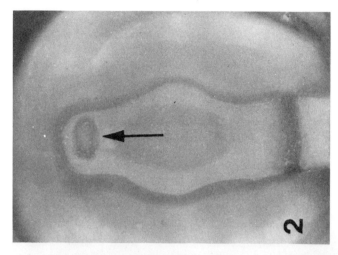

Fig. 1-101

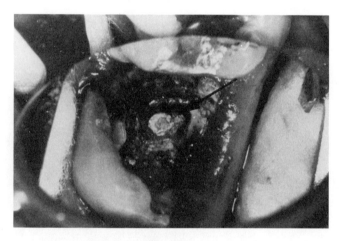

Fig. 1-102

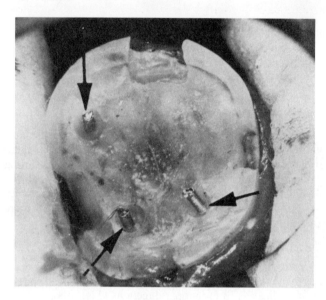

Fig. 1-103

They may be parallel or non-parallel, vertical or horizontal, threaded or cemented.

E. Triangular areas (see chapter on direct gold restorations) are placed within the dentin and are laterally located without undermining overlying enamel plates.

F. Etching or acid conditioning (Fig. 104) of enamel (and sometimes dentin) is done with certain acids. This creates mechanical locks and increases surface areas of contact between tooth structure and the restorative material. In certain situations it can be considered a principal retention mode.

G. Cement, or luting agents, is the least effective auxiliary means of retention. Cement occupies the space between a restoration fabricated outside the mouth and the adjacent tooth structures.

H. If the restoration is designed so that occlusal loading (Fig. 74) is directed to seat the restoration rather than to displace it, it is an ideal auxiliary retention form. It is sometimes

considered a principal means of retention, e.g., for cemented type restorations.

IV. Obtaining the Convenience Form

Convenience form is defined as that shape given to a tooth preparation or modifications added to the preparation or its instrumentation, which enable the operation to be completed conveniently. Ideally, a tooth preparation fulfilling all requirements for outline, resistance, and retention forms will be convenient to instrumentation. The most effective way to obtain the convenience form is by proper control of the field of operation and by adequate training and familiarity with the armamentarium.

There is no excuse for unnecessary involvement of sound tooth structure simply for the sake of speedy, convenient access to the internal details of a preparation. Presently available operative instruments are quite efficient in creating indicated tooth

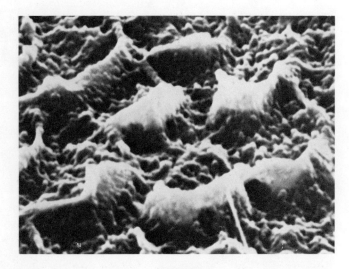

Fig. 1-104

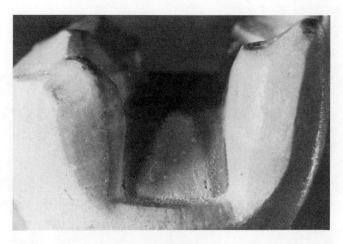

Fig. 1-105

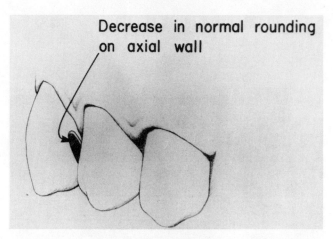

Decrease in normal rounding on axial wall

Fig. 1-106

preparations with no further extension than that necessitated by the three previously described forms. However, situations do arise that require one or more of the following modes to obtain convenience form.

A. Modifications in tooth preparation for convenience form

These modifications include flaring some walls more than otherwise necessary for resistance or retention form in order to decrease distortion errors in intermediate materials during restoration fabrications (castings) (Fig. 105), decreasing the roundness of some walls more than normally needed (Fig. 106), and extending margins (walls or finishing lines) more than otherwise necessary (Fig. 107).

B. Instrument modification for convenience form

Contra-angling, bayonetting, or the addition of several angles to the shank of an instrument facilitates access and enables force application in the proper directions (Fig. 108).

C. Separation

Wedging teeth away from each other can be the most radical way to make interproximal instrumentation convenient. However, the use of wedges interproximally during proximal surface instrumentation is the most indicated convenience form to be used (Fig. 109).

V. Removal of Carious Dentin

This process is defined as the mechanical and/or chemical actions resulting in complete elimination of the diseased, non-reparable portions of dentin. The process almost always necessitates the removal of undermined enamel in order to expose carious dentin in a backward decay situation. Usually, with the completion of the previous steps, the carious dentin has been removed. Sometimes, however, the caries activity is deep, and the normal depth of the preparation does not involve the dentin caries cone. As a result, diseased carious dentin remains axially or pulpally. A separate step becomes necessary in order to eliminate these undesirable tissues.

If the decay is soft (always acute), removal should be done

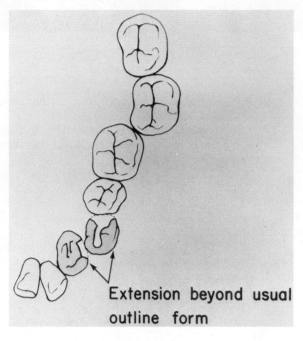

Extension beyond usual outline form

Fig. 1-107

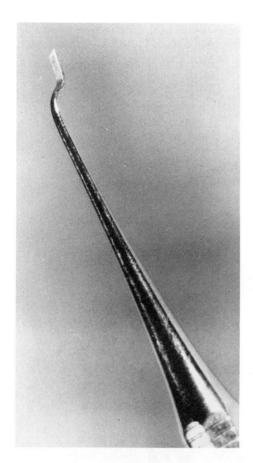

Fig. 1-108

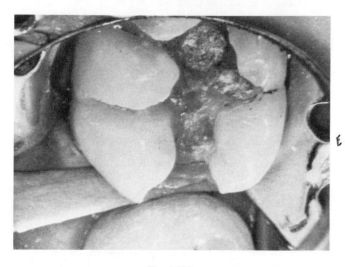

Fig. 1-109

with the broadest discoid or spoon/excavator suitable for the cavity size, directing it with scooping actions from the cavity peripheries to the center. Trying to move the excavator from the center to the peripheries will concentrate pressure on the thinnest cross-section of the dentin bridge, incurring the possibility of pulp chamber involvement.

If the decayed dentin is hard (always chronic decay), the excavator may not be sufficient to remove the diseased tissue.

In addition, a large round bur (preferably dull), revolving slowly, should be moved in brushing strokes from the peripheries of the cavity preparation to the center. These strokes should be done with minimal pulpal or axial pressure and with a lot of water coolant, in order to minimize thermal irritation to the nearby pulp tissues.

To be sure of the complete removal of carious dentin, there are available disclosing agents, e.g., 0.2-0.5% basic fuschsin, which can be applied to the prepared dentin, and which will stain areas with irreparable decay, indicating the necessity for their removal.

For proper instrumentation and treatment of carious dentin, one has to differentiate between acute and chronic decay. Although a more detailed mention of this subject is made in chapter 13, a brief introduction is in order here.

Acute caries is defined as decay in which the acids dissolving the tooth structure are preceding the microorganisms producing them, in relation to the pulp (Fig. 25). *Chronic caries* is defined as decay in which the microorganisms are preceding the acids produced by them or are at the same level pulpally as these acids. (Fig. 26). The two types of decay have the following comparative characteristics:

1. Duration is longer for chronic decay (years); and shorter for acute decay (months).

2. The consistency of chronic decay is hard and somewhat resistant to scooping by excavators, whereas acute decay is soft and easily scooped.

3. The color of chronic decay is dark brown to blackish, the color of stained decalcified dentin and acute decay is usually straw yellow.

4. Although odor is the least reliable criterion, chronic decay is usually noticeably foul-smelling, while there is no odor in acute decay.

5. Chronic lesions affect older ages more often than acute lesions, as there is greater resistance and possibility of repair from the affected teeth in chronic than in acute decay.

6. Usually there is a reparative reaction of the pulp to chronic decay, but little or no repair in acute decay.

The most important information from this brief description of acute and chronic decay is that the deepest dentinal layer in acute decay can be considered sterile, as it contains just acids with no microorganisms. On the contrary, in cases of chronic decay, where the microorganisms are totally impregnating the carious dentin and even penetrating some sound dentin, the entire carious mass can be considered infected. In the chapter on management of deep carious lesions we will discuss and apply this information in greater detail.

VI. Configuration and Correlation of Enamel Walls

The "configuration" of enamel walls is the shape, dimension, location, and angulation of enamel components in a final tooth preparation. The "correlation" is the relationship of the enamel configuration to surrounding tooth preparation and restoration details. It should be emphasized that although enamel is the hardest tissue in the human body, it comprises one of the weakest points in a preparation wall, especially when it loses its dentinal support. The enamel (prism) rods are stronger than the interprismatic enamel. So, whenever enamel is stressed, it tends to split along the length of the rods. This splitting is easier when the enamel rods are parallel to each other (like a straight-grained pine). If the rods are interlaced and twisted together, this splitting will be somewhat difficult (like the pine-knot). Fortunately, the enamel prisms are interlaced and twisted upon each other in the inner one-half to two-thirds of their thickness, while in the remaining outer portion of the enamel, they are parallel. For an *ideal* enamel wall, Noy devised certain structural requirements. These requirements tend to take full advantage of the enamel's hardness and strength, and avoid the disadvantages of the enamel's splitting characteristics.

A. Structure requirements

1. *The enamel wall must rest upon sound dentin* (Fig. 110), i.e., all carious dentin must be removed and the enamel cut back until it is supported by sound tooth structure. Otherwise, there would be some portion of the enamel left standing that has been weakened by the dissolution of its minerals in backward caries. This enamel would most likely break down

under the stresses of mastication after a restoration was placed (refer back to Mechanical Properties of Undermined Enamel).

2. *The enamel rods which form the cavosurface angle must have their inner ends resting on sound dentin* (Fig. 111). Noy suggests that when this condition is established, the dentin, which is elastic, gives the enamel, which is brittle, a certain degree of elasticity, which is very important at the margins of a restoration.

3. *The rods which form the cavosurface angle must be supported, or be resting, on sound dentin and their outer ends must be covered by the restorative material* (Fig. 112). This provides the strongest wall possible but it can only be produced by a bevel of the cavosurface angle. The second strongest configuration is when the plane of the enamel wall is made parallel to the length of the rods. The first situation can only be applied when the restorative materials are stronger and tougher than tooth structure. The second situation is the maximum that can be expected when the restorative material is weaker and more brittle than the tooth structure.

4. *The cavosurface angle must be so trimmed or bevelled that the margins will not be exposed to injury in condensing the restorative material against it* (Fig. 112). This rule is applied particularly to Class I cavities and to occlusal portions of Class II, i.e., in narrow occlusal cavities where the enamel rods are inclined inward so that the cavosurface margin will be very sharp. The latter pattern can make the enamel rods extremely susceptible to injury, so they have to be trimmed or bevelled to prevent this type of marginal failure.

The above are the ideal requirements for a proper enamel wall. However, there are certain restrictions in applying the last two rules, from the restorative material point of view, since not all materials can perform well if placed in a cavity with such enamel walls. The primary example is amalgam. However, these rules should be applied as feasibly often as possible.

B. General principles for formulation of enamel walls

As will be shown in the discussion of different designs of a tooth preparation, the direction of the enamel rods is one of the most influential factors in dictating the number of planes,

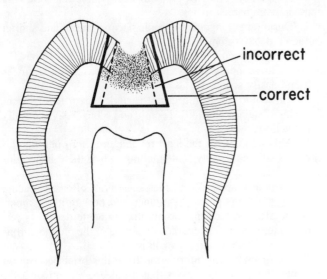

Fig. 1-110

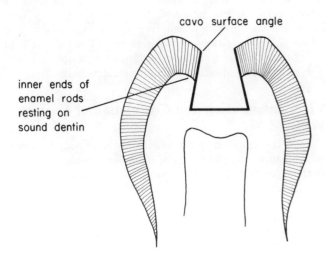

Fig. 1-111

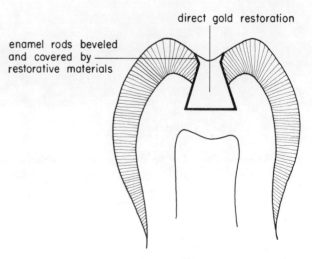

Fig. 1-112

angulation, configuration, and correlation of a wall which has enamel as part of its structural components. In addition to Noy's structural requirements for an ideal cavity wall, the following are some additional guidelines. Others will be presented with each design of tooth preparation.

1. The enamel portion of a wall should be the smoothest portion of the preparation anatomy, if it is not going to be etched. Any roughness, besides interfering with the proximity of tooth to the restorative material, will increase the possibilities of frail, loosely attached enamel rods. Such frail enamel rods will be detached during function, increasing the leakage space in this critical marginal area.

2. Junctions between different enamel walls should be very rounded, even if the junctions between the inner parts of the wall (dentinal) are angular. This will improve adaptability of the restorative material at the preparation corners, in addition to decreasing stress concentration there. Furthermore, such rounding decreases the possibility of any frail, unsupported, easily detachable enamel rods at the corners.

3. If inclining a preparation wall to follow the direction of the enamel rods will nullify its resistance and retention capabilities, different planes for that wall should be established. Still, this should be accomplished with the most peripheral planes formed of enamel supported by dentin, following the direction of the enamel rods there in three dimensions.

4. When the preparation margins come to an area of abrupt directional changes of enamel rods or an area where no rules for enamel rods direction exist, this area should be included in the preparation, and the margins placed in areas of a more predictable rod pattern. This provides for a wall with predictable behavior.

From this discussion one can appreciate that good knowledge and understanding of the enamel pattern, especially the direction of enamel rods in three dimensions, is very important for a proper formulation of cavity details containing enamel.

C. Enamel pattern

1. The direction of the enamel rods (prisms) in different parts of the crowns of the teeth.

Generally, the enamel rods (prisms) in the outer one-third to one-half project in straight lines from the DEJ to the enamel surface. For a clear, understandable illustration of the direction of the enamel rods, one should have a reference of a fixed plane. This can be either the long axis of the crown (Fig. 113, A and B), or the enamel surface itself, i.e., the tangent of the surface at the point of the examination (Fig. 113, A and B).

Directions of the enamel rods relative to the long axis of the crown (Fig. 114) may be described as follows:

The rods at the center of the occlusal surfaces always lean to pits or fissures towards the long axis of the crown. The stronger the inclination of the cusps, the greater the degree of such slants. On the periphery of the occlusal surfaces, i.e., near the tips of the cusps and crests of the marginal ridges, the rods are inclined toward those tips and crests, away from the long axis of the tooth crown. In between, the rods are parallel to this axis.

The rods on the axial surfaces are perpendicular to the long axis of the crown only in the middle third. They incline incisally or occlusally in the incisal or occlusal third, making an average of plus 36° (plus means toward incisal or occlusal) with the perpendicular to the long axis at this area. In the gingival third, they incline by an average of minus 13° (toward the gingival) from the perpendicular to the long axis of the crown in this area.

Enamel rod inclination relative to the tangent to the enamel surface is the most feasible way, in practice, to understand the enamel rods' direction. The rods stand perpendicular to the tangent of the enamel surface in only two areas: the middle third of all axial surfaces (Fig. 115) and the middle third of the distance from the tips of cusps and crests of ridges to their adjoining fossae occlusally. For directions in other locations, see details in (Fig. 115).

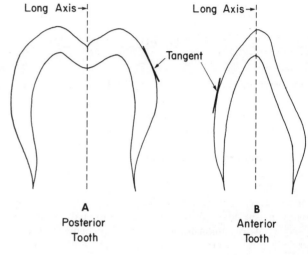

A
Posterior Tooth

B
Anterior Tooth

Fig. 1-113

INCLINATION ON OCCLUSAL SURFACE

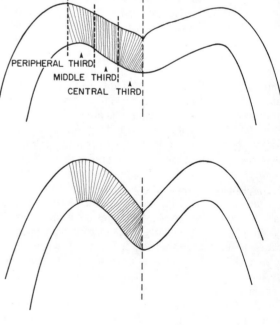

PERIPHERAL THIRD
MIDDLE THIRD
CENTRAL THIRD

Fig. 1-114

THE DIRECTION OF ENAMEL RODS RELATIVE TO TANGENTS

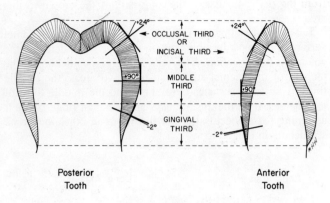

Fig. 1-115

Cusp tips:
fanning of enamel rods

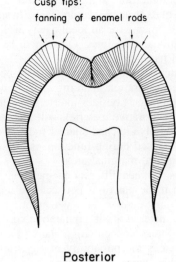

Posterior Tooth

Fig. 1-116

The rods in occlusal enamel generally radiate their heads toward cusp tips and ridge crests at the outer third. At the center of the tips of the cusps and crests of ridges they open their heads making an onion-like section (Fig. 116). So the change in enamel rod direction from the occlusal surface to the axial surface is abrupt at the intervening cusp tip or ridge crest. At the inner third they lean toward the occlusal pits.

In anterior teeth, the rods change their direction suddenly on the incisal edge, from the labial to lingual surface (Fig. 117A), showing onion-like sections. The change in direction takes place rather gradually on the incisal angles from incisal to proximal, if the incisal angle is round (Fig. 117B). In square incisal angles, the change in direction will be abrupt from proximal to incisal surfaces (Fig. 117B). Extremely abrupt changes in direction can also be noticed over pronounced marginal ridges and pointed cuspid tips.

On the axial surface, the rods will make a right angle to the tangent of the enamel surface just at their middle thirds (Fig. 115). In their incisal or occlusal thirds, they lean incisally or occlusally, making an angle on the average of plus 24° with the perpendicular to the tangent of the enamel surface in this area (Fig. 115).

In the gingival third, the enamel rods lean gingivally, making an angle of −2°, on the average, with the perpendicular to the tangent of the enamel surface at this area (Fig. 115).

The inclination of the enamel rods around the teeth in the circumferential direction is generally perpendicular to the tangent of the surface at any particular point there (Fig. 118A). An exception to this is at the approach to and over the mesio- and disto-lingual marginal ridges on anterior teeth (Fig. 118B). Here, the enamel rods incline somewhat toward the marginal ridges, but in passing over these ridges their directions change very abruptly and irregularly, i.e., there are no rules for the direction of the enamel rods there. Therefore, when the margin of a proximal cavity preparation reaches this lingual marginal ridge, cut sufficiently past it to be certain of the direction of the enamel rods at the margin formed.

On facial or lingual grooves or concavities, the enamel rods surface ends radiate toward the center of these concavities mesio-distally and sometimes inciso (occluso)-gingivally.

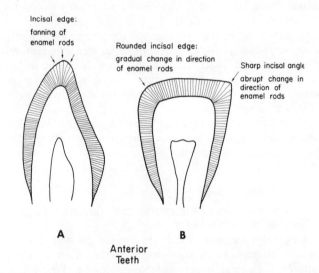

Anterior Teeth

Fig. 1-117

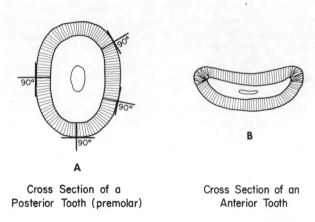

Cross Section of a Posterior Tooth (premolar)

Cross Section of an Anterior Tooth

Fig. 1-118

2. Thickness pattern of enamel in different areas of the tooth crown (Fig. 89)

The enamel will have its maximum thickness at the tips of the cusps, and at the crests of triangular, marginal, and crossing ridges. It diminishes in thickness going occlusally to the depth of the pits, fissures, and grooves. At the inner one-third of the occlusal inclined plane it may have a thickness of 0.2-0.5 mm. At the depth of the pits and fissures there is no enamel coverage in most cases.

Enamel also diminishes in thickness going gingivally on the axial surfaces, with its least thickness at the CEJ. At the cervical third of the axial surfaces, the thickness may be as low as 0.2 mm. There are certain areas of enamel thickening axially, e.g., the axial angle and the axial height of contour, the occlusal one-third of facial surfaces of lower molars and the lingual surface of upper molars.

For anterior teeth, the maximum dimension of enamel is at the incisal ridge (slopes in the canine) and it diminishes gingivally to the CEJ on the axial surfaces.

The lingual enamel plates are generally thinner than the facial, a pattern more apparent in anterior teeth than in posterior ones. At grooves on the facial and lingual surfaces of molars, the enamel coverage thins to their center, but not to the extent of discontinuation, except in a pit, if one is present there.

With increasing age, enamel is decreased in thickness at the occluding areas as a result of attrition. Also, enamel mineralization and dehydration increase by age, increasing the brittleness and crazing tendency of enamel.

VII. Debridement of the Preparation

This is the act of freeing the preparation walls and margins from objects that may interfere with the proper adaptability and behavior of the restorative material. There are three main objectives for debriding the preparation:

A. The first is the freeing of all preparation walls, floors, and margins from enamel and dentin chips resulting from excavation and grinding. In addition to occupying a space that is supposed to be filled with the restorative material and interfering with its proximity to preparation details, this dentin and enamel debris may be sequestrated at a future time, resulting in increased microleakage space, greater possibilities of restoration micromovement, and decay recurrence around and under the restoration. Several agents are used to dislodge and free these debris particles, most of them are mainly mild detergents.

B. Drying the preparation walls, floors, and margins from any introduced moisture (i.e., any moisture other than dentin's own moisture, e.g., saliva, blood, exudate, etc.) is a prerequisite for the proper setting and behavior of any restorative material that will be inserted into a preparation. It is not only necessary to dry moisture, but also to completely remove the dried residue from different preparation details, as this residue can interfere with the tooth structure-restorative material interface, increasing the dimension of leakage space.

C. Sterilization of preparation walls and floors was one of G.V. Black's instructions. He advocated surgical sterilization of dentinal walls before insertion of restorative materials. But, given our present knowledge of the dimensions of the microleakage space around and under any restoration, it is impossible to maintain any sterile conditions once the restoration is exposed to the oral environment. Also, it is doubtful that surgical sterilization can be attained in preparation walls and floors without endangering the vitality of the pulp and dentin tissue.

So, until the introduction of a restorative material that can chemically bond with tooth structure, gross disinfection of the preparation before inserting the restorative material is the best that can be achieved.

Methods for Debridement and Their Effectiveness

A. Water, air, or combinations of air-water jets, using the water-air syringe, or the water and air accompanying any rotary cutting with a high speed handpiece, may be very efficient in removing gross debris, but there may also be some danger of overdrying of the dentin with consequent desiccation (see Biologic Form).

B. Dry cotton pellets are a very efficient and infinitely safer way to dry preparation details.

C. Cavity cleaners, which are solutions of very low concentration of citric, ascorbic and acetic acids (1-10%), are sometimes used to dislodge debris from preparation details. These should be used in shallow cavities, and they should be followed with a long period (at least 60 sec.) of water-jet rinsing. Some investigations imply that such cleaning solutions can irritate the P-D organ when they are used at certain depths. A dilute solution of hydrogen peroxide is a very efficient debris dislodging agent when rubbed in the preparation with a small cotton pellet. Sometimes, the liquid of certain cement restorative materials (polycarboxylate cement), when placed on a piece of cotton and rubbed in the cavity details, is a good cleaning agent.

D. Scraping preparation walls, floors and margins with sharp hand instruments, preferably chisels, is the most effective way of freeing lodged debris, which may then be washed away with running water.

E. Using preparation disinfectant has been almost discontinued in modern dental practice. In the past, dentists used phenolic and antibiotic compounds to sterilize the cavity preparation, but this is no longer acceptable. It is quite sufficient to irrigate the cavity with chloramine, saline or hydrogen peroxide solution before drying it, partially with air and finally with cotton pellets.

F. Whichever debridement technic is used a microscopic layer of dentinal smear will always be present on cut dentin. It could not be eliminated except with a 10% E.D.T.A. solution, a procedure needed only for chemically adhesive restorations.

VIII. Observing and Practicing the Biologic Form

Biologic form consists of the modifications added to the procedures of tooth preparation instrumentation to insure minimum irritation to the pulp-dentin organ and the investing periodontium. To observe and practice the biologic form, it is essential to know the biologic basis of the pulp-dentin organ and the periodontium, as well as to recognize the possible avenues of irritation to these tissues.

The Biologic Basis of the Pulp-Dentin Organ as Related to Operative Procedures

This section has been contributed by
Dr. A. H. El-Kafrawy, Professor,
Department of Oral Diagnosis and Medicine,
Indiana University School of Dentistry

Introduction

Embryologically and physiologically, dentin and pulp are so intimately related that dentin can be considered as the peripheral calcified portion of the dental pulp. Embryologically, both dentin and pulp are derived from the ectomesenchymal dental papilla. Physiologically dentin protects the pulp; conversely, dentin owes its vitality to the pulp. This intimate relation between dentin and pulp extends beyond embryologic and physiologic considerations. It has important clinical implications. It implies that the pulp would react whenever dentin is injured, whether the injury is caused by caries, attrition, abrasion, erosion, or operative procedures. Remember that dentin is permeated by the dentinal tubules, and that exposure of 1 mm square of dentin actually means exposure of about 30,000 dentinal tubules. Imagine then the number of dentinal tubules which will be exposed by full crown preparation. The nature of the pulp reaction which follows peripheral injury of the dentin depends on the nature of the causative agent and its proximity to the pulp. With mild irritation, reparative dentin will form beneath the damaged tubules. With more severe injury pulp inflammation would ensue.

Embryologic Considerations

While both dentin and pulp are derived from the ectomesenchymal dental papilla, this is, in turn, of neural origin. The neural crest is an important structure which forms in the embryo on each side of the neural tube. The neural tube and the neural crest are the two components of the neuroectoderm, which in turn is derived from the surface ectoderm under the inductive effect of the notochord and the paraxial mesoderm. The neural crest gives rise to a variety of derivatives including sensory and autonomic ganglia, the adrenal medulla, C cells of the thyroid glands, melanocytes, Schwann cells, and ectomesenchyme. Ectomesenchyme, then, is mesenchyme which is derived from the mesoderm. It is well to remember that most of the mesenchymal derivatives of the craniofacial region, including the dental papilla and the dental sac are of neural crest origin.

While tooth development will not be reviewed here in any detail, certain salient features should be considered. Tooth development starts at an early stage of embryonic life. The first sign of tooth development begins when the embryo is about 6 weeks of age. At this stage, the embryo is about 11 mm in length. By this time, ectomesenchyman cells from the neural crest already have migrated and populated the developing facial processes and pharyngeal arches. In the region of the developing jaws, ectomesenchymal cells induce the overlying oral epithelium which is ectodermal in origin to proliferate, thus forming the dental lamina. At localized points, the dental lamina proliferate to form the enamel organs. The enamel organs are initially spherical, but later through differential growth they will assume the shape of a cap, and then the shape of a bell. Meanwhile, ectomesenchymal cells underneath the enamel organ proliferate to form the dental papilla. Ectomesenchymal cells around the dental papilla and enamel organ also proliferate to form the dental sac. The enamel organ, dental papilla and dental sac constitute the tooth germ, the primordium of a developing tooth.

The enamel organ is the formative organ of enamel. It is also essential for differentiation of the odontoblasts. The dental papilla is the formative organ of dentin, and is the primordium of the dental pulp. The dental sac is the formative organ of cementum, and the periodontal ligament. There is recent evidence that the alveolar bone proper is also formed by the dental sac.

At the bell stage, the cells of the enamel organ would already have differentiated into the outer enamel epithelium, the stellate reticulum, the stratum intermedium, and the inner enamel epithelium. The cells of the inner enamel epithelium induce the adjacent ectomesenchymal cells of the dental papilla to differentiate into odontoblasts. Upon their differentiation, the odontoblasts start their synthetic and secretory activities and deposit the organic matrix of dentin. Thus, dentin is the first hard dental tissue to form during tooth development. With the deposition of a thin layer of dentin, the cells of the inner enamel epithelium, which already have differentiated into the ameloblasts, start their synthetic and secretory activity and deposit the enamel matrix. As they do so, they recede from the matrix which they have deposited. Tomes' processes are conical projections at the secretory pole of the ameloblasts. Enamel matrix formation is followed by initial mineralization, whereby 25% to 30% of the total mineral content of enamel is deposited. Maturation of the enamel matrix later follows through crystal growth so that ultimately, mature enamel, which is the hardest tissue in the human body, contains about 96% mineral, chiefly, calcium hydroxyapatite. Obviously, room has to be provided for the crystals to grow. To provide this, the ameloblasts resorb over 90% of the matrix which they initially deposited.

Meanwhile, the odontoblasts have been depositing the organic matrix of dentin. As they do so they recede towards the future pulp, leaving behind cytoplasmic processes (Tomes' fibers) within the dentinal tubules, Organic matrix formation is followed by mineralization; however, mineralization lags behind matrix formation and a layer of uncalcified matrix or predentin is found in mature teeth with healthy pulps on the pulpal surface of dentin. Dentin is less hard than enamel, and its mineral content is about 65% to 70% of the weight of dentin.

At the cervical region of the enamel organ, the outer and enamel epithelium form the cervical loop. Proliferation of the latter gives rise to Hertwig's epithelial root sheath. The cervical loop marks the future cementoenamel junction. Hertwig's epithelial root sheath forms a mold which determines root morphology. It also exerts an inductive effect on the adjacent ectomesenchymal cells of the dental papilla to differentiate into odontoblasts, which form the radicular dentin.

When root dentin formation has begun, the newly deposited dentin is separated from the adjacent ectomesenchymal cells of the dental sac by Hertwig's epithelial root sheath. The continuity of the latter is soon lost (programmed cell death). With partial disintegration of the root sheath, ectomesenchymal cells of the dental sac come in contact with the root dentin and differentiate into cementoblasts. The latter deposit cementum in two stages. An organic matrix is first deposited (cementoid). Calcification of cementoid then follows. Cementum is the softest dental tissue and it has a mineral content of about 45% to 50% by weight.

When enamel formation is completed, the outer cells of the enamel organ form a stratified squamous epithelium, the reduced enamel epithelium which covers the entire surface of the crown. The reduced enamel epithelium protects enamel from contact with adjacent mesenchymal cells prior to tooth eruption. If the reduced enamel epithelium separates from the enamel surface or if it prematurely degenerates, mesenchymal cells from the dental sac come in contact with enamel and deposit afibrillar cementum over the enamel surface. This happens frequently over the cervical portion of the crown where in 60% to 65% of instances, the cementum overlaps enamel in the region of the cementoenamel junction. With tooth eruption, the reduced enamel epithelium fuses with the oral epithelium. Once the tip of the crown has emerged through the oral mucosa, the reduced enamel epithelium becomes the primary junctional epithelium. The latter is attached to the tooth surface by means of a basal lamina with associated hemidesmosomes. Gradually, the primary junctional epithelium is replaced by the secondary junctional epithelium, which is derived from the oral epithelium. Like the primary junctional epithelium, the secondary junctional epithelium is attached to the tooth surface by a basal lamina with associated hemidesmosomes.

Histologic Considerations

The histology of dentin and pulp will not be reviewed here in any detail. Only certain features will be considered.

Dentin is permeated by the dentinal tubules. The tubules are about 3 to 4 microns in diameter towards their pulpal ends, and they taper to about 1 micron peripherally. Peritubular dentin surrounds the dentinal tubules. Peritubular dentin is harder and more heavily mineralized than the adjacent intertubular dentin. With age and in response to irritants, e.g., slowly progressing caries, the dentinal tubules may become obliterated through deposition of minerals inside them. This results in dentin sclerosis and, eventually, in calcific barrier.

Histologically, the pulp is a special type of connective tissue, and as such it is made up of cells and intercellular substance. It is richly supplied with blood vessels and nerves. The existence of lymphatic vessels in the pulp has long been the subject of considerable controversy. It is now recognized that lymphatic vessels exist in the pulp.

The cells of the pulp can be classified into formative cells, defense cells, and reserve cells. The formative cells are the odontoblasts and fibroblasts, which are involved in the formation of dentin and components of the intercellular substance of the pulp, respectively. The defense cells are occasional histiocytes and occasional lymphocytes. The reserve cells are undifferentiated mesenchymal cells. The latter, which bear morphologic similarity to quiescent fibroblasts, are found mainly in perivascular location and in the cell rich zone of the pulp. They are pluripotent and can differentiate into odontoblasts and fibroblasts.

The odontoblast consists of a cell body located on the pulpal surface of the dentin, and a cytoplasmic process (Tomes' fiber) which extends inside the dentinal tubules. How far inside the tubules Tomes' fibers does extend has recently been debated. The classive view is that Tomes' fibers extend throughout the entire length of the tubule. However, some recent studies have shown that Tomes' fibers are restricted to the pulpal portion of the dentinal tubule. Nevertheless, at one time in tooth development, the fibers have been present throughout the entire length of the tubule. Whether Tomes' fibers undergo regressive changes in their peripheral portion, as recent studies suggest, or whether they extend throughout the length of the tubules must await further investigation. More studies are needed to answer this important question in pulpal biology.

When active in dentin formation, the odontoblastic perikaryon show all features of cells active in protein synthesis and secretion: a well-developed granular endoplasmic reticulum, a well-developed Golgi complex, and numerous mitochondria. By contrast, Tomes' fibers show only a few organelles and a granular endoplasmic reticulum is absent. This indicates that the organic matrix of the peritubular dentin is formed within the odontoblastic cell bodies and is then transported via Tomes' fibers to be released extracellularly. The odontoblasts synthesize and secrete the components of the organic matrix of dentin, chiefly type I collagen and proteoglycans. They appear to play a role in matrix calcification, through the formation and release of matrix vesicles containing alkaline phosphatase, and calcium and phosphate ions. Whether they play a role in dentin sensitivity is debatable. Odontoblasts are end cells, being incapable of mitosis.

Pulpal fibroblasts, when active, show all features of cells active in protein synthesis and secretion. They synthesize and secrete components of intercellular substance of the pulp, namely type I and type III collagen and glycosaminoglycans of the ground substances, chiefly hyaluronic acid.

Occasional histiocytes are found in the normal pulp, chiefly in perivascular locations. A recent view is that connective tissue histiocytes are derived from blood monocytes which have migrated from the circulation. The occasional lymphocytes found in the normal pulp are also hematogenous in origin. It is now recognized that lymphocytes, particularly T lymphocytes, are highly migratory cells. They undergo constant recirculation, leaving the blood to reside transiently in lymph nodes and other lymphoid organs and then they return to the blood. They also migrate from the blood to connective tissue of various organs in the body. The reason for this constant lymphocyte shuttle is to monitor the body for antigens.

The dental pulp has a rich vascular supply. The major blood vessels of the pulp enter and exit through the apical foramen, as well as through accessory foramina which are frequently present in the apical region. The pulpal blood vessels are quite unique, in that even the larger blood vessels have thin walls in relation to the size of their lumen. The terminal ramification of the pulpal blood vessels are present adjacent to the odontoblasts, but are seldom found among them. This anatomical feature is of clinical importance, since in deep cavities it is possible to have a microscopic pulp exposure without clinically detectable bleeding.

The dental pulp has a rich nerve supply. Both myelinated and unmyelinated nerve fibers enter through the apical foramen. The unmyelinated fibers belong to the sympathetic division of the autonomic nervous system. They supply the smooth muscle cells in the walls of the larger blood vessels, and they regulate blood flow through the pulp. The myelinated fibers as their name indicates possess a myelin sheath, which is derived from the plasmalemma of Schwann cells which has been wrapped around the axon during development. The myelinated fibers ultimately lose their myelin sheath and some terminate close to the odontoblastic perikaryon, and gap junctions have recently been demonstrated between them. This is a type of intercellular junction, which permits intercellular communication through interchange of ions and small molecules between cells at the site of the junction. The demonstration of this type of junction in the pulp between nerve endings and odontoblastic cell bodies have implications in dentin sensitivity; they indicate that the odontoblasts and the nerve endings may be electrotonically coupled. Some unmyelinated nerve fibers enter the dentinal tubules; however, the proportion of tubules that contain nerve fibers has been estimated to range from 1:10 to 1:2000. The nerve fibers of the pulp belong to the Aδ and C type of fibers. These fibers transmit pain sensation. The dental pulp responds to any stimulus regardless of its nature, whether thermal, electrical, or mechanical by pain and pain only. The reason for this is that the pulp contains only free nerve endings which are receptors for pain. Encapsulated nerve endings such as Meissner's corpuscles, Krause's end bulbs or Ruffini's corpuscles are not present in the dental pulp.

Physiologic Considerations

I. Dentin Sensitivity

Dentin is a highly sensitive tissue, and the pulp is responsible for dentin sensitivity. However, the mechanism of sensation transmission through dentil still remains obscure.

There is no doubt that dentin is innervated. Unmyelinated nerve fibers have been demonstrated within the dentinal tubules, where they lie in a concavity in Tomes' fibers. However, these fibers are limited to the pulpal one-third of some dentinal tubules. They are not present in the peripheral portion of the dentinal tubules; nor at the dentino-enamel junction wich reputedly is the most sensitive part of the dentin. The role of the intratubular nerve fibers in dentin sensitivity is obscure; it is not known whether these fibers are sensory or autonomic. It has been suggested that these fibers are involved in regulation of dentinogenesis.

The concept that the odontoblast, with its cytoplasmic process, serves as a receptor has been advanced. The morphology of the odontoblast with a perikaryon and a ctyoplasmic process is somewhat reminiscent of that of a neuron. Furthermore, the odontoblasts are of neural crest origin, and they may retain some neurogenic properties. However, the resting membrane potential of the odontoblast is too low for the cell to be considered highly excitable. The resting membrane potential of the odontoblasts has been estimated to be about $-35mv$. Compare that to the resting potential of a neuron ($-70mv$). In addition, chemicals which are known to elicit pain when applied to exposed nerve endings (e.g., histamine and bradykinin) do not produce pain when applied to exposed dentin. Lastly, the possibility that Tomes' fibers are restricted to the pulpal portion of the dentinal tubules will cast further doubt

on the role of the odontoblasts in sensation transmission through the dentin. On the other hand, the presence of gap junctions between nerve endings and the odontoblastic perikaryon would suggest that they are electrotonically coupled, and that the odontoblast may transmit signals (ions) through the junctions, thus exciting the nerve endings in the pulp.

Finally, it has been suggested that sensation transmission through dentin is a hydrodynamic phenomenon, involving fluid movement in the dentinal tubules. Such fluid movement can occur as a result of dehydration of dentin, heat, or application of sugar or salt solution to dentin. It is known that dentin contains fluid which originates from the interstitial tissue fluid in the pulp. The fluid movement in the tubules would lead to minute changes in intrapulpal pressure, exciting sensory nerve endings in the pulp. If this is the case, the pulp has to be considered as a mechanoreceptor, sensitive to minute volume changes.

II. Dentin Permeability

There is constant interchange of fluid between dentin and pulp. Radioactive iodine applied to exposed dentin has been found to reach the pulp. Phosphoric acid labelled with radioactive phosphorous and applied to dentin surface penetrates dentin and reaches the dental pulp.

III. Dentinogenesis

Dentinogenesis has been reviewed earlier. Dentinogenesis occurs throughout the life span of teeth with healthy pulps. Dentin has been classified into primary, secondary, and tertiary categories. Primary dentin is that which is formed during tooth development. With apical closure, formation of primary dentin is complete. Dentinogenesis continues thereafter at a slow rate. This secondary dentin formation occurs in the absence of any external stimulus. It occurs in unerupted teeth. Tertiary dentin forms as a result of peripheral injury to the dentinal tubules. It is localized underneath the tubules which have been damaged. Since tertiary dentin is a reparative phenomenon in response to injury, tertiary dentin has also been designated as reparative dentin. The term secondary dentin has been used in the past rather loosely to designate reparative or tertiary dentin.

The rate of reparative dentinogenesis has been investigated in men and monkeys. In men the average daily rate was 1.5 microns. In monkeys the average daily rate is about 4 microns. The rate of reparative dentinogenesis is similar under materials of different irritational potential.

Reparative dentin is an effective protective barrier. In a study of pulp reactions to silicate cement, cavities which were left exposed to the oral environment for three months to induce reparative dentinogenesis were later restored with silicate cement. Such teeth showed no pulp inflammation. On the other hand, silicate cement placed in freshly cut cavities showed pulp inflammation, the intensity of which varied with remaining dentin thickness. This study indicates that greater pulp reaction will occur when sound dentin is cut beyond carious dentin for extension for prevention or in crown preparation.

Pathologic Considerations

The most common cause of pulp injury is progression of dental caries. Pulp injury may also be iatrogenic in origin. Iatrogenic pulp injury will be considered later. Caries destroys dentin at a rate that has been estimated to be about one mm/ six months. As caries progresses, the pulp attempts to defend itself by deposition of reparative dentin under the tubules which have been damaged. Without treatment, pulpitis eventually develops.

There is a difference of opinion as to the point in caries progression at which pulpitis ensues. There are studies which indicate that foci of pulp inflammation develop when caries is still restricted to the superficial portion of dentin. Other studies showed that significant pulp inflammation occurs only when caries is within 750μm from the pulp. More studies are needed in this important area of pulp biology. But regardless of the point in time at which pulpitis ensues, early detection and treatment of dental caries is the best measure for prevention of irreversible pulp disease.

It is significant to note that pulpitis ensues before actual invasion of the pulp by bacteria from the carious dentin. The pathogenesis of such pulpal lesions could be bacterial acid metabolites and other irritant products of bacterial metabolism, bacterial enzymes, bacterial toxins, and irritant by-products of tissue degradation. Some of these products may serve as antigens and elicit an immune response. The inflammatory infiltrate which develops in such pulpal lesions, prior to actual bacterial invasion is predominately mononuclear (lymphocytes, plasma cells and macrophages). With actual invasion of the pulp by bacteria, polymorphonuclear neutrophil leukocytes will accumulate in significant numbers at the site of invasion.

While the inflammatory process will not be reviewed here in any detail, certain salient features will be considered. Inflammation can be defined as a series of morphological and biochemical changes which occur in a living tissue in response to a sublethal injury. Such injury can be due to physical agents, e.g., traumatic injury to the pulp if it is accidentally exposed during cavity preparation, pressure generated during condensation of amalgam or gold foil, or heat generated during cavity preparation. It can be due to chemical irritants such as phosphoric acid in silicate cement or zinc phosphate cement, or residual monomers in resin restorations. The injury can be due to infection with microbiologic agents, e.g., invasion of the pulp by bacteria from carious dentin, or it can be a consequence of immunologic reactions, e.g., those which involve the formation and deposition in tissues of immune complexes, or the development of sensitized T lymphocytes. But regardless of the causative agent, the inflammatory process is stereotyped.

The essence of inflammation is to mobilize to the site of injury the humoral and cellular defense elements of the body, with the object of elimination and destruction of the irritant, removal of the cells which have been damaged, and, ultimately, repair of the damage which has been done. Inflammation, therefore, generally serves a useful purpose. However, inflammation can be harmful and destructive. Witness the destruction which accompanies the progression of pulpitis to periapical pathoses and the destruction of tooth supporting tissues which occur in untreated chronic inflammatory periodontal disease.

The defense elements of the body which are mobilized to the site of injury are present in the blood. To achieve their mobilization, changes occur in the microcirculation of the injured area. Without going into any detail, these vascular and hemodynamic changes are dominated by vasodilatation, and increased vascular permeability (due to contraction of the endothelial cells). The vascular and hemodynamic changes are mediated by a variety of chemical substances which are released in the injured area. These include histamine (from mast cells and basophil leukocytes), serotonin (from the dense granules of blood platelets), the kinins (peptides formed through cleavage of kininogens by kininogenases), the anaphylatoxins (cleavage of the third and fifth components of the complement system releasing the anaphylatoxins C_3a and C_5a, which in turn release histamine from mast cells and basophils), and the prostaglandins and the leukotrinenes (arachidonic acid derivatives).

Exudation develops as a result of the increased vascular permeability. Leukocytes which have marginated adjacent to the vascular endothelium and adhered to the endothelial cells send pseudopods through the gaps between the endothelial cells and escape from the vascular lumen. Once outside the endothelial cells, they migrate towards the area of injury under the influence of chemotactic factors, which are both bacterial and endogenous in origin. The latter include C_5a, the triple complex C_{567}, and lymphokines released from both T and B lymphocytes.

Neutrophils are the first leukocytes to arrive at the site of injury. They constitute a primary line of defense against infection. They are the predominant cells of acute inflammation. However, virtually any type of injury results in initial accumulation of neutrophils. Neutrophils are motile, phagocytic, and efficient bacterial killers. Marked increase in the metabolic activity of the neutrophils accompanies phagocytosis. This involves a respiratory burst with increase in oxygen consumption, activation of the hexose monophosphate shunt, and generation of reactive oxygen radicals (superoxide and hydrogen peroxide). The latter are bactericidal. Furthermore, H_2O_2 in the presence of myeloperoxidase (enzyme present in the primary granules of neutrophils) and a halogen (e.g., chloride or iodide) lead to the generation of a hypohalite (hypochlorite, hypoiodite) which damages the bacterial cells. Lactoferrin (an iron binding protein present in the specific granules of the neutrophils) binds iron and deprives bacteria of this essential element. Lysozyme (present in both the primary and specific granules of the neutrophils) breaks down the cell walls of certain bacteria.

Neutrophils are end cells, being incapable of mitosis. Their life span in the circulation is limited, with half-life of about 6 hours. The primary granules of the neutrophils are of the nature of lysosomes. These membrane-bound organelles contain a variety of enzymes which can digest virtually every cellular constitutent. Release of such enzymes leads to tissue injury. Such release follows neutrophil death; it follows phagocytosis of crystalline particles, and it occurs when the neutrophils attempt to phagocytose particles that are too large to ingest (frustrated phagocytosis).

Whereas the neutrophils are the predominant cells of acute inflammation, macrophages, lymphocytes, and plasma cells are the predominant cells of chronic inflammation. What leads to chronicity is the persistence of the irritant, or the development of a delayed hypersensitivity reaction or both.

Macrophages are derived from the monocytes of blood. Monocytes are not end cells. Their half-life in the circulation is about one day. They leave the circulation and form the different components of the mononuclear phagocyte system (histiocytes, Kupffer cells, alveolar and peritoneal macrophages, etc).

Macrophages are efficient phagocytes. Not only do they

phagocytose bacteria, but they also ingest tissue debris (hence the name scavengers) to clean up the area in preparation for repair. They also play an essential role in the development of immune reactions through antigen processing and antigen presentation to lymphocytes. They have a secretory function. Among their secretory products are the antibacterial enzyme lysozyme, the antiviral protein interferon, certain components of the complement system, and collagenase.

Lymphocytes are the essential cells of the immune system. Two major types are recognized: T and B lymphocytes. T lymphocytes are the essential cells of cell-mediated immunity. B lymphocytes are the essential cells of humoral immunity. Intricate interactions take place between T and B lymphocytes and T helper cells are essential for the induction of a humoral immune response to certain antigens. T supressor cells regulate both humoral and cell mediated immune reactions.

Plasma cells are derived from B lymphocytes. They synthesize and secrete immunoglobulins. The function of lymphocytes and plasma cells in areas of nonspecific chronic inflammation has long been a mystery. Their known role in immune reactions suggests that antigens are released locally, eliciting a local immune response.

Eosinophils may be encountered in inflamed tissues, including inflamed pulps. They are prominent in allergic inflammation. They phagocytose antigen antibody complexes. They contain enzymes which inactivate many of the chemical mediators which are released in areas of injury. They are end cells, with a half-life in blood of 2 to 5 hours.

The cardinal signs of inflammation are redness, swelling, heat, pain and loss of function. Keep in mind that these signs are evident when inflammation affects an area of the body that is accessible to inspection. Neither redness, swelling nor heat are evident on clinical inspection of a tooth with pulpitis. Furthermore, whereas pain is one of the cardinal signs of inflammation, inflammation can be present without pain being experienced by the patient. Painless pulpitis is a well recognized clinical entity.

Biological Aspects of Dental Materials

Historically, biological evaluation of dental materials lagged behind evaluation of their physical and chemical properties, despite the fact that the biological aspects of dental materials are just as important as their physical and chemical properties. Currently, numerous tests are available for evaluation of the biocompatibility of materials used in dentistry. These tests can be classified into screening tests and usage tests. Screening tests can be further classified into *in vitro* tests, which rely mainly on cell culture methods for evaluation of the cytotoxicity of the material, and *in vivo* tests, which rely mainly on subcutaneous implantation of the material in small laboratory animals, for evaluation of the irritational potential of the material. Screening tests are also available for assessing acute systemic toxicity, mucosal irritation, and the allergenic and carcinogenic potential of dental materials. In the usage tests, the materials are evaluated in suitable laboratory animals, preferably subhuman primates, under conditions simulating the clinical use of the material. If the screening tests and usage tests in animals show that the material is safe, the material would then be ready for evaluation in humans.

Clinical Considerations

"DO NO HARM" is a basic principle which should be followed by all members of the health professions. The dentist, during his restorative procedures, can elicit pulp injury. The precautions to avoid this are quite simple. First, it is important to recognize the potential causes. Iatrogenic pulp injury can occur during the preparation and restoration of the tooth due to: a) the inherent irritational potential of the material used for restoration b) residual bacteria left after cavity preparation c) bacteria which gain access to the cavity after restoration through microleakage d) undetected microscopic exposure of the pulp (Dentin is a vital tissue; the fact that it is a hard tissue that does not bleed on cutting might give rise to a false sense of security) e) heat generation and dentin dessication during cavity preparation.

Heat dissipation and prevention of dessication can both be accomplished through the use of a water coolant. With the present-day high-speed instrumentation, the use of a water coolant is mandatory. So the first principle to eliminate two sources of iatrogenic pulp injury (heat and dessication) is *Never Cut Dry*.

Iatrogenic pulp injury can also occur during the insertion of the restorative material. Pressure generated during condensation of gold foil and amalgam can lead to transient pulpitis. Such lesions are reversible, barring the presence of a microscopic exposure of the pulp.

As mentioned above, pulp injury can be due to the inherent irritational potential of the material used for restoration. In this regard, the most critical factor in determining the intensity of pulp reaction is the remaining dentin thickness; however, another important factor is the presence or absence of reparative dentin beneath the cut dentinal tubules. For most materials, 2mm of remaining dentin affords adequate pulp protection. Since it is difficult to determine clinically the cavity floor thickness, the use of a protective base is mandatory with restorative materials which are known to be chemically irritating. Every cavity to be restored with composite resins, whether chemically-cured or photoactivated, or with silicate cement, should have a protective base before the insertion of the restorative material. Furthermore, such protective bases should be inserted in every deep cavity regardless of the type of restorative material to be used, since there is always the possibility in such deep cavities of the presence of an undetected microscopic exposure.

The "ideal" protective base should possess the following characteristics: 1). It should be well tolerated by the dental pulp. 2). It should promote reparative dentinogenesis in case of accidental pulp exposure. 3). It should provide adequate pulp protection, preventing irritant components in the restorative material from reaching the pulp. 4). It should have adequate physical properties to withstand forces incidental to the insertion of the restorative material. 5). It should have antibacterial properties to eliminate any residual bacteria left in the cavity. Such antibacterial properties should prefereably be sustained, so that in the event of microleakage, bacteria that would reach the cavity floor would be promptly killed or their growth inhibited. 6). It should have an obtundent effect on the pulp. 7). It should be compatible with the restorative material used, so that the restorative material will not discolor or in any way be altered through interaction with components of the base.

Unfortunately, the ideal protective base which fulfills all of these criteria has yet to be developed. However, both calcium hydroxide, either in pure chemical form mixed with water, or as a component of one of the proprietary preparations, and also zinc oxide and eugenol fulfill many of these criteria. In most cases, both calcium hydroxide and its preparations, and zinc oxide and eugenol, are well tolerated by the pulp when placed in cavities with an intact floor. Both afford adequate protection and both have antibacterial properties, but whether the antibacterial effect is sustained is doubtful and should await further investigation. Zinc oxide and eugenol has an obtundent effect on the pulp (eugenol inhibits prostaglandin synthesis). However, zinc oxide and eugenol does not readily stimulate reparative dentinogenesis in cases of microscopic exposure; on the contrary, when placed in direct contact with the pulp, it could elicit a low grade chronic inflammation in the vicinity of the exposure. (This subject will be discussed in full detail in a chapter on intermediary bases and basing).

There has been considerable discussion as to the role of bacteria in pulp irritation under restorative materials. In fact, the concept has been advanced that pulp irritation under restorative materials is primarily bacterial in origin. However, while bacteria may contribute to pulp irritation, particularly in deep cavities, they cannot be considered solely responsible for pulp irritation to the exclusion of the inherent irritational potential of the restorative material itself.

For a long time, an exposed pulp was considered a doomed pulp. However, no longer can this be considered to be true, for numerous studies have shown that the pulp has remarkable reparative potential. The importance of bacterial infection in determining the ultimate fate of exposed pulps has been well demonstrated in studies with germ-free animals. In these studies, pulp exposure is followed by repair, without the application of any medicament to the exposed pulp. On the other hand, similarly exposed pulps in conventional animals developed inflammation, necrosis and periapical pathosis.

Numerous agents have been advocated for pulp capping. However, calcium hydroxide or one of its proprietary preparations have been most widely used for this purpose. These preparations are well tolerated by the dental pulp. They induce reparative dentinogenesis over the exposure, resulting in dentinal bridging of the exposure. The mechanism by which calcium hydroxide or one of its preparations exert this salutary effect on the pulp is rather obscure. It is known that such preparations are basic in the freshly mixed state (pH about 11), but basicity cannot be entirely responsible for their favorable effect, as compounds which are equally basic elicit persistent pulpitis. Furthermore, studies with ^{45}Ca labelled calcium hydroxide showed that calcium ions in calcium hydroxide are not utilized in the calcification of the bridge.

Histological studies have shown that calcium hydroxide mixed with water and applied over exposed pulps elicits a superficial zone of coagulation necrosis. New odontoblasts then develop through differentiation of undifferentiated mesenchymal cells in the pulp. Bearing in mind that odontoblasts are end cells, being incapable of mitosis, differentiation of odontoblasts from the undifferentiated mesenchymal cells of the pulp in preparation of reparative dentinogenesis is one of the most fascinating aspects in pulp biology. During tooth development, odontoblasts differentiate under the inductive influence of epithelium, i.e., the inner enamel epithelium in the case of odontoblasts that form coronal dentin, and Hertwig's epithelial root sheath for odontoblasts that deposit radicular dentin. How an inorganic compound can elicit, directly or indirectly, similar cell differentiation is obscure. One might speculate that some of the undifferentiated mesenchymal cells of the pulp have already been induced under epithelial influence during tooth development. In other words, these cells could be predestined for odontoblastic differentiation. It should be mentioned that odontoblastic differentiation also occurs in formation of reparative dentin under cavities with intact floors. Following cavity preparation and restoration, odontoblasts may get displaced inside the dentinal tubules (aspiration of odontoblasts). These displaced odontoblasts degenerate, and new odontoblasts develop from the undifferentiated mesenchymal cells of the pulp.

There has been widespread concern among dentists that calcium hydroxide preparations applied over exposed pulps exert a persistent stimulating effect on reparative dentinogenesis, sometimes resulting in eventual pulp obliteration. This is not the case if calcium hydroxide is brought in contact with a pulp-dentin organ that has not undergone any degeneration. In an experimental study of pulp reactions to three capping agents, the rate of reparative dentinogenesis under a calcium hydroxide preparation (Dycal) was investigated. An initial high rate of reparative dentinogenesis was noticed. That rate of formation declined with time, and none of the pulps capped by this preparation showed obliteration after a follow-up period of 880 days. Interestingly, with this calcium hydroxide preparation, reparative dentin was often noticed to be directly in contact with the material. Of further interest, is that one of the other materials used in this study (an antibiotic) proved to be highly irritating. Many of the pulps capped with this antibiotic showed severe inflammation, and many underwent necrosis, but a few survived with persistent inflammation. These persistently inflamed pulps showed evidence of pulp obliteration. Thus, the stimulus for eventual pulp obliteration is apparently persistent inflammation, rather than the direct effect of any medicament applied to the pulps.

Direct Irritation to the Pulp-Dentin Organ

The pulp tissues of the tooth may be directly endangered or injured either by its exposure (Fig. 119), especially in large pulp chambers of young persons, or by involvement of its recessional lines. Both situations allow direct access for the oral flora and other irritating ingredients to reach the pulp and root canal system.

I. Recessional Lines

Recessional lines of the pulp horns are the lines along which the pulp has receded during the growth of the dentin. They are also lines in which unusually long pulpal extensions are found, which are often exposed when these lines are cut. In its early growth, the full size of the crown of the tooth presents as the junction of the enamel plates of several lobes of tooth. At this juncture, a very thin layer of dentin is formed on the inner

DIRECT PULP EXPOSURE

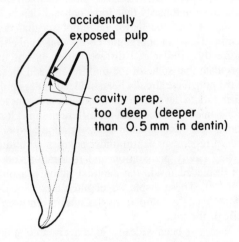

accidentally
exposed pulp

cavity prep.
too deep (deeper
than 0.5 mm in dentin)

Fig. 1-119

RECESSIONAL LINES

Older Patient   **Young Patient**

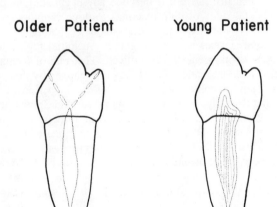

Fig. 1-120   **Fig. 1-121**

surface of the enamel cap. Practically speaking, the whole dentin of the tooth crown is represented within the pulp tissues. Because the dentin grows from the dentino-enamel junction inwards, the pulp recedes and becomes smaller as this dentin is formed. This growth is comparatively rapid during childhood, and, under normal conditions, gradually slows until age 40. Under abnormal conditions, e.g., irritation from caries, erosion, or abrasion, the process is more rapid, and it may progress to complete obliteration of the pulp chamber. During both normal and abnormal recession of the pulp, the pulpal horns become shorter and shorter (Fig. 120). The path of this recession of the horns of the pulp has been named the recessional lines of the pulpal horns. Frequently, a pulp horn will persist as a slender thread of tissues near the point of a cusp, even when the rest of the pulp chamber has become quite small (Fig. 121). These tiny remnants of the pulp horns, although continuous with the pulp tissues proper, cannot be seen in all

cross-sections of the tooth, and they are definitely not visible in a radiograph of the tooth.

The recessional lines travel from the axio-occlusal margin or crest of the pulp near its corners, towards the tip of each of the cusps of the tooth (Fig. 121). Although this line is nearly straight, it may have a little bend following the concavity of the occlusal surface. Therefore, tooth cutting should not cross this path, in order to avoid directly involving the pulp. The vascularity of these pulp threads is very limited, so there will usually be no bleeding if they are inadvertently involved in the cavity preparation.

II. Anatomy of the Pulp in Situ

It is not the intention in this presentation to describe in detail the anatomy of the pulp chamber and pulp horns, but to point out only certain salient aspects of that anatomy.

Maxillary incisors (Fig. 122) have four pulp horns, three in the mesio-distal direction and one in the labio-lingual direction. The one closest to the surface is the cingulum pulp horn. The pulp chamber is lingually deviated in the labio-lingual direction, but centrally placed in the mesio-distal direction.

Maxillary lateral incisors (Fig. 123) are similar to maxillary central incisors, but the pulp horns are more blunt, and the pulp chamber is larger, relative to the tooth size.

Maxillary canines (Fig. 124) have two pulp horns. The closest to the surface is the one within the cingulum. The pulp chamber is lingually deviated in the labio-lingual direction but centrally placed in the mesio-distal direction. Compared to the central incisors, the canine pulp chamber is smaller relative to the crown size.

Maxillary first premolars (Figs. 125 and 126) have two pulp horns. The most pronounced and the one closest to the surface is the buccal horn. The pulp chamber is centrically located within the tooth structure, but elongated in the bucco-lingual direction.

Maxillary second premolars (Fig. 127) are similar to the maxillary first prelars, but the pulp horns are less pronounced.

Maxillary first molars (Fig. 128) have four pulp horns. Each corresponds to a cusp. The one closest to the surface is the mesio-buccal horn. The one furthest from the surface is the disto-lingual horn. The pulp chamber walls are convex internally. The pulp chamber and pulp horns are mesio-buccally deviated.

Maxillary second molars (Fig. 129) are similar to the maxillary first molars but they present less pronounced pulp horns.

Maxillary third molars have the youngest relative pulpal age of *all* maxillary teeth. If this tooth is quadritubercular, it will have similar pulpal anatomy to the first and second molars, except for a larger pulp chamber and more pronounced pulp horns, a more occlusally deviated pulp chamber with more funnel shape towards the roots, and the whole tooth crown and pulp are disto-buccally tilted.

If this tooth is tritubercular, there will be one pulp horn for each cusp, with the previously mentioned variations. However, each tooth should be examined individually, both clinically and radiographically, in order to estimate the location of the pulp chamber and horns, as it may vary.

Mandibular central incisors (Fig. 130) have three pulp horns, two in a mesio-distal direction and one lingually at the cingulum. Although the horns are more blunt than those of

Maxillary Central Incisor

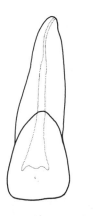
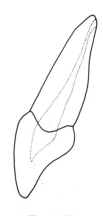
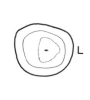

L

Fig. 1-122

Maxillary Lateral Incisor

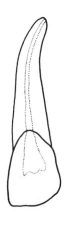
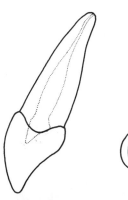

L

Fig. 1-123

Maxillary Canine

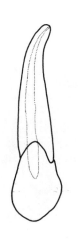
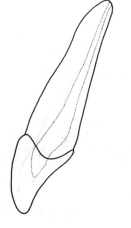

L

Fig. 1-124

Maxillary 1st Premolar

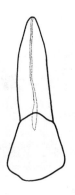
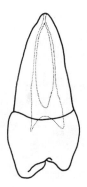

Fig. 1-125

Maxillary 1st Premolar

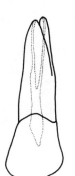
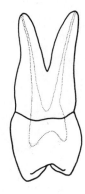

Fig. 1-126

Maxillary 2nd Premolar

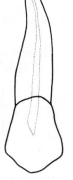
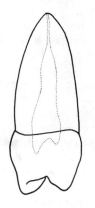

Fig. 1-127

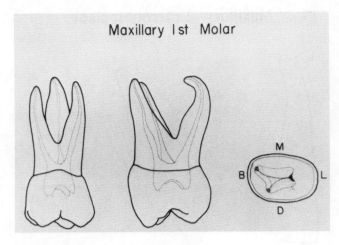

Fig. 1-128

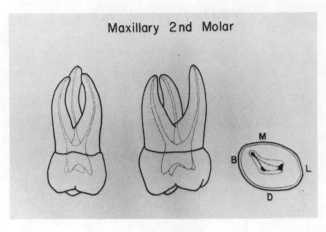

Fig. 1-129

maxillary incisors, the pulp chamber size is very large relative to the tooth size. The pulp is larger in the mesio-distal direction than in the labio-lingual direction at its incisal half, but the reverse is true at its gingival half.

Mandibular lateral incisors (Fig. 131) are very similar to the mandibular centrals, but they possess a more fan-shaped pulp and crown.

Mandibular canines (Fig. 132) are very similar to the maxillary canines, except they have a very compressed pulp chamber in the mesio-distal direction.

Mandibular first premolars (Fig. 133) usually have only one pulp horn buccally, but sometimes there may be two pulp horns —a very pronounced buccal horn, and a minute, blunted lingual horn. The pulp chamber is rounded and always centrically placed within the tooth.

Mandibular second premolars (Fig. 134) vary, depending on whether they are bicuspid or tricuspid. A bicuspid second premolar will be similar to a first premolar, with two pulp horns. A tricuspid premolar will have three pulp horns. The more pronounced of these is the buccal horn, and the least pronounced is the disto-lingual horn. The pulp chamber and horns will be slightly mesio-buccally deviated, so that the pulp horns are not exactly under the tip of each cusp.

Mandibular first molars (Fig. 135) usually have five pulp horns, each corresponding to a cusp. The most pronounced of these is the mesio-buccal pulp horn. Because the entire pulp chamber is mesio-buccally deviated, the closest pulp horn to the surface is the mesio-buccal horn. The walls of the pulp chamber are concave internally and generally triangular in shape, with the base towards the mesial.

Mandibular second molars (Fig. 136) usually have four pulp horns, each corresponding to a cusp. The pulpal anatomy is similar to that of the first molar.

Mandibular third molars also vary, depending on the number of cusps. If the tooth is quadritubercular, pulpal anatomy will be similar to that of the second molar. If it is quantitubercular, pulpal anatomy will resemble that of the first molar, with the following variations:

1. The third molar, the youngest tooth in the quadrant, will have a relatively large pulp chamber and more pronounced pulp horns.

Mandibular Central Incisor

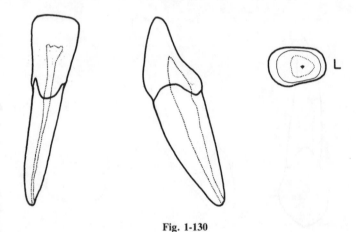

Fig. 1-130

Mandibular Lateral Incisor

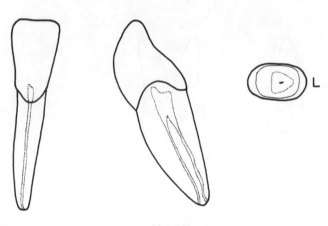

Fig. 1-131

Mandibular Canine

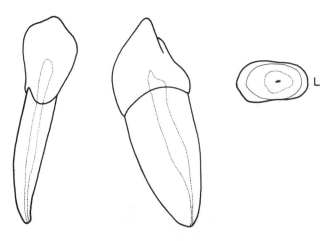

Fig. 1-132

Mandibular 1st Premolar

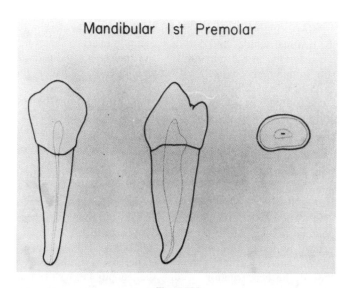

Fig. 1-133

Mandibular 2nd Premolar

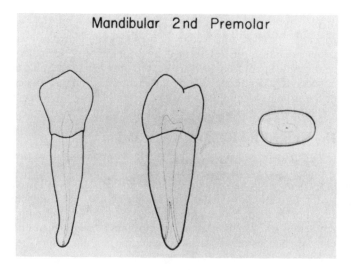

Fig. 1-134

Mandibular 1st Molar

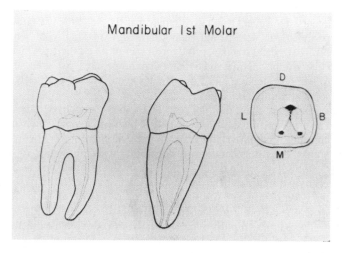

Fig. 1-135

Mandibular 2nd Molar

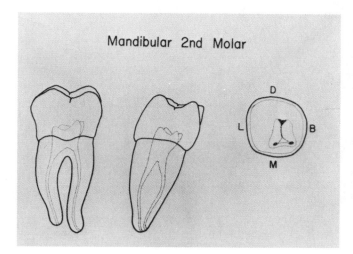

Fig. 1-136

2. The pulp chamber is occlusally deviated and constricted apically.
3. The entire crown and pulp are mesio-lingually tilted.

If the tooth has more or less than five, or, four cusps, it should be evaluated individually, both radiographically and clinically.

Indirect Modes of Irritation to the Pulp-Dentin Organ

Anatomically and physiologically, the dentin and the pulp are considered as one organ, which is the pulp-dentin organ. This is because Tome's fibers (which are the protoplasmic extensions of the odontoblasts) constitute one-third of the dentin substance. The cytoplasm of one Tome's fiber constitutes three-fourths of the cytoplasm of the odontoblast. It is no wonder that irritation of the dentin causes a definite reaction in the pulp!

Most irritating toxins or chemicals penetrate the dentin via the dentinal tubules and not via the dentin matrix. Therefore, the reactions in the odontoblasts and underlying tissues will still initially be confined to the area directly pulpal to the irritated dentinal fibrils.

The odontoblasts responsible for the formation, metabolism and innervation of the primary and secondary dentin are very specialized, delicate, and easily irritated cells. If an irritation is mild, the odontoblasts can remain vital, prompting Tome's fibers to form more peritubular dentin peripherally. Such peritubular dentin is highly calcified in contrast to the remaining intertubular dentin matrix and is called *dentin sclerosis*. This is the first defensive mechanism against irritation to the pulp-dentin organ. If further irritation occurs, the more peripheral dentinal tubules will be completely obliterated by peritubular dentin, replacing the ends of Tome's fibers. This is called a *calcific barrier*, which is the second defensive mechanism. If indeed, further irritation occurs, the odontoblasts will completely degenerate, leaving their protoplasmic fibers in the dentin. As these fibers disintegrate, a *dead tract* is formed. The dead tract was formerly thought to be a defensive mechanism for the pulp, as it was believed to be impervious to irritating agents. However, it is now known that the dead tract is *more* permeable to detrimental chemicals and toxins than vital dentin. Also, dead tracts deprive the dentin of its elasticity, which is very important for some restorative procedures. So, contrary to being protective, dead tracts may be considered destructive for the pulp-dentin organ.

It is seen, then, that the pulp, like other connective tissues, has a powerful reparative capacity. This demonstrates itself in correctly diagnosed and properly treated conditions. For example, after degeneration of odontoblasts and formation of a dead tract, the pulp tissue (especially the undifferentiated mesenchymal cells and the fibroblasts), can assume the work of the odontoblasts and form a reparative, irregular type of dentin to seal itself off from the irritation.

The peripheral pulp tissues, namely, the odontoblastic, sub-odontoblastic, and layer of Weil, are completely or partially avascular. Even if capillaries are present, their lumens are so narrow and torturous as to restrict free passage of red and white corpuscles. (Fig. 137) Therefore, when a mechanical insult to the pulp is restricted to these layers, no hemorrhage will occur, although the pulp is actually exposed (Fig. 138, A, B, and C). Hemorrhaging occurs only when the pulp tissues proper are contused (Fig. 139, A, B, and C), and this usually constitutes massive destruction (Fig. 139C).

The first sign of a pulp exposure is the oozing of the dental pulp fluid (Fig. 140, A, B, C) via microscopic discontinuities (cracks) (Fig. 140D) in the dentin. This sign cannot be detected macroscopically.

The nearer a source of irritation is to the pulp tissues (i.e., the less the effective depth of dentin bridge), the more severe is the reaction of the pulp-dentin organ.

The pulp-dentin organ may react against any stimulation or irritation in one of the following ways.

I. Healthy Reparative Reaction

This is the most favorable response, and it consists of stimulating the P-D organ to form sclerotic dentin and/or calcific barriers. These are followed by normal secondary dentin, containing dentinal tubules formed by odontoblasts. Secondary dentin is different from primary dentin, only in that the tubules of secondary dentin are slightly misangulated from the tubules of the primary dentin. The healthy reparative reaction occurs without any disturbances in the pulp tissues.

II. Unhealthy Reparative Reaction

This may be considered to be only fairly favorable. It begins with degeneration of the odontoblasts, either by being poisoned or by being aspirated into the dentinal tubules. This is followed by the formation of the dead tract in the dentin, and complete cessation in the formation of secondary dentin. The unhealthy reparative reaction is accompanied by mild pathological and clinical changes of a reversible nature in the pulp tissues, re-

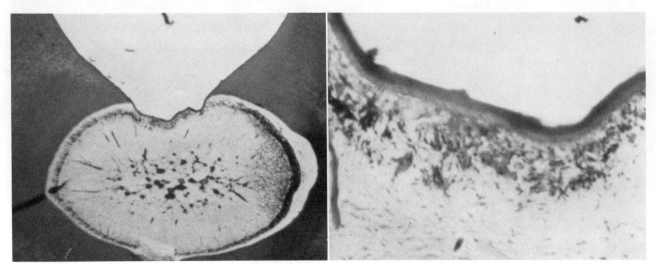

Fig. 1-137. A, Histologic cross-section showing the relative narrowness and absence of blood vessels in the peripheral three layers of the pulp tissues. **B,** High magnification showing a dentin bridge thickness of 12 microns, with no evidence of fluid seepage from the cavity floor.

sulting in the formation of an irregular type of tertiary dentin (irritation dentin) replacing the degenerated odontoblasts. Such tertiary dentin is the product of the formative action of the undifferentiated mesenchymal cells and fibroblasts. Tertiary dentin deposits continue until they seal the dead tracts and counteract the irritation. Eventually, the odontoblasts will pave over this reparative dentin, and start the formation of normal secondary dentin. The tertiary dentin is considered to be the function of the pulp tissue proper, and as such, it is a clear indication of the massive recuperative capacity of the pulp. However, tertiary dentin has certain limitations. It is not completely impervious like the calcific barrier. Also, the rapid formation of tertiary dentin will lead to the occupation of part of the pulp chamber with tissues other than those normally responsible for further repair, metabolism and innervation. Therefore, tertiary dentin may be said to "age the pulp," reducing its capacity for further defensive action against future irritation. This is very important clinically, because if this reaction occurs as a result of a carious process, the restoration of this tooth may not be favorably received by the P-D organ. Finally, tertiary dentin is less elastic than the primary dentin, which is an important mechanical characteristic of the dentin in certain restorative procedures.

III. A Destructive Reaction

This is the most unfavorable pulpal response to irritation. It begins with the loss of odontoblasts and the outer protective layer of the pulp. The insult eventually involves the pulp tissue proper, exceeding its reparative capacity. The resulting tissue reaction will be inflammation, which may progress to abscess formation, phlegmonous or chronic inflammation, or, finally, complete necrosis of the pulp. In any event, the pulp tissues cannot recuperate from these pathologic changes, and removal of these tissues or the whole tooth becomes necessary.

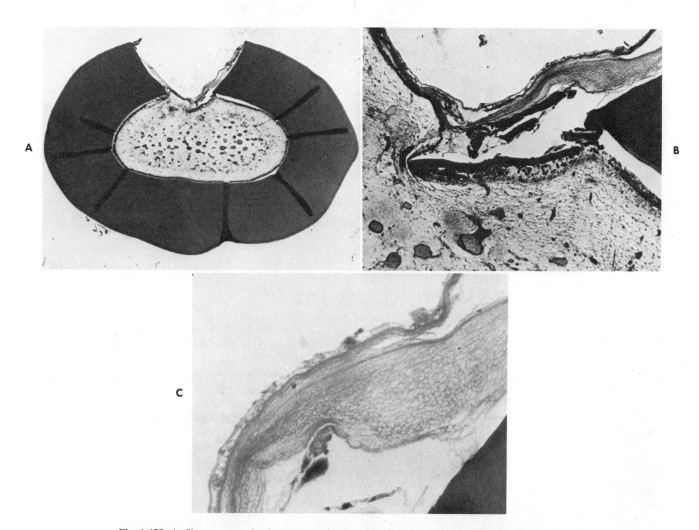

Fig. 1-138. A, Shows an actual pulp exposure with the cavity floor depressed into the pulp tissues as far as the layer of weil, fibrinous material (coagulated dental pulp fluid) along the walls of the preparation. The pulp tissues are otherwise normal. Pulp exposure is 1500 microns. **B,** High magnification of **A** at the 1500 micron exposure site. **C,** Higher magnification of the coagulated fibrinous fluid. The fibers are arranged more or less parallel, i.e. they do not cross one another. There is no beading at interlacing points, like that in a true blood serum clot. It is stained with hematoxylin and it contains no blood cells.

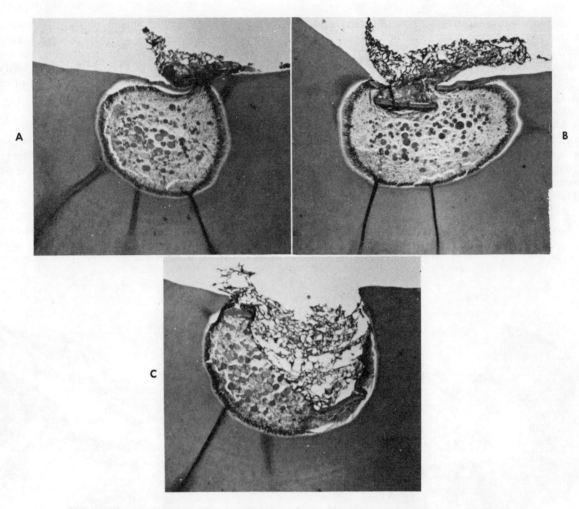

Fig. 1-139. The serial histologic sections of the same tooth which showed up at the site of the exposure (absorbed by gel-foam plus classical beading at the interlacing points of the fibrinous material). The situation shown in **A** could hardly create any bleeding. That shown in **B** may not have caused bleeding. Bleeding occurred mainly from situation shown in **C** where the preparation dentin bridge (floor) has been pressed all the way across the pulp tissues to the other side of the pulp chamber.

Irritants to the Pulp-Dentin Organ: Caries Irritation

Sometimes, the pulp-dentin organ will react to caries as early as enamel penetration. For proper treatment, we have to correctly diagnose the extent of the pulp-dentin organ response. This response is influenced by:

I. The type of decay, i.e., the more acute the decay is, the more destructive is the response. Chronic caries is usually accompanied by a reparative reaction, provided there is no pulp exposure.

II. The duration of decay, i.e., the longer the duration is in acute decay, the more massive is the destruction; but the longer it is in chronic decay, the more chances there are for repair, provided that the pulp is not actually directly involved.

III. The depth of involvement by decay, i.e., the deeper the carious cavity is, the nearer is the source of irritation to the pulp, so the destruction is worse.

IV. Pathogenecity of the microorganism in the caries cone, i.e., the more virulent the microorganisms (streptococci) are, the more destructive is the pulpal reaction.

V. Individual responses of the pulp depend upon its own resistance to irritation. Variables include age, cellularity, vascularity and other individual differences.

VI. The tooth's resistance to the carious process, which might be influenced by mineralization, tooth location, and other factors could increase the chances of a P-D organ's defense against irritation and decrease the possibility of a destructive response.

Irritating Agents of Tooth Preparation

A tooth preparation introduces a number of irritating factors to the pulp.

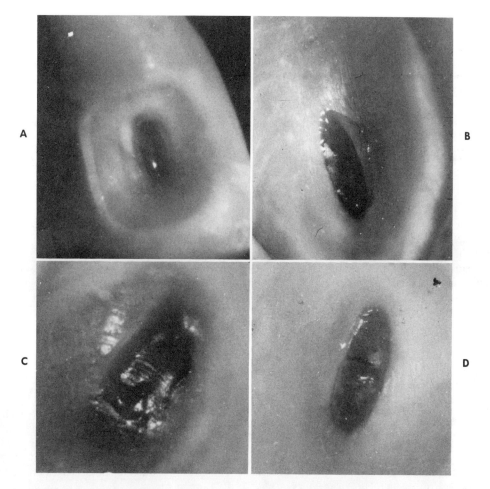

Fig. 1-140. A and B, 50-time magnification showing the clear colorless dentinal pulp fluid. **C,** 200-time magnification of the cavity floor covered with the dental pulp fluid. **D,** Shows the crack in the same tooth through which the fluid was oozing.

I. The actual cutting of dentin, in as much as every square mm contains 30,000 to 45,000 dentinal tubules, can irritate many millions of odontoblasts.

II. The pressure of instrumentation on exposed dentin characteristically causes the aspiration of the nuclei of the odontoblasts or the entire odontoblasts themselves or nerve endings from pulp tissues into the dentinal tubules. This will obviously stimulate them, disturb their metabolism and may lead to their complete degeneration and disintegration. This can occur by excessive pressure of hand or rotary instruments, especially in decreased effective depths.

Sometimes this pressure may drive some microorganisms from an infected cavity floor or wall into the pulp, leading to its irritation.

III. The type of cutting instruments used has variable irritating factors. Sharp hand-cutting instruments wherein the energy used with them is completely dissipated in the actual cutting, instead of crushing the vital dental tissues, are the most biologically acceptable cutting instruments.

Rotary cutting instruments (burs) are also biologically acceptable, if used over effective depths of 2 mm and more, and with proper coolants. This is truer with carbide than with steel burs, as the former are more cool-cutting than the latter.

Rotary abrasive instruments (stones) are not recommended for cutting in vital dentin, as their abrasive action, especially without sufficient coolants, will elevate the temperature of surrounding dentin. This is because the energy used to abrade, which is far more than that used to cut, is dissipated in the form of heat. Rotary abrasive instruments may also crush vital dentin much more than any other cutting instruments. Therefore, abrasive actions should be confined to the enamel and the superficial 1 mm of dentin, as much as possible.

IV. The depth of the cavity is the most detrimental irritating factor to the pulp. Most important is the thickness of the dentin bridge between the floor of the cavity and the roof of the pulp chamber, called the *effective depth*. The less this effective depth, the nearer the irritating ingredients to the pulp, so the more destructive the pulpal reaction will be.

V. Heat production is the second most detrimental factor. If the pulp temperature is elevated by 11° F, definite destructive reactions will occur even in a normal, vital P-D organ. Lesser temperatures can precipitate similar responses in already irritated organs, depending on the extent of prior irritation. Unfortunately, it is not uncommon to arrive to such temperatures during ordinary cavity preparations. Remember that "heat" is a function of:

1. RPM's. i.e., the more the RPM's, the more the heat production. It is more so with abrasive than cutting heads. The most deleterious speed is from 3000 to 30,000 RPM. In deep penetrations of dentin without using coolants, e.g., pin holes, the cutting speed must not exceed 3000 RPM.

2. Pressure, which is directly proportional to heat generation. Whenever the RPM's are increased, pressure must be correspondingly reduced. Instrumentation pressure should not be more than four ounces when using high speed and twelve ounces when using low speed.

3. Surface area of contact, which is related to the size and shape of the revolving tool. The more the contact between the tooth structures and the revolving tool, the more the heat generation. Whenever the RPMs are increased, the size of the cutting instrument's head must be correspondingly reduced.

Heat not only creates destruction in the pulp tissues, but it can also coagulate protoplasm, and even char, dentin if the temperature is sufficiently elevated. Even the enamel can be charred and lose cohesion if overheated. These affected parts of the enamel and dentin may remain as a part of the preparation walls, but eventually they will be sequestrated, for they have no cohesion to the underlying tooth structure.

VI. Desiccation, if occurring in vital dentin to the extent that some moisture (water) in the protoplasm of Tome's fibers is eliminated, will create a disturbance in the osmotic pressure of those dentinal tubules, resulting in the aspiration of the nuclei of the odontoblasts, or the odontoblasts themselves, into the tubules. The subsequent disturbances in their metabolism may lead to their complete degeneration. Also, desiccation will increase the permeability of the vital dentin to any subsequent irritant, e.g., microorganisms or elements in restorative materials. So, whenever, possible, a prepared tooth must be kept in a fairly sterile hydrous field during preparation. If air alone is applied to the vital dentin, care must be taken to remove only debris and additional moisture from the field of operation, and not the dentin's own moisture.

VII. Coolants, as stated previously are essential for any cutting that involves dentin. As explained above, air can do more harm than good. A spray of air and water is an acceptable coolant, if it is mainly used to dislodge attached debris. Plain water coolant is the most effective, and should be the coolant of choice. To be effective, the water should be delivered directly at the point of contact between the rotary cutting head and the tooth. Frequently, a handpiece, containing only one aperture for water, is unable to fulfill this requirement.

When cross-cut fissure burs or diamond stones, which produce immense heat, are used, coolant water should strike the bur or stone at several different levels, thereby keeping wet the entire area of contact between the revolving tool and the tooth.

In high speeds, the centrifugal force of the revolving head will create an area of turbulence which tends to deflect the water from the dentin being prepared. Therefore, a jet of water with sufficient power and velocity to penetrate this turbulence is necessary for proper cooling.

There can be no excuse for not using water coolants, given our present day availability of high-speed suction. Coolant sprays should be used even in non-vital or devitalized tooth structures, since, as previously mentioned, the heat will burn

tooth structures, and these burnt areas will be sequestrated later, leaving a space around the restoration where failures can occur.

VIII. Vibrations, which are measured by their amplitude or their capacity and frequency (the number/unit time), are an indication of eccentricity in rotary instruments. The higher the amplitude is, the more destructive may be the response of the pulp. The reaction is very characteristic and is called the *rebound response*. It is thought to be the result of the ultrasonic energy induced, and it takes the form of:

1. Disruption of the odontoblasts in the opposite side of the pulp chamber from where the cavity is prepared.
2. Edema.
3. Fibrosis of pulp tissues proper.
4. Change in ground substance.
5. Reduction in the predentin formation all around the pulp chamber.

Besides affecting the pulp tissues, vibration can create microcracks in enamel and some non-elastic dentin. These cracks may propagate and interconnect, directly joining the oral environment with the delicate pulp and periodontal tissues. At the very least, they increase the permeability of the dentin and enamel to oral diffusants. In both situations, of course, detrimental results can be precipitated in these delicate tissues.

IX. The extensiveness of the preparation, or the duration of the preparation time is directly proportional to the extensiveness of the reaction of the P-D organ, e.g., a crown preparation will cause more response than a Class I preparation. Less time used in preparing a cavity using a biologically sound procedure keeps the reaction of the P-D organ less acute. Knowing the beginning and the end of every stroke used in a tooth preparation is essential before applying any instrument to a tooth. This prevents wasting some strokes crushing and irritating the P-D organ.

X. Not all persons will have the same reaction towards the same irritant. Indeed, individual variations in pulpal response can occur. In fact, teeth in the same person can react differently towards the same irritant. This is due to both known factors, e.g., cellularity, vascularity (of the pulp), age, heredity, etc., and also to unknown factors.

XI. Modifications. The last picture of the reaction of the P-D organ cannot be due to one factor only. It is due to a cumulative effect, which starts by decay, then cavity preparation instrumentation, then the restorative materials and procedures. So during a tooth preparation it should always be remembered that the P-D organ has been already irritated before the present instrumentation and is going to be irritated more by the restoration.

The Biologic Basis of the Periodontium as Related to Operative Procedures

This section was contributed by
Dr. A.H. El-Kafrawy, Professor,
Department of Oral Diagnosis and Medicine,
Indiana University, School of Dentistry.

In the previous section, some biological aspects of operative dentistry were considered. Emphasis was placed on maintenance of pulp integrity; after all, a perfect restoration will be useless, if pulp integrity is impaired through unjudicious operative procedures. In the present section, some aspects of the biology of the periodontium will be considered. Emphasis will be placed on maintenance of periodontal health; after all, a restoration will be of little value, if it creates an environment that is conducive in the long run to periodontal destruction. The fact is simple: the long-term success of any restoration is dependent on the maintenance of the integrity of the pulp and the periodontium.

Anatomical and Histological Considerations

The periodontium constitutes the tooth-supporting tissues. Its components are the gingiva, the dentogingival junction, the peridontal ligament, the cementum and alveolar bone. In health and in disease, the components of the periodontium constitute a continuum.

The gingiva is a part of the oral mucosa. Classically, the oral mucosa is divided into masticatory, specialized and lining mucosa. The masticatory mucosa is so designated since it is subjected to mechanical stresses during mastication; it comprises the gingiva and the mucosal covering of the hard palate. The specialized mucosa comprises the mucosal covering of the lingual dorsum; it is so designated since it carries the lingual papillae and taste buds. The lining mucosa constitutes the remainder of the oral mucous membranes. Topographically, the gingiva can be divided into marginal, attached and interdental gingiva. The marginal or free gingiva forms the soft tissue wall of the gingival sulcus or crevice. The gingival sulcus is the shallow space between the marginal gingiva and the tooth surface. Ideally, sulci should be non-existent; in health their depth should be minimal and should not exceed 3mm.

The attached gingiva in health is firm in consistency, pink in color (although the color shows variation and is influenced by the presence of physiologic melanin pigmentation), has a stippled surface texture, and is firmly attached to the underlying alveolar bone. The interdental gingiva in health fills the interdental space to the contact areas. In anterior teeth the interdental gingiva is pyramidal in shape; in posterior teeth it has a vestibular and an oral peak, joined by a depression, the interdental col.

Histologically, the marginal gingiva consists of a core of connective tissue and is covered with stratified squamous epithelium. The epithelial covering of the outer surface of the marginal gingiva is parakeratinized or orthokeratinized or it may show alternating areas of para- and orthokeratinization. It has prominent rete ridges. The epithelial covering of the inner surface of the marginal gingiva forms the sulcular or crevicular epithelium. In man, monkeys and dogs, the sulcular epithelium is nonkeratinized, in rodents and rabbits the sulcular epithelium is keratinized. The interface between the sulcular epithelium and the adjacent connective tissue is normally flat and rete ridges are absent. The sulcular epithelium is continuous apically with the junctional epithelium, a component of the dentogingival junction.

In gingiva that appears clinically healthy, foci of inflammatory cells, chiefly lymphocytes and plasma cells, are often present in the lamina propria of the marginal gingiva beneath the sulcular epithelium. The presence of these chronic inflammatory cells is a response to irritant products of bacteria in the gingival sulcus.

Like the marginal gingiva, the attached gingiva is covered with stratified squamous epithelium, which is histologically similar to the epithelium covering the external surface of the marginal gingiva. The lamina propria of the gingiva is rich in collagen fibers. Both type I and type III collagen are present, with type I predominating. The dentogingival junction attaches the gingiva to the tooth surface. It has an epithelial and a connective tissue component. The epithelial component is the junctional epithelium which is nonkeratinized stratified squamous epithelium, and is attached to the tooth surface by a basal lamina with its associated hemidesmosomes. The connective tissue component which provides mechanical strength to the dentogingival junction is composed of collagen fibers, which originate in the cervical portions of the cementum and radiate coronally into the lamina propria of the gingiva.

The periodontal ligament attaches the tooth to the alveolar bone. Its principal fibers consist of bundles of collagen fibers which extend from the cementum to the alveolar bone. The portion of the principal fibers embedded in cementum and alveolar bone constitute Sharpey's fibers. Collagen is a fibrous protein with remarkable tensile strength. A collagen fiber 1mm in diameter can support a load of 10-40 Kg before reaching its breaking point. This high tensile strength of collagen is comparable to that of steel. Thus, collagen is ideally suited for the construction of ligaments. The principal fibers of the periodontal ligament are well adapted to withstand masticatory stresses. Epithelial cells are present in the periodontal ligament. These are the cell rests of Malassez, which are remnants of Hertwig's epithelial root sheath. They form a network in the periodontal ligament. Although no definite function has yet been assigned to the cell rests, it has been suggested that they may play a role in maintenance of the integrity of the periodontal ligament, by serving as an ankylosis inhibitor.

Cementum is the hard tissue which covers the root surface; it often overlays enamel for a short distance in the region of the cemento-enamel junction. Cementum is an integral component of the periodontium; it provides a medium for the insertion of the principle fibers of the periodontal ligament. Cementum is thinnest over the cervical portion of the root, where it is about 20 to $50\mu m$ thick (about the thickness of a hair). It progressively increases in thickness towards the apex. The fact that cementum is so thin over the cervical portion of the root, and that cementum is the softest of the hard dental tissues, explains the cervical sensitivity which often accompanies gingival recession. Exposed cementum is readily abraded, exposing the highly sensitive dentin.

The alveolar bone forms and supports the tooth sockets. Its components are the alveolar bone proper which provides a medium for the attachment of the principal fibers of the periodontal ligament, and the supporting bone which supports the alveolar bone proper and consists of vestibular and oral cortical plates and spongy bone which intervenes between the cortical plates and the alveolar bone proper. Bone is well adapted to withstand mechanical stresses with minimal amount of bone tissue. Disuse atrophy affects the periodontium in teeth which have been out of function as a result of loss of opposing teeth. This will be manifested by reduction in alveolar bone mass and thinning of the periodontal ligament.

Pathological and Immunological Considerations

Chronic inflammatory periodontal disease is world-wide in distribution. It is the most common cause of tooth loss in individuals past the age of 35 years.

Numerous epidemiologic studies have shown a strong positive correlation between plaque accumulation and chronic inflammatory periodontal disease. Studies of experimental gingivitis in man have shown that young adults with healthy gingiva who abstained from their oral hygiene measures developed gingivitis concomittant with plaque accumulation. Resumption of the oral hygiene measures was followed by resolution of the gingival inflammation. What are the possible mechanisms by which plaque induces its damaging effects? Before attempting an answer to this question, the microscopic changes in the gingiva which follow plaque accumulation will be reviewed briefly.

As gingivitis develops, changes occur in the sulcular epithelium and in the underlying connective tissue. The sulcular epithelium shows areas of proliferation manifested by the development of rete ridges; remember, the interface between the sulcular epithelium and the underlying connective tissue is normally flat. The epithelium may also show areas of ulceration. The underlying connective tissue shows an inflammatory infiltrate composed chiefly of lymphocytes and plasma cells. Neutrophils are present in substantial numbers in the sulcular epithelium, in their way towards the gingival sulcus. Apparently, they are attracted by chemotactic factors in the sulcus (both bacterial in origin, as well as chemotactic factors generated through activation of the complement systems). At the ultrastructural level, the sulcular epithelium shows widening of the spaces between the epithelial cells with decrease in the number of the junctions that join the epithelial cells (desmosomes, intermediate and tight junctions).

The widened intercellular spaces contain leukocytes, lysosomes, and cellular debris. Whereas bacteria are present in large number on the surface of the epithelium, they are not seen invading the epithelium or the connective tissue. Thus bacterial invasion of the gingival tissues is not a feature of chronic inflammatory periodontal disease.

There are several mechanisms by which plaque can induce damage to the periodontium without actual bacterial invasion. Bacterial metabolites such as hydrogen sulfide, ammonia and organic acids are chemical irritants. Bacterial enzymes such as hyaluronidase, collagenase and other proteolytic enzymes can produce tissue degradation. Endotoxin can produce direct cell injury, can activate the alternative pathway of the complement system, can serve as a T-independent antigen with the production of IgM antibodies with subsequent activation of the classical pathway of the complement system, can serve as a B-cell mitogen, can stimulate release of collagenase from macrophages, and can stimulate osteoclastic bone resorption.

Endotoxin is a lipopolysaccharide component of the cell wall of gram negative bacteria. It is a large molecule, with a molecular weight exceeding 10^6. Can such a large molecule penetrate an intact sulcular epithelium to produce injury and initiate inflammation? Studies with rabbits showed that endotoxin cannot penetrate the sulcular epithelium unless the epithelium has been previously scarified. Studies with dogs showed that endotoxin labeled with tritium can penetrate an intact sulcular epithelium. Remember that the sulcular epithelium is keratinized in rabbits and is nonkeratinized in dogs.

In addition to endotoxin, other antigenic components of plaque bacteria may reach the gingival tissues and initiate immune reactions of both humoral and cell-mediated types.

There is no doubt that immune reactions take place in patients with chronic inflammatory periodontal disease. Several observations attest to this fact. First, the gingival tissues have a rich vascular supply which make it possible to mobilize to the site the elements needed for the induction of an immune response. Second, the gingival tissues are exposed to numerous antigens. Third, numerous studies have demonstrated immunoglobulins of the different classes in the gingival fluid and in inflamed gingivae. IgG, IgM, IgA and possibly IgE have been shown to be present. IgA in the gingival fluid and inflamed gingivae is of the monomeric serum type and is not of the dimeric secretory type. Likewise, different components of the complement system have been demonstrated in the gingival fluid and in inflamed gingiva. Furthermore, lymphocyte transformation tests have shown that peripheral blood lymphocytes of patients with chronic inflammatory periodontal disease have been sensitized to plaque antigens. Fourth, the inflammatory infiltrate in chronic inflammatory periodontal disease consists chiefly of lymphocytes, plasma cells and macrophages. These are the cells which are known to participate in immune reactions. Last, but not the least, experimental animal studies have shown that immune reactions of both humoral and cell mediated types can be induced through gingival administration of antigens.

While the development of immune reactions in patients with chronic inflammatory periodontal disease is universally accepted, the role of such reactions have been extensively debated. Are they primarily destructive? Are they primarily protective? Or, are they primarily protective, with local tissue destruction due to chronicity of the process, being the price paid for protection?

The demonstration of IgG and IgM and complement components in the inflamed gingivae suggest that immune complexes may deposit locally with activation of the complement system with all of the consequences of complement activation, e.g., anaphylatoxin generation, leukocyte chemotaxis, stimulation of prostaglandin synthesis, release of lysosomal enzymes with subsequent tissue injury. The demonstration of IgE would suggest mast cell activation with degranulation and release of preformed mediators which are stored in their granules such as histamine, and synthesis of unstored mediators such as the leukotrienes and platelet activating factor. The demonstration of sensitized lymphocytes indicate that a variety of lymphokines could be released locally. Among these are lymphotoxin which produces cell injury and the osteoclast activating factor which stimulates bone resorption. In this regard, it should be remembered that both T and B lymphocytes produce lymphokines.

One should not lose sight of the fact that the immune system has evolved for the preservation of self and that immune reactions are primarily protective. One should also remember that plaque has a definite pathogenic potential. It seems that immune reactions in chronic inflammatory periodontal disease are primarily protective, preventing invasion of the gingival tissues by plaque bacteria and thus limiting what potentially can be a serious infection. Local tissue destruction due to chronicity of the process (since the inflammatory and immune reactions cannot eliminate the irritants without therapeutic intervention) will then be the price paid for protection. If left untreated, chronic gingivitis would ultimately progress to periodontitis. Gingival sulci will deepen to form periodontal pockets, with apical migration of the junctional epithelium. Alveolar bone loss occurs. Among the factors which have been shown to stimulate osteoclastic activity are endotoxin, lipoteichoid acid, prostaglandins and the osteoclast activating factor.

In the previous discussion the importance of plaque in the causation of periodontal disease has been emphasized. Plaque is the archenemy of the periodontium. Calculus deposits mechanically irritate the gingival tissues; the rough surface of calculus favors plaque accumulation. Faulty restorations with overhangs, open contacts and improper contours are conducive to periodontal destruction. In a recent study, 46% of proximal restorations were found to be involved with calculus or overhanging margins.

Clinical Considerations

(For further details, see chapter on single tooth restorations and the periodontium.)

Whenever possible, margins of restorations should be placed coronal to the gingival margin. If esthetics indicate, they should be placed at the gingival margin. Placement of the margin subgingivally, particularly with resin and silicate restorations, is to be avoided. Since these restorations cannot be finished to a perfectly smooth surface, they provide a favorable surface for plaque accumulation. Glazed porcelain and well polished gold and alloy restorations are better tolerated by the gingiva than silicate or resin restorations. Avoid overhangs; these are conducive to periodontal destruction. The open contact is deleterious; not only does it lead to food impaction, but it also encourages plaque accumulation with attendant inflammation and ultimate tissue destruction. Avoid overcontouring and undercontouring of restorations; the former is conducive to plaque accumulation, whereas the latter may lead to traumatic injury of the gingiva during mastication. Proper occlusion is important; an interfering restoration serves as an improperly constructed orthodontic appliance. Whereas, occlusal trauma does not lead to gingival inflammation or pocket formation, it may influence the extension of inflammation, if inflammation is already present.

Irritating Factors to the Periodontium

Although the entire relationship of single tooth restorations and the periodontium will be presented in detail in chapter #15, the following is a brief mention of the factors that may irritate the periodontium during preparation instrumentation.

I. Mechanical trauma, be it cutting, contusion, or crushing of periodontium components, can result from any type of instrumentation. Hand instruments, however, afford the operator more control and are therefore less likely to cause injury than rotary instruments.

II. Excessive pressure during instrumentation, especially if not applied parallel to the long axis of the tooth, could tear some of the periodontal ligament fibers.

III. Vibrations from rotary instrumentation could, at the very least, tear periodontal attachments (see chapter on single tooth restoration and the periodontium).

IV. Thermal trauma from rotary instrumentation, especially abrasive instruments, can create ulcerations and burns in the adjacent periodontium.

V. Air coolants or air accompanying rotary instruments can detach the periodontal organ from the tooth at its dentino-gingival junction, if brought close to it and applied in sufficient velocity and amount. This becomes more likely if the attachment is not strong to begin with. Undoubtedly, loss of the attachment could lead to numerous periodontal problems,

VI. By the actions mentioned in (I) and (V), plaque materials and microorganisms close to the periodontium could be driven apically past the gingival sulcus, starting or accelerating a periodontal break-down.

From this discussion one should conclude that every effort should be made to protect the periodontium during operative instrumentation. Most important, in this regard, is proper training in handling and controlling operative armamentarium. In addition, establishing a physical barrier between the areas on the tooth being cut and the adjacent periodontium is also a safe and sure measure to pursue, e.g., rubber dam and/or wedges, etc.

BIBLIOGRAPHY

American National Standards Institute/American Dental Association Document No. 41. Recommended Standard Practices for Biological Evaluation of Dental Materials. Council on Dental Materials and Devices. American Dental Association, 1979.

Baum et al.: Operative Dentistry. Philadelphia, Saunders, 1981.

Benaceraf, B., and Unanue, E.R.: Textbook of immunology. Baltimore, Williams and Wilkins, 1979.

Bhaskar, S.N.: Orban's oral histology and embryology. 9th ed. St. Louis, C.V. Mosby Co., 1980.

Black, G.V., and Black, A.P.: A work on operative dentistry. Vol. I and II, 6th ed. Chicago, Medico-Dental Pub., 1924.

Braden, M.: Heat conduction in normal human dentin. Arch. Oral Biol. 9, p. 479, 1964.

Brannstrom, M.: The hydrodynamics of the dentin: its possible relationship to dentinal pain. Int. Dent. J. 22:219, 1972.

Brannstrom, M., and Nyborg, H.: Cavity treatment with a microbicidal fluoride solution. Growth of bacteria and effect on the pulp. J. Prosth. Dent. 30:303, 1973.

Caranza, F.A., Jr.: Glickman's clinical periodontology. 5th ed. Philadelphia, W.B. Saunders Co., 1979.

Charbeneau et al.: Principles and practice of operative dentistry. Philadelphia, Lea and Febiger, 1980.

Craig, R.G., and Peyton, F.A.: Elastic and mechanical properties of human dentin. J. D. Res. 37:710 Aug. 1958.

Diamond, M., and Weinmann, J.P.: The enamel of human teeth. New York, Columbia Univ. Press, 1940.

Dickey, D.M., Miller, C.H., Kafrawy, A.H., and Phillips, R.W.: Bacterial survival under restorative materials. IADR Program and Abstracts, No. 1158, 1979.

Finn, S.B. (editor).: Biology of the dental pulp organ: a symposium. Birmingham, University of Alabama Press, 1968.

Fudenberg, H.H., Stites, D.P., Cladwell, J.I., and Wells, J.V.: Basic and clinical immunology. 3d ed. Los Altos: Lange Medical Publications, 1980.

Gilmore, H.W., et al.: Operative Dentistry. 3d ed. St. Louis, C.V Mosby Co., 1977.

Grant, D.A., Stertn, I.B., and Everett, F.G.: Periodontics in the tradition of Orban and Gottlieb, 5th ed. St. Louis, C.V. Mosby Co., 1979.

Hancock, E.B., Mayo, C.V., Schwabb, R.R., and Wirthlin, M.R.: Influence of interdental contacts on periodontal status. J. Periodontol. 51:445, 1980.

Hausmann, E.: Potential pathways for bone resorption in human periodontal disease. J. Periodontol. **45:**338, 1974.

Horton, J.E., Oppenheim, J.J., and Mergenhagen, S.E.: A role of cell-mediated immunity in the pathogenesis of periodontal disease. J. Periodontol. **45:**351, 1974.

Howell, A.H., and Manly, R.S.: An electronic strain gauge for measuring oral forces. J.D. Res. 27. Dec. 1948, p. 705.

Kafrawy, A.H.: Biology of the dental pulp. Indiana University School of Dentistry Alumni Bulletin, p. 4-10. Spring Issue, 1978.

Kafrawy, A.H. and Mitchell, D.F.: Pulp reactions to open cavities later restored with silicate cement. J. Dent. Res. 42:874, 1963.

Kakehashi, S., Stanley, H.R., and Fitzgerald, R.: The effects of surgical exposure of the pulps in germ-free and conventional laboratory rats. Oral Surg. **20:**340, 1965.

Langeland, K., Dowden, W.E., Tronstad, L., and Langeland, L.K.: Human pulp changes of iatrogenic origin: In Siskin, M. (editor): The biology of the human dental pulp. St. Louis, C.V. Mosby Co., 1973.

Larson, T.D., Douglas, W.H., and Geistfield, R.E.: Effect of prepared cavities on the strength of teeth. Operative Dentistry 6, page 2, 1981.

Loe, M., Thelaide, E., and Jensen, S.B.: Experimental gingivitis in man. J. Periodontol. **36:**177, 1965.

Mahler, D.B., and Terkla, L.G.: Analysis of stress in dental structures. D. Clin. N. America, p. 789, Nov. 1958.

Marzouk, M.A.: Effect of deep cavity preparation on the dental pulp using the operating microscope as well as serial histologic sections. Thesis submitted to Indiana University, School of Dentistry, in partial fulfillment of the Master of Science degree in Operative Dentistry, 1963.

Marzouk, M.A.,: Strong, M.E., and Diemer, R.: Introduction to operative dentistry. Self-instructional package. Washington University, School of Dental Medicine, 1977.

Marzouk, M.A., and Van Huysen, G.: Pulp exposure without hemorrhage. JDR, March-April, 1966.

McGhee, W.H., True, H., and Inskipp, F.E.: A textbook of operative dentistry. New York, McGraw-Hill Book Co., 1956.

McWalter, G.M., Kafrawy, A.H., and Mitchell, D.F.: Long-term study of pulp capping monkeys with three agents. J. Amer. Dent. Assoc. **93:**105, 1976.

McWalter, G.M., Kafrawy, A.H., and Mitchell, D.F.: Pulp capping in monkeys with a calcium hydroxide compound, an antibiotic and a polycarboxylate cement. Oral Surg. **36:**90, 1973.

McWalter, G.M., Kafrawy, A.H., and Mitchell, D.F.: Rate of reparative dentinogenesis under a pulp capping agent. J. Dent. Res. **56:**93, 1977.

Mitchell, D.: The irritational qualities of dental materials. JADA. 59, Nov 59, p. 954.

Moore, K.L.: The developing human. Clinically oriented embryology. 2nd ed. Philadelphia, W.B. Saunders Co., 1977.

Newbrun, E.: Cariology. Baltimore, Williams and Wilkins, 1978.

Nisengard, R.: Immediate hypersensitivity and periodontal disease. J. Periodontol. **45:**344, 1974.

Nisengard, R.J.: The role of immunology in periodontal disease. J. Periodontol. **48:**505, 1977.

Randolph, K.V.: Principles of mechanical retention of restorations, West Virginia D. J. **38:**2, 1964.

Robbins, S.L. and Cotran, R.: Pathologic basis of disease. 2nd ed. Philadelphia, W.B. Saunders Co., 1979.

Roitt, I.M. and Lehner, T.: Immunology of oral diseases. St. Louis, C.V. Mosby Co., 1980.

Seltzer, S. and Bender, I.B.: The dental pulp, biologic considerations in dental practice. 2nd ed. Philadelphia, J.B. Lippincott Co., 1975.

Spouge, J.D.: A new look at the rests of Malassez. A review of their embryological origin, anatomy and possible role in periodontal health and disease. J. Periodontol. 51:437, 1980.

Stanford, J.W. et al.: Compressive properties of hard tooth tissues and some restorative materials. JADA. 60, June 1960, p. 746.

Stanford, J.W. et al.: Determination of some compressive properties of human enamel and dentin. JADA. **57:**487 Oct 1958.

Stanley, H.R.: Human pulp response to operative dental procedures. Gainesville, Storter Printing Co., Inc., 1976.

Stanley, H.R., White, C.D. and McCrea, L.: The rate of tertiary (reparative) dentin formation in the human tooth, Oral Surg. **21:**180, 1966.

Stibbs, G.D.: Operative Dentistry. JADA, **64:**645-655, 1962.

Sturdevant et al.: The art and science of operative dentistry. New York, McGraw-Hill Book Co., 1968.

Schwartz, J., Stinson, F.L., and Parker, R.B.: The passage of tritiated bacterial endotoxin across intact crevicular epithelium. J. Periodontol. **43:**270, 1973.

Swartz, M.L., Niblack, B.F., Alter, E.A., Norman, R.D., and Phillips, R.W.: In vivo studies of penetration of dentin by constituents of silicate cement. J. Amer. Dent. Assn. **76:**573, 1968.

TenCate, A.R.: Oral histology, development, structure and function. St. Louis, C.V. Mosby Co., 1980.

Vale, W.A.: Cavity preparation and further thoughts on high speed. B.D.J. 107, p. 333, 1959.

Vale, W.A.: Cavity preparation. Irish D. Rev. 2, p. 33, 1956.

Weissman, G.: Advances in inflammation research. Vol. I, New York, Raven Press, 1979.

Wheeler, R.: Pulp, cavities of the permanent teeth. Philadelphia, Saunders Co., 1976.

CHAPTER 2

Operative dentistry armamentarium

Instruments for operative dentistry procedures can generally be classified as those used for exploration, those used for removal of tooth structure, and those used for the restoration of teeth.

Exploring Instruments

Physical exploration of dental lesions requires the following procedures:

A. Dry the area on the tooth. This necessitates the use of an air syringe and a pair of tweezers (cotton pliers) (Fig. 1) which carry and hold cotton pellets, to dry the tooth, and cotton rolls, to isolate the area around the tooth. Both come in different sizes to fit various needs.

B. Illuminate the area to be examined. A source of light could be either an overhead fixture supplying non-reflecting light or an intra-oral light. These devices can be battery operated lights, built-in lights attached to the dental unit, or lights attached to a mirror or a handpiece. The latter two could be carried by a fiber optic bundle built into the instrument. Light can be introduced directly from one or more of these devices, or indirectly by reflecting it on the field via a mirror used as a viewing device (Fig. 2).

C. Retract the soft tissues that may interfere with proper exploration. The hand mirror is usually used to move the tongue and the cheek away, but some of the blunt-bladed restoring instruments (plastic instruments) may help in this retraction. Tongue depressors-retractors are sometimes helpful for this procedures. (See chapter on control of the field of operation).

D. Probe the potential lesions. This is the actual physical identification of tooth lesions. Explorers are used for this. Any explorer is formed of three parts (Fig. 3): the handle which is straight with serrations, the shank which is smooth and may carry a curvature or one or more angles, and the exploring tip which is the terminal portion of the explorer. The tip is pointed and should be checked and sharpened frequently.

There are four types of explorers for operative dentistry use:
1. The straight explorer has a shank which is straight except for a slight curvature near the exploring tip (Fig. 4).
2. The right-angled explorer has a shank with a right angle,

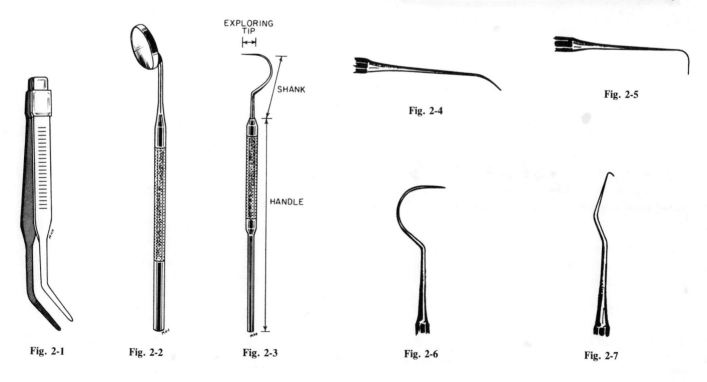

EXPLORING TIP

SHANK

HANDLE

Fig. 2-1   Fig. 2-2   Fig. 2-3   Fig. 2-4   Fig. 2-5   Fig. 2-6   Fig. 2-7

placing the exploring tip at a right angle to the handle (Fig. 5).

3. The arch explorer, with the shank curved in a semi-circle like an arch, also has the exploring tip at a right angle to the handle (Fig. 6).

4. The interproximal explorer, with its shank consisting of two or more angles, has the exploring tip pointing toward the handle. This instrument is specific for detecting proximal lesions (Fig. 7).

E. Separators are also infrequently used to verify the presence of proximal lesions. These are described in the chapter on contact and contour.

Armamentarium and Instruments for Tooth Structure Removal

To restore a tooth it first must be prepared, which involves the removal of both diseased and sound tooth structure. Currently there are three sets of instruments for tooth structure removal:

I. Hand cutting instruments
II. Rotary cutting and rotary abrasive instruments
III. Ultrasonic instruments

I. Hand Cutting Instruments

It is not the intention of this chapter to describe all hand cutting instruments, as there are a great number of them. An effort will be made to describe the instruments used in regular operative procedures. Specialized instruments will be described in discussions of operative procedures necessitating their use.

Every hand instrument has the following parts (Fig. 8):

The shaft, which is used as a handle, is straight, and is usually without variations in size. It may be serrated to increase friction for hand gripping.

The shank, which connects the shaft with the blade or working point. It usually tapers from its connection with the shaft to where the blade begins. It is here where any angulation in the instrument can be placed.

The blade is that part of the instrument bearing the cutting edge. It begins at the angle if one angle is present in the shank; or at the last angle, if more than one angle is present in the shank; or at the point which terminates the shank. The blade ends in the cutting edge.

The cutting edge is the working part of the instrument. It is usually in the form of a bevel with different shapes.

The blade angle (Fig. 9) is defined as the angle between the long axis of the blade and the long axis of the shaft.

The cutting edge angle (Fig. 9) is defined as an angle between the margin of the cutting edge and the long axis of the shaft.

A. Instrument nomenclature

G.V. Black described a way to name dental instruments which is similar to zoological classification:

1. The order denotes the purpose of the instrument, e.g., excavator, scaler.

2. The suborder denotes the position or manner of use of the instrument, e.g., push, pull.

3. The class describes the form of the blade, e.g., hatchet, chisel.

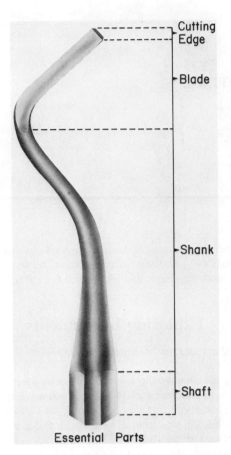

Essential Parts

Fig. 2-8

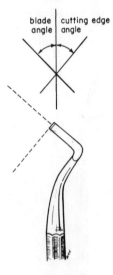

blade angle | cutting edge angle

Fig. 2-9

4. The angle denotes the number of angles in the shank. If the instrument contains one angle in its shank, it is called monangle (Fig. 10). If it contains two angles, it is called binangle (Fig. 11). If it contains three angles, it is called tripleangle (Fig. 12). Four angles are called quarternary-angle. Naming of the instruments usually moves from 4 to 1. For example, a binangle hatchet push excavator. In most cases, the suborder describing the position or manner of use is variable and non-

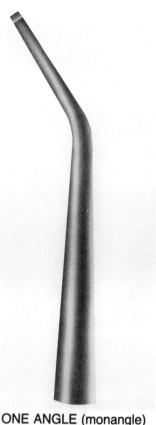

ONE ANGLE (monangle)

Fig. 2-10

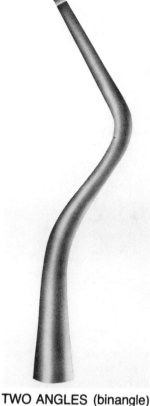

TWO ANGLES (binangle)

Fig. 2-11

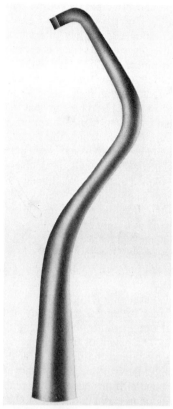

THREE ANGLES (triple angle)

Fig. 2-12

specific, and for practical purposes it is usually omitted. Identifying the working end and the purpose of the instrument is sufficient, e.g., binangle hatchet excavator.

B. Instrument formula

According to this identification method, in order to describe the parts of an instrument accurately, it is necessary to give three measurements, all expressed in the metric system. These are carved on one side of the instrument's shaft, in the following sequence:

1. The width of the blade in tenths of millimeters (Fig. 13)
2. The length of the blade in millimeters (Fig. 13B)
3. The blade angle in centigrade (Fig. 9)

These three measurements are sufficient for describing a great percentage of instruments. However, for instruments with their cutting edges at an angle other than a right angle to the long axis of the blade, a fourth unit, cutting edge angle, (Fig. 9) is added to the basic three-unit formula. This additional number is expressed in centigrade degrees and represents the angle formed between the cutting edge and the long axis of the handle. It is placed in the second position of the formula, i.e., before the length of the blade.

C. Instrument design

Hand instruments are made of stainless steel, carbon steel, or blades of tungsten carbide soldered to a steel handle. Carbon steel is able to keep a cutting edge better than stainless steel. Carbide blades, however, are the most efficient in cutting, even though they are somewhat brittle.

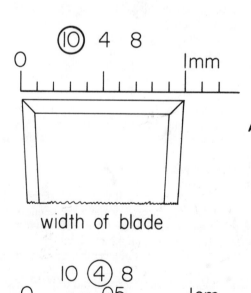

width of blade

A

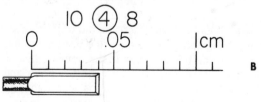

length of blade

B

Fig. 2-13

The main principle of cutting with hand instruments is to concentrate forces on a very thin cross-section of the instrument at the cutting edge. Thus, the thinner this cross-section, the more the pressure that is concentrated and the more efficient the instrument will be (Fig. 14).

1. Direct Cutting and lateral cutting instruments

A direct cutting instrument is one in which the force is applied in the same plane as that of the blade and handle. It is called a "single-planed" instrument. Lateral cutting instruments are those in which the force is applied at a right angle to the plane of the blade and handle. These usually have a curved blade and are called "double-planed" instruments. The single-planed instruments, although they may have two or more curves or angles in their shanks, all are in the same plane as the handle. Double-planed instruments have an angle or curve in a plane at a right angle to that of the handle. Single-planed instruments can be used in direct and lateral cutting (provided that they are contrangled). However, double-planed instruments can only be used in lateral cutting (all should be contrangled).

2. Contrangling (Fig. 15)

In order to gain access, many instruments have the shank bent at one or more points to angle the blade relative to the handle. The extent of this arrangement depends on the length of the blade and the degree of angulation in the shank. Accordingly, the working point is moved out of line with the axis of the handle. If this occurs to more than 3 mm from the handle axis (its imaginary continuation), the instrument will be out of balance in lateral cutting motions, and force will be required to keep the instrument from rotating in the hand (compare a knife and a cleaver in lateral cutting strokes). To solve this problem, modern instruments are designed to have one or more angles in the shank placing the working point within 3 mm from the axis of the handle. This principle of design is called contrangling (Fig. 15). A short blade and small blade angle requires only binangle-contrangling, while longer blades and greater blade angles require triple angle-contrangling. The length of the blade required is determined by the depth of the cavity and the blade angle is determined by the accessibility requirements. It follows, then, that greater angles are necessary for more posterior teeth and incisal portions of proximal cavities in anterior teeth. So, in addition to balance, contrangling will provide better access and a clearer view for the field of operation.

3. Right and left instruments

Direct cutting instruments are made either right or left by placing a bevel on one side of the blade. If the instrument is held with the cutting edge down and pointing away from the operator and the bevel is on the right side, it will be a "right" instrument. If the bevel is on the left, it will be a left instrument (Fig. 16A). As mentioned before, these are single-planed instruments, and for direct cutting acts the non-bevelled side of the blade should be in contact with the wall being shaved. For lateral cutting acts, always move the instrument in a scraping action from the bevelled side to the non-bevelled side of the blade. Lateral cutting instruments are made left and right by having the curve or angle, which is at a right angle to the principal plane (shaft plane), either on the right or on the left (Fig. 16B). Holding the instrument with its blade down and cutting edge pointing away, the instrument having that curve

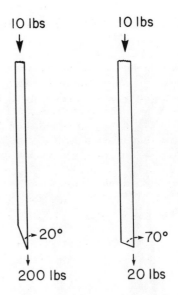

Relationship of cutting edge to force

Fig. 2-14

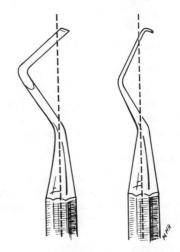

Fig. 2-15

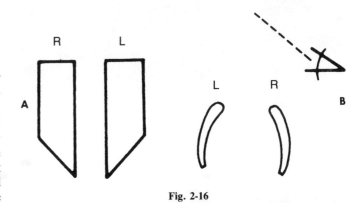

Fig. 2-16

of the blade directed to the right is a right instrument and vice versa for the left (Fig. 16B).

4. Single bevelled instruments

These are all single-planed instruments with the cutting edge at a right angle to the long axis of the shaft. They all are designed like carpenter's chisels. If they are regularly bevelled on the side away from the shaft, they are called "distally bevelled" (Fig. 17A). If they are bevelled on the side of the blade towards the shaft, they are called "mesially bevelled" (Fig. 17B). When these types of instruments have no angle in the shank (Fig. 17C), or an angle of 12° or less (Fig. 28), they are used in push (direct cutting) and scraping motions (bevelled to non-bevelled side). If this angle in the shank exceeds 12°, the instruments could be used in pull (distally bevelled) and push (mesially bevelled) motions. Understandably, right and left single-planed instruments having their blades parallel to the long axis of the shaft are single-bevelled instruments (Fig. 18).

5. Bibevelled instruments

Only hatchets and straight chisels can be bibevelled. The blade is equally bevelled on both sides (Fig. 19), and they cut by pushing them in the direction of the long axis of the blade.

6. Triple-bevelled instruments (Fig. 20)

Bevelling the blade laterally, together with the end, forms three distinct cutting edges. Most modern single-planed instruments, especially the small ones, are triple bevelled, affording the instrument an additional cutting potential which is very useful.

7. Circumferentially bevelled instruments

A circumferential bevel usually occurs in double-planed instruments where the blade is bevelled at all peripheries (Fig. 21).

8. Single-ended and double-ended instruments

Most modern instruments are double-ended, incorporating the right and left or the mesial and distal form of the instrument in the same handle. Single-ended instruments are confined now to those types of instruments having only one specific function.

Single-planed instruments with no angle in the shank have the potential for five cutting movements—vertical (parallel to the long axis of the blade), right, left, push, and pull. A right-left single-planed instrument with one or more angles in the shank will have four potential cutting movements. They are vertical, push, pull, then right or left, depending on the location of the bevel. For the mesially and distally bevelled single-

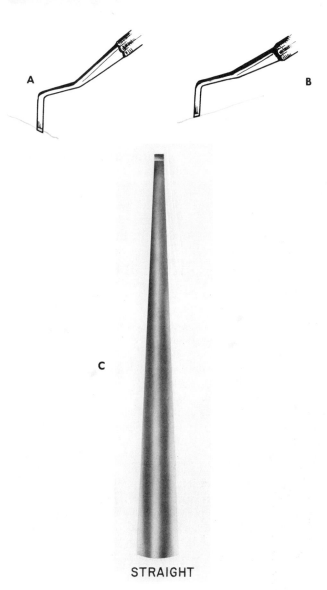

STRAIGHT

Fig. 2-17

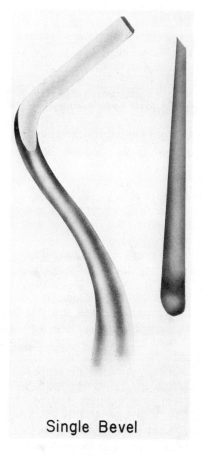

Single Bevel

Fig. 2-18

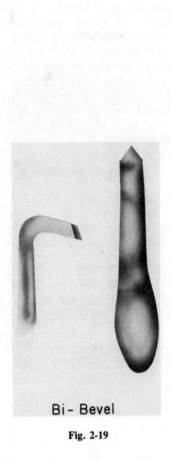

Bi - Bevel

Fig. 2-19

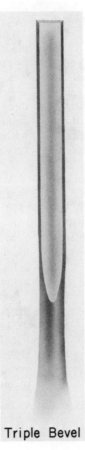

Triple Bevel

Fig. 2-20

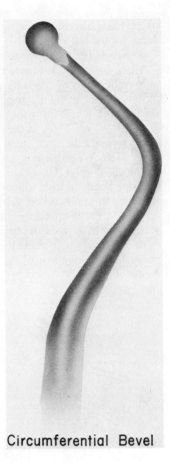

Circumferential Bevel

Fig. 2-21

planed instruments the four movements are vertical, right, left, and push or pull, depending on the location of the bevel.

D. Types of hand cutting instruments

Hand instruments are classified into three groups:

1. Excavators
2. Chisels
3. Special forms of chisels

1. Excavators are designed for the excavation and removal of carious dentin and for the shaping of the internal parts of cavities. There are five types:

a. Hatchet excavators (Fig. 22) have the edge of the blade running in a direction parallel with the handle. They are usually single-planed bibevelled instruments. They cut by being pushed or pulled in the direction of the blade. They may shave a wall by being inclined toward the wall and moved vertically, or they may be used laterally with a scraping motion. This form of excavator is used for delicate cutting within preparations, especially in incisors.

b. Hoe excavators, where the bevel runs at a right angle to the shaft. They may come with the edge of the blade bevelled on the side distal to (away from) the shaft, i.e., distally bevelled (Fig. 23A). Also, it may be mesially bevelled, i.e., bevelled toward the shaft (Fig. 23B). These are used for cutting mesial and distal walls of premolars and molars. They are single-planed instruments with four possible cutting movements—

vertical, pull (push), right, and left. Both hatchets and hoes are used to remove harder varieties of caries as well as to give form to the internal parts of the cavity preparations.

c. Spoon excavators (Fig. 24) are made in pairs with the blade of one curved to the right, and the blade of the other curved to the left. The cutting edge is ground to a semi-circular circumferential bevel and sharpened to a thin edge. The direction of the curve of the blades makes the instruments lateral cutting instruments. They are used for removal of decayed dentin. The spoon excavator is a double-planed instrument with right or left cutting movements only.

d. Discoid (disclike) excavators (Fig. 25) have a blade which is circular in shape, with a cutting edge extending around the periphery except where it is joined to the shank. This circular blade is placed at an angle with the shaft. It is used for the same purpose and in the same manner as a spoon excavator (removal of carious dentin). It is a double-planed instrument with right or left cutting movements only.

e. The cleoid (clawlike) excavator (Fig. 26) is essentially a spoon excavator except the blade comes to a point. It resembles a claw, hence the name "cleoid". It is used in carving amalgam and in excavating decay from areas of difficult access. The cleoid excavator is a double-planed instrument with lateral cutting movements only.

2. Chisels

These are instruments designed after ordinary carpenter's

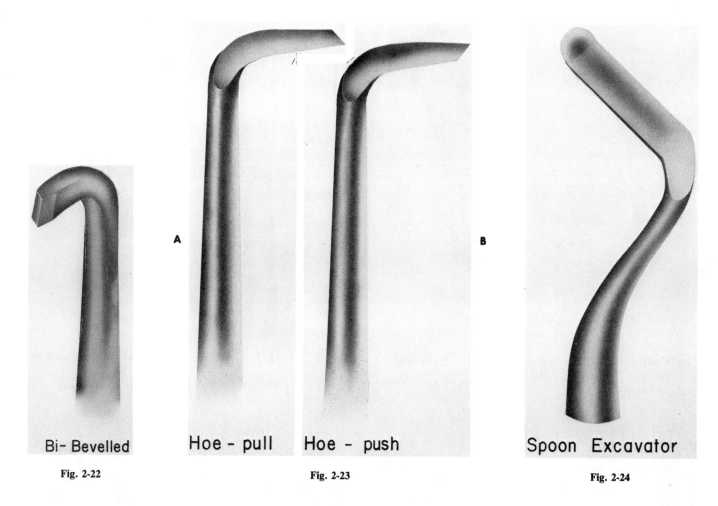

Bi- Bevelled   Hoe - pull   Hoe - push   Spoon Excavator

A   B

Fig. 2-22   **Fig. 2-23**   **Fig. 2-24**

tools and are intended for cutting enamel. They are usually bevelled on one side only, and there are four types available:

a. Straight chisels (Fig. 27) have a straight blade in line with the handle and shank. The cutting edge is on one side only, with the bevel of the blade running at a right angle to the shaft. They are single-planed instruments with five possible cutting movements.

b. Monangle chisels (Fig. 28) are similar to straight chisels, except the blade is placed at an angle to the shaft. It may be mesially or distally bevelled.

c. Binangle chisels (Fig. 29) where the chisel blade is placed at a slight angle with the shaft as in the hoe. Like all chisels, it may be mesially or distally bevelled. As the name indicates, there are two angles between the shaft and the blade. The three aforementioned chisels are all used to cleave or split undermined enamel.

d. The triple-angle chisel (Fig. 30) has three angles in its shank and is usually used to flatten pulpal floors. It may also be mesially or distally bevelled.

The monangle, binangle, and triple-angle chisels are single-planed instruments. All possess three possible cutting movements: vertical, right, and left. The mesially bevelled chisels can cut in push movements, while the distally bevelled ones can cut in pull motions.

3. Special forms of chisels are chisels designed to perform specific functions.

a. Enamel hatchets (Fig. 31)

The hatchet shank has one or more angles or curves. The blade is in the same plane as this angle or angles, parallel with the shaft. The cutting edge is in the form of a bevel parallel to the shaft. These instruments are either paired, one with a left and the other with a right bevel, or they may be bibevelled. Hatchets are used for splitting or cleaving undermined enamel in proximal cavities and on buccal and lingual walls where it is not possible to use a chisel. The smaller sizes are primarily used in anterior teeth, although they are useful in bicuspids and molars. Larger sizes are mainly used in posterior teeth. Hatchets are single-planed instruments with four potential cutting movements: vertical, push, pull, and either right or left lateral cutting.

b. Gingival margin trimmers (Fig. 32, A, B, and C)

These instruments are similar to spoon excavators in both their curves and the dimensions of their blades (Fig. 32A). Although the cutting edge is similar to the single-bevelled hatchet, it makes an angle with the entire length of the blade. There are two pairs of these instruments constituting a set of four. In a given size each pair has a right and a left bevelled instrument. The cutting edges of one pair make an acute angle with that edge of the blade furthest from the handle. These are distal gingival margin trimmers. The cutting edge of the other pair makes an acute angle with that edge of the blade nearer to the handle. These are mesial gingival margin trimmers. A

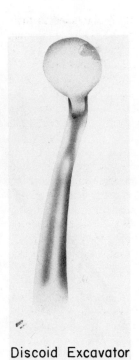

Discoid Excavator

Fig. 2-25

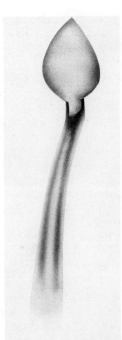

Cleoid Excavator

Fig. 2-26

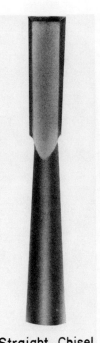

Straight Chisel

Fig. 2-27

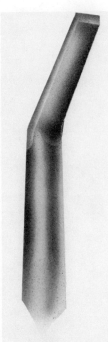

Monangle Chisel

Fig. 2-28

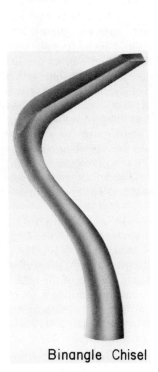

Binangle Chisel

Fig. 2-29

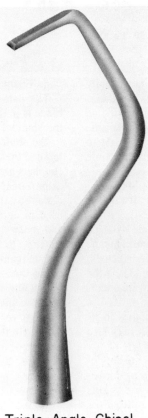

Triple Angle Chisel

Fig. 2-30

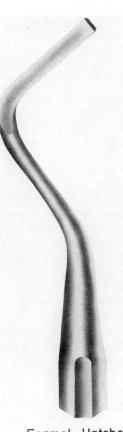

Enamel Hatchet

Fig. 2-31

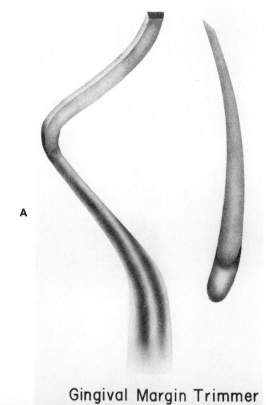

Gingival Margin Trimmer

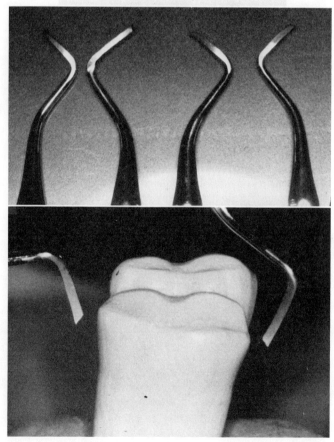

Fig. 2-32

figure for the cutting edge angle should be included in their instrument formula. They are convenient for trimming the margins of various walls of a cavity preparation, and especially in creating the proper bevel of the gingival floors (Fig. 32C). They are also used for forming sharp angles in internal parts of cavity preparations. They are primarily lateral cutting instruments, since the cutting edge is in a plane other than that of the shaft. Occasionally, they are used in pull and push motions to sharpen point and line angles.

c. Angle formers (Fig. 33)

These instruments are made by grinding the bevel at an angle of 80° with the shaft, thus forming an acute angle with the long axis of the blade. This creates a pointed and a linear cutting edge. They are used to cut line and point angles. Being single-planed instruments, with right (Fig. 33A) or left (Fig. 33B) bevelling, they share three cutting potentials: vertical, push and pull. The right ones can also cut from right to left while the left ones can cut from left to right.

d. Wedelstaedt chisels (Fig. 34)

The Wedelstaedt is like a straight chisel, but with a slight vertical curvature in its shank (the blade does make a real angle with the shaft). It is bevelled on one side of the blade only. If this bevel is on the side toward the curvature of the shank, it is mesially bevelled; if it is on the side of the blade away from the curvature, it is distally bevelled. Wedelstaedt chisels are used for cleaving undermined enamel and for shaping walls. They are single-planed instruments, with three cutting motions: vertical, right, and left. The mesially bevelled can be used in push movements, and the distally bevelled can be used in pull motions.

e. Off-set hatchets (Fig. 35, A, B, and C)

The off-set is like the regular hatchet, except the whole blade is rotated a quarter of a turn forward or backward around its long axis (Fig. 35C). These are single-planed instruments with the same cutting potential as regular hatchets. They may be right or left (Fig. 35B). However, there are two for both the right and left—one with the whole blade rotated forward and the other with the whole blade rotated backward.

They are useful to create and shape specific angulations for cavity walls, especially in areas of difficult access.

f. Hatchets or off-set hatchets with cutting edges making an angle, other than a right angle, with the long axis of the shaft (Fig. 36).

These are like ordinary hatchets or off-set hatchets, but the cutting edges of the blade are designed exactly like the cutting edge of the gingival margin trimmer. They are cut so that one pair will have the cutting edge make an acute angle with the edge of the blade nearer to the handle (mesial), while the other pair will make an acute angle with the edge of the blade further from the handle (distal). So, like gingival margin trimmers, these hatchets will have right and left pairs, and each pair will have a distal and mesial type. Accordingly, there are eight types of off-set hatchets (Fig. 36).

g. Triangular chisel (Fig. 37)

This chisel has a blade which is triangular in shape, with the base of the triangle away from the shaft. It has a terminal cutting edge like the straight chisel.

h. Hoe chisel (Fig. 38)

This is very similar to a hoe excavator, but it has a sturdier blade.

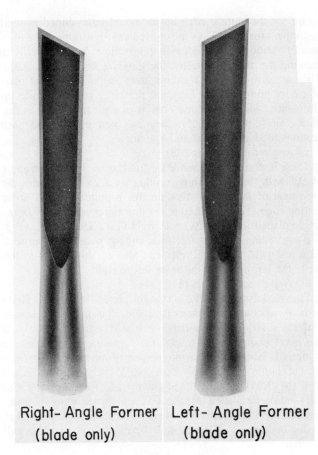

Right- Angle Former   Left- Angle Former
(blade only)   (blade only)

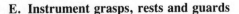

Fig. 2-33

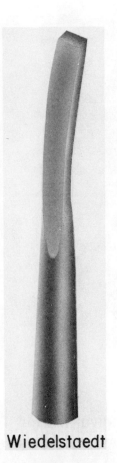

Wiedelstaedt

Fig. 2-34

E. Instrument grasps, rests and guards

a. Pen grasp

This method of holding an instrument allows the application of considerable force with very accurate control. While the instrument is held like a pen between the thumb and the first two fingers, care must be taken that the second finger, not the index finger, applies the pressure to the instrument. This way, due to the greater length of the second finger, the application point for the force will be nearer the working point of the instrument.

b. Inverted pen grasp

This is similar to the pen grasp, but the hand is rotated so that its palm is facing upwards. It is usually used in upper teeth. In both the aforementioned types of grasps the third or preferably the third and fourth fingers are held firmly against the adjacent tooth of the same jaw. This is called a "rest" and it is used to steady the hand and prevent the slipping of instruments. The pen grasp is probably the most effective and most universally used grasp because it can be used equally well with all instruments whether the applied force is in the direction of the handle axis; at an angle to the axis, but in the same plane of the shank; or in a lateral direction.

c. Palm and thumb grasp

Using this method, the instrument is held in a manner similar to that employed in holding a knife to whittle a piece of wood. The handle of the instrument is held in the palm of the hand and is grasped by the four fingers, with the thumb resting on

an adjoining surface. It may be useful on maxillary teeth, particularly the right side, when working from the right rear chair position. This form of grasp is usually necessary where the rest support for the thumb is at some distance from the point of operation, so that the thumb itself must be extended and hence cannot be used for gripping.

d. Modified palm and thumb grasp

When the rest can be obtained on the same or on an adjoining tooth, greater freedom of movement and delicacy of control may be obtained by a modification of the previous grasp. In this modified form, the handle of the instrument is in contact with the tips of the four fingers on one side, opposed to which are contacts with the mesial end of the first phalanx of the thumb. The hand is only about half closed, instead of being fully closed as in the case of the usual palm-thumb grasp. The end of the thumb is used for the rest.

The original type of palm and thumb grasp is a remnant of techniques employed with older large-handled instruments. The force potential with it is very limited and ineffective; the support rest is unstable and not proximate to the operating area. However, the modified palm and thumb grasp not only permits greater freedom and ease of movements, but also gives a delicacy of control, comparable to the pen grasp while preventing instrument slippage during a thrusting stroke.

With the grasps just described there is no need for a guard, which is created by using the thumb and first one or two fingers of the left hand (for a right-handed operator) to steady the

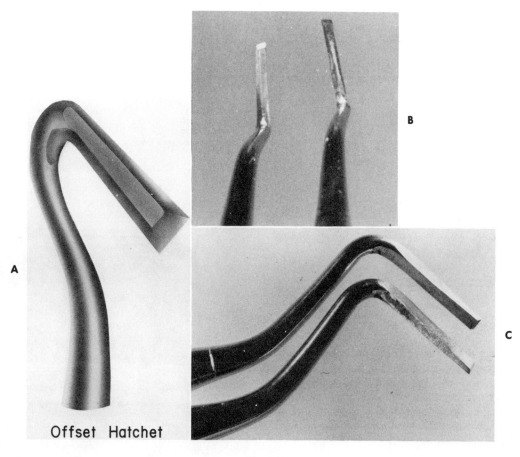

Offset Hatchet

Fig. 2-35

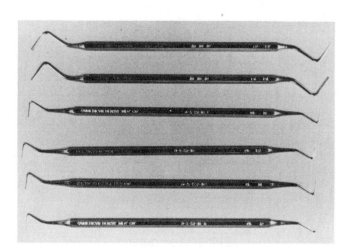

Fig. 2-36

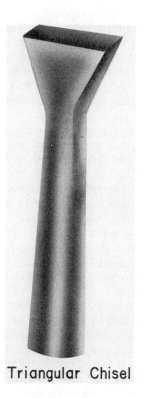

Triangular Chisel

Fig. 2-37

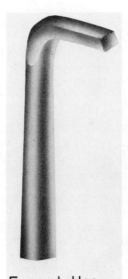

Enamel Hoe

Fig. 2-38

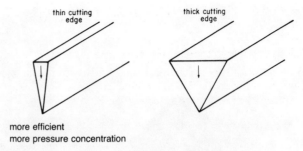

Fig. 2-39

more efficient
more pressure concentration

thin cutting edge   thick cutting edge

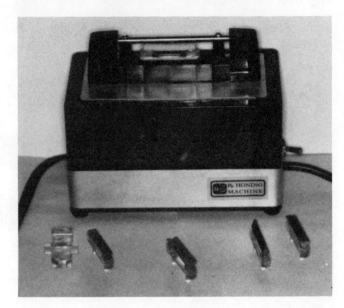

Fig. 2-40

instrument and protect the tissues. Where firm rests on adjoining teeth of the same jaw are available, the operator can apply substantial force and still have remarkable control of the instrument. Where teeth are not available and the rest must be put on soft tissues and/or on the opposite jaw, a guard should be used. Even then, however, the control is not reliable enough to permit much force.

F. Sharpening of hand instrument

Instruments are dulled by repeated contact with tooth tissues and by frequent sterilization. So, the frequency with which dental hand cutting instruments should be sharpened is determined by the extent of their use. Magnifying lenses are useful in evaluating the condition of their cutting edges.

Sharpening is done by reducing the bulk of the metal at the cutting edge, following the original configuration of the bevel (Fig. 39).

For sharpening hand instruments, one may use either a soft, wheel-shaped Arkansas stone rotated at a slow speed, or a sharpening machine with different shapes and sizes of cutting edges, moving in rotary or back and forth motions. The sharpening machine has a specific blade for each shape and angulation of the instrument's cutting edge (Fig. 40); or free-hand application of the instrument to an Arkansas stone where the instrument is moved in one direction with the bevel in contact with the stone surface. In any sharpening technique oil should be used as a lubricant.

Hand cutting instruments have several advantages. They are self-limited in cutting enamel, i.e., they will not cut sound enamel, but will cut only enamel undermined by loss of dentin. (Fig 41). They can remove large pieces of undermined enamel quickly, thus saving time and effort. No vibration or heat accompanies the cutting, making it painless and with no adverse effects on the tooth tissues. They are the most efficient means for precise intricate cutting, especially when cutting is needed adjacent to important anatomy. They can create the smoothest surface of all cutting instruments. They have the longest life

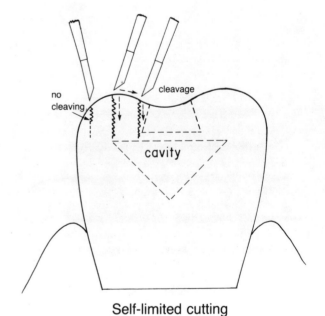

no cleaving   cleavage

cavity

Self-limited cutting

Fig. 2-41

span of all cutting instruments inasmuch as they can be re-sharpened.

II. Rotary Instrumentation

Rotary instruments are the most universally used instruments for gross removal of tooth structure. The following are the characteristics of rotary instrumentation.

A. Speed

An explanation of the term speed is needed for a more complete understanding of rotary instrumentation. Speed refers not only to the revolutions per minute, but also to the surface feet per unit time of contact that the tool has with the work to be cut (Fig. 76).

According to industrial investigation, the maximum cutting efficiency of a cutting tool of uniform width ranges between 5000-6000 surface feet per minute. Since the surface feet per minute is controlled mainly by the RPM and the size of the revolving tool (length and diameter), it is important to consider the size of the working tool in relation to the speed of operation. A rotary tool should be large in diameter when used with low speeds to approach the optimum surface feet per unit time. In the ultra-high speed range, the diameter of a cutting tool should be reduced to approximate the limits of maximum cutting efficiency.

For dental purposes we classify speeds as follow:
a. Ultra-low speed (300-3000 RPM)
b. Low speed (3000-6000 RPM)
c. Medium high speed (20,000-45,000 RPM)
d. High speed (45,000-100,000 RPM)
e. Ultra-high speed (100,000 RPM and more)
Some dental equipment can actually produce up to 500,000 RPM.

B. Pressure (P)

Pressure is a resultant effect of two factors under the control of the dentist.
1. Force (F): The gripping of the handpiece and its positioning and application to the tooth.
2. Area (A): The amount of surface area of the cutting tool in contact with the tooth surface during a cutting operation. Pressure relates as follows:

$$P = \frac{F}{A}$$

Using the same force F, smaller tools (burs or stones) will apply more pressure to the point of contact than larger tools. To have both small and large tools cut at the same pressure, it is necessary to reduce the force applied with the smaller ones (constant RPM). If the constant force is reduced on the smaller tool so that there is equal pressure on the tooth (constant RPM), obviously the larger tool will remove more tooth structure, since there is more surface feet per minute contact. To have the smaller tool remove the same amount of tooth structure as the large one, it is necessary to increase the surface feet per minute contact of the smaller tool by increasing the RPM.

The net result obtained is a cutting tool smaller in size with less force required by the operator and running at greater revolutions per minute. The pressure at the point of contact is the same as with larger tools, but we have reduced the forces to

be applied in controlling and operating the instrument. It has been observed clinically that low speed requires 2-5 pounds force, high speed requires less force (1 pound) and ultra-high speed still less force (1-4 ounces) for efficient cutting. One of the most desirable features of higher speed rotary operation is better control with less fatigue on the part of the operator, and greater patient comfort. All these are due to reduction of forces on the tool and more efficient removal of tooth structure.

C. Heat production

Heat is directly proportional to:
1. Pressure
2. RPM
3. Area of tooth in contact with the tool
Therefore, if any of these factors is increased, heat production is increased. Since heat production will cause pulps of teeth to be permanently damaged if a temperature of 130° F is reached, heat must be carefully controlled. Even a temperature of 113° F within the pulp can produce inflammatory responses that could result in pulpitis and eventual pulp necrosis. It has been shown that when the area of the cutting tool is reduced, but the speed of rotation is increased, it is an absolute necessity that coolants be employed to eliminate pulpal damage. This can be accomplished by various coolants such as flowing water, a water-air spray, or air. For cutting dentin using rotary instruments in the range of high speed or faster, it is the author's opinion that flowing water is the only adequate coolant. Because pressure is a result of applied force, a reduction of this force will minimize heat production. Since higher speeds call for less force and if coolants are used, heat production could be eliminated or at least minimized.

D. Vibration

Vibration is not only a major annoying factor for the patient, but it also causes fatigue for the operator, excessive wear of instruments and, most importantly, a destructive reaction in the tooth and supporting tissues. Vibration is a product of the equipment used and the speed of rotation. The equipment, primarily the handpieces and the various revolving cutting tools, all contribute to the quantity and quality of vibration.

The deleterious effects of vibration are two-fold in origin:
1. Amplitude (Fig. 42)
2. Undesirable modulating frequencies (Fig. 44)
Minimizing or eliminating these factors can reduce the undesirable effects of vibration.

1. Amplitude

A wave of vibration consists of frequency and amplitude. At low speed the amplitude is large but the frequency is small. At higher speeds the reverse is true. The greater harm is caused by the amplitude; it is the factor most destructive to instruments and it not only causes the most apprehension in the patient but also the greatest fatigue for the dentist. By increasing the operating speed the amplitude and its effects are reduced as well as its sequelae.

Vibration waves are measured in cycles per second. It has been shown that rotation of approximately 6000 RPM sets up a fundamental vibrational wave of approximately 100 cycles per second. This has been demonstrated to be the range most annoying to the patient and the dentist.

As the RPMs are increased, the cycles per second of the

fundamental vibration waves are increased until at 100,000 RPM there is an average vibration of 1600 cycles per second. In experiments conducted in vivo, it has been demonstrated that at a wave vibration over 1300 cycles per second, vibrations are practically imperceptible to the patient. This is due to the fact that stimulations occur during the refractory period of recovery of the perception mechanism (Fig. 43). In other words, at vibration cycles of 1300 cycles/sec. and more, no apparent stimulation will be evident. Thus it can be concluded that higher RPMs produce less amplitude and greater frequency of vibrations. As a result, perception will be lost in the ultra-high speed ranges of 100,000 RPM or more. It has to be emphasized that the no-perception status does not mean that the effect of these vibrations on the involved vital dental tissues is not present or prevented.

2. Undesirable modulating frequency (Fig. 44)

The second deleterious effect of vibration is caused by improperly designed, or poorly maintained, equipment. Although there must be a fundamental vibrational wave, improper equipment use or care allows modulating frequencies to be established so that a series of vibrations (in different directions) are perceived by the patient and the dentist. The end result is again apprehension in the patient, fatigue for dentist and accelerated wear of cutting instruments. The fundamental vibration wave is set up when the handpiece turbine is running. Each piece of the remaining attachment (handpiece) will vibrate, depending upon the amount of wear or eccentricity in its moving parts. Each will set up a modulating frequency, or "overtone", accompanying the fundamental vibrational wave, so that the patient and the dentist are subjected not only to the basic wave but also to other accompanying vibrations. It should be the objective of the operator to eliminate these by having the equipment free from any such defects. He should supply himself with a true running energy source, centrically cutting tools, and handpieces manufactured to run true at high speeds.

E. Patient reaction

The factors that cause patient apprehension consist primarily of heat production, vibrational sensation, length of operating time, and number of visits. The proper understanding of the instrument being used and the speed at which it is being used allows the operator to counteract these potentially irritating stimuli. The use of coolants, intermittent applications of a tool to the tooth; sharp instruments, etc., all aid greatly in minimizing both patient discomfort and unnecessary irritation to the oral structures. In instances where irritation is unavoidable (e.g., drilling pin channels in vital teeth), the patients should be forewarned and properly anesthetized.

F. Operator fatigue

The major causes for fatigue are: duration of operation, vibration produced in the handpiece, forces needed to control the rotating instrument, apprehension on the part of the dentist regarding the possibility of producing a pulp exposure or injuring adjacent oral, intra- and paraoral tissues, and lack of patient cooperation.

High speed rotary instrumentation minimizes fatigue by decreasing both the vibrations and the time of the operation. Proper balancing (contrangling) of the handpiece and reduction of its weight will minimize the forces needed to control the

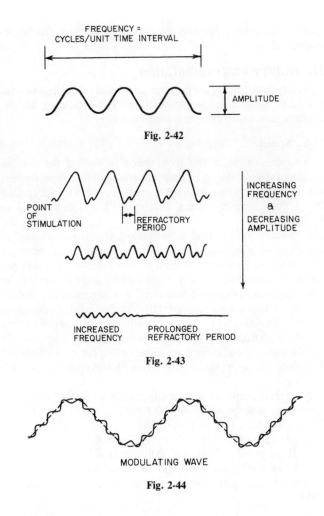

FREQUENCY = CYCLES/UNIT TIME INTERVAL

AMPLITUDE

Fig. 2-42

POINT OF STIMULATION

REFRACTORY PERIOD

INCREASING FREQUENCY & DECREASING AMPLITUDE

INCREASED FREQUENCY   PROLONGED REFRACTORY PERIOD

Fig. 2-43

MODULATING WAVE

Fig. 2-44

instrument. Operator confidence and patient cooperation can be enhanced only by proper training and experience on the part of the operator.

G. Sources of power

The introduction in the 1950's of the air-turbine as a power source changed the shape of dental practice. The belt driven handpiece was rendered obsolete for operatory use. The air turbine remains the main power source.

H. Instrument design

Instrument design for rotary instrumentation should be evaluated in two parameters: one, the handpiece, which will hold and provide power for the cutting tool; and two, the cutting tool itself (bur, stone, etc).

1. Handpiece

Handpieces come in a variety of sizes and shapes: straight, contra-angled, and right-angled. Each is designed for a specific range of functions. They will retain the cutting tool by a screw-in, latch, or friction grip type of attachment. The following criteria should be used in evaluating handpieces.

a. Friction

Friction will occur in the moving parts of a handpiece, especially the turbine. This becomes critically important at speeds of high speed or above. If the heat from friction is not prevented or counteracted, the handpiece will be unsuitable for dental use. For this reason, handpieces are equipped with bearings: ball bearings, needle bearings, glass and resin bearings, etc., the life spans of which will vary.

b. Torque

Torque is the ability of the handpiece to withstand lateral pressure on the revolving tool without decreasing its speed or reducing its cutting efficiency. Torque is dependent upon the type of bearing used and the amount of energy supplied to the handpiece.

c. Vibration

As previously discussed, vibration is a very deleterious aspect of rotary instrumentation. While some vibration is unavoidable, care should be taken not to introduce it unnecessarily. Excessive wear of the turbine bearings, for example, will cause eccentric running which creates substantial vibration. It is best to always follow the manufacturers' recommendations for use and maintenance of handpieces to minimize turbine wear.

2. The rotary tools for the removal of tooth structure

These are the units actually responsible for the removal of tooth structure and may be one of two types: *burs,* which are cutting tools, and *stones,* which are abrading tools.

a. Dental cutting burs

i. Composition and manufacture

Dental burs can be classified by their composition into two types: steel burs and tungsten carbide burs. Steel burs are cut from blank steel stock by means of a rotary cutter that cuts parallel to the long axis of the bur. The bur is then hardened and tempered until its Vicker's hardness number is approximately 800.

Tungsten carbide burs are the product of powder metallurgy, i.e., a process of alloying in which complete fusion of the constituents does not occur. The tungsten carbide powder is mixed with powdered cobalt under pressure and heated in a vacuum. A partial alloying or sintering of the metals takes place. A blank is then formed and the bur is cut from it with a diamond tool. This cutting process is better controlled than the cutting of steel burs. Sometimes, only the cutting head is tungsten carbide, welded or soldered to a steel shank. The Vicker's hardness number of this type of bur is in the range of 1650-1700.

ii. General design of dental burs

The dental bur is a small milling (cutting) instrument. A common design is displayed in Fig. 45, with the standard nomenclature:

A. Bur tooth: This terminates in the cutting edge, or *blade.* It has two surfaces, the tooth face, which is the side of the tooth on the leading edge; and the back or flank of the tooth, which is the side of the tooth on the trailing edge.

B. Rake angle (Fig. 46): The rake angle is the angle that the face of the bur tooth makes with the radial line from the center of the bur to the blade. This angle can be negative if the face is beyond or leading the radial line (referring to the direction of rotation). It can be 0 if the radial line and the tooth face coincide with each other (radial rake angle). The angle can also be positive if the radial line leads the face, so that the rake angle is on the inside of the radial line.

C. Land: The plane surface immediately following the cutting edge (Fig. 48).

D. Clearance angle (Fig. 45): The angle between the back

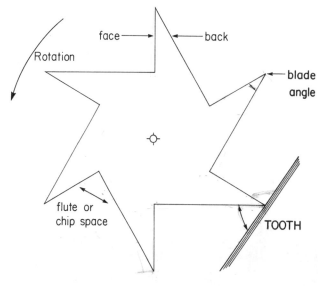

Fig. 2-45

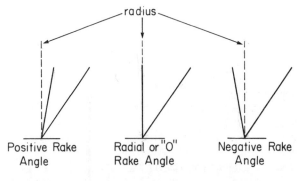

Fig. 2-46

of the tooth and the work. If a land is present on the bur, the clearance angle is divided into: primary clearance which is the angle the land will make with work, and (Fig. 48) secondary clearance, which is the angle between the back of the bur tooth and work. When the back surface of the tooth is curved, the clearance is called radial clearance (Fig. 47).

E. Tooth angle: This is measured between the face and back. If a land is present, it is measured between the face and land (Figs. 45, 46).

F. Flute or chip space: The space between successive teeth (Fig. 45).

The number of teeth in dental cutting burs is usually 6-8. Every bur will have three parts (Fig. 49): the head—the portion carrying the cutting blades, the shank—the portion connecting the head to the attachment part, and the shaft or the attachment part—the portion which will be engaged within the handpiece.

According to their mode of attachment to the handpiece, dental burs can be classified as either latch type or friction grip type. Also, they may be classified according to the handpiece they are designed for, i.e., a contrangle bur or a straight handpiece bur. They can also be classifed as right and left. The most common ones are the right, which cut when they revolve clockwise.

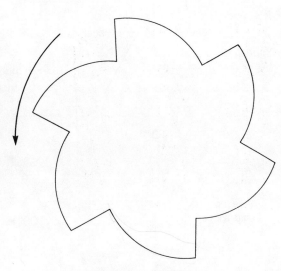

Bur with Radial Clearance

Fig. 2-47

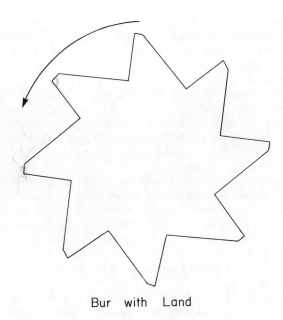

Bur with Land

Fig. 2-48

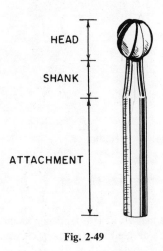

HEAD

SHANK

ATTACHMENT

Fig. 2-49

Burs can be classified as long, short (pedominiature) or regular, according to the length of the head. They may be classified as cutting burs or those used to finish and polish restorations.

According to their shapes and sizes, they may be classified as follows:

Round burs (Fig. 50)

They are numbered from ¼, ½, 1, 2, to 10. They are round in shape and used for initial tooth penetration and for the placement of retention grooves.

Wheel burs (Fig. 51)

They are numbered as 14 and 15. They are wheel shape and are used to place grooves and for gross removal of tooth structure.

Inverted cone burs (Fig. 52)

They are numbered from 33¼, 33½, 34, 35, to 39. As the name indicates, they are an inverted cone shape, used mainly for cavity extension and occasionally for establishing wall angulations and retention forms.

Plain cylindrical fissure bur (Figs. 53, 54, 55)

They are numbered from 55 to 59. The bur teeth can be cut parallel to the long axis of the bur, which are designated straight (Fig. 53) or cut obliquely to the long axis of the teeth (for better unclogging), which are called spiral (Figs. 54, 55).

Cross cut cylindrical fissure bur (Figs. 56, 57)

They are numbered from 555, 556, to 560. Their teeth can also be cut parallel to the long axis of the bur (straight) or obliquely (spiral). All four types of cylindrical fissure burs are used for gross cutting, cavity extension and creation of walls.

Plain tapered fissure bur

They are numbered from 168, 169, to 172. They have a tapered cylindrical head; their teeth can be straight (Fig. 58) or spiral (Fig. 59).

Cross-cut tapered fissure bur

They are numbered from 699, 700, to 703. They also can be straight (Fig. 60) or spiral (Fig. 61). The four types of tapered fissure burs are the most universally used burs in operative dentistry.

Round nose fissure burs

All eight types of fissure burs can be round-ended. The number 1 will be added to previous numbering to denote round nosing, e.g., round-nose plain cylindrical fissure burs will have the number from 156 to 159 (Fig. 62). Round-nose cross-cut cylindrical fissure burs (Fig. 63) will have the numbers from 1555 to 1559, etc. Round-nose tapered fissure burs (Figs. 64 and 65) will have numbers from 1169 to 1172 and from 1700 to 1702. (It is impossible to round-nose the smaller tapered fissure burs because of the narrow diameter at the end of the bur.)

Pear-shaped burs (Fig. 66)

As the name indicates, they are shaped like pears. They are numbered from 229 to 333 and are mainly used in pedodontics.

End cutting burs (Fig. 67)

They are cylindrical in shape, with just the end carrying blades. They are very efficient in extending preparations apically without axial reduction. They are numbered from 900 to 904.

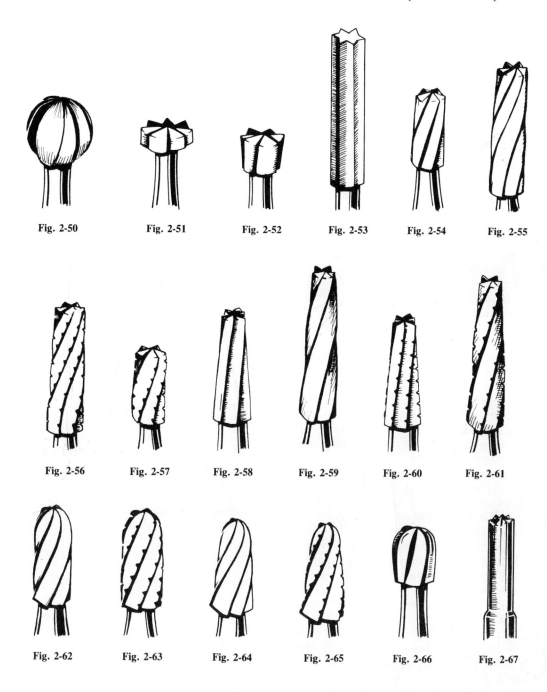

Fig. 2-50   Fig. 2-51   Fig. 2-52   Fig. 2-53   Fig. 2-54   Fig. 2-55

Fig. 2-56   Fig. 2-57   Fig. 2-58   Fig. 2-59   Fig. 2-60   Fig. 2-61

Fig. 2-62   Fig. 2-63   Fig. 2-64   Fig. 2-65   Fig. 2-66   Fig. 2-67

iii. Factors influencing the cutting efficiency of burs

A. Influence of design and manufacturing

1. Rake angle

The more positive that the rake angle is, the greater is the bur's cutting efficiency (Fig. 68). Also, burs with radial rake angles cut more effectively than designs with negative rake angles. However, with a negative rake angle the cut chip moves directly away from the blade edge and often fractures into small bits or dust (Fig. 68). This is in contrast to burs with a positive rake angle where the chips are larger and tend to clog the chip space (Fig. 68). There are practical objections to the use of positive rake angles in dental burs, particularly steel burs, because the positivity of the rake angle decreases the size of the bur tooth and its tooth angle, thus decreasing its bulk (Fig.

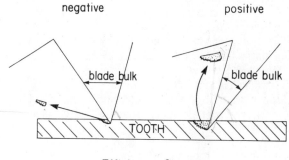

Fig. 2-68

68). As a result, there is a great possibility that bur teeth will be curved, flattened or even fractured during cutting. The positive rake angle can be used with tungsten carbide burs where the greater hardness and strength of the material allow sacrifice of bulk to obtain a more efficient cutting edge. Even with carbide burs a negative rake angle or radial clearance with a short bur tooth height is employed to contribute to a longer bur life.

2. Clearance angle

As its name implies, this angle provides clearance between the work and the cutting edge to prevent the tooth back from rubbing on the work. There is always a component of frictional force on any cutting edge as it rubs against the surface, following the dislodgement of the chip (Fig. 69).

Any slight wear of the cutting edge will increase the dulling perceptibility. However, it is possible that large clearance angle may result in less rapid dulling of the bur.

3. Number of teeth or blades and their distribution

The number of teeth in a dental bur is usually limited to 6-8. Since the external load is distributed among the blades actively cutting, as the number of blades is decreased, the magnitude of forces at each blade increases and the thickness of the chip removed by each flute correspondingly increases (Fig. 70). Under certain conditions, nearly the same amount of material can be removed by either 8, 7 or 6-fluted burs, i.e., the product of the chip thickness removed by each tooth and the number of flutes may be nearly a constant. The reason for constructing burs with a fewer number of bur teeth arises from the possible increased space between the bur teeth which decreases their clogging tendency (Fig. 71). Inasmuch as each bur tooth is removing more material, the tendency for bur tooth wear should be greater and the cutting life reduced. Furthermore, it has been shown that a fissure bur with *straight flutes* produces less temperature rise than one with *spiral flutes*. This may be due to the formation of large chips by the straight fluted bur. That chip then carries some heat energy with it. Therefore, a bur with fewer flutes would be cooler operating. It is apparent then, that the number of blades on the bur and the size of the flutes are definitely related.

As might be expected, the fewer the number of bur teeth, the greater the tendency for vibration. However, if there are two or more blades in contact with the work at one time, this effect would not be of great importance, particularly as related to the difference between a six or eight-tooth bur. If the bur teeth are cross-cut, the tendency is to increase the number of teeth, based on the assumption that the cross-cutting reduces the friction in cutting and provides more chip space. Some burs will have 10-12 or even up to 40 blades. Understandably, they are not designed for cutting. They are used only for finishing and polishing of a dental restoration.

4. Run-out

Run-out refers to the eccentricity or maximum displacement of the bur head from its axis of rotation while the bur turns (Fig. 72). The average value of clinically acceptable run-out is about 0.023 mm. Run-out will depend not only on the eccentricity of the bur itself, but also on the precision of the dental handpiece. If the shaft or collar holding the bur wobbles during rotation, the effect will be magnified at the bur head according to the length of the bur shank (Fig. 73). The efficiency in cutting of the bur is definitely affected by its run-out. If the bur moves away from the tooth periodically, all of

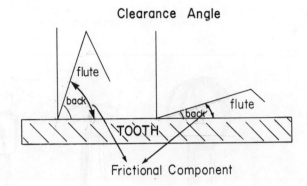

Clearance Angle

Fig. 2-69

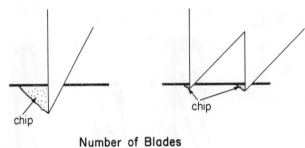

Number of Blades on Bur

Fig. 2-70

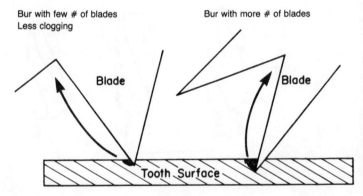

Fig. 2-71

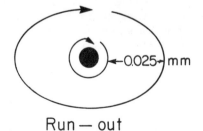

Run — out

Fig. 2-72

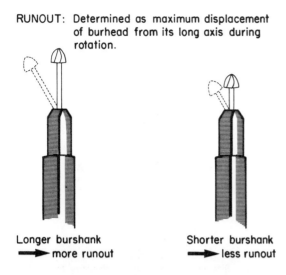

RUNOUT: Determined as maximum displacement of burhead from its long axis during rotation.

Longer burshank
➡ more runout

Shorter burshank
➡ less runout

Fig. 2-73

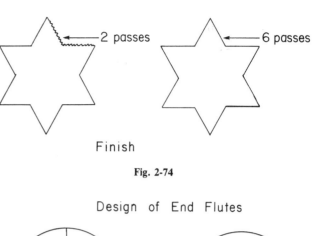

—2 passes   —6 passes

Finish

Fig. 2-74

Design of End Flutes

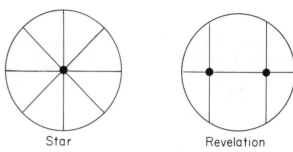

Star   Revelation

Fig. 2-75

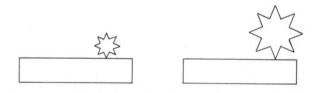

Surface area of Contact/Unit Time —Diameter

Fig. 2-76

the blades will not cut equally. If the operator senses this lack of cutting, he will probably exert greater force on the bur. The result will be that at one stage of revolution the bur and the work tend to be pushed apart, only to be driven together at the next half-revolution, resulting in disagreeable vibration. As far as the rate of removal of tooth structure is concerned, although it may appear to be increased during such vibration, the structure is removed by a shattering rather than cutting process. Such a method of tooth removal is inefficient, inaccurate, and increases heat generation.

5. Finish of the flutes

The dental bur is formed by cutting each flute into the bur blank with a rotating cutter while it progresses nearly parallel to the axis of the bur. During the first cut or pass of the cutter the flute is roughly formed. The second cut places a cutting edge on the bur flute. However, considerable roughness (Fig. 74) along the flute will remain. This roughness may be removed by making subsequent passes or cuts on the bur flute (Fig. 74). Tests for cutting efficiency were done on different types of burs undergoing two, four, and six flute cuts. Those cut six times were the most efficient while those cut two times were the least efficient.

6. Heat treatment

Heat treatment is used to harden a bur that is made of soft steel. This operation preserves the edge placed on the bur flute by the cutter, and hardens the bur to increase its cutting life. (This operation is not needed with tungsten carbide burs).

7. Design of flute ends

Dental burs are formed with two different styles of end flutes: the revelation cut, where the flutes come together at two junctions near a diametrical cutting edge (Fig. 75), and the star cut, where the end flutes come together in a common junction at the axis of the bur (Fig. 75). The revelation type shows some superiority in cutting efficiency, but in direct cutting only. In lateral cutting both types prove to be of equal efficiency.

8. Bur diameter

Generally, the forces on each bur tooth from external load do not depend on the diameter of the bur, but rather on the number of flutes or teeth and their rotational position (Fig. 76). The average linear displacement per revolution and length of cut does not depend upon the diameter of the bur. It follows that because the length of the cut is constant the volume of material removed will vary directly with the bur diameter as will as the torque and the amount of mechanical energy that the power source is required to supply.

9. Depth of engagement (depth of cutting)

As the depth of engagement is decreased, the force intensity on each small portion of the bur tooth still cutting is correspondingly increased and accordingly the average displacement per flute revolution should also be increased. This increase is so great that the volume of material removed by a shallow cut exceeds that of deeper cuts (Fig. 77).

10. Influence of load

Load signifies the force exerted by the dentist on the tool head and not the pressure or stress induced in the tooth during cutting. The force or load exerted is related to the rotational speed of the bur of a given design. The exact amount of force generally employed is not known, but is has been estimated as being equivalent to a maximum of 1000 gm (2 pounds) for low rotational speed and from 60-120 gm (2-4 ounces) at high rotational speed. Actually the dentist operates according to the variables encountered. Generally speaking, every range of

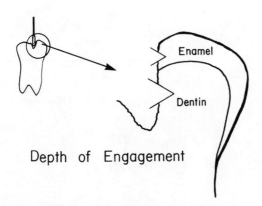

Depth of Engagement

Fig. 2-77

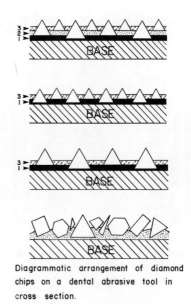

Diagrammatic arrangement of diamond chips on a dental abrasive tool in cross section.

Fig. 2-78

speed at which the bur is rotating has a minimum force or load under which the cutting efficiency of the bur used is decreased. It also has a maximum force or load over which the cutting efficiency of the bur is decreased too, because of torque. The minimum and maximum loads for low speed are 1000-1500 gm, while the minimum and maximum loads for high speed are 60-120 gm.

11. Influence of speed

With a given load the rate of cutting increases with the rotational speed, but this increase is not in direct proportion. The rate of increase in cutting at rotational speed above 30,000 RPM is greater than that below this speed. However, it has been found at very high speeds, 150,000 and above, that the time required for the removal of the same weight of tooth structure is very nearly the same as at still higher speeds. Such a conclusion appears to indicate that no time is saved by the dentist when rotation speeds are employed higher than 150,000 RPM. There is, however, a minimum rotation speed for a given load below which the tool will not cut. The greater the load, the lower this minimum rotational speed. The correlation between the load and the minimum rotation speed depends upon whether enamel or dentin is being cut, the design and composition of bur, and similar factors. Here, again, the tactile sense of the dentist, acquired by experience, is the controlling factor.

b. Dental abrasive stones

i. Designs

Abrasive particles are held together by means of a ''binder'' (base) of variable nature (Fig. 78). A ceramic binder is used in many cases, particularly for binding diamond chips. Also, an electroplating process providing a metallic binder may be used. For soft grade stones, rubber or shellac may be used. The latter types wear rapidly, but they are useful when delicate abrasion is required.

The type of binder is intimately related to the life of the tool in use. With most abrasives, the binder is impregnated throughout with abrasive particles of a certain grade so that as a particle is wrenched from the binder during use, another will take its place as the binder wears. Furthermore, the abrasive should be distributed so that the surface of the tool wears evenly. The wide spacing between the particles provides room for the resultant debris with less chance for packing or clogging. Some abrasives are glued to paper to form discs that can be attached to a handpiece via certain mounting tools. According to the composition of the abrasive particles, dental stones can be classified as follows:

A. Diamond stones

They are the hardest and most efficient abrasive stones for removing tooth enamel. The diamond chips are bound together with either a ceramic binder or a more efficient metallic binder.

B. Carbides

They may be silicone carbides or boron carbides, both of which are manufactured by heating silicone or boron at a very high temperature to affect their union with carbon. The carbides are sintered or pressed with a binder into grinding wheels, discs or stones.

C. Sand

Sand and other forms of quartz (cuttle) can be bound and mounted into different shapes of discs, stones, and strips.

D. Aluminum oxide

Natural or extracted pure aluminum oxide is one of the most efficient abrasives for stones in fine cutting.

E. Garnet

These particles contain a number of different minerals which possess similar physical properties and crystalline forms. Stones made of these can be used for finishing and polishing of dental appliances.

ii. Factors Influencing the Abrasive Efficiency of Dental Stones

A. Irregularity in shape of abrasive particles (Fig. 79)

An abrasive should be irregular in shape so that it presents a sharp edge, i.e., a round smooth particle would possess poor abrasive properties. Similarly, cubical particles which would always present a flat face to the work would not be as efficient in abrasion as would irregularly shaped particles.

Therefore, the more irregular the particles, the greater the abrasive efficiency of the stone.

B. Hardness of the abrasive material relative to that of the work

If the abrasive cannot indent the surface to be abraded, it cannot remove any of that material. In such a case the abrasive

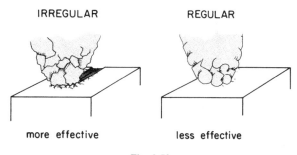

IRREGULAR   REGULAR

more effective   less effective

Fig. 2-79

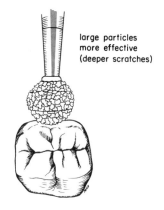

large particles
more effective
(deeper scratches)

Fig. 2-80

will dull or wear. The harder the abrasive material relative to the hardness of the work, the more the abrasive efficiency of the stone.

C. Impact strength of the abrasive material

During rotation the abrasive particles strike the work suddenly. If it shutters the instant it contacts the work, it will be ineffective. If it engages but never fractures, its edge may become dull in time. Accordingly, the efficiency of the abrasive will be reduced. In fact, the abrasive should fracture rather than dull so that sharp edges are always present. Fracture of the abrasive is also helpful in shedding the debris accumulated from the work. Although diamond stones will cut almost any type of tooth structure or restorative material, the diamond particles do not fracture, but rather lose substance at the tip. Furthermore, they are likely to become clogged when ductile or soft substances are abraded. They are most efficient if they are used in removal of the very hard and brittle tooth enamel.

D. Size of the abrasive particles (Fig. 80)

The larger the particles, the deeper the scratches on the surface of the work and the faster the work will be worn away.

E. Pressure and RPM

The same factors are involved here as discussed with rotary cutting instruments.

iii. Types of dental stones

Dental stones can be mounted, i.e., the abrading head (Fig. 81) (similar to the cutting head in a bur) is permanently welded to the shank and attachment part (Fig. 81). They can also be unmounted, i.e., the abrading head is supplied separately and may be mounted on an appropriate mandrel (Fig. 82).

Mounted dental stones are provided in short (miniature), regular or long lengths. They also may be either in latch or friction grip form (attachment part) (Figs. 83, 84, 85).

Dental stones can be produced in countless shapes: cylinder, wheel, cone, inverted cone, tapered, doughnut, round, filamentous, V-shaped, hour glass, etc. At the present there is no standardized numbering system for dental stones; rather, every manufacturer has his own nomenclature according to size and shape.

Advantages and limitations of rotary instruments

As previously mentioned, rotary instruments are the most efficient tools for gross removal of tooth structure, especially of sound tooth structure.

Dental stones, especially diamonds, have the highest efficiency in removing enamel (brittle material), whereas carbide burs have the highest efficiency in removing dentin (elastic material). Removal of tooth structure using any stone should be confined to enamel and perhaps the superficial 0.5-1 mm

ABRADING HEAD

SHANK

ATTACHMENT

Fig. 2-81

Fig. 2-82

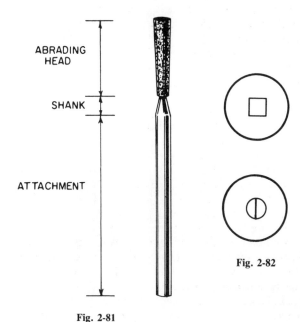

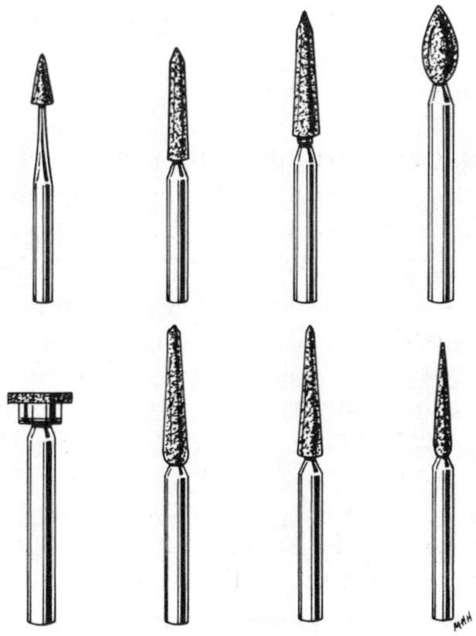

Fig. 2-83

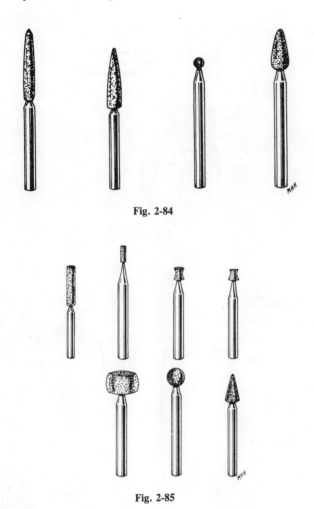

Fig. 2-84

Fig. 2-85

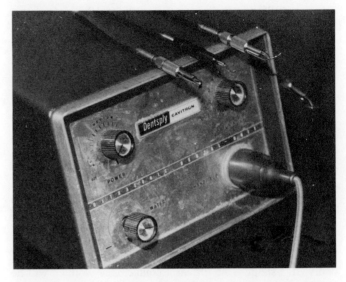

Fig. 2-86

of dentin. It is hazardous to use them in preparations deeper than that (see chapter 1).

For removal of dentin 2 mm or more from the pulp, burs are efficient. However, in areas deeper than that or for removal of carious dentin use of hand instruments is highly advised. Coolants are essential for tooth removal with all rotary instruments, with the exception, perhaps, of ultra-low speed rotary instrumentation.

III. Ultrasonic Instruments (Fig. 86)

The ultrasonic dental unit consists of an ultrasonic generator separate from a magnetostrictive transducer located within the handpiece. The generator delivers the energy to the transducer which in turn creates vibrations used to remove hard substances. In addition, a water cooling system is incorporated into the equipment for controlling heat generated in the handpiece. Another type of system direct a water-borne abrasive or slurry against the working point while providing an additional water jet for irrigation.

Energy used for removal of enamel and dentin is generated within the handpiece. Electric current causes the transducer of the handpiece to slightly contract and expand. The amplitude of this movement is determined by the number of watts delivered to the handpiece and may be variable. The desirable amplitude depends on the length and thickness of the working point and is under the control of the operator.

Working points used for removal of enamel and dentin are constructed to tolerate greater amplitudes.

Generally speaking, ultrasonic instruments are not universally used for cavity preparations; they are mostly used for calculus and stain removal from teeth and restoration surfaces.

Restoring Instruments

By no means will this be a description of all instruments used for restoring teeth. An effort will be made to classify them and give examples of each class. The description of each restorative technique will elaborate upon its instruments and instrumentation.

Each restoring instrument is composed of three parts (Fig. 87): the handle, which is like the handle for the previous types of hand instruments, the shank, as found in exploring and hand cutting instruments, and the nib, which is the working end of the instruments. The nib may be present in different dimensions, shapes, and surface configurations, according to its specific use. It is equivalent to the blade in hand cutting instruments and carries the face of the instrument, which, in turn, is equivalent to the cutting edge in hand cutting instruments.

A. Mixing instruments (Fig. 88)

Insofar as most dental materials used for restorations to be fabricated directly inside the mouth are originally made of powder and liquids, we need instruments to mix them. The most common of these instruments are the spatulas which have flat and wide nibs with blunt edges. Their shank is straight. Spatulas come in different sizes and different degrees of stiffness in their nibs to suit various uses. They may be made of stainless steel, ivorine or plastic. (The armamentarium for mechanical mixing will be described specific techniques, e.g., amalgam, gypsum, etc.)

B. Plastic instruments (Fig. 89)

Within this class are an enormous number of instruments. They all differ mainly in the shape of their nibs and angulation or curvature in their shanks. They all can be used for carrying

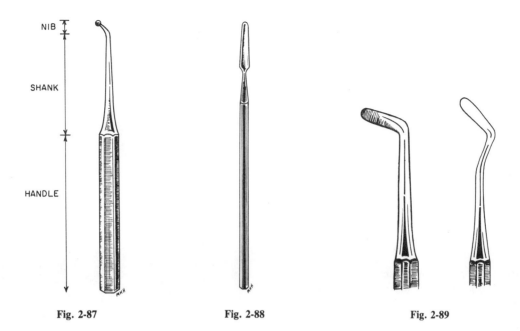

NIB

SHANK

HANDLE

Fig. 2-87   Fig. 2-88   Fig. 2-89

and handling materials after mixing while the materials are in their plastic stage. They all have a flat-sided nib with blunt edges and corners. They may be made of stainless steel, ivorine or plastic. They also can be plated with teflon to minimize material adhesion and to facilitate easy cleaning.

C. Condensing instruments (Fig. 90)

Any material that needs condensation during its insertion into the cavity preparation has a specific set of condensing instruments. Depending upon the material they are used with, they will differ from one another in the surface configuration of the nib-face, e.g., amalgam requires smooth-surfaced faces, gold foil requires serrated-surfaced faces. Most of these instruments have angles and curvatures in their shanks. The nibs have different shapes, e.g., rounded, triangular, diamond, rectangular, parallelogram, etc. They are also supplied in different sizes for each shape and shank angulation.

D. Burnishing instruments (Fig. 91-96)

Because burnishing is an essential act for the fabrication of all metallic restorations, this necessitates numerous types of burnishers. Their nibs can be ball-shaped (Fig. 91), egg-shaped (Fig. 92), apple-shaped (Fig. 93), beaver-tail-shaped (Fig. 94), conical (Fig. 95), hour-glass-shaped, fish-tail-shaped, bullet-shaped, etc. Naturally, they may have different angulations and curvatures in their shanks. Their nibs are smooth-faced. There are burnishers for specific operations, e.g., Sprateley burnishers (Fig. 96), which are used for proximal gingival marginal burnishing of metallic restorations. Burnishers can be in the form of burs (Fig. 93), i.e., burs with perfectly smooth heads that perform a burnishing operation by rotary action.

E. Carvers (Fig. 97)

These are basically cutting instruments with their blades (nibs) either bevelled or knife-edged (elongated bibevelling). The most universally used carvers are Hollenback carvers (Fig. 97), which posses double-sided knife-edged, point-edged nibs,

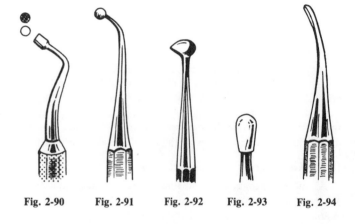

Fig. 2-90   Fig. 2-91   Fig. 2-92   Fig. 2-93   Fig. 2-94

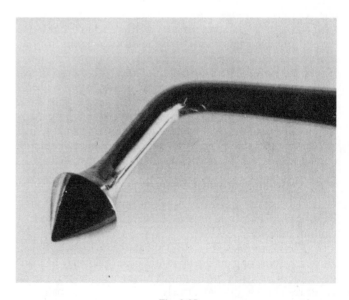

Fig. 2-95

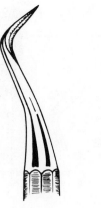
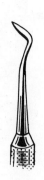

Fig. 2-96   Fig. 2-97

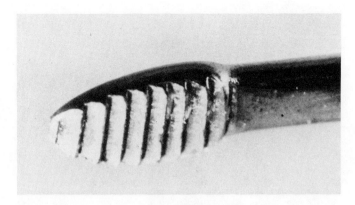

Fig. 2-98

with curved monangled or binangled shanks. They are very efficient in carving both amalgam and wax. The discoid and cleoid excavators can be used as amalgam and gold carvers. There are a considerable number of special forms of carvers, such as those with triangular nibs, or diamond-shaped nibs. Both have bibevelled cutting edges (faces). All carvers are used in the same way hand instruments are used—in direct or lateral cutting motions.

F. Files (Fig. 98)

Very few files are used in restorative dentistry. They are always used for margination of restorations if knifes and carvers will not suffice. The nibs of the file can be foot-shaped, hatchet-shaped or parallelogram-shaped. The serrations on the face of the nib can be directed away from the handle, making a push file, or directed toward the handle, making a pull file.

G. Knives (Figs. 99,100 and 101)

As the name indicates, the nibs of these instruments carry knife-edged faces on one of their sides only. The most universal is the Bard-Parker knife, which has several shapes.

Black's knives have the nibs almost at a right angle to the handle, with the cutting edge (face) away from the handle in one set (push cutting), and toward the handle in another set (pull cutting). Some other versions of Black's knives have the nib at different angulations from the shaft, ranging from an acute to an obtuse angulation (Fig. 99). The above mentioned knives are universal for a variety of restorative procedures. Some knives are made for specific purposes, e.g., Wilson's knife (Fig. 100), which has the nib in a plane at a right angle to that of the shaft, so they can be introduced interproximally for proximal and gingival manipulation of the restorative materials. Stein's knife (Fig. 101), which has a trapezoidal nib, is used mainly for direct gold contouring and margination.

H. Finishing and polishing instruments

Most of these are rotary type instruments: burs, stones, paper-carried abrasives, brushes, rubber (wheel cups or cones), cloth or felt, etc.

2. Finishing burs (Fig. 102) should be at least 12-fluted. However, some of them are up to 40-fluted. They may be made of stainless steel (for amalgam) or tungsten carbide (for composite resins). They do not grossly cut the restorative materials,

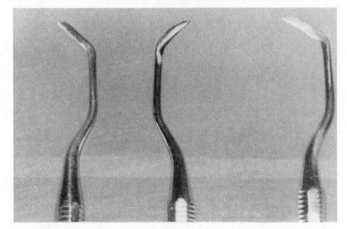

Fig. 2-99

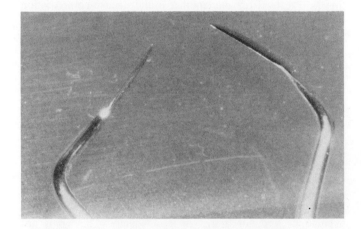

Fig. 2-100

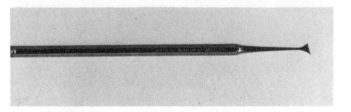

Fig. 2-101

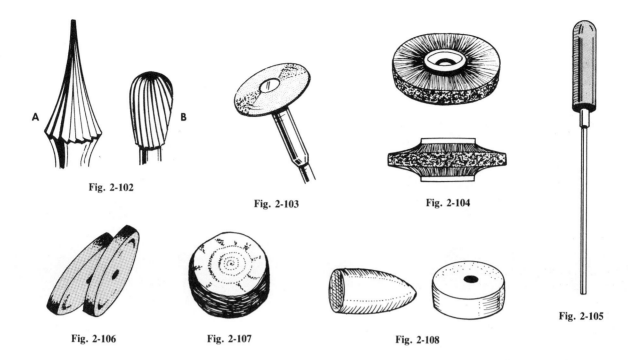

Fig. 2-102

Fig. 2-103

Fig. 2-104

Fig. 2-105

Fig. 2-106   Fig. 2-107   Fig. 2-108

but only remove excesses, creating a smoother surface. Such burs come in different shapes, e.g., rounded, apple-shaped, pear-shaped (Fig. 102B), flame-shaped (Fig. 102A), tapered, cylindrical, inverted cone. Furthermore, each can be furnished in different sizes.

3. Paper-carried abrasives (Fig. 103)

These are usually sand, cuttle, garnet or boron carbide, glued to paper discs or strips. The paper discs should be attached to a mandrel (screw-in or square-headed) (Fig. 82) for rotary finishing. The paper-strip carried abrasives are used by hand in a back and forth motion similar to a shoe-polishing action.

4. Brushes (Fig. 104)

They come in different forms, e.g., wheels, cylinders, cones, etc. They can be screwed in the handpiece (in the opposite direction of their revolution), attached to a mandrel, or have their own frictional attachment extension. Brushes can be used alone or with intermediate abrasive pastes. Most have synthetic bristles, but some have wire bristles for polishing cast restorations.

5. Rubber (Fig. 105, 106)

Plain, rubber-ended rotary tools are essential for any polishing procedure. They come in a variety of shapes, e.g., cups, wheels, cones, etc. They can be attached to the hand-piece either via a mandrel, a screw-in device, or their own frictional or latch extension. They are furnished in different sizes and frequently are used with other abrasives or polishing pastes.

6. Cloth (Fig. 107)

Cloth, carried on a metal wheel, is used in the final stages of polishing, either with or without a polishing medium.

7. Felt (Fig. 108)

To obtain lustre for metallic restorations, different shapes of felts, e.g., wheels, cones, and cylinders are used, usually with a polishing agent. Felt can be attached to the handpiece in the same way rubber tools are attached.

BIBLIOGRAPHY

Baum et al.: Operative Dentistry. Saunders, 1981.

Black, G.V.: A work on operative dentistry. Vol. II, Chicago, Medico-Dental Pub., 1924.

Bryton and Skinner.: Cutting effectiveness of dental burs as related to designs. JDR. 33, p. 993, 1954.

Charbeneau et al.: Principles and practice of operative dentistry. Philadelphia, Lea and Febiger, 1980.

Craig et al.: Restorative dental materials. St. Louis, The C.V. Mosby Co., 1981.

Eames, W.B., and Nales, J.L.: A comparison of cutting efficiency of air-driven fissure burs. JADA, 86, 412-415, 1973.

Gilmore et al.: Operative dentistry. St. Louis, The C.V. Mosby Co., 1977.

Henry, E.E.: Influence of design factors on performance of inverted cone burs. JDR. 33, p. 704, 1956.

Lammie, G.A.: A comparison of cutting efficiency and heat production of tungsten carbide and steel burs. BDR, May 1951, p 231.

Lammie, G.A.: A study of some different tungsten carbide burs. Dental Records. 22, p. 283, 1952.

Marzouk, M.A., Strong, M.E., Gross, R.D., and Diemer, R.: Operative dentistry instruments and instrumentation. Self-Instructional Package, Washington University, School of Dental Medicine, 1980.

McGehee et al.: A textbook of operative dentistry. New York, McGraw-Hill Book Co., 1956.

Peyton, F.A.: Modern methods of shaping cavities in teeth, Fort. Rev. Chicago Dental Society. 34:11-17, 1957.

Peyton and Henery.: The relationship between design and cutting efficiency of dental burs. JDR, vol. 33, p. 281, 1954.

Phillips, R.W.: Skinner's science of dental materials. Philadelphia, Saunders, 1979.

Schuchard, A., and Watkins, E.C.: Cutting effectiveness of tungsten carbide burs and diamond points at ultra-high rotational speeds. Journal of Prosthetic Dentistry, 18, 58-65.

Skinner, E.: Temperature rise in teeth developed by rotary instruments. JADA, vol. 50, p. 629, 1955.

Stanley, H.R.: Traumatic capacity of high speed and ultrasonic dental instrumentation. JADA **63**:749-766, 1961.

Stanley, H.R., and Swerdlow, H.: Reaction of the human pulp to cavity preparation: results produced by eight different operative grinding technics. JADA **58**:49-59, 1959.

Sturdevant et al.: The art and science of operative dentistry. New York, McGraw-Hill Book Co., 1968.

CHAPTER 3

Control of the field of operation

The complexities of the oral environment certainly present obstacles to physical diagnosis and mechanical treatment of dental and oral tissues. As the patient is usually conscious during dental operations, the cooperative efforts of the dentist, his assistant(s) and the patient are required to control that field and allow the necessary treatment with the least trauma to involved and surrounding tissues.

The term ''oral environment'' refers to the following items, which require proper control to prevent them from interfering with the execution of any restorative procedure.

A. Saliva

With six major salivary glands excreting it (four under the tongue in the floor of the mouth, and two each opposite the facial surface of the upper second molar), there must be a way to remove saliva, either by mechanically evacuating it, by allowing the patient's own swallowing mechanism to do the job, or by chemically reducing its secretion. All these procedures are important because saliva in the operating field may obstruct proper vision and access, interfere with and detrimentally affect the setting and adaptability of restorative materials, modify or negate the effect of medicaments, and may be sprayed with rotary instruments to propagate infection in the office atmosphere.

B. Moving organs

The tongue, whose movements should be minimized, since it cannot be immobilized, should be retracted from the field of operation, in order to avoid injuring it. The tongue retraction and partial immobilization, together with the actual tooth instrumentation, should be done in a manner that avoids stimulating gagging mechanisms via receptors located primarily at the posterior half of the tongue.

The patient's head should be stabilized and immobilized to prevent unpredictable and unwanted engagement of instruments with tissues intraorally and extraorally, and, also, so the operator can have correct orientation to the operating field and its details.

The mandible, held open and stable, is essential for access, instrument support, and procedures oriented with the field of operation. Of course, this stability helps prevent accidental tissue involvement by operating instruments.

The patient's body itself, should be in a stable, comfortable resting position, to minimize movements that may create the same problems as moving the head or mandible.

C. Lips and cheek retraction is necessary to better expose the teeth being operated on. The sole act of opening the mouth and stabilizing the mandible will partially retract them, but for complete retraction, we have to mechanically pull the lip and cheeks, trying not to exceed the stretching limit of their tissues. These retractions away from the operating field are necessary not only to visualize it, but also to avoid traumatizing these tissues during mechanical and chemical procedures.

D. The periodontium, especially gingival tissue, can interfere with tooth instrumentation when the extent of the lesion might involve trauma to these tissues. The same procedures used to control the periodontium prior to taking impressions for cast restorations may be used in this situation. It should also be emphasized that any periodontal infections that are not going to be corrected by the placement of a restoration should be successfully treated *before* any operative procedure is attempted.

E. Contacting teeth or restorations, adjacent to proximal tooth preparations, carry the danger of mechanical or chemical injury during operative procedures. Thus, procedures for tooth preparations should be designed to avoid cutting movements directed towards these contacting surfaces and, if possible, to protect them (e.g., by matrix bands, wedges or any other resistant coverage).

F. Facial and lingual sulci, floor of the mouth and palate, although they are relatively stable, they have possible impinging capability on the operating area (e.g., the floor of the mouth being in close proximity to the cervical area on the lingual surfaces of lower molars). Very rarely will the soft and hard palate interfere with any operative procedure, except as locations for stimulating reflexes that may move musculature otherwise immobilized during the procedure.

G. Respiratory moisture can precipitate on reflecting and viewing instruments, obstructing the field of operation. This is most apparent when the patient is breathing through his mouth due to a temporary or permanent nasal obstruction.

H. Usually, dental operations are performed without the dentist wearing surgical gloves or masks. A diseased oral environment contains multiple, countless pathogens, so visible gross infectants like plaque and the materia alba should be mechanically removed. As mentioned, saliva carrying these pathogens should be rerouted away from the operating field. If it is possible, disinfect the mouth and especially the areas to be operated upon before performing the procedure. Wearing masks and even surgical gloves is indicated with susceptible patients and in seasons of climate changes. This is done not only for the sake of the operator, but also to prevent spread of these pathogens from one area of the mouth to another.

I. Deposits interfering with proper isolation of the field and the recognition and extent of the lesion are mainly calculus, stains, or other foreign bodies. The tooth to be operated upon should be completely cleansed of these visual and tactile interferences, so the operative procedure can be done efficiently.

J. Patients with certain systemic disorders should be managed differently, as dictated by their physical and mental conditions. Modification of regular procedures may even be to the extent of doing procedures in multiple stages and visits, or doing multiple procedures at one visit under sedation or general anesthesia.

K. Ground up solid debris, medicaments, excess filling materials and cooling fluids should be recovered from the mouth quickly to avoid the possibility of ingestion or inhalation.

Bearing in mind all of these variables of the oral environment, their control should start with the patient as a whole, psychologically controlling his apprehension and anxieties, seating him comfortably and explaining in simple terms the ensuing procedures and the operation's objectives. *The complete cooperation of the patient during the procedures is essential.*

The actual mechanisms of controlling the complexities of the operating field involve the following:

    I. Patient seating
    II. Dentist and assistant seating
   III. Role of the assistant and dentist in each quadrant
   IV. Rubber dam

    V. Fluids and debris evacuating mechanisms and equipment
   VI. Fluid absorbing mechanisms and materials
  VII. Tissue retraction and protection
 VIII. Mouth probes
   IX. Use of medicaments in controlling the field of operation
    X. Mechanical and chemical elimination of intraoral deposits when deemed to be biologically hazardous and/or interfering with proper execution of the operation
   XI. Illumination and viewing
  XII. Possible complications and corrective measures

I. Patient Seating

The lounge chair is the most advisable chair for four-handed (six-handed) dentistry. The patient should be seated, so that all parts of his body are properly supported. Dental chairs are usually contoured for that purpose. Most importantly, the neck and head muscles should be in the most unstrained position to help control the operating field and obtain correct occlusal records, if these are contemplated during the operation. Usually, the chair's back and base are adjusted separately. Frequently, the head rest may also be adjusted to attain the most comfortable position. Preferably, the patient's head should be in line with his back, while the chair base is usually parallel to or making a slight angulation with the floor.

Using mirror vision for all upper teeth, the patient is preferably seated in a supine position (Fig. 1A), with the back of the chair almost in line with its base and parallel to the floor. For an even more comfortable arrangement, the back may be angulated from 150° to 170° with the base (Fig. 1B). Using

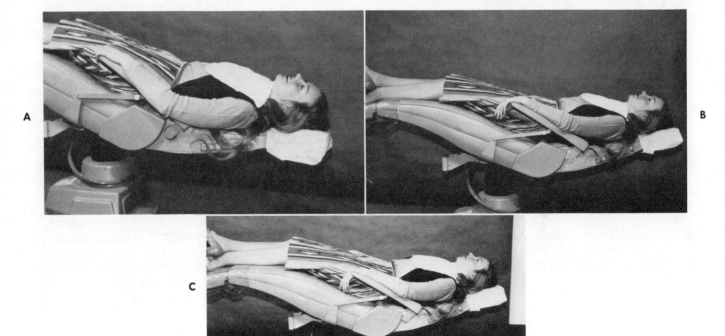

Fig. 3-1

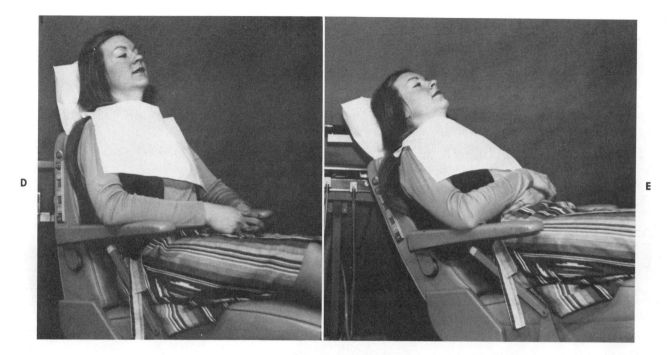

Fig. 3-1—cont'd.

direct vision for all upper teeth, the chair back could be put at 130° to 140° with the base. This position is usually used for right facial and left lingual operations (Fig. 1C). For the lower right quadrant the chair back should make almost 90 to 100° with the base (Fig. 1D), while for lower left quadrant the chair back should make 110 to 130° with the base (Fig. 1E). The chair should be positioned as low as possible to facilitate direct vision in the lower arch and mirror vision in the upper arch.

These arrangements are merely guidelines which may be adjusted and modified according to many factors, including the physical conditions of the dentist, the assistant and the patient, any abnormality in tooth location, the method of controlling facial and masticatory musculature, office space and adjustability of equipment, etc.

II. Dentist and Assistant Seating

The following arrangements are for right-handed operators, and the exact reverse should be applied for left-handed operators.

Using a clock-like arrangement, when operating in the lower right quadrant, the dentist always assumes a position at 7-9 o'clock and the assistant assumes a position at 2-4 o'clock. The same position may be assumed by the dentist for operations in the lower front sextant (Fig. 2A). For operations in the lower left quadrant, the dentist assumes a 10-11 o'clock position, and the assistants will assume a 3 o'clock position. The same position may be taken for the upper and lower front teeth (Fig. 2B). For operations in the upper arch, using mirror vision, the dentist assumes a position at 11-12 o'clock and sometimes at 1 o'clock. The assistant will assume a 3-5 o'clock position (Fig. 2C). For the right facial and left lingual areas in the upper arch, using direct vision, the dentist may assume the 7 o'clock-10 o'clock position.

The dentist should be seated with his (her) feet flat on the

floor, preferably with his (her) lower leg making 90° angle with his (her) upper leg (Fig. 2D). The dental chair should be elevated and tilted so the patient's head is level with the dentist's elbow. This will (Fig. 2E) prevent straining of the dentist's arm and back muscles. The dentist should be seated with his (her) back straight, and with at least 6 inches between his (her) eye and the field of operation. There should be an unobstructed straight line view of the field of operation or its image in the mirror.

The assistant should be seated at a higher position on her stool, so her knees will be level with the patient's head (Fig. 2E), with her feet resting on the foot rest of her chair. She should be seated with her back straight (Fig. 2F) and with an unobstructed straight line view of the field of operation.

These positions are not inflexible, rather they can be adjusted

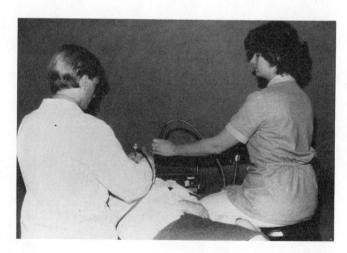

Fig. 3-2

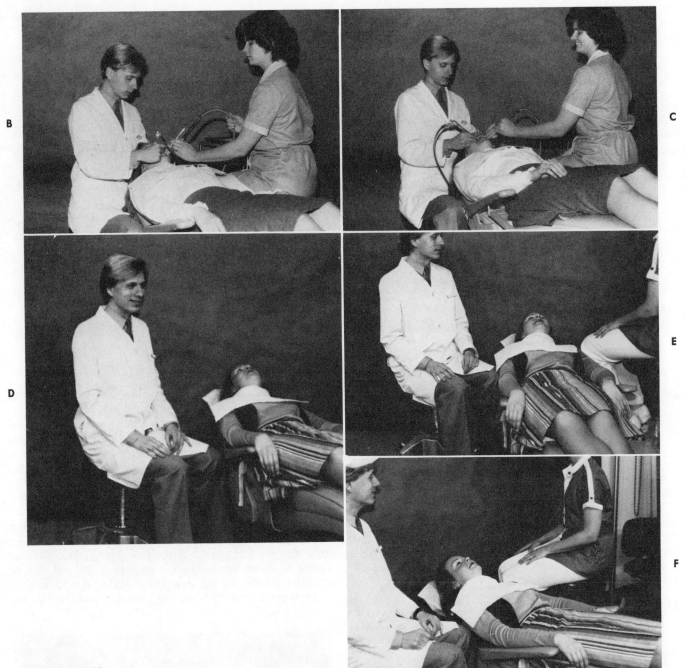

Fig. 3-2—cont'd.

and modified according to specific needs. Generally, however, most operations can be performed in these positions, depending on the patient's controlability, the equipment adjustability, and the possibility of mirror (indirect) vision, etc.

III. Role of the Assistant and the Dentist in Each Quadrant

After positioning the patient and soliciting his cooperation, it is the joint effort of the assistant and the dentist that will put the field of operation under control.

In addition to evacuating cut debris, cooling fluids and saliva from the lower right quadrant, the assistant controls tongue movements using the high speed evacuating tip. The tip is usually bevel-ended, so that the bevel will face the tooth being operated on. The remainder of the suction tip can help retract the tongue by locating the tip between the lingual surface of these teeth and the tongue (Fig. 3A), always with a positive pressure toward the tongue. For a very active and/or large tongue this pull by the evacuator may not be sufficient retraction so the assistant should use a mirror or tongue retractors also (Fig. 3B). The dentist can control the cheek and lips by retracting them away from his cutting instruments, using a mirror in his left hand with a positive pressure away from the teeth (Fig. 3, A and B).

In the lower left quadrant (Fig. 3C), the assistant can manage the lip and cheeks by putting the bevel of the high speed evacuating suction tip toward the buccal surfaces of these teeth, with the rest of the suction tip pulling the lip and cheeks away from the tooth being operated on. In cheeks with a sizable buccal pad of fat or strong unyielding musculature, the assistant can use a mirror or a cheek retractor also. The dentist can manage the tongue by retracting it with his mirror towards the right of the patient (Fig. 3C).

For the operations in the upper right quadrant, the assistant should use the evacuator and sometimes other retracting items in a similar manner as in the lower right. In addition, her pull against tongue should be with a downward pressure, to prevent its elevation into the field of operation. Using mirror vision,

the dentist will have his (her) left hand busy holding the viewing mirror, which should be angulated for optimum viewing without obstructing the assistant's vision and access, and avoiding excess water coolants accumulated on its surface (Fig. 3D). The dentist's right hand, holding the cutting instruments, will have the thumb and first two fingers operating the instruments. The third and fourth fingers are used for support. The tips of these fingers only should be involved in these activities, while the phalanges are used to retract the cheek away from the area being operated upon. Using direct vision, the same arrangement as for lower right quadrant is optional.

For operations in the upper left quadrant (Fig. 3E) the as-

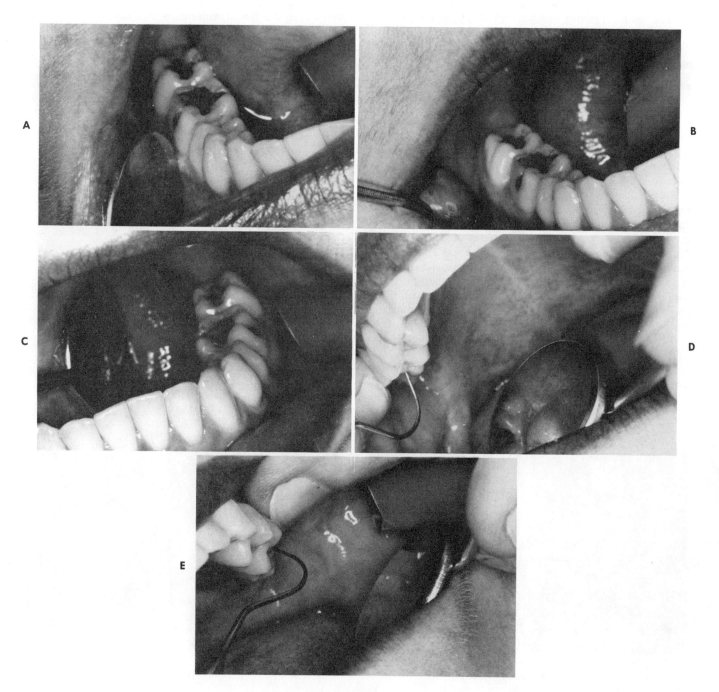

Fig. 3-3

sistant should perform the same role as for the lower left quadrant, except that her evacuator and retracting instruments might engage the cheek more loosely.

Using mirror vision, the dentist will also perform the same role, except that the phalanges of his (her) fingers, especially the third and fourth fingers, are used to drop the tongue down and to act as a barrier between it and the area being operated upon. Also, even though the mirror is primarily a viewing tool, in that position it can help the assistant retract the lip and cheek (Fig. 3E). Using direct vision, the dentist will perform the same role as in the lower left quadrant.

In the extremely difficult access to the facial of the upper left quadrant, the dentist should assume a 12-1 o'clock position, and use his (her) mirror to retract the cheek, helping the assistant there. This facilitates direct vision facially.

Additional roles for the assistant and the dentist will be mentioned in the subsequent sections.

IV. Rubber Dam

Without any doubt, the rubber dam is the most effective way for controlling the field of operation. The goals achieved by rubber dam application, in isolating the field of operation, are a combination of most of the goals achieved by all other isolation methods taken together. Sometimes it even exceeds these goals.

Rubber dam material (Fig. 4) is usually latex rubber. It may be supplied in rolls, 5 and 6 inches wide, from which the appropriate size pieces are cut. It may also be supplied precut in 6″ × 6″ or 5″ × 5″ squares. The rubber can be one of four different thicknesses ranging from light to extra heavy. The heavy and extra heavy are the most suitable for operative procedures, while the light and medium are adequate for endodontic therapy. The rubber also comes in different colors for operative procedures, but, preferably, it should be a contrasting color: dark brown, green or black.

A. Anchoring devices

For the rubber dam to be securely attached to the area being isolated, there are several devices and methods.

1. Anchoring clamps (Fig. 5)
Each clamp consists of:

a. A jaw (Fig. 5) on each side carrying the tooth attachment blades and sometimes dam-engaging projections (wings).

b. A bow (Fig. 5), which connects the two jaws and which should be elastically strainable and resistant enough to impart a gripping force on the attaching blades against the teeth.

According to the type and shape of the tooth attachment blades, clamps can be:

a. Those with four-point contact blades (Fig. 6), i.e., the blade portions of the jaw point inwards at each corner, so that all the gripping forces will be applied on these four points only. Usually they contact the axial angles of the tooth and create a very secure attachment with the tooth. These types of clamps are indicated when the retaining curvature of the tooth surfaces is not present (newly erupting teeth) or is insufficient for the

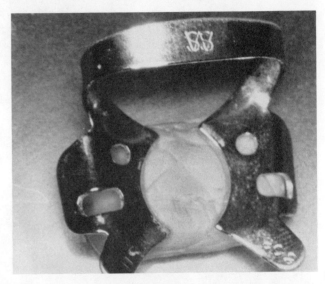

Fig. 3-5

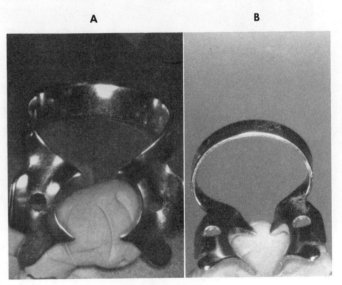

Fig. 3-6

Fig. 3-4

amount of rubber stretching that is expected. Also, they are used in single tooth isolation when all the rubber stretching will be on the clamp, itself, with no other anchoring mechanism. The major danger from this type of clamp is its possible traumatic effect on weakened undermined tooth structures.

b. Clamps with circumferential contact blades (Fig. 7), i.e., the blade portion has no projections and will contact the tooth surface evenly throughout its length. This type is less retentive, but it could also be less traumatic, it is to be used when the axial angles are lost or do not coincide with the corners of the four-point contact clamps, and when the axial convexity of the tooth surface is sufficient for anchorage. Besides, the clamped tooth should be fully erupted and the rubber stretching should be resisted by several other anchoring devices.

Clamps also can be classified as winged clamps (Fig. 8) and wingless clamps (Fig. 9) according to whether or not they have a dam-engaging projection in their jaws. Those having wings can be attached to the rubber dam before application so the dam may be released after the clamp has engaged the tooth. These are always bulkier than wingless clamps, and sometimes they cannot be used in last molars when the surrounding anatomy will not allow sufficient room for these relatively large clamps.

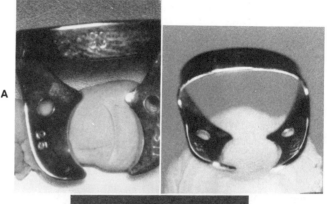

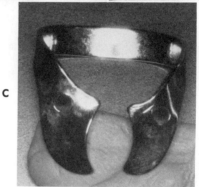

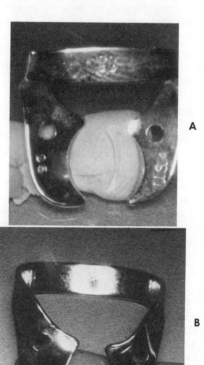

Fig. 3-7

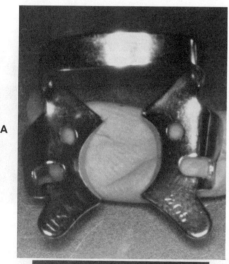

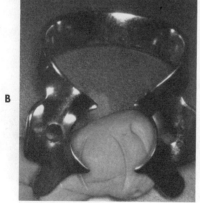

Fig. 3-8

Fig. 3-9

2. Retracting-anchoring clamps

These are clamps especially designed to other functions besides anchoring the dam to the tooth. Examples:

a. The 212 clamp series (Fig. 10) consists of double bowed clamps, specifically designed for retracting the facial or lingual gingiva away from Class V cavity preparations. The clamp jaws are usually circumferentially bladed with the blade portion in different sizes (213, 214, etc.) to coincide in dimension with the mesio-distal width of the tooth surface cervically. They are usually used in addition to a regular anchoring clamp, and they are stabilized using compound between their bows and the occlusal surfaces of the adjacent teeth.

b. The Schultz clamp series (Fig. 11) resembles the 212 clamp, but are split in half facio-lingually making them a gingivally retracting clamp with one bow only. Their use and attachment is very similar to that of the 212 clamps, but they are especially useful where a second bow cannot be accommodated due to a lack of space or limited access.

c. Cervical retracting clamps (Fig. 12) may be single- or double-bowed, but the jaws with their blades are movable, even after attaching the clamp to the tooth. By moving these blades apically, the gingiva can be retracted more apically or vice versa.

d. Some clamps have long guard extensions which retract and protect the cheek and tongue. Some even have tube-like, perforated extensions which hold cotton rolls in the adjacent sulci.

3. A piece of cut rubber dam (Figs. 13 and 30), if wedged between contacting teeth, can be used to anchor the dam, especially proximal to the most anteriorly isolated tooth.

4. Interceptal rubber (Figs. 13 and 30), if it is of sufficient dimension and is placed between intact teeth or properly restored teeth, will be a very effective locking mechanism against rubber dam displacement.

5. Compound, in addition to being used for immobilization of certain clamps by engaging their bows with adjacent teeth (Fig. 31), can also be used on the facial, occlusal and lingual surfaces of the anchoring tooth to increase the tooth's facial and lingual convexities for locking the dam. For the later purpose etched enamel retained resin could be used.

6. Wooden wedges (Fig. 30 B), placed between teeth, can be used to immobilize the interceptal rubber. Sometimes they can be used alone to anchor the dam at its most anterior end. Also, they can be utilized to momentarily anchor the dam if the anchoring clamp is displaced or dislodged during the operation. They are also used successfully in isolating bridge pontics and abutments (Fig. 33 A).

7. A dental floss (tape) tied around a piece of cylindrical rubber which could be an anesthetic carpule rubber plunger or any piece of rubber or cork with the same dimension. It can be wrapped or tied around the axial surface(s) to lock the dam apical to the rubber cylinder. This could be used when there is no holding convexities on the axial surfaces of a terminal anchoring tooth (Fig. 14).

8. Dental tape or floss is not indicated to anchor the rubber dam, if the gingiva and surrounding periodontium are not at the same horizontal level circumferentially. However, if the gingival crest is at the same level on all tooth surfaces, and will be in contact with the dental floss or tape (e.g., after considerable gingival recession), we can use dental floss or

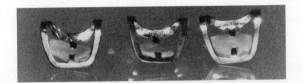

Fig. 3-10

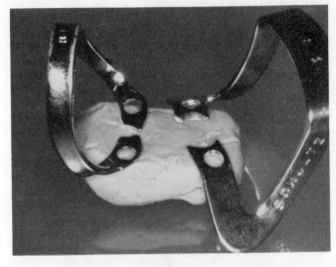

Fig. 3-11

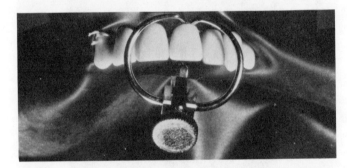

Fig. 3-12

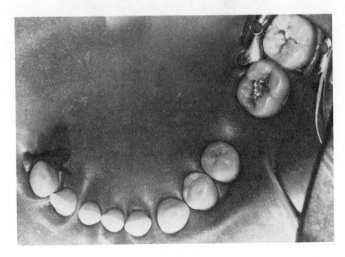

Fig. 3-13

tape, tied around the neck of the tooth, to retain the dam apically.

B. Rubber dam punch (Fig. 15)

This instrument is used to cut the holes in the rubber which will encompass the teeth to be isolated. It has a lever type plunger and a rotatable table containing holes of different diameters. The edges of the holes are very angular. The appropriate hole in the table is moved to coincide with the plunger, and the rubber is placed in-between the plunger and the table and the appropriate hole is punched. Usually the larger holes accommodate molars, medium size holes are for premolars, upper cuspids, and sometimes for upper incisors, and the smallest holes are for lower incisors. Of course, the proper size hole for the diameter of the tooth to be isolated should be matched and used.

C. Rubber dam clamp forceps (Fig. 16)

This instrument is a modified forceps which retracts the jaws of a clamp away from each other, allowing the clamp to overcome the occlusal diameter of the tooth and to be seated apical to the height of the axial contour. Each clamp has holes or grooves in each of its jaws to accommodate this forceps.

D. Rubber dam napkins (Fig. 17)

These are absorbant paper or cloth towels that can be applied between the rubber dam and the patient's face to absorb fluids leaking from the mouth or perspiration fluids from the skin, and to prevent frictional movements of the rubber against the patient's skin.

E. Rubber dam holders (Figs. 18 and 19)

There are a variety of holders for the rubber dam, but their main objectives are to keep the peripheries of the dam out of the mouth, stretch the applied dam in four directions, to retract the tongue, cheek and lips, and to clear the operation field for further procedures. They can be classified as:

1. Strap type (Fig. 18, A and B), which depends on the back of the patient's head for anchorage. It should be attached to the dam at its corners and sides. From these attachments come belts, which stretch and pull the rubber toward the occipital parts of the head. E.g., Woodbury holder (Fig 18A) Wizzard holder (Fig. 18B).

These are most convenient for the operator because they do not obstruct the field of vision in any direction. They may need a weight (Fig. 18C) to keep the dam from wrinkling.

2. Hanging frame holders (Fig. 19) are U-shaped, elliptical or rectangular metal or plastic frames, with multiple prongs at their peripheries. The prongs can engage the stretched rubber, thus retracting both the dam and the musculature engaged by the dam. These are the most popular holders; their advantages are ease of application and allowance for minimal contact of the rubber with the skin. Their disadvantage is that they may be in the access for the field of operation.

F. Preparing the mouth for rubber dam application

Rubber dams are the safest means of isolating the field of operation, but they need the following mouth preparations to assure their safe, speedy and effective application.

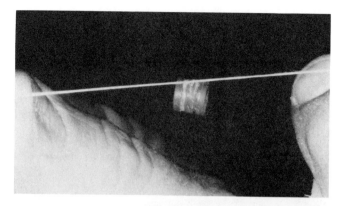

Fig. 3-14

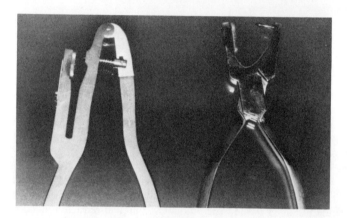

Fig. 3-15

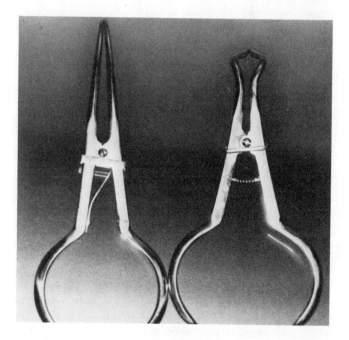

Fig. 3-16

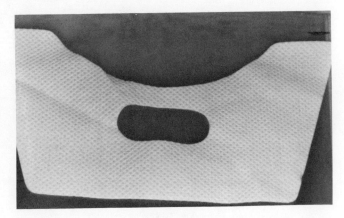

Fig. 3-17

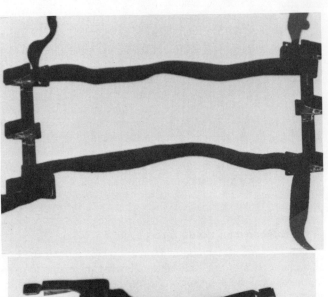

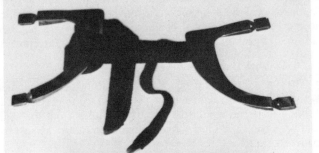

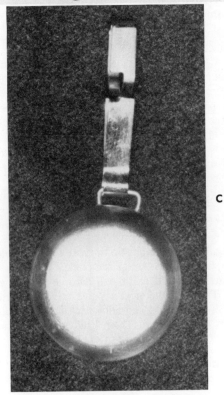

Fig. 3-18

All deposits on the involved teeth should be removed, in order to avoid tearing the dam during insertion or forcing these deposits deeper into the peridontium. Contact areas should be tested with dental tape to evaluate their tightness and the presence of deposits or sharp lesion edges. If tightness is substantial, separation may be needed during seating the dam. If the contact area is to be included in the preparation, it should be primarily involved in the tooth preparation before dam application. If the lesion margins tear the tape, the proximal part of the preparation should be prepared before the dam application.

For the tooth to receive a rubber dam, the periodontium should be sound, otherwise the application might aggravate the inflamed tissue. The amount of gingival retraction needed should be predetermined so the proper thickness of dam material can be chosen (the heavier, the more the retraction). The patient should be properly anesthetized before applying the rubber dam.

Vulnerable and previously irritated soft tissues inside the mouth should be covered with insoluble emollients (petroleum jelly). Extraorally the vermix of the lips, corners of the mouth, and cut or ulcerated areas that will be under the dam should also be covered with a suitable emollient.

G. Preparing the rubber for application

First the proper location of the holes should be predetermined. Several ways can be used, e.g., a template (Fig. 20) to mark the location of the holes for any tooth in either arch. Although this is a speedy way, results are not consistent, as the templates are for average tooth locations, and in human dentitions there are many deviations from the norm. However, these marks can be used as guidelines, modifying them according to the actual locations of teeth in each mouth.

Another method is to place the area of the rubber dam to be punched on the teeth (whether in the mouth or on study models) and marking them directly for punching (Fig. 21, A, B, C). Also, the patient may be asked to bite on a piece of softened baseplate wax, which is then chilled and applied over the area of the rubber to be punched. The rubber is then marked by penetrating teeth locations in the wax with a pin (Fig. 22). These two methods are the most feasible and always have consistent, efficient results.

For operative procedures it is advisable to isolate, from at

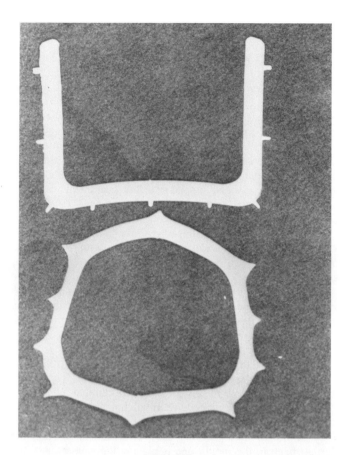

Fig. 3-19

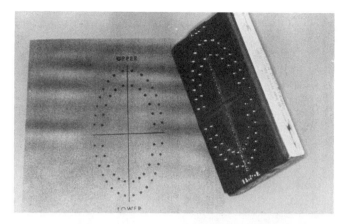

Fig. 3-20

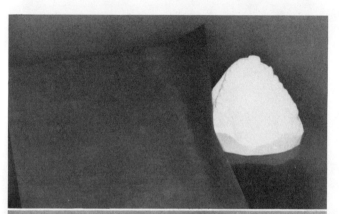

A

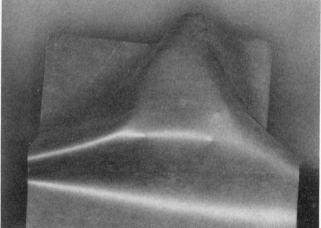

B

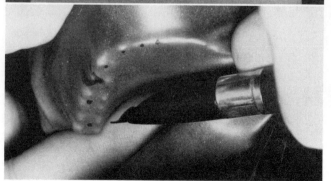

C

Fig. 3-21

least one tooth behind, the one being operated on over to the opposite canine, so that the anterior teeth are always isolated (Fig. 30A). This is to standardize the process for the operator and make it a feasible and routine procedure. In addition, this will assure that the finger support during instrumentation (which is usually involving anterior teeth) is on dry, isolated tooth structures with maximum security. This arrangement will prevent the lips from coming between the rubber and anterior teeth subjecting them to trauma from instrumentation. This is especially important during lower operations when the lip is anesthesized and the patient is not able to attract the operator's attention to any possible injury.

For operations on anterior teeth, an isolation from canine to canine is quite sufficient (Fig. 30B), and usually is without clamps. Wedges or wedged pieces of rubber distal to the cuspid are adequate to retain the dam.

Hole punching should allow for at least 2 inches of intact rubber peripheral to lower anterior teeth and lateral to upper and lower posterior teeth on each side. Also, 1-1.5 inches of intact rubber should be left peripheral to the upper anterior teeth. Holes for anterior teeth usually follow a curve. Those for premolar teeth follow a straight line paralleling the midline. Holes for molar teeth follow a straight line, slightly inclined to the midline. These rules are for normally aligned teeth and for lesions other than cervical ones. For Class V lesions necessitating a clamp in the 212 series, the hole for the tooth having the lesion should be deviated 2-3 mm away from the normal arch line facially or lingually, depending on whether it is a facial or lingual lesion.

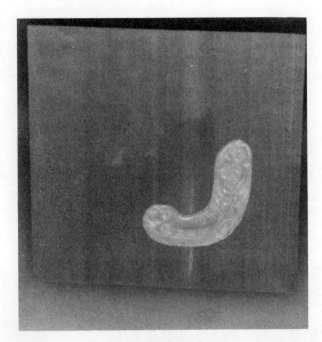

Fig. 3-22

The interceptal rubber should have an average of 4-5 mm width. This would increase, of course, if there is a missing tooth (teeth) or a highly arching interdental papillae or diastema. On the contrary, this distance should be decreased in the presence of square teeth with minimal interdental papillae. It is better to midjudge with increased width than with decreasing width, as increasing the width of the interceptal rubber will only lead to buckling or curling of the rubber occlusally, where it might be caught in rotary instruments and obstruct the field of operation. Decreasing the width of the interceptal rubber will lead to compression of the interdental gingiva, or separation of the gingiva from the tooth and/or strangulation of the gingiva. Any of these can effect permanent changes in the interdental col.

It is helpful to cut off one of the upper corners of the dam and to keep it aside. The cut area will help orient the operator as to the proper location of the dam in the mouth, and the cut piece may be used to anchor the dam anteriorly.

H. Attaching the dam to the anchor teeth

After choosing the indicated safe anchor clamps, eight inches of dental floss or dental tape are tied to the bow of the clamp. This will enable quicker recovery of an ingested or inhaled clamp.

There are four ways to attach the dam to the anchor tooth after this initial step:

1. The lateral edges of the anchor tooth's hole are attached to the dam-engaging projection of a wing type clamp, being sure they are not covering the blades of the jaws. The clamp is gripped by a clamp forceps so that its bow is facing occlusally and distally. With the forceps, the clamp is opened and slipped over the occlusal end of the anchor tooth, slightly tilting the clamp lingually. Apical to the height of contour lingually, the blades (the points) of the clamp are brought in contact with the tooth surface. The clamp is then pushed apically on the facial surface of the tooth, over the height of contour there. The remaining jaw blade(s) is (are) brought in contact with the tooth surface. The clamp is then released from the forceps and the forceps is removed in an occlusal direction, trying not to disturb the established relationship between the clamp and the tooth (Fig. 23). After making sure of the stability of the clamp, the dam hole edges are disengaged from the clamp wings and directed apical to the clamp components.

2. A wingless clamp is attached to the anchor tooth in the same way as previously mentioned but without the dam. The hole for the anchor tooth in the rubber is then stretched on both sides laterally and slipped over the bow and jaws of the clamp and anchored apical to the clamp jaws.

3. Also, the hole for the anchor tooth in the dam may first be stretched laterally and slipped over the height of contour of the anchored tooth apically and kept there with two fingers. Then the clamp can be applied occlusally to it, as indicated above (Fig. 24).

4. Finally, the dam can be attached to the bow of a wingless clamp by the edges of its anchor tooth hole. Then the clamp is anchored to the tooth and the rubber can be slipped apical to its jaws (Fig. 25).

These various methods of attachment can be done with the frame rubber dam holder already attached to the rubber, a procedure that may improve handling of the dam. The choice between any of these means is a matter of clinical judgement. Generally speaking, procedures involving attachment of the dam to the clamp before anchoring are the most tolerated, but they cannot be used in every case. It is safe to say that the further back in the mouth one is placing the rubber dam, the more frequently one would apply the clamp and the dam separately.

I. Seating the rubber dam

The mouth surface of the dam should be lubricated with a water soluble lubricant (sometimes the saliva may be sufficient for such lubrication).

The hole for the most anteriorly isolated tooth is stretched over its corresponding tooth while the edge nearest the next tooth is teased through the contact area in between. The piece of rubber, previously cut from the corner of the dam, should then be used to anchor the dam anteriorly (Fig. 26). A dental floss can also be used (Fig. 28).

Each hole is oriented occlusal to its tooth and loosely engaged there, at least through the mesial and distal occlusal embrasures (Fig. 27). Concurrent drying of the tooth with air will help. The rubber dam holder should be preliminarily placed at this time.

The interceptal rubber is now forced interproximally past the contact areas by stretching the rubber bucco-lingually with apical pressure, while drying each tooth with a continuous stream of air. In most cases this will seat the interceptal rubber. If not seated, then pass waxed dental floss over both proximal sides of the tooth ahead of the interceptal rubber. If this will not seat it, use a wedge between the teeth to create sufficient separation for the interceptal rubber to go in between.

To invert the edge of the dam's holes in the gingival crevice, simply use a blunt-nobbed instrument to guide the dam into the crevice, while drying the tooth surface of the crevice. (Fig. 29A). If this does not work, tease a dental floss (tape) to

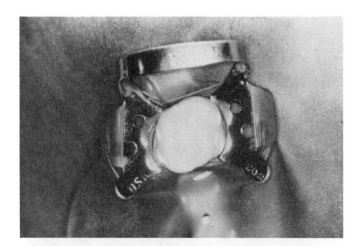

Fig. 3-23

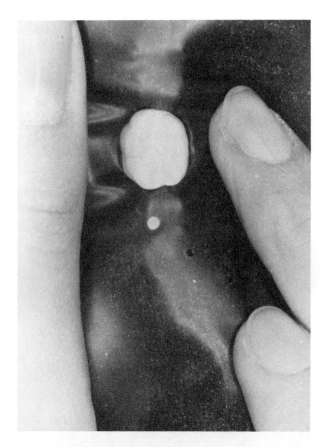

Fig. 3-24

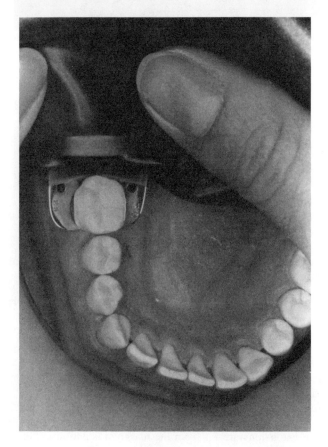

Fig. 3-25

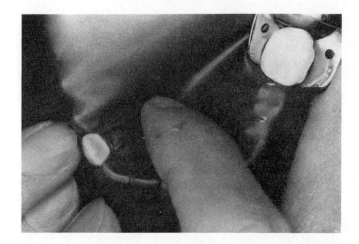

Fig. 3-26

surround the neck of the tooth, and with a blunt instrument gently push the dental floss with the involved edges of the rubber holes into the gingival crevice (Fig. 29B). After the rubber edges are inverted there, remove the dental floss. If this does not invert the dam into the crevice, the dental floss loose ends are crossed buccally and in gentle sawing actions, both ends are pulled, one end at a time, with a very gradual and gentle apical force (Fig. 29C), inverting the edges of the dam apically into the crevices.

J. Attachment of the rubber dam holder

A rubber dam napkin is slipped under the rubber dam after removing the preliminarily applied holder; then the attaching prongs or clips of the holder are engaged to the dam, stretching the dam between holding prongs. Any excess unattached rubber should be directed downwards, away from the holder perimeters, to prevent wrinkling in the rubber around the mouth. Any excess rubber under the nose which obstructs nasal breathing should be cut away. Be sure that the napkin is not wrinkled

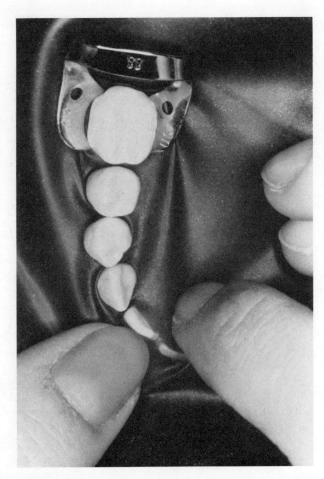

Fig. 3-27

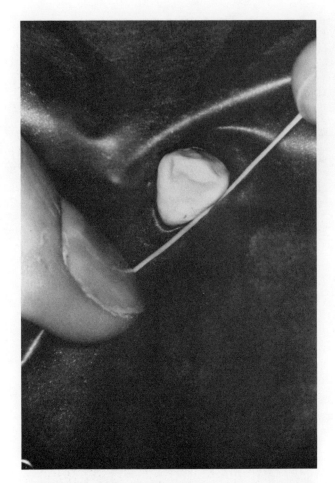

Fig. 3-28

and is stable. Fluid evacuating mechanisms should be introduced at this time, according to the designated location to be described later (Fig. 30, A and B).

K. Special rubber dam applications

For Class V lesions, the rubber dam is applied in a conventional way, and, after being inverted, a suitable size 212 series clamp is chosen and seated on the tooth, so that its jaws displace the gingiva and the rubber away from the lesion's margins. The clamp blades should not be wider or narrower than the width of the tooth at its area of contact, and the clamp jaws may be ground to obtain this relationship. After being sure of the stability of the clamp and its non-impingement on the opposite (facial or lingual) surface gingiva, tempered compound is placed between the clamp bows and occlusal surfaces of the adjacent teeth (Fig. 31). This compound braced clamp, in addition to retracting the gingiva, will distribute forces applied to the tooth during the restorative procedures to at least two other teeth, allowing greater resistance to these forces (Fig. 31).

Clamp jaws and blades can be adjusted by grinding to suit any unusual tooth form. Sometimes the facial Class V lesions are very apically located, accompanied by more recession of the gingiva facially than lingually. If we were to apply one of

the regular 212 clamp series, the lingual jaws would encounter the gingiva, to compensate the clamp may be softened by heating it to red hot, then working it with two pliers, moving the lingual jaw occlusally and the facial jaw gingivally. The clamp is then allowed to bench cool to regain its gripping resilience.

Single tooth isolation (Fig. 32) is used for endodontic therapy, but sometimes it is useful for operative procedures, especially on teeth undergoing vital bleaching or receiving bonded type restorations. Isolation for cast restoration-cementation may involve different techniques for different circumstances. If the cavity preparation has no surface extensions or any surface extensions are far from the margins, isolation is done in a conventional manner. However, if the surface extension has margins at the gingiva, in addition to the regular isolation, a clamp is also applied onto the tooth receiving the casting. If the bows of this additional clamp interfere with the position of the original clamp, it may be placed on the tooth backwards, i.e., with the bows facing each other occlusally and mesially.

Isolation of a cemented abutment tooth may be achieved by several means. First, there may be isolation with no holes in the positions of the pontics. The dam is seated so that the rubber will actually be located occlusal to the abutment. Suitable size wedges are inserted interproximally between the pon-

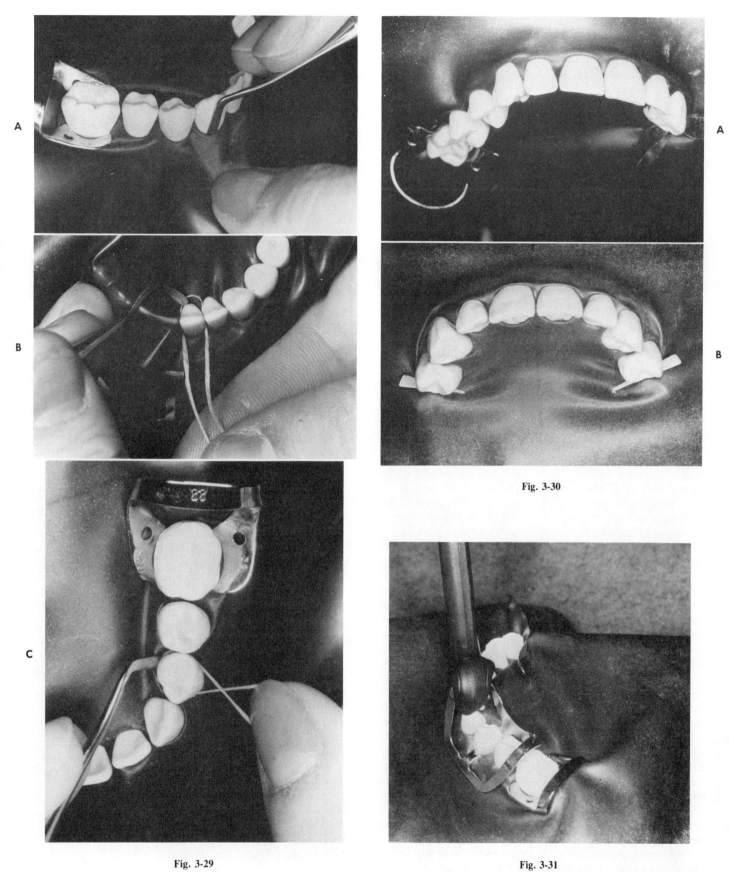

Fig. 3-29

Fig. 3-30

Fig. 3-31

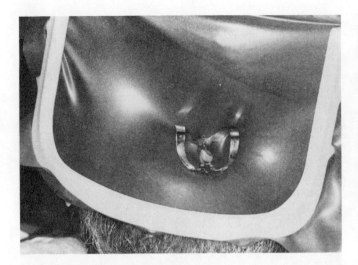

Fig. 3-32

tic and the abutment tooth, to retain the rubber apically. Softened compound is added to stabilize these wedges against the rubber (Fig. 33A). The second technique is similar, except that a piece of pipe cleaner is used instead of the wedges. This may also be stabilized with compound (Fig. 33B).

A third technique involves punching a hole in the dam for each abutment tooth, then punching a small hole 2 mm from each side of the abutment hole. After applying the dam as usual, use a large curved needle (upholstery needle), to thread floss in the abutment hole under the bridge joint, keeping one end of the floss buccally. Then thread the lingual end of the floss through the two-sided holes linguo-buccally, and tie the two buccal ends very tightly. The piece of rubber between the abutment hole and the side holes will be pushed under the joint sealing it (Fig. 33C).

Finally, one may punch the usual holes in the dam, then cut the interceptal rubber in the position of the pontic mesio-distally. Punch several holes 2 mm from this mesio-distal cut facially and lingually. The dam is then applied in the usual way, tucking the split portion of dam under the pontic, and using the side holes to thread dental floss and tie the two pieces of rubber together in a continuous suture fashion (Fig. 33D).

L. Removal of the rubber dam

After the completion of operative procedures, all used wedges, corner pieces of rubber, pipe cleaners, etc. should be removed first. Then, the interceptal rubber is stretched facially and the stretched rubber is cut with a pair of straight scissors (Fig. 34). A finger placed under the rubber will prevent cutting the patient's underlying tissues with the scissors. The clamps are then removed. If isolation involved placing compound for one reason or another, it may be split with a sharp chisel and dislodged with pressure. The clamp forceps is engaged in the clamp and activated laterally to open the clamp over the tooth's maximum convexity. The holder is detached, the dam removed, and the napkin is used to wipe saliva and/or perspiration from the patient's face. After the mouth is rinsed, dental floss should be passed between all the teeth that had been isolated or involved in the rubber dam anchoring, to assure

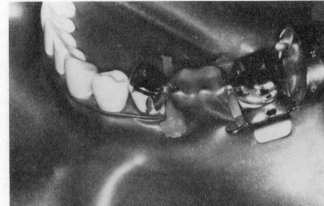

A

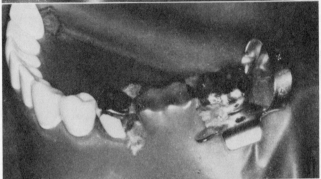

B

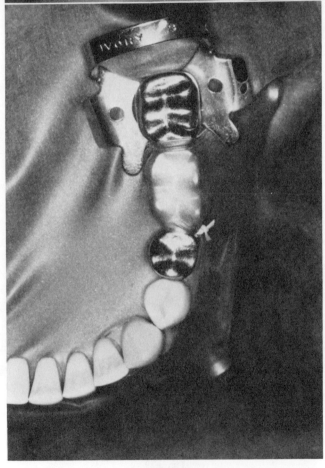

C

Fig. 3-33

that there are no remaining pieces of rubber dam. The gingiva may then be massaged to counteract any ischaemia.

V. Debris and Fluid Evacuation Mechanisms and Equipment

Most of the modern dental units are supplied with two types of vacuum systems, one usually being stronger than the other. The "high volume" evacuation vacuum systems are usually operated by the dentist or the dental assistant. The "low volume" system is usually attached to a saliva ejector which may remain in the mouth during the procedure.

The following are some examples of these evacuating systems:

A. Equipment to be left in the mouth during the procedure

1. Saliva ejectors may be a metallic type, which are autoclavable. These should have a rubber tip to avoid irritating the delicate tissues on the floor of the mouth. More frequently used are disposable plastic types. Certain requirements must be observed when using any saliva ejector (Fig. 35).

a. Always mold it so the tip end will be facing backward with a slight upward curvature. The floor of the mouth should not directly contact the openings in the tip, as the delicate mucous membrane will be aspirated into these holes and badly traumatized by the vacuum energy.

b. Always cover the floor of the mouth under the saliva ejector with a piece of gauze or cotton rolls to further prevent injury to the tissue.

c. As it approaches the mouth, the saliva ejector should be formed so that its side will not rub against the corners of the mouth. If such contact cannot be avoided, a lubricant applied at the corner of the mouth will reduce frictional irritation in that area.

d. Remove the saliva ejector periodically, in order to change the gauze or cotton rolls, and to check for any irritations.

e. Avoid pushing the saliva ejector during instrumentation to prevent injuring the soft surrounding tissues. Instead, it should always be removed if it interferes with instruments.

f. When used with a rubber dam, it is most convenient to make a hole for it to pass through the rubber, instead of placing it under the rubber. Also, the hole through the rubber will stabilize the ejector laterally.

g. The saliva ejector cannot be used as the sole evacuating device, for it is inefficient in removing coolant water during tooth cutting.

2. High speed devices (e.g., vacu-rinse) (Fig. 36)

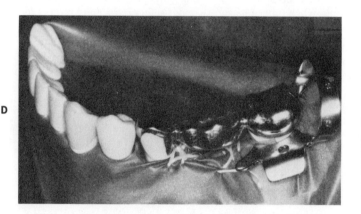

Fig. 3-33 D

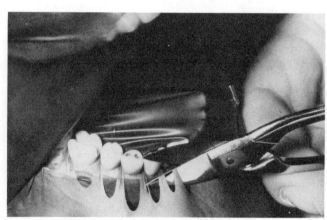

Fig. 3-34

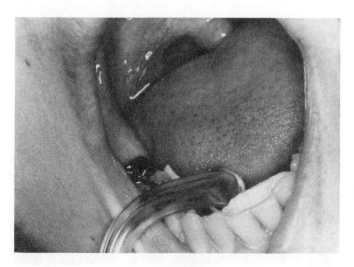

Fig. 3-35

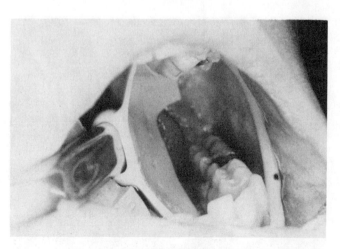

Fig. 3-36

This equipment is always attached to the high speed, high volume suction system of the unit. It consists of circular hoses perforated by multiple orifices. When applied intraorally, it circumvents the quadrant being operated on. Typically, such devices have plastic or metallic guards for the cheeks, the floor of the mouth, and the tongue (i.e., retracting them away, so as not to be drawn in the vacuum stream). Each device is attached to the patient's chin using holding clamps, made of rubbery or resinous material. These devices are so efficient that they can replace the rubber dam during cast restoration procedures. Because there is a hazard of overdrying or dehydrating the involved and/or adjacent tissues with the continuous high volume evacuation, it is advisable to eliminate the vacuum when not cutting to allow tissues to rehydrate.

B. Equipment to be intermittently used by the dentist or assistants (Fig. 3).

This usually consists of the high speed evacuator with a plastic, disposable or metallic autoclavable tip. The tip is usually bevelled, with the flat surface facing the area being cut and having the maximum opening possible to evacuate cooling fluids, secretions, and debris. Usually the assistants hold these tips, and they should not push the soft tissues or rest on them. These devices allow high speed cutting of teeth with the prescribed amount of water coolant to be carried out in an efficient, practical manner.

VI. Fluid Absorbing Mechanisms and Materials

These materials should be used mainly to absorb salivary secretions. Three typical materials which are used for this purpose are:

A. Cotton rolls (Fig. 37), which are furnished in different diameters, cut to a variety of lengths, and have either plain or woven surfaces, to improve their compactness. Cotton rolls are applied and stabilized sublingually with specific holders or with an anchoring rubber dam clamp. Also, they can be applied without a holder, over or lateral to salivary glands orifices, e.g., in the floor of the mouth under the tongue, or in the upper buccal vestibule in the molar area. Cotton rolls are usually used in conjunction with other fluid control devices, such as the rubber dam, or the saliva ejector.

B. Gauze (Fig. 38), may be supplied in pieces 2″ × 2″ or larger, and they perform the same function as cotton rolls. However, they are better suited for covering larger areas than cotton rolls. Also, they are better tolerated by delicate tissues, as their adhesion to dry tissues is much less than that of cotton rolls.

C. Absorbant paper pads or wafers (Fig. 39) are supplied in different shapes to fit various locations in the mouth. These are more absorbant than cotton rolls and gauze and they are well tolerated by the oral tissues.

VII. Tissue Retraction and Protection, Types and Modes of Actions

The best tissue retractor and protector of oral tissues is a properly applied rubber dam. Auxillary procedures include wedges, inserted interproximally during proximal preparations (Fig 40). They compress the gingiva apically, and retract it from the gingival margins of the lesions as well as physically guard it against any misdirected instrument strokes. Another auxiliary procedure is laying a flap with a vertical releasing incision to reflect the nearby gingiva until the operative procedure is completed. Of course, this procedure is necessitated only when other measures cannot safely retract and protect the gingiva.

As mentioned before, the tongue, cheek, and lips are retracted and protected jointly by the dentist and the assistants, if the rubber dam is not used. In addition, there are certain devices that can be left in the patient's mouth during the operative procedure. These include:

A. Tongue guards, which create a wall between the tongue and the operating field with an adjustable space (Fig. 36). These are usually metallic, autoclavable, or plastic disposable.

B. Tongue depressors (Fig. 41), i.e., the wooden disposable type, which can help lower the elevation of the tongue during the operative procedure. Also, they can help with the tongue retractor and mirrors, mentioned before, to control the tongue away from the field of operation. They can also be used to retract the cheek along with the other devices.

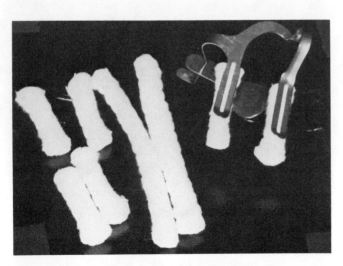

Fig. 3-37

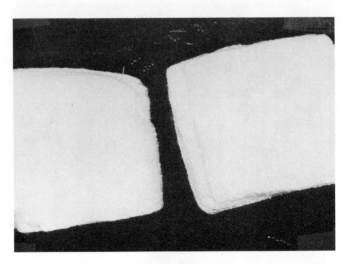

Fig. 3-38

C. Cheek and lip retractors (Fig. 42, A and B), which fit half of the upper and lower lips including the mouth corner held in a grooved partition of the device, are used to pull both lips and cheeks backwards and outwards, exposing the facial surfaces of the teeth. Some of these devices fit one lip with the adjacent corner of the mouth to retract and expose the facial surface of one quadrant only. Others are designed to engage the whole peripheries of the upper and lower lips, so as to expose the facial surfaces of all teeth. These are usually used for photographic purposes (Fig. 42A).

A cotton roll in the buccal vestibule during cervical facial or lingual tooth preparation is a secure protective mechanism against sudden accidental movements of the vestibular tissues,

especially lower lingual ones, or unpredictable apical strokes of cutting instruments. To forcefully retract the vestibular tissues away from the field of operation, a piece of gauze continuously pressed apically by the operator or his (her) assistant is very effective.

Covering adjacent teeth with a metallic band during proximal preparation is a very effective way of preventing unplanned cutting strokes from encountering the adjacent intact or restored proximal surfaces. Also, use of safe-sided discs proximally with the non-cutting surface facing the intact adjacent tooth (or restoration) is a safe, effective way of cutting proximal surfaces for cast restorations.

Preparing the proximal parts of a preparation inside its own proximal plate of enamel, as will be described in Class II cavity preparation for amalgam, is the most efficient way to protect adjacent teeth from proximal cutting injuries.

VIII. Mouth Probes

Patients, having difficulty keeping their mouth open during the operative procedure, may require certain rigid rubbery devices to facilitate their remaining open. Such devices are triangular in shape with blunted corners. They have multiple

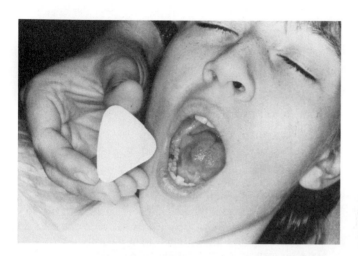

Fig. 3-39

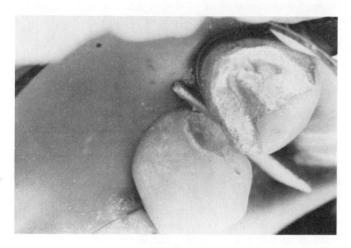

Fig. 3-40

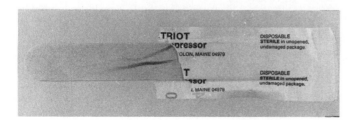

Fig. 3-41

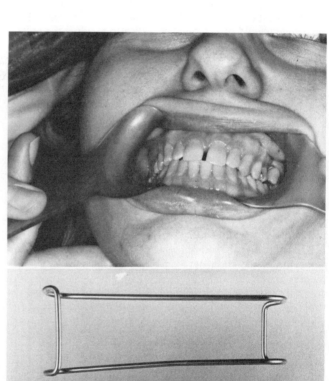

Fig. 3-42

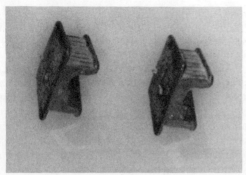

Alse consider madill sublunated and nosage Tu *muscles.*

Fig. 3-43

serrations along their side surfaces to stabilize them on the occlusal surfaces of opposite teeth. The device is inserted between the teeth on the unoperated side, with the narrow end directed distally (Fig. 43). The further posteriorly it is placed, the more mouth opening will occur. After its insertion the patient is asked to bite on it in order to keep it between the teeth.

It is advisable not to push the device too far posteriorly, as it may strain the masticatory muscles beyond their limits. Also, the device should be removed periodically to allow the patient to bite and relax. *Don't use equilibrit teeth who wy probe because pseudo feelig always tell y the patient has hy contact*

IX. Use of Medicaments

Occasionally, it is necessary to resort to medicaments administered orally or parenterally, to control the operating field or to prevent complications from the operative procedures. Examples include:

A. Anti-sialogogues. These medications are rarely used. However, occasionally a patient whose salivary flow is extremely excessive requires medicaments such as atropin (5 mgm a half-hour before the appointment). This will substantially decrease the salivary flow, but should be avoided in patients with high ocular pressure or with cardio-vascular problems.

B. Anti-anxiety, anti-apprehension medicaments. To improve the cooperation of the patients during the dental procedures it is sometimes necessary to premedicate them with drugs like valium (5-10 mgm) or barbiturates (Seconal) 24 hours before the appointment. Since these drugs are habit forming, they should be given only for short periods and to selected patients.

C. Muscle relaxants.

D. Antibiotic premedications.

Patients with a history of heart problems require such medications to prevent complications from the possible driving of oral microbia into the blood stream during the mechanotherapy. The American Heart Association recommendations for such prophylactic premedication should be reviewed and followed precisely.

E. Medicaments used in controlling the gingiva (see chapter on Control of the Periodontium prior to taking the impressions for cast restorations).

F. Pain control medicaments.

Undoubtedly pain is the major factor in creating an uncooperative patient. However, with modern techniques and medicaments there is no reason for excessive pain experiences during dental operations. Generally, there are four categories of pain controlling medications, i.e., local anesthesia, general anesthesia, analgesia (nitrous oxide-oxygen mixture), and psychosomatic medicaments.

X. Mechanical and Chemical Elimination of Intraoral Deposits and Undesirable Solids

Any deposit which is deemed to be biologically hazardous and/or interfering with proper execution of the operation (e.g., plaque, food substrate, calculus, stains, and old restorations) should be mechanically removed before the operative procedure begins.

Scaling and polishing of teeth using ultrasonic equipment may be necessary. Irrigating the mouth with antiseptic solutions under air pressure may be needed to control microbial activities before rotary instrumentation, which may spread them into the surrounding atmosphere. Sometimes irrigating the mouth with a deodorizing solution may be necessary to control foul odors from diseased areas so that the procedure can be done under tolerable circumstances.

XI. Illumination and Viewing

Illumination of the operating field can be achieved through overhead lights (Fig. 44) or lights attached to the instruments used in the procedures (e.g., handpiece or mirrors) (Fig. 45). The overhead light should be positioned so that the light rays will travel unobstructed to the area being operated upon. Reflecting mirrors for this light should be checked and cleaned frequently, to obtain the maximum light intensity.

There are certain rules for intraoral viewing:

A. Ideal viewing occurs when light comes directly from its source to the operating field, which is being viewed directly. Every effort should be made to establish this arrangement, if possible.

B. In areas where the overhead light is obstructed by certain immovable anatomy, the hand mirror should be used to reflect some of the overhead light on the unilluminated area. Direct vision can still be used.

C. In areas, where the light from the available lamp is unavoidably obstructed and the operated areas must be viewed in a mirror, position the mirror so that it will reflect lights to the operating field while simultaneously allowing the field to be viewed in the mirror. This situation occurs in the upper right molar area (for right-handed operator).

D. One of the assistant's jobs should be to clean the dentist's viewing mirror from debris and cooling water by continuously applying a stream of air on the mirror and washing it with water periodically while it is in the mouth.

To facilitate cleaning the viewing mirror the dentist should position and angulate the mirror so that the cooling water will not cover its reflecting surface, or apply certain hydrophobic antimoisture agents (waxes) to the mirror surface. These temporarily prevent accumulation of moisture but must be applied several times during the procedure.

Some mirrors have a battery or air-activated revolving viewing surface that will eliminate water accumulation by the centrifugal force of its spinning action. To prevent condensation moisture deposition it is helpful to warm the mirror by running hot water on it.

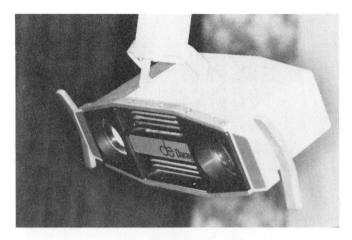

Fig. 3-44

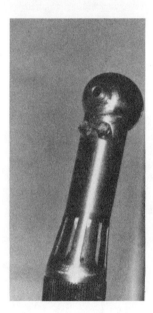

Fig. 3-45

The most non-obstructed illumination is a light attached to an instrument like the handpiece (fiber optics) (Fig. 45). Such light illuminates the exact field being operated upon, and when using direct optics, it is unnecessary to reflect light by mirrors.

For critical evaluation and precise cutting magnifying devices may be used. These may be magnifying loupes to be worn by the dentist, magnifying mirrors for intricate viewing, or magnifying lenses that may be placed clost to the tooth.

XII. Possible Complications and Corrective Measures for the Procedures of Controlling the Field of Operation

The most usual hazards of field of operation control are:

A. Injury to soft tissues from mechanical retractors, or dentist's or assistant's movements, or from adhered cotton rolls.

Any resultant bleeding should be controlled by pressure application and/or sutures. The wound should be debrided, infection should be safeguarded against by applying mild antiseptics, and the patient should be advised regarding the use of warm salt water mouth rinses. Antibiotics may be prescribed as deemed necessary.

B. Swallowing or inhaling debris or foreign objects. Immediate retrieval with high speed vacuum should be attempted. If this is impossible, place the patient in an upright position to avoid inhalation of the foreign object. Chest and abdominal x-rays should be ordered to detect location of the object. Usually swallowed items of dental origin are eliminated through the bowel, but in the case of inhaled items the patient must be referred to ENT or chest specialists for proper treatment. *The best safeguard against this hazard is the use of the rubber dam.*

3. Strained muscles. Light massage, applications of hot, moist heat, or even muscle relaxants may be necessary to alleviate muscle spasm.

4. Painful TMJ. This is usually a sequela of prolonged use of a mouth prop. Subluxation, resulting from overstretching of the mandible protractors, especially the external ptergoid and the TMJ ligaments may also occur. In the case of the latter, the mandible should be manipulated backwards and upwards rehousing its condyle into the fossae. Simple overstretching of the muscles and ligaments, without the condyle leaving its fossae housing, requires application of moist heat and resting immobilization of the masticatory muscles.

5. Facial emphysema. This is usually due to air blown facially at an area of minimal, weakly attached gingiva. The patient should be comforted and informed that, with time, the condition will resolve itself. Ice bags may be used for the first few days to minimize its spread. Closure of the opening through which the air passed to the facial surgical spaces should be accomplished. Antibiotics should be prescribed routinely.

6. Complications from rubber dam applications. Leftover pieces of rubber dam in the gingival crevice should be removed, and any periodontal defect created must be corrected by whatever means is deemed necessary.

7. Complications of local anesthesia, general anesthesia, and analgesia.

8. Gagging. This problem is of psychological origin with minimal physical etiology. The patient's apprehension should be controlled before trying any direct gagging control measures. These include:

a. The application of topical anesthetic solution or ointment on the posterior half to two-thirds of the tongue.

b. Avoiding contact with the posterior tongue during the procedure.

c. Injecting local anesthesia in the tongue.

d. Distracting the patient's attention by asking him (her) to concentrate on some extraneous procedure such as slightly raising his (her) feet during the procedure that promotes the gag reflex, applying a salt solution on the side of his (her) tongue, or involve him (her) in minor exercises by the finger, toes, etc.

Sometimes patients showing a gagging tendency are very difficult to treat and it may be necessary to resort to general anesthesia, hypnosis or bio-feedback in order to perform any dental procedures on them.

BIBLIOGRAPHY

Barbakow, A.Z.: The rubber dam; a 100 year history. J. Am. Acad. Gold Foil Oper. **8:**13, 1965.

Castano, F.A., and Alden, B.A.: Handbook of expanded dental auxiliary practice. Philadelphia, J.B. Lippincott Co., 1973.

Daniel, D.: Suction tip placement and manipulation. JADAA May, 1973, 26.

Ingraham and Koser: An atlas of gold foil and rubber dam procedures. Los Angeles. Section of operative dentistry. Univ. of Southern California School of Dentistry, 1980.

Kilpatrick, Harold C.: Functional dental assisting. Philadelphia, W.B. Saunders Co., 1977.

Murray, M.J.: Value of the rubber dam in operative dentistry. J. Am Acad. Gold Foil Operators **3:**25, 1960.

Prime, J.M.: Inconsistencies in operative dentistry (fifty reasons for using the rubber dam), Am. Dent. A. J. & Dent. Cosmos. **24:**82, 1937.

Schwarzrock, S.P., and Jensen, J.R.: Effective dental assisting. 5th ed. Dubuque, Wm. C. Brown Co., Publishers, 1978.

Wolfson, E.: Four-handed dentistry for dentists and dental assistants. St. Louis, The C.V. Mosby Co., 1974.

CHAPTER 4

Dental amalgams

Almost 80% of tooth restorations are fabricated from amalgam. This is probably due to the fact that the material is relatively inexpensive, and also offers a lot of technical advantages. Two of these advantages are that the material possesses an excellent sealing ability which tends to improve with age, and that the material can, to some extent, absorb and mask some manipulative errors without undue clinical consequences.

As with other dental materials, the operator actually fabricates the multiphased amalgam restoration. By his manipulation, he permanently establishes the nature of the component phases, their composition, and their relationship with each other. This, of course, determines the physical, mechanical and biological behaviors of the final restoration.

So, even with the crudest amalgam material, a proper understanding of its material science, metallurgic and manipulative variables is mandatory if the quality of the restoration is to be predictable.

Definition and Classification of Dental Amalgams

By definition, amalgam is an alloy which has mercury as one of its components. Amalgam, as used in dentistry, is a powder and liquid. The liquid is mercury; the powder is a silver-based alloy with variant types and combinations. The powder can be classified and described in different ways:

I. According to the Number of Alloyed Metals

These include binary alloys (e.g., silver-tin), ternary alloys (e.g., silver-tin-copper), and quaternary alloys (e.g., silver-tin-copper, indium).

II. According to Whether the Powder Consists of Unmixed or Admixed Alloys

Certain amalgam powders are only made of one alloy. Others have one or more alloys or metals physically added (blended) to the basic alloy, e.g., adding copper to a basic binary silver-tin alloy.

III. According to the Shape of the Powdered Particles

The alloy particles may have a spherical (smooth-surfaced spheres) shape, or irregular shapes ranging from spindles to shavings (lathe-cut), or in between shapes, e.g., spherical with irregular surfaces (spheroidal).

IV. According to the Powder's Particle Size

Although the particle diameter can be used to classify alloys, it is the least used classification. However, by this method, alloys may be microcut, fine cut, coarse cut, etc.

V. According to the Copper Content of the Powder

Due to the extremely influential effect of copper on the properties of amalgam, alloys with a copper content of 4% or less are called "low copper" alloys. Those containing more than 10% Cu are considered "high-copper" alloys. In concentrations below 4%, copper can be an admixture, without adverse effect on the alloy properties; above 4%, however, copper should be alloyed with the rest of the powder components or at least with some of them in order to avoid undesirable properties in the final set amalgam.

VI. According to the Addition of Noble Metals

When metals such as palladium, gold, or platinum are alloyed to the powder, the resulting amalgams may be classified as "noble-metal alloys". To date, palladium has proven to be the most effective noble metal addition to modern alloys.

The composition of amalgam alloy powder is best understood in an historical perspective. In this vein, it proves most expeditious to refer to the various types of alloy according to compositional changes of succeeding "generations" of amalgam. The first generation of amalgam, for example, was that studied and recommended by G.V. Black. Popular for more than 80 years, this first generation amalgam was a basic three part silver and one part tin, peritectic alloy.

The alloy is a product of the reaction between the beta-phase of solid solution of tin in silver with the liquid phase of silver and tin. This is defined as gamma-phase, which is one of the ordered solutions of tin in silver. To this basic formula, copper was added (admixture) up to 4% to decrease the plasticity and to increase the hardness and strength of the alloy. Traces of zinc (up to 1%) were also added to act as a deoxidizer or scavenger for the alloy and to decrease its brittleness. The addition of copper and zinc gave rise to the newer, second generation amalgam.

Although silver can make three types of ordered, solid solution alloys (alpha, beta, and gamma) and one eutectic alloy with tin, its manufacturers aim to have only one type of solid solution, namely gamma, because it possesses the most favorable properties for dental use. However, there will definitely be some traces of the two other ordered solid solutions (alpha and beta) and the eutectic alloy, even after proper aging and homogenization heat treatment during the manufacturing process.

In recent years, new compositions for amalgam alloy powder have been introduced. The admixture (blending) of a spherical Ag_3-Cu eutectic alloy to the original alloy powder creates a very interesting and valuable effect in the final product (to be described later in this chapter). This silver-copper eutectic containing alloy may be classified as the third generation amalgam.

The alloying of copper to silver and tin, in a percentage up to 29%, forms a ternary alloy, in which most of the tin is firmly bonded to the copper. This development was the fourth generation amalgam.

The alloying of silver, copper, tin and indium together, creating a true quaternary alloy in which almost none of the tin is available to react with the mercury when mixed with the powder, was the fifth generation amalgam to be developed.

Finally, the alloying of palladium (10%), silver (62%), and copper (28%), to form a eutectic alloy, which is lathe-cut and blended into a first, second, or third generation amalgam in a ratio of 1:2. The set amalgam exhibits the highest nobility of any previous amalgam and has been the most recent (sixth) generation of amalgam to be developed.

A description of the setting reaction of amalgam and the properties of each phase in the set will emphasize why all efforts have been aimed at eliminating or at least minimizing the availability of tin to react with mercury. Although first and second generation amalgams are seldom used now, understanding their reaction products is basic to an understanding of the newer generations of amalgam. In fact, certain of these reaction products continue to be integral parts of reactions of generation 3-6 alloys.

The amalgamation reaction in the first generation (G.V. Black) alloy occurs when the powder is mixed with mercury and dissolution of the powder particles in the mercury takes place. However, this dissolution will not be total since only the particle surface is attacked by the mercury. Before this is complete, two reaction products, namely the mercury-silver phase and the mercury-tin phase, will form and precipitate within, joining together what is left of the silver-tin particles. This forms a coherent mass into which the unreacted mercury and other unreacted ingredients are trapped. So the multiphase nature of the product becomes apparent. It contains the following component phases and their properties (Fig. 1):

A. The Original Gamma Phase (i.e., Ag_3Sn or the alloy powder) which has not been completely dissolved in mercury. Mechanically, this is the strongest phase, and for this reason it should occupy the maximum available space in the volume of the restoration.

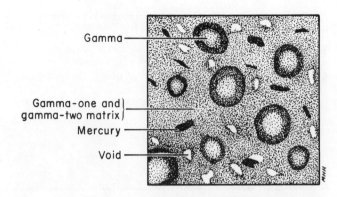

Fig. 1 Microstructure of a set first generation amalgam

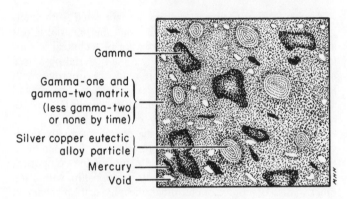

Fig. 2 Microstructure of a set second generation amalgam

B. The Gamma-1 Phase (i.e., silver-mercury phase, or Ag_2Hg_3) is one of the amalgamation products that forms part of the matrix, joining the original Ag_3Sn particles. Comparatively, it is the noblest phase, i.e., the most resistant to tarnish and corrosion, and every effort is made to allow this phase to occupy the maximum available space in the bonding matrix of the final product.

C. The Gamma-2 Phase, the tin-mercury phase (Sn_7Hg_8), is also a product of the amalgamation reaction, forming part of the bonding matrix. It is the least resistant to tarnish and corrosion, and every effort should be made to minimize its volume percentage in the matrix. It is a well documented fact that most of the amalgam restoration failures are due to this phase, which is specifically prone to corrosion and creep.

D. The Mercury Phase, i.e., unreacted, residual mercury, will be present in isolated areas within the amalgam mass. Although it will continue to diffuse and react with the gamma-phase or any other present or future phases, this reaction rate is very slow and incomplete. Mechanically, this is the weakest phase in the product mass, and when it exceeds a certain volume limit, there will be a drastic drop in the strength and hardness properties of the amalgam, in addition to an increase in the flow and creep of the restoration.

E. The Voids (Pores) Phase occurs as the process of building the amalgam restoration traps air bubbles despite the most meticulous procedures to avoid this problem. Such voids act as nidi, not only for internal corrosion, but also for stress concentration and propagation. Both lead to early failure of the structure of the restoration.

F. The Trace Element Phases, in which copper and zinc might be found either as separate phases or combined (alloying) with tin, silver, or mercury. It depends on how much of each element is present, the solubility limit of one in another, and on the dimensions and nature of their surface area. Although present only in trace amounts in the final product, these elements are very influential in the behavior of amalgam. As mentioned before, copper can increase strength, brittleness, hardness, and the proportional limits of amalgam. Zinc can increase deformability, ultimate strengths, and resistance to oxidation of the final product. Its presence will also predispose to an interesting reaction in the presence of moisture (to be described later in the chapter).

G. The Interphases, in terms of the serviceability of the final restoration, are the most important components of the mass. This especially applies to the interphases between the three main components, namely, between gamma, gamma-1 and gamma-2. In the final restoration, the more continuous (uninterrupted) they are and the less their dimensions (closer together), the better is the bonding between these primary phases. Consequently, the more coherent and the more resistant to environmental variable the restoration will be.

As mentioned previously, third generation alloys are composed mainly of Ag_3Sn, but they also contain an admixture of silver-copper eutectic (spherical particles of silver-copper eutectic with 71.9% Ag and 28.1% Cu). These are blended with a basic silver-tin gamma-composition alloy. When the resultant admixtured powder is mixed with mercury, the immediate reaction will be exactly as mentioned for first and second generation alloys, i.e., between the Ag_3Sn and mercury, forming gamma-1 and gamma-2 alloys, joining together what is left of the original gamma-particles. However, the spherical, silver-copper eutectic particles will be left lodged in the mass for almost one to two weeks, at which time a solid state reaction occurs at mouth temperature. The gamma-2 (tin-mercury) phase reacts with the silver-copper eutectic alloy, forming a more stable tin-copper alloy (Cu_6Sn_5), which is more corrosion resistant than gamma-2. Furthermore, mercury is released from the gamma-2, and silver from the eutectic alloy. These react to form more gamma-1 (relatively, the most noble phase). The transformation reaction will continue until almost all of the gamma-2 is replaced by gamma-1. The remainder of the spherical eutectic alloy particles are covered with the tin-copper alloy and the silver-mercury alloy, binding them to the rest of the neighboring phases.

It should be obvious from the description of this reaction, that the end product in third generation alloys is more noble than the end product of the earlier Ag_3Sn + Hg amalgamation. Also, due to the difference in shape of the space lattices of the late-forming copper-tin alloys from the already present space lattices in the solid mass, in addition to the formation of more new phases within a solid mass without its changing dimension, lattice distortion and strain-hardening can be expected to occur. Furthermore, the bonding of the spherical particles to the rest of the phases in the mass will improve due to the solid state reaction. All three of these microstructural changes will improve the restoration's mechanical properties. In summary the end product here will differ from the first two generations of amalgam in that it will have almost no gamma-2 phase. Instead, it will have two additional phases—Ag_3Cu

eutectic phase original particles, and a less corroding Cu_6Sn_5 phase. The Ag_3Cu is as strong as the Ag_3Sn. The Cu_6Sn_5 phase is as noble as the Ag_3Sn phase. The set product will continue to have the usual residual mercury, voids, trace phases and interphases as previously described.

Fourth generation (ternary) alloys of silver, tin and copper (Ag_2CuSn), when mixed with Hg, will have a tendency to release silver only to react with more mercury, as the affinity of tin for copper is greater than its affinity for mercury. Therefore, the final product will have the binding matrix phase formed almost completely of gamma-1, the noblest of all component phases. The main bulk of the set mass will be the original Ag_2CuSn alloy particles, the strongest of all the phases. In addition to gamma-1 in the matrix, the other components (Hg, interphases, trace elements, and voids) will be present, exerting the same effect on the amalgam's behavior as previously described.

Though the tin, in a fourth generation amalgam is very well bound to copper, a limited percentage of it can react with mercury to create traces of gamma-2.

A fifth generation of amalgam was developed to overcome this problem. In these quarternary alloys, binding of tin more to the original alloy is accomplished by alloying indium to the other three primary elements. The same reaction as in third generation alloys can be expected when mixing quarternary alloys of silver, tin, copper and indium with mercury. Primarily, silver will be released for reaction with mercury, resulting in a bonding, gamma-1 matrix surrounding the original silver, tin, copper, and indium alloy particles. Furthermore, the indium will improve the plasticity of the mass as well as act as a de-oxidizer.

In sixth generation amalgams a nearly eutectic alloy consisting of silver (62%), copper (28%) and palladium (10%) is dispersed in a first, second or third generation amalgam in a ratio of 1:2 (dispersed:dispersion phase). When mixed with mercury, a reaction will occur which resembles that of the first three generations of amalgam. Then, within a one to two week period, the previously described solid state reaction will occur, producing Cu_6Sn_5 and gamma-1. However, two additional solid state reaction activities will occur. First will be the precipitation of a Cu_3Pd phase within the gamma-1 and Cu_6Sn_5 phases. Second, will be the increased possibility of eliminating gamma-2. The resulting presence of this disordered palladium-containing phase (which is more noble than gamma-1) and the greatly diminished presence of gamma-2 create a final product with improved mechanical and inert properties. Of course, the other reaction products as in third generation amalgams (especially the solid state phases) continue to be present, although in much lesser concentrations.

Behavior of Amalgam

Amalgam behavior can best be described in terms of its (I) dimensional stability, (II) strength properties, and (III) flow and creep.

I. Dimensional Changes

During setting, amalgam undergoes three distinct dimensional changes. These are most clearly visualized by studying the graph in Fig. 3. Stage 1, called the initial contraction,

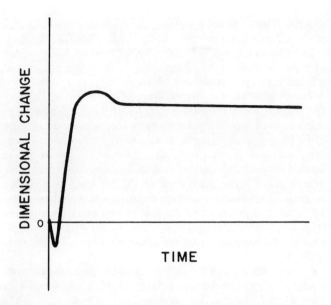

Fig. 4-3. Dimensional change pattern during normal setting of an amalgam.

results from the absorption of the mercury into the interparticular spaces of the alloy powder. This is followed by the expansion of Stage 2, due to the formation and growth of the matrix crystals. This expansion reaches a plateau with the cessation of matrix crystal formation. In Stage 3, there is a limited, delayed contraction of the mass resulting from the absorption of unreacted mercury.

The apparent expansion or contraction of amalgam will depend not only on the amalgamation stage at which the measurement is done, but most importantly, on what stage of amalgamation the cavity preparation was completely filled. According to ADA specification #1 for amalgam, -20 to $+20$ micron/cm dimensional changes are acceptable.

The following are the most probable factors that affect the dimensional changes of amalgam within and beyond acceptable limits:

A. Constituents

The more the basic gamma-phase or its equivalent contains traces of beta-phase, the greater is the possibility of expansion. Greater traces of tin produce less expansion.

B. Mercury

More Hg in the amalgam mix produces a more prolonged second stage of amalgamation (expansion). A greater amount of matrix crystals (gamma-1, or gamma-1–gamma-2), also produces more expansion.

C. Particle size

Smaller particle size indicates more surface area of the particles per unit volume. So, when they are mixed with mercury, the dissolution of the first stage will occur more rapidly and more efficiently than if the particles are large, thus leading to marked contraction. The second stage will also occur very fast, which may neutralize the original contraction. The expansion plateau may be achieved too early (before the cavity is filled), so the apparent expansion may not be noticed. On the contrary, the contraction of stage 3 may be more noticeable.

D. Trituration

The more energy used for trituration, the smaller the particles will be made, yet more mechanical force will be present pushing mercury in between the particles. Both situations will discourage expansion. Also, the more the trituration energy there is, the greater will be the distribution of the forming matrix crystals all over the mix, preventing them from the outwards growth which creates the expansion of the second stage. Furthermore, the more the energy of trituration is, the faster the amalgamation process proceeds, so the plateau part of the expansion curve might occur before completely filling the cavity preparation. This results in no apparent expansion and possibly a limited contraction.

E. Condensation

The more energy used in condensing the amalgam into the cavity preparation, the closer the original particles of the powder are brought together at the expense of the expanding matrix-crystals. Increased condensation energy also squeezes more Hg out of the mix. Both situations lead to less formation of the growing matrix crystals, inducing more contraction.

F. Particle shape

The more regular the particle shape is and the smoother its surfaces are, the faster and more effectively the mercury can wet the powder particles. This makes a faster amalgamation process in all its stages; so most of the time, the maximum expansion occurs before filling the cavity, with no apparent expansion.

G. Contamination

The primary contaminant affecting dimensional stability is moisture, especially as it affects zinc-containing amalgam. If brought in contact with water from any source (saliva, blood, respiration, etc.), zinc in an amalgam will react with water, producing ZnO and hydrogen gases. The reaction takes place 24-72 hours after amalgam insertion into the cavity preparation. Hydrogen gases within the amalgam accumulate in considerable amounts, exerting pressure sometimes estimated to be 2000 PSI (pound/inch^2). Many complications result from such gases, including protrusion of the entire restoration out of the cavity, increased microleakage space around the restoration, restoration perforation, blister formation on the restoration surface, increased flow and creep, and pupal pressure pain. The most obvious detrimental effect is a delayed expansion up to 400 micron/cm^3.

II. Strength

Set amalgam has a very weak tensile and a very high compressive strength. Generally speaking, if properly fabricated, amalgam strengths are adequate for normal situations within the oral cavity. However, these amalgam strengths can be drastically reduced by manipulative factors. Besides, amalgams cannot be strain-hardened by deformation at mouth or room temperature, as these temperatures are above the recrystallization temperature of amalgam. The following factors may affect the strengths of amalgam:

A. Temperature

Amalgam loses about 15% of its strength when its temperature is elevated from room temperature to mouth temperature.

It loses 50% of its room temperature strength when its temperature is elevated to 60° C (as when hot coffee or soup flows over it).

B. Trituration

The more trituration energy used, the more continuous are the interphases between the amalgam matrix crystals and the original particles, and the more evenly distributed are these matrix crystals over the mix. Consequently, this more coherent mass contributes to a greater strength pattern in the restoration. On the other hand, if trituration is continued after complete formation of the matrix crystals, the excess energy will create cracks in these crystals and their interphases, leading to a drop in the strength of the set amalgam.

C. Mercury

Because it is the weakest phase of the amalgam mass, residual mercury in amalgam restorations drastically affects the strength of these restorations. As it is fluid at room and mouth temperature, mercury cannot resist any slip or dislocation within the amalgam caused by external loading. It is a well documented fact that increasing the mercury content of an amalgam mix even from 53% to 55%, causes a drop in compressive strength of more than 50%.

D. Condensation

The more energy is used in condensation, the less will be the residual mercury, resulting in a higher relative percentage of the strong original particles in the restoration. Also, as previously mentioned, the more continuous will be the interphase between the original particles and the forming matrix. Furthermore, one can expect a more even distribution of the gamma-1 or gamma-1–gamma-2 matrix crystals throughout the restoration. All of this will lead to a greater, more consistent strength throughout the restoration mass. Condensation of an amalgam mass after formation of the matrix crystals does not diminish the strength properties as trituration does, because there is more resistance to the crystal displacement during condensation than during trituration.

E. Porosity

Although porosity cannot be avoided in an agglomerated mass such as amalgam, it is very important to minimize the number and size of the pores, as well as to keep them away from critical areas in the restorations, e.g., margins and surfaces. Pores facilitate stress concentration, propagation of cracks, corrosion, and fatigue failures of amalgam structures. Porosity of only 1% can be as detrimental in reducing amalgam strengths as 10% excessive mercury. Porosity results from the fact that the different phases of the amalgam do not completely wet each other simultaneously during the amalgam fabrication. Therefore, porosity can be expected and increased by undertrituration, undercondensation, irregularly shaped particles of the alloy powder, miscalculated diameter varieties of powder particles to occupy available spaces, insertion of too large increments into the cavity preparation, delayed insertion after trituration or a generally non-wetting, non-plastic mass of amalgam.

F. Particle shape

Alloy particles which are more regular and smooth are more wettable. Therefore, they will react and combine more efficiently. The resultant, less interrupted interphases create a more coherent and strong mass.

G. Interparticle distance (Fig. 4, A and B)

The closer the original particles of the amalgam alloy are to each other, the stronger the end product will be. It has been estimated that, in terms of compressive strength, there is a noticeable increase in 24 hour specimens when the average

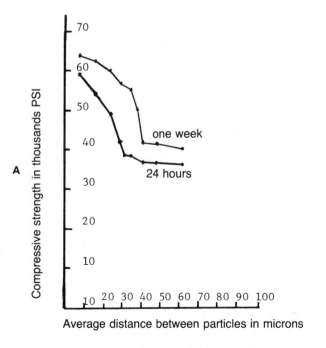

A

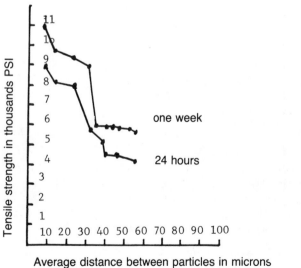

B

Fig. 4-4

interparticle distance is 38 microns or less (Fig. 4A). For one week specimens, the noticeable strength increase occurs when the average interparticle distance is 32 microns or less (Fig. 4A). In terms of the tensile strength, 24 hour specimens demonstrate a marked increase (Fig. 4B) when the average interparticle distance is 28 microns or less. For one-week specimens, the incresae in tensile strength is exhibited when the average interparticle distance is 39 microns or less (Fig. 4B).

H. Particle size (Fig. 5, A and B)

It is a well established fact that the smaller the diameter of the original particles is, the greater will be the strength of the set amalgam. In terms of compressive strength, one-day specimens will show a substantial increase in strength when the average particle diameter is 12 or less microns (Fig. 5A). One week specimens show this substantial increase when the average particle diameter is 16 microns or less (Fig. 5A). In terms of tensile strength, one-day specimens exhibit marked increase in strength when the average particle diameter is 18 microns or less (Fig. 5B), and the one-week specimens show the same increase when the average particle diameter is 12 microns or less (Fig. 5B).

I. Dispersion

As previously stated, amalgam cannot be strain-hardened by cold working. However, a solid-state dispersion within the amalgam mass of another phase, preferably one which has a different shape and dimension than the original phases, can distort the original space lattices, precipitating interferences with slip and consequently increasing the amalgam strengths. This has been done, as mentioned before, by the addition of copper, or by the addition of silver-copper eutectic, or, most

recently, by the addition of silver-copper-palladium near-eutectic alloys. All of these are capable of solid state modifications and/or precipitation of new phases within the amalgam without changing its dimension. The net result, of course, is greatly enhanced strength.

J. The Gamma-2 Phase

Mechanically, gamma-2 is the second weakest phase. This fact, combined with its corrosion ability, makes it almost as influential in the strength behavior of amalgam as mercury and porosity. Its reduction, or the prevention of its formation can definitely increase the strength of amalgam, especially the age strength.

K. Corrosion

Decreasing the corrosion activity within an amalgam restoration will protect the adhesive integrity between the multiple phases, thus preventing the strengths from deteriorating.

III. Flow and Creep Properties of Amalgam

The phenomenon of flow is measured during the setting of an amalgam and reflects the change in dimension of the amalgam under load. Creep, on the other hand, is usually measured *after* amalgam setting, and it reflects the constant change in dimension under either static or dynamic loading (the most meaningful measurement is under dynamic, cyclic loading which simulates occlusal loading). Creep is defined as incremental deformation. It is markedly pronounced above a specific temperature called the equicohesive temperature, when the grain boundaries change their mode from termini to dislocations, to pathways for dislocation movements, facilitating the visible deformation of the material. This equicohesive temperature of amalgam is lower than the mouth temperature. It is an established fact that the more energy is used in condensation, the less will be the creep. Mercury excess, on the other

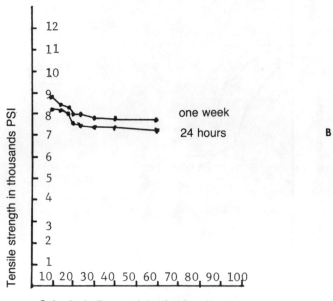

A

Comprehensive strength in thousands PSI

one week
24 hours

Spherical alloy particle size in microns

Tensile strength in thousands PSI

one week
24 hours

B

Spherical alloy particle size in microns

Fig. 4-5

hand, will drastically increase the creep. It has been estimated that creep of an amalgam mix of 53% mercury is 1.5 times that of a mix of 48% mercury. Dispersion can reduce creep. Also, elimination of gamma-2 or any process which increases the nobility of amalgam can substantially reduce the creep.

There is recent evidence that the clinical performance of amalgam is closely related to its creep values: the less the creep is, the better will be the amalgam restoration's marginal integrity and, consequently, its longevity.

IV. Rate of Attaining Strength Properties

Amalgam restorations, especially those restoring more than one surface of a molar or premolar, should possess sufficient strength by the time the patient is dismissed in order to resist cracking or fracturing during normal functional use. Therefore knowing the rate of attaining these strengths is essential in order to avoid such accidents. As long as there is residual mercury (always present) in the amalgam restoration, the amalgamation process is never complete; but, generally speaking, more than 90% of the amalgam strength is attained within 24 hours. The rate of attaining strength is dependent on two major factors: the maturity (or complete crystallization) of the matrix phase(s) and completion (or attainment of maximum continuity) of the interphases between the matrix phase(s) and the original particles. This rate can be accelerated by the following factors:

A. Reduction of the particle size
B. Regularity and smoothness of the particle shape and surfaces
C. More trituration energy
D. More condensation energy
E. Homogenization heat treatment of the powder alloy during manufacture
F. Minimal amount of mercury in the mix allowing it to be workable
G. Constituents in the original alloy particles that have good affinity to mercury, e.g., gamma-phase

V. Techniques for Amalgam Restoration Fabrication

For building an amalgam restoration the following steps should be involved:

A. Choice of the alloy and mercury
B. Proportioning
C. Trituration
D. Mulling
E. Matricing
F. Condensation
G. Burnishing
H. Carving
I. Finishing and polishing

A. Choice of the alloy and mercury

It is mainly the operator who causes the amalgam restoration to be a success or a failure, so the alloy choice is a personal preference. Generally speaking, the basic lathe-cut alloy Ag_3Sn without any additive or modification is seldom used nowadays, having given way to the dispersed phases, ternary and quaternary as well as noble-phased alloys. The choice between spher-

ical, spheroidal or lathe-cut alloy particles can be related to the type of patient population the dentist is involved with. If quick attainment of amalgam strength is necessary, the best choice will be the spherical particle alloys, but they require a fast operator to use them. It should be realized, however, that the spherical alloys exhibit more flow and deformation with time. All in all, manufacturers can supply amalgam alloys that need trituration time ranging from 2 seconds to 20 seconds and amalgam alloys that will lose their plasticity and carvability after 2 minutes or after 20 minutes. Amalgams can have ultimate compressive strength of 40,000 PSI, or 75,000 PSI, if properly manipulated, etc. Understandably, these variations can be made by metallurgical modifications in the constituents, heat treatment, particle size and shape, and surface texture. So the clinician is the one who determines his situation and needs and ultimately chooses the proper alloy suitable for his situation. However, it should be certified for use by the ADA and FDA. Several well controlled clinical studies have shown that after 5-10 years of clinical service, different amalgams of the third through sixth generation behaved similarly, provided they were manipulated properly during placement.

The choice between zinc-containing and zinc-free alloys is controversial, and personal clinical judgement is also the major factor here. Definitely, a zinc-containing alloy in the presence of moisture will create major problems as mentioned before. However, amalgams not containing zinc or any of its substitutes will tend to be less plastic and less workable and more susceptible to oxidation. So non-zinc alloys should be chosen only for cases where it is clinically impossible to eliminate moisture from the field of the operation (e.g., root apices and very subgingival lesions). Indium containing alloys are the exception to this rule, as indium performs the same functions as zinc in addition to diminishing the gamma-2 phase.

There can be no decision in the choice of mercury, except that it follow the USP specifications.

B. Proportioning of the alloy and mercury (Fig. 6)

One must choose between two mercury concentration techniques. In the high-mercury technique (increasing dryness technique), the initial amalgam mix contains a little more Hg than needed for the powder (52-53% Hg), producing a very plastic

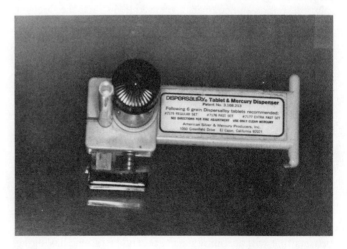

Fig. 4-6

mix. It is necessary to continue squeezing the mercury out of the mix increments being introduced during build-up of the restoration, so that each increment will be dryer than the previous one. Another, more popular technique is the minimum mercury or 1:1 (Eame's technique). The initial amalgam mix contains equal amounts of mercury and powder alloy; but it is still necessary to squeeze mercury out of the mix during the incremental build-up of the restoration. Using this technique one can assume that 50% or less mercury will be in the final restoration, with obvious advantages.

In deciding which technique to use, one must consider the manufacturer's recommendation, which is based upon the metallurgical condition, thermal treatment and powder particle specification, and the type of the restoration. For example, restorations to be retained with multiple auxillary means of retention (pins, internal boxes, grooves, etc.) need the most wetting (plastic) consistency of amalgam. This indicates increasing dryness technique. A very large restoration which needs more than one mix also might indicate use of the first technique, if the second (due to metallurgical difference) cannot guarantee the proper bonding between successive increments from different mixes. Finally, the operator training and ability is the most important criterion in making the decision, as either technique can give the same results, if properly executed by trained personnel in the specific technique.

Regarding proportioning of the alloy and mercury, bear in mind that proportioning should be done by weight if possible, and not by volume. Volume proportioning may be misleading because of trapped air and voids in the mass, especially in the powder mass.

Proportioning steps also involve a choice between preweighed, preproportioned alloy-mercury capsules or doing the weight-proportioning oneself in the office. This choice, also, involves a personal decision, to be made after considering many factors. For example, if restoration output is fairly large in number with a lot of personnel involved in dispensing of amalgam (e.g., dental schools or other clinics, where there are multiple shifts of dentists and auxillary), to prevent unavoidable disproportioning, preweighed, preproportioned capsules are the best method of quality control. By contrast, when the operation is fairly small, with the dentist or trained personnel proportioning every mix to be used, preproportioned capsules may present an unnecessary expense. If, in fact, the decision is made to proportion in the office, there are still several choices available. For example, preweighed tablets of the alloy, where a specific weight of the powder has been pressed to create tablets, might be chosen. It should be noted here, that the induced stresses in the powder during such tablet formation may increase the affinity of the powder to mercury. There are several dispensers that can accommodate preweighed tablets and mercury containers. Usually, by pressing on a lever, one tablet with the appropriate volume of mercury can be dispensed into mixing capsules. Using this system, mercury is proportioned by volume, not weight, as there is little or no chance of trapping air or voids in the liquid mercury. In these dispensers it is possible to adjust the mercury percentage from 48% to 55% (Fig. 6).

If this system is not desirable, one may choose to use dispensers that will accommodate two containers, one having Hg and the other containing the powder. By pressing a lever, the specific volume (always equal volumes) of the powder and mercury will be dispensed into a capsule. Being a volumetric proportioning there is great tendency to have less powder (than planned) relative to the mercury, as the powder can trap more voids and air than the mercury. Therefore, this method entails a greater possibility of having a wetter mix than desirable. If this is considered during the adjustment of the dials for the powder and mercury proportioning, one can arrive to a workable consistency mixture.

C. Trituration

There are six objectives of the trituration process. They are:

1. To achieve a workable mass of amalgam within a minimum time, leaving sufficient time for its insertion into a cavity preparation and carving to the predetermined tooth anatomy.

2. To remove oxides from the powder particle surface, facilitating direct contact between the particles and the mercury.

3. To pulverize pellets into particles that can be easily attacked by the mercury.

4. To reduce particle size so as to increase the surface area of the alloy particles per unit volume, leading to a faster and more complete amalgamation.

5. To dissolve the particles or part of the particles of the powder in mercury, which is a prerequisite for the formation of the matrix crystals.

6. To keep the amount of gamma-1 or gamma-1–gamma-2 matrix crystals as minimal as possible, yet evenly distributed throughout the mass for proper binding and consistent, adequate strength.

Fulfilling these objectives, either wholly or in part, results from the trituration energy supplied. Mechanical trituration, which is used universally today, necessitates a plastic or metal capsule to contain the powder and mercury during the trituration process. Some of these may have a metal or plastic pestle or ball within the capsule with the amalgam while mixing. There are three basic movements of mechanical triturators (Fig. 7):

A. The mixing arm carrying a capsule moves back and forth in a straight line. Such movement can occur at varying speeds (Fig. 7).

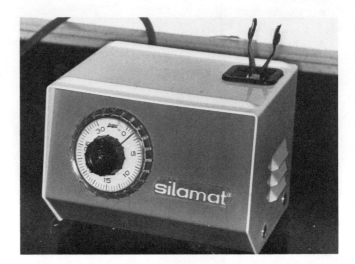

Fig. 4-7

B. The mixing arm travels back and forth in a figure 8, also at varying speeds.

C. The mixing arm travels in a centrifugal fashion.

Each of these movements is effective in fulfilling the mechanical objectives of trituration.

Trituration energy is correlated to five factors. These are:

1. The speed or the number of unit movements per unit time, e.g., the number of figure 8 movement/second that there are for the second type.

2. The thrust of the movement, e.g., the more the distance that the mixing arm travels from one part to another to be repeated over and over, the more energy there is. Also, the more complicated the pathway of the mixing arm is, the more energy there is (straight line versus Fig. 8).

3. The weight of the capsule and/or the pestle, e.g., the more weight there is, the more energy there will be.

4. The time involved in trituration, e.g., the more time is used, the more precipitated energy there will be.

5. The difference in size between a pestle (ball) and the encasing capsule, e.g., the greater this difference is, the more the distance the pestle (ball) can travel within the capsule, so more energy will be expended.

All triturators are supplied with timers to stop the action at predetermined time. For those supplying high energy (high speed or centrifugal, etc.) it is not necessary to use a pestle within the capsule, as this may cause overtrituration. The same thing is true for alloys with very short amalgamation time due either to metallurgical or other reasons. It is advisable to use threaded capsules instead of the friction fit ones as the latter may create mercury aerosol in the office atmosphere (Fig. 8).

Commonly, mistakes occur in reusing non-disposable capsules. For example, leaving remnants of previous mixes in the capsule will cause these to be incorporated into a new mix without proper binding or plasticity, weakening the final product. Also, scratches in the capsules may trap mercury or traces of old mixes, compromising the quality of the amalgam product. Cracks in the capsule that leak mercury will pollute the office and reduce the mercury in the mix, sometimes with undesirable effects.

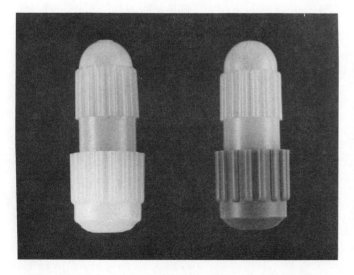

Fig. 4-8

D. Mulling

Mulling is actually a continuation of trituration. Although it is a remnant of the old morter-and-pestle trituration technique, the step can still be used following mechanical trituration to improve the homogeneity of the mass and to assure a consistent mix. It can be accomplished in two ways;

1. The mix is enveloped in a dry piece of rubber dam and vigorously rubbed between the first finger and thumb; or the thumb of one hand and palm of another hand. This process should not exceed 2 to 5 seconds.

2. After trituration the pestle (ball) can be removed from the capsule, and the mix triturated in the pestle-free capsule for an additional 2 to 3 seconds. In addition to fulfilling the objectives of mulling, which is homogeneity of the mix, this will also assure cleaning of the capsule walls of remnants of the amalgam mix, thereby delivering the mix in one single, coherent, and consistent mass.

E. Matricing

If a cavity preparation for amalgam involves more than one surface, in order to have the required four surrounding walls and a floor for the amalgam condensation into the cavity, a matrix should be adapted to the tooth. Further details of the procedure are explained in chapter #12.

F. Condensation

Condensation of the amalgam into the cavity preparation is, in effect, a continuation of the trituration process. As such, it serves to complete the objectives of trituration, as well as to encourage the conclusion of the amalgamation.

Condensation squeezes unreacted mercury out of the increments building up the restoration, thereby preventing entrapment of residual mercury as well as the formation of weak matrix crystals. This mercury squeezed to the surface also initiates the binding effect of successive increments. The forces used during condensation bring the strongest phase of the amalgam (the original particles) closer together, and by increasing the percentage composition of these particles, condensation, in effect, boosts the final strength of the restoration. Only efficient condensation can adapt the plastic amalgam mix to cavity walls and margins, assuring retention and minimizing microleakage. This effect is enhanced if condensation force creates elastic deformation of the dentin. In addition to the previously mentioned effect of increasing the percentage of original particles, condensation also reduces the size and number of voids and keeps matrix crystals to minimal dimensions while maximally continuous around the original particles. For amalgam that undergoes a solid state reaction, condensation brings the reactant phases close together (e.g., Ag_3Cu and Sn_7Hg_8) to start the reaction.

Condensation should occur immediately after trituration. Usually only three to three and one-half minutes of condensation time is possible for a given amalgam mix. Further condensation efforts may create cracks in the already formed matrix. These will remain permanently within the restoration, and future fracture, corrosion and leakage failure can be expected. Not only is it impossible to squeeze residual mercury from a mix over 3 minutes old, but such a mix loses sufficient plasticity to prevent adaptation to cavity details. As can be expected, enhanced microleakage and diminished retention of the restoration will result. Because of these problems, amalgam mixes should be discarded after 3.5 min. Large restorations may, in fact, need several mixes to complete them.

Amalgam mixes should be squeezed out of their excessive mercury just before the incremental insertion into the preparation. This is particularly necessary for increasing dryness technique, and may be necessary for 1:1 technique. The squeezing is done in a piece of gauze (squeezing cloth) in a twisting action.

Energy applied in the proper direction and location is the major factor involved in satisfying the objectives of condensation. This energy can be supplied by hand or mechanically. There is evidence to indicate that mechanical condensation is superior in terms of fulfilling the objectives of condensation; consistency of results is at least more predictable using mechanical condensation, especially if the operator builds multiple restorations daily.

Condensers are profivied in different shapes and sizes (Fig. 9), e.g., round, parallelogram, diamond, etc., as well as in various angulations to facilitate access. The face or "nib" of the amalgam condenser should be flat and smooth.

It has been shown that the pressure applied by the condenser nib is inversely proportional to the square of its surface area. Therefore, an equal force will apply more pressure with a smaller condenser than with a larger one. In any event, a force of at least six pounds should be used to condense amalgam or the objectives of condensation will not be completely fulfilled.

All amalgams, with the exception of spherical particle alloy, should be inserted in small increments and condensed with small condensers. This will maximize the elimination of voids and the binding of increments together, as well as facilitate the filling of small details within the cavity preparation. As the surface of the preparation is reached, larger condensers should be used in order to avoid undue pressure on the enamel at the cavosurface. It is wise, if possible, to utilize condensers that conform, in shape, to cavity details.

For non-spherical amalgams, condensation forces should be applied at 45° to walls and floors, i.e., bisecting line angles

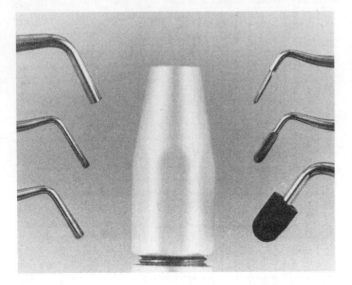

Fig. 4-9

and trisecting point angles (Fig. 10). Subsequent increments should be condensed at 90° to the previous portion to avoid shear forces that may displace the already condensed amalgam. Each portion of amalgam should be condensed from its center to its periphery, in an effort to avoid overlapping or bridging of voids at critical areas. Finally, each portion of amalgam should be condensed until the following features appear:

A concave amalgam surface faces the condenser, indicating the proper angulation and application of force.

The condensed increment is not indented by further condensation efforts, indicating coherence of the mass.

Mercury comes to the surface to prevent trapping it in the restoration and to act as a binder for the next increment in the building of the restoration. Excess mercury or splashy amalgam which appears on the surface should be excavated and discarded before inserting another increment.

The condensation of spherical alloy amalgam differs from the nonspherical ones in two ways:

1. It is necessary to use increments large enough to fill the entire cavity or a large part of the cavity. In this situation the condenser will be acting as a moving roof against amalgam confined within four surrounding walls and floors, with the condenser moving toward the floor.

2. It is necessary to use the largest condenser that will fit the cavity or part of it. This will prevent the lateral escape of the spherical particles during condensation pressure toward the cavity floor (Fig. 11).

These differences in condensation pattern are necessitated by the spherical shape particles which have a tendency to roll over each other. The high wetting ability of most of the component phases and the amalgam mass as a whole will compensate for the less energy used in condensing these types of amalgam.

With either type of amalgam, after completely filling the cavity preparation and covering the cavosurface anatomy, an overdried amalgam mix (made by squeezing off mercury in a squeezing cloth) is condensed heavily over the restoration using the largest condensers possible for the involved tooth. This mix is called the blotting mix. It serves to blot excess mercury from the critical marginal and surface area of the restoration and to adapt amalgam more intimately to the cavosurface anatomy. This mix is excavated and discarded after it achieves these two functions.

Following application of the blotting mix, the matrix should be removed. The condensed amalgam can now be exposed to moisture without any undue harm.

G. Burnishing or surfacing

Immediately after discarding the blotting mix a large rounded burnisher (Fig. 12) is used in light strokes proceeding from the amalgam surface to the tooth surface on the occlusal and other conspicuous portions of the restoration. Inaccessible areas, such as the proximal portion of the restoration, should be similarly burnished using a beaver-tail burnisher and/or Sprately burnisher. This process has four objectives:

1. It is a continuation of condensation, in that it will further reduce the size and number of voids on the critical surface and marginal areas of the amalgam.

2. It brings any excess mercury to the surface, to be discarded during carving.

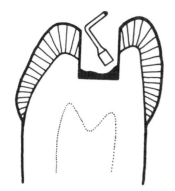

Fig. 4-10. Condensing pattern for non-spherical alloy.

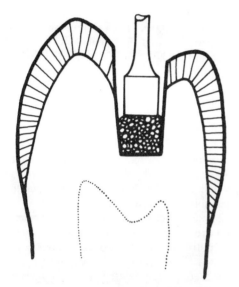

Fig. 4-11. Condensing pattern for spherical alloy.

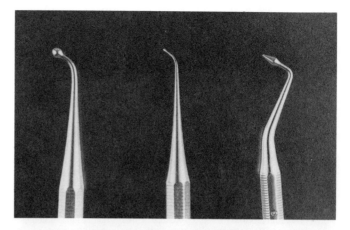

Fig. 4-12. From left to right, two sizes ball burnishers and a cone-shaped one.

3. It will adapt the amalgam further to cavosurface anatomy.

4. It conditions the surface amalgam to the carving step.

If any defect in the amalgam at the margins is discovered at this stage, addition of a fresh mix is indicated, provided the area has not been contaminated by moisture.

H. Carving

Carving is the anatomical sculpturing of the amalgam material. There are eight objectives to this process:

1. To produce a restoration with no underhangs, i.e., all marginal details of the cavity preparation are completely covered with amalgam without any shouldering or shelving of tooth structure there.

2. To produce a restoration with the proper physiological contours.

3. To produce a restoration with minimal flash, i.e., not to the extent of overhangs. Flashes can be easily removed with the finishing and polishing operation.

4. To produce a restoration with functional, non-interfering occlusal anatomy.

5. To produce a restoration with adequate, compatible marginal ridges.

6. To produce a restoration with the proper size, location, extent, and interrelationship of contact areas.

7. To produce a restoration with physiological compatible embrasures.

8. To produce a restoration not interfering in any way with the integrity of the periodontium, enhancing its health and amenable for plaque control.

Amalgam carving should be accomplished using sharp instruments (Fig 13) and with strokes either proceeding from tooth surface to amalgam surface, or laterally, along the tooth-amalgam interface.

After burnishing and before removing the matrix, all accessible embrasures and non-gingival peripheries should be established in the restoration. This is accomplished with a sharp explorer or the lateral edges of a Hollenbeck carver. Not only will this procedure establish the parameters of the future restoration and help prevent fracturing of the condensed mass during matrix removal, but it will also facilitate the discovery of any discrepancies in the amalgam mass. Since the matrix is still in place, these discrepancies can be corrected by adding additional amalgam.

The next step in the carving procedure is to create the triangular fossae, using discoid/cleoid carvers. This, coupled with the previous step, will erect and define the marginal ridges. The matrix is then removed, and the process of margination is begun. This involves the use of discoid carvers, Hollenbeck carvers, or other sharp lateral cutting instruments to remove as much marginal flash of amalgam as possible. With movements from tooth surface to amalgam, this procedure also should "rough in" the outline of the occlusal anatomy. A second burnishing may be performed here if margination exposed voids, either on the surface of the amalgam or at the cavosurface.

If non-proximal axial surfaces are involved in the restoration, they should be carved at this stage. Frequently, matricing fails to reproduce these surfaces adequately, so carving is required to establish physiologic contours both vertically and horizontally. In addition, facial and lingual grooves should now be formulated to correspond in location, dimension, and interrelationship with the involved and opposing tooth. All of this may be accomplished using Hollenbeck carvers, cleoid/discoid carvers, chisels, etc.

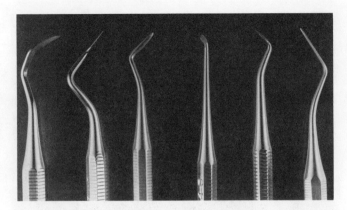

Fig. 4-13. From left to right—Inter-proximal knives (right & left) Hollenback carver, discoid, cleoid & Hollenback carver.

With the occlusal surface parameters having been defined by margination and the establishment of axial contours, the cusp ridges and inclined planes as well as the occlusal fossae and grooves can be carved. Using sharp Hollenbeck carvers or cleoid carvers placed concurrently on amalgam and adjacent occlusal tooth surface, move the instrument laterally, cutting the amalgam while guided by intact tooth. It is also possible to use a sharp binangle hatchet or chisel in direct movements from tooth surface to amalgam to create a predetermined configuration of the occlusal anatomy. All embrasures, fossae, marginal ridges, inclines and grooves may be refined by utilizing the same instruments but in lighter, more rapid cutting strokes.

It is necessary, next, to remove excessive occlusal contacts during centric loading and excursive mandibular movements. To do this, it is preferable to start with an overoccluding restoration which can be carved to the desirable occlusal patterns. It is almost impossible to effectively add amalgam at this stage in an effort to create the desirable occlusion. With a marking ribbon placed between the tooth, guide the mandible to a centric occlusion position, then remove the marked amalgam at verified noncentric stops and relieve any heavy appropriate centric stops. Then, utilizing a different color marking ribbon between the teeth, guide the mandible through excursive movements. Marked areas on the restoration which are inappropriate contacts during these movements should be carved away. Following this procedure, it may be necessary to refine anatomies that have been changed and to round-off the junctions between the different anatomical parts of the restoration.

The final stage of the carving process is a third burnishing or surfacing. This is, perhaps, the most important of the burnishing steps, as it removes scratches and irregularities on the amalgam surface, facilitating easier and more efficient finishing and polishing.

I. Finishing and Polishing

A. Objectives

Unfortunately, finishing and polishing of new amalgam restorations is the most forgotten step in the fabrication of these restorations. It should, in fact, be considered as important as condensation, and it does continue the objectives of carving. Through this process, amalgam flash that was left behind after carving is removed. In addition, major overhangs are removed, and minor enamel underhangs are corrected, thus assuring the continuity between tooth surface and amalgam surface. A further objective of the finishing and polishing procedure is the conversion of the superficial amalgam into a relatively inert layer galvanically. This minimizes electrolytic corrosion which is a normal phenomenon due to the complex, multiphasic nature of amalgam materials.

The most important objective of finishing and polishing is the removal of superficial scratches and irregularities. If this is accomplished properly, it will minimize fatigue failure of the amalgam under the cyclic loading of mastication. This failure occurs in the form of surface cracks which propagate inwards. If such cracks join together, or subsequently connect with internal voids or flaws, they can precipitate gross fracture and increase corrosion and microleakage. The scratch and irregularity free surface layer created by the polishing procedure not only minimizes concentration cell corrosion which could begin in these surface irregularities, but also prevents the adherance of plaque, with all of its sequelae.

B. Principles and procedures for finishing and polishing amalgam restorations

There are multiple, acceptable procedures which fulfill the objectives of finishing and polishing, so this text will concentrate on general principles that can help the operator derive a technique suitable for his own needs.

Usually, 24 hours should pass after amalgam insertion before any finishing and polishing commences. However, some newer alloys can be polished after 8-12 hours; still others require only a 30-minute wait after insertion. For empirical reasons, finishing can be defined as the process which continues the carving objectives, removes flash and overhangs, and corrects minimal enamel underhangs. Polishing, on the other hand, is the process which creates a corrosion resistant layer by removing scratches and irregularities from the surface.

All accessible areas of an amalgam restoration should be finished and polished. The process should begin with the removal of gross overhangs and flash using periodontal files and finishing burs. Care should be taken not to traumatize the periodontium. The movement of these instruments should be precise, with the only objective to see or feel the continuity of the original outline.

The relief in diameter and depth of areas contraindicated for occlusal contact should be the second step in the procedure. These unwanted contacts may have been overlooked during the occlusal adjustment of the carving process. They usually appear as shiny areas in the amalgam.

Removing superficial scratches and irregularities, and the conversion of the surface layer of amalgam to an amorphous nature, are accomplished simultaneously. This is done using descending grade abrasives, either in impregnated rubber mounted stones, or carried to the tooth on rotary brushes or rubber cups. The combination of frictional heat and pressure with these materials achieves the desired results. For contact areas and gingival embrasures, abrasives may be carried on linen polishing strips or dental tape. Very little work should be necessary in these areas; since the amalgam was inserted against a smooth metallic matrix, the contact area and gingival embrasure accommodate few scratches and irregularities.

The final polishing act, i.e., obtaining a metallic lustre, is always done with a polishing agent (e.g., precipitated chalk, tin or zinc oxide) applied with a rubber cup. This lustre will not materialize, however, unless the previous finishing and polishing steps have been accomplished.

One should bear in mind throughout these procedures that overabrading can cause a loss of anatomy or contact or contour. Likewise, too much friction can produce overheating, which may endanger the P-D organ as well as adversely affect the mechanical properties of amalgam, dentin, and enamel.

The Biologic Form of Amalgam Restorations

This text will attempt to explore the "biologic form" not only of each restoration per se, but also of their associated technique. As with all other materials and techniques to be described in this text, the "biologic form" of amalgam will be evaluated through answers to the following questions.

Question 1: Is the amalgam irritant to the pulp-dentin organ?
Answer: Yes.
Question 2: What are the irritating ingredients and characteristics?
Answers:

A. Mercury

Residual mercury, especially in large build-ups requiring the use of high mercury mixes of amalgam, can diffuse from the restoration to the surrounding dentin. Eventually, it can penetrate the pulp tissues via the dentinal tubules. This process of mercury ion migration can be energized or accelerated by galvanic currents, and sometimes thermal or mechanical energy. Such mercury has been reported to poison odontoblasts, subsequently reducing predentin and secondary dentin formation. At the very least, discoloring of involved dentin occurs.

B. Galvanism

These small electrical currents are especially present when dissimilar metal restorations are in contact or in occlusion with amalgam. Galvanism is, in fact, inherent in an amalgam restoration, due to its multi-phased nature and the facts that certain areas will be stressed more than others during condensation, and certain areas on the surface will contain scratches and irregularities even after scrupulous finishing and polishing. Galvanism, per se, has a limited effect on the pulp-dentin organ (unless the restoration is very close to the pulp tissues). The major effect of galvanism is secondary; i.e., it drives corrosion products, mercury, and some salivary ions pulpally, thereby creating interference with the metabolism, and consequently the formative and reparative capacities of the pulp-dentin organ.

C. Thermal conductivity

As with any metal, amalgam has the ability to transmit thermal energy, which can be very detrimental to the dentin and pulp. This effect is especially harmful when the restoration is close to the pulp chamber or root canal system peripheries. In addition to its direct effect, thermal energy can also act secondarily to accelerate the diffusion of irritating ions from the oral environment and restoration toward the pulp.

D. Energy of condensation

The detrimental limits of condensation energy differs not only from individual to individual, but also from tooth to tooth. If the "effective depth" (see below) of the cavity preparation is very limited, excessive condensation can cause a disruption in the paving continuity of the odontoblasts, or aspiration of the odontoblasts or their nuclei into the dentinal tubules. In rare instances, cracking of the dentin bridge can occur. Naturally, all of these irritations will have detrimental effects on the physiology of pulp-dentin organ.

E. Heat of finishing and polishing

During the finishing and polishing of amalgam restoration, the generated frictional heat may be readily transmitted through the restoration to the underlying pulp-dentin organ. Local burn lesions, varying in their extent, are created. Because of the enhanced possibility of bacterial deposition in this burned area through anachoresis, the destructive effect may be magnified, and the reaction of the pulp-dentin organ may be either a reversible or an irreversible pulpitis.

F. Delayed expansion

Moisture contaminated amalgam can create an expansion of such magnitude that it may not always be directed toward the outer surface of the restoration. Axially or pulpally directed expansion will exert tremendous pressure in the pulp-dentin organ. This can precipitate changes in the position and the environment of odontoblasts and surrounding tissues, a situation that may lead to interference with the normal physiologic (reparative) activity of the P-D organ.

G. Corrosion products

These chemical by-products of the corrosive process include tin-oxide, copper-oxide, and silver sulfides. Unfortunately, they are unavoidable in any amalgam restoration, and any factor which enhances corrosion will consequently increase the by-products. All of them are free to migrate toward the pulp tissues if the pulp-dentin organ is left unprotected or if diffusion activity is increased by galvanic and thermal energy.

H. Induced stresses

Micromovement of amalgam restorations can result from, among other things, an ill-designed cavity preparation. If the stresses induced by such movement exceed certain limits or concentrations at thinned areas of the dentin bridge, they may be transmitted to the underlying pulp tissues in a way that would interfere with the natural functions of the P-D organ.

I. Plaque adhesion

Owing to its surface roughness, amalgam is an adherend for bacterial plaque. When this occurs at the tooth-amalgam interface, it can create sufficient toxins to diffuse toward the pulp. In some instances, the resulting irritation is irreversible.

J. Loose restoration

As a result of deficient retention or interfacial failure, loose restoration may pump several environmental irritants into the P-D organ with the expected sequelae.

Question 3: What is the effect of amalgam and amalgam placement procedure at different effective depth?

Answer: The effective depth of a preparation may be defined as the thickness of the bridge of dentin and enamel separating the floor of a cavity preparation at its greatest depth from the contents of the pulp chamber at their highest location. The information that follows has been rounded off to the nearest figure. These figures result from an experiment performed on sound, vital teeth—i.e., they are not subjected to any pathologic process, including decay. No protective bases were used under the amalgam restorations. In applying this data clinically, the reader should consider the irritating factors of cavity preparation as well as preexisting disease, before he attempts to predict the reaction of the pulp-dentin organ to the amalgam procedure:

A. Generally, with an effective depth of 2.5 mm or more, the pulp-dentin organ will respond with a healthy reparative reaction.

B. With an effective depth of 1-2 mm, the P-D organ will usually respond with an unhealthy reparative reaction.

C. With an effective depth of less than 1 mm, the P-D organ will usually undergo destruction.

Question 4: What intermediary base protection should be utilized to promote the biocompatibility of amalgam and the P-D organ?

Answer: Varnishes should be routinely used on all walls and floors of a cavity preparation when there is an effective depth of 2 mm or more. This applies whether this depth is created solely by a dentin bridge, or by a combination of dentin bridge and overlying base. As is mentioned in chapter 13, varnish will not only seal, to some extent, the dentinal tubules, but it will also diminish microleakage around amalgam restorations.

In cavity preparations with effective depths of 1-2 mm, a base of modified ZOE is to be placed in specified locations, followed by generous varnish over all walls and floors.

In cavity preparations with an effective depth of 1 mm or less, and with questionable soundness, diminished reparative capacity or a history of degenerative changes of the P-D organ, a subbase of unmodified ZOE, followed by a base of modified ZOE is indicated. This treatment is also warranted when calcium hydroxide as a subbase is contraindicated. Again, all walls and floors, including the ZOE base, should be covered with varnish.

In cavity preparations with an effective depth of less than 1 mm, and with high probability of a sound P-D organ (no history of degeneration, all clinical and radiographic signs and symptoms indicate adequate reparative capacity), calcium hydroxide cement can be used as a base. Care must be taken, however, not to place calcium hydroxide at an area where tertiary dentin deposition will interface with pulp circulation. In extensive cavity preparations, where calcium hydroxide cement is likely to be subjected to excessive condensation forces, it would behoove the operator to utilize calcium hydroxide as a subbase, to be covered with a base of modified ZOE. Whatever base is used along with surrounding walls and floors should be covered with varnish before amalgam insertion.

BIBLIOGRAPHY

Allan, F.C., Asgar, K., and Peyton, F.A.: Microstructure of dental amalgam. J. Dent. Res. **44**:1002, 1965.

Anderson, L.D.: Mechanical adaptation and condensation of dental amalgams. Iowa Dental Bulletin **40**:130-134, 1954.

Asgar, K.: Amalgam alloy with a single composition behavior similar to Dispersalloy. J. Dent. Res. **53**:60, 1974.

Asgar, K., and Sutfin, L.: Brittle fracture of dental amalgam. J. Dent. Res. **44**:977, 1965.

Black, G.V.: Operative Dentistry, vol. 2. Technical procedures in filling teeth. ed. 4, Chicago, Medico-Dental Publishing Company, p. 329, 1920.

Blackwell, R.E.: G.V. Black's Operative Dentistry. 9th ed. vol 2, p. 287. South Milwaukee: Medicon-Dental Publishing Company.

Caul, H.J., Langton, R., Sweeney, W.T., and Paffenbarger, G.C.: Effect of rate loading, time of trituration and temperature on compressive strength values of dental amalgam. J. Am. Dent. Assoc. **67**:670, 1963.

Chan, K.C., Edie, J.W., and Bayer, D.B.: Microstructure of amalgam surfaces. J. Pros. Dent. **36**:644-648, 1976.

Charbeneau, G.T.: A suggested technique for polishing amalgam restorations. J. Mich. Dent. Association **47**:320-05, 1965.

Craig (Editor): Restorative dental materials. Sixth ed. St. Louis, The C.V. Mosby Co., 1980.

Duperon, D.F., Nevile, M.D., and Kasloff, Z.: Clinical evaluation of corrosion resistance of conventional alloy, spherical-particle alloy and dispersion phase alloy. J. Prosth. Dent. **25**:650-656, 1971.

Eames, W.B.: A clinical view of dental amalgam. Dental Clinics of North America, 20, 385-395, 1976.

Eames, W.B.: Factors influencing the marginal adaptation of amalgam. Journal of the American Dental Association, 75, 629-637, 1967.

Eames, W.B.: Preparation and condensation of amalgam with a low mercury-alloy ratio. J.A.D.A. **58**:78, 1959.

Eames, W.B.: Status report on amalgamators and mercury/alloy preparations and disposable capsules. J.A.D.A. **85:** 1972.

Eames, W.B., and Cohen, K.S.: A dispersed phase amalgam. J. Georgia Dent. Assoc., Spring, 1974.

Eames, W.B., Mack, R.M., and Auvenshine, R.C.: Accuracy or mercury/alloy proportioning systems. J. Amer. Dent. Assoc. **18**:137-141, 1970.

Eames, W.B., and MacNamara, J.F.: Eight high-copper amalgam alloys and six conventional alloys compared. J. Operative Dentistry **1**:98-107, 1976.

Eames, W.B., Tharp, L.G., and Hibbard, E.D.: The effects of saliva contamination on dental amalgam. J.A.D.A. **86**:1973.

Eden, G.T., and Waterstrat, R.M.: Effects of packing pressures on the properties of spherical alloy amalgams. J. Am. Dent. Assoc. **74**:1024, 1967.

Greener, E.H.: Anodic polarization of new dental amalgams. J. Dent. Res. **55**:1142, 1976.

Gronka, P.A., Bobkoskie, R.L., Tomchick, G.J., Bach, F., and Rakow, A.B.: Mercury vapor exposures in dental offices. Journal of the American Dental Association, 81, 923-925, 1970

Gruber, R.G., Skinner, E.W., and Greener, E.H.: Some physical properties of silver-tin amalgams. J. Dent. Res. **46**:497-502, 1967.

Guthrow, C.E., Johnson, C.B., and Lawless, K.B.: Corrosion of dental amalgam and its component phases. J. Dent. Res. **46**:1372, 1967.

Healey, H.J., and Phillips, R.W.: A clinical study of amalgam failures. J. Dent. Res. **28**:439-446, 1949.

Hefferren, J.J.: Mercury surveys of the dental office: equipment, methodology, and philosophy. Journal of the American Dental Association, 89, 902-904, 1974.

Holland, G.A., and Asgar, K.: Some effects on the phases of amalgam induced by corrosion. J. Dent. Res. **53**:1245, 1974.

Hood, J.A.A., and Challis, G.A.: Marginal seal of amalgam restorations. Abstract. J. Dent. Res. **50**:731, 1971.

Innes, D.B.K., and Youdelis, W.V.: Dispersion strengthened amalgam. Journal of the Canadian Dental Association, 29, 105.

Johnson, L.B., and Lawless, K.R.: Corrosion under stress of materials composing dental amalgams. J. Biomed. Mater. Res. 3, 569, 1960.

Jorgensen, K.D.: Adaptability of dental amalgams. Acta Odont. Scand. **23**:257-270, 1965.

Jorgensen, K.D.: Bond strength of repaired amalgam. Acta Odont. Scand. **26**:605-615, 1968.

Jorgensen, K.D.: The mechanism of marginal fracture of amalgam fillings. Acta Odont. Scand. **23**:347-387, 1965.

Jorgensen, K.D., Esbensen, A.L., and Borring-Moller, G.: The effect of porosity and mercury content upon the strength of silver amalgam. Acta Odont. Scand. **24**:535-553, 1966.

Jorgensen, K.D., and Nielsen, M.R.: The influence of the condensation pressure upon crushing strength and mercury content of amalgam. Acta Odont. Scand. **22**:539-545, 1964.

Jorgensen, K.D., and Okuda, R.: Mercury leakage of amalgam capsules. Acta Odont. Scand. **29**:461-469, 1971.

Jorgensen, K.D., Otani, H., and Kanai, S.: The influence of temperature on the crushing strength of dental amalgams. Acta Odont. Scand. **22**:547-556, 1964.

Jorgensen, K.D., and Saito, T.: Structure studies of amalgam - V. The marginal structure of occlusal amalgam fillings. Acta Odont. Scand. **25**:235-246, 1967.

Jorgensen, K.D., and Wakumoto, S.: Occlusal amalgam fillings; marginal defects and secondary caries. Odont. T. **76**:43-54, 1968.

Kanai, S.: Structure studies of amalgam-II. Effect of burnishing on the margins of occlusal amalgam fillings. Acta Odont. Scand., **24**:47-53, 1966.

Kato, S., Okuse, K., and Fusayama, T.: The effect of burnishing on the marginal seal of amalgam restorations. J. Prosth. Dent. **19**:393-398, 1968.

Koran, A., and Asgar, K.: A comparison of amalgams made from a spherical alloy and from a comminuted alloy. J. Am. Dent. Assoc. **75**:912, 1967.

Leinfelder, K.F., Sluder, T.B., Strickland, W.D., and Taylor, D.F.: Two year clinical evaluation of burnished amalgam restorations. AADR Annual Meeting, Las Vegas. June, 1977.

Lind, V., Wennerholm, G., and Nystron, S.: Contact caries in connection with silver amalgam, copper amalgam and silicate fillings. Acta Odont. Scand. **22**:333-341, 1964.

Mahler, D.B.: Microprobe analysis of a dispersant amalgam. Abstracted IADR program and abstract of papers No. 14, 1971.

Mahler, D.B.: Plasticity of amalgam mixes. J. Dent. Res. **46**:708-713, 1967.

Mahler, D.B.: Slow compressive strength of amalgam. J. Dent. Res. **51**:1394, 1972.

Mahler, D.B., Adey, J.D., and Marantz, R.L.: Creep versus microstructure of gamma 2 containing amalgams. J. Dent. Res. **56**:1493, 1977.

Mahler, D.B., Adey, J.D., and Van Eysden, J.: Quantitative microprobe analysis of amalgam. J. Dent. Res. **54**:218-226, 1975.

Mahler, D.B., and Mitchem, J.C.: Effect of precondensation mercury content on the physical properties of amalgam. J. Amer. Dent. Assoc. **71**:593-600, 1965.

Mahler, D.B., and Mitchem, J.C.: Transverse strength of amalgam. J. Dent. Res. **43**:121-130, 1964.

Mahler, D.B., Terkla, L.G., and Reisbick, M.H.: Marginal fracture vs. mechanical properties of amalgam. J. Dent. Res. **49**:1452-1457, 1970.

Mahler, D.B., Terkla, L.G., and Van Eysden, J.: Marginal fracture of amalgam restorations. J. Dent. Res. **52**:832-837, 1973.

Mahler, D.B., Terkla, Vay Eysden, J., and Reisbick, M.H.: Marginal failure vs. mechanical properties of amalgams. J. Dent. Res. **49**:1452-1457, 1970.

Mahler, D.B., Terkla, L.G., Van Eysden, J., and Reisbick, M.H.: Marginal fracture vs. mechanical properties of amalgam. J. Dent. Res. **49**:1452-1457, 1970.

Mahler, D.B., and Van Eysden, J.: Dynamic creep of dental amalgam. J. Dent. Res. **48**:501-508, 1969.

Malhotra, M.L., and Asgar, K.: Physical properties of dental silver-tin amalgams with high and low copper contents. J. Am. Dent. Assoc **96**:444, 1978.

Marek, M., and Hochman, R.F.: In vitro corrosion of dental amalgam phases. J. Biomed. Mater. Res. **10**:789, 1976.

Markley, M.R.: Amalgam restoration distal surfaces of cuspid teeth. North-West Den 31.

Markley, M.R.: Restorations of silver amalgam. J.A.D.A. **43**:133, Aug. 1951.

Marzouk, M.A.: Compressive and tensile strengths of amalgams as governed by particle diameter and interparticle distances. Paper presented in the I.A.D.R. meeting, Washington D.C., March 1973.

Massler, Maury, and Barber, T.K.: Action amalgam on dentin. J.A.D.A. **47**:415 Oct. 1953.

Mateer, R.S., and Reitz, C.C.: Galvanic degradation of amalgam restorations. J. Dent. Res. **51**:1546-1551, 1972.

Mateer, R.S., and Reitz, D.C.: Phase identification and quantitive metallographic procedure for dental amalgams. J. Dent. Res. **50**:551-558, 1971.

Mathewson, A.E., Retzlaff, A.E., and Porter, D.R.: Marginal failure of amalgam in deciduous teeth: a two year report. J.A.D.A., vol. 88, Jan. 1974.

McDonald, R.E., and Phillips, R.W.: Clinical observations on a contracting amalgam alloy. J. Dent. Res. **29**:482-485, 1950.

Moffa, J.: Unpublished data. U.S. Public Health Service.

Mueller, H.J., Greener, E.H., and Crimmins, D.S.: The electrochemical properties of dental amalgam. J. Biomed. Mater. Res. **2**:95, 1968.

Murphy, H.A.: The constitution of the alloys of silver and tin. J. Inst. Metals **35**:107, 1926.

Nadal, R., Phillips, R.W., and Swartz, M.L.: Clinical investigation on the relation of mercury to the amalgam restoration: II. J. Amer. Dent. Assoc. **63**:488-496, 1961.

Nagai, K., Ohashi, M., Habu, H., Makino, K., Usui, T., Matsuo, M., Hawa, M., and Kawamoto, M.: Studies on the tensile strength of dental amalgams by the application of diametral compression test. Part 2. Effects of manipulative variables. J. Nihon Univ. Sch. Dent. **13**:21-26, 1971.

Nagai, K., Ohashi, M., Habu, H., and Hemoto, K.: Study on the initial hardening time of amalgam mix - an analysis of the so-called "setting time of amalgam". Journal of Nihon Univ. School of Dent. 10, 115-135, 1968.

Nagai, K., Ohashi, M., and Hasegawa, K.: Comparative study on the marginal strengths of conventional and spherical amalgam alloys. J. Nihon Univ. School Dent. **9**:49-66, 1967.

Ohashi, M., Ware, A.L., and Docking, A.R.: A comparison of methods for determining setting rate of amalgam. Australian Dental Journal, 20, 176-182, 1975.

Osborne, J.W., et al.: Clinical performance of ten amalgam alloys. J. Dent. Res. **56**: Special issue B, 250, Abstract, 1977.

Osborne, J.W., et al.: Three-year clinical comparison of three amalgam alloy types emphasizing an appraisal of the evaluation methods used. J. Am. Dent. Assoc. **93**:784, 1976.

Osborne, J.W., Phillips, R.W., Crale, E.N., and Binon, P.P.: Three-year clinical comparison of three amalgam alloy types emphasizing an appraisal of the evaluation methods used. J.A.D.A. **93**:984-989, 1976.

Osborne, J.W., Phillips, R.W., Norman, R.D., and Swartz, M.L.: Static creep of certain commercial amalgam alloys. J.A.D.A. **89**:620, 1974.

Phillips, R.W.: Physical properties of amalgam as influenced by the mechanical amalgamator and pneumatic condenser. J.A.D.A., 31, 1308-1323, 1944.

Phillips, R.W.: Skinner's Science of Dental Materials. 7th edition. Philadelphia, W.B. Saunders, 1973.

Phillips, R.W., and Boyd, D.A.: Importance of the mercury-alloy ratio to the amalgam filling. J.A.D.A. **34**:451 April 1, 1947.

Phillips, R.W., Boyd, D.A., Healey, H.J., and Crawford, W.H.: Clinical observations on amalgam with known physical properties, final report. J.A.D.A. **32**:325-330, 1945.

Phillips, R.W., and Swartz, M.L.: Effect of moisture contamination on the compressive strength of amalgam. J.A.D.A. **49**:436, 1954.

Ryge, G., Dickson, G., Smith, D.L., and Schoonover, I.C.: Dental amalgam: the effect of mechanical condensation on some physical properties. J.A.D.A. 45, 269-277.

Ryge, G., Fairhurst, C.W., and Fischer, C.H.: Present knowledge of the mechanism of the setting of dental amalgam. Int. Dent. J. **11**:181-195, 1961.

Sarkar, N.K., and Greener, E.H.: Absence of γ_2 phase in amalgams with high copper concentration. J. Dent. Res. **5**:1511, 1972.

Sarkar, N.K., and Greener, E.H.: Detection and estimation of the gamma 2 phase of dispersalloy by electro-chemical techniques. J. Dent. Res. **51**:1675, 1972.

Schoonover, I.C., Souder, W., and Beall, J.R.: Excessive expansion of dental amalgam. J.A.D.A. **29**:1825, 1942.

Schoonover, I.C., and Souder, Wilmer: Corrosion of dental alloys. J.A.D.A. **28**:1278, Aug. 1941.

Sockwell, C.L., Leinfelder, K.F., and Taylor, D.F.: Two year clinical evaluation of experimental copper additive amalgams. AADR Annual Meeting. Las Vegas. June, 1977.

Svare, C.W., and Chan, K.C.: Effect of surface treatment on the corrodibility of dental amalgam. J. Dent. Res. **51**:44-47, 1972.

Swartz, M.L., and Phillips, R.W.: Residual mercury content of amalgam restorations and its influence on compressive strength. J. Dent. Res. **35**:458-466, 1956.

Taylor, N.O., Sweeney, W.T., Mahler, D.B. and Dinger, E.J.: The effects of variable factors on crushing strengths of dental amalgams. J. Dent. Res. 28, 228-241, 1949.

Teixeira, L.C., and Deneby, G.E.: Burnishing: A technque for improving the amalgam restoration. J. Ind. Dent. Assoc. **55**:14-17, 1976.

Terkla, L.G., Mahler, D.B.: Clinical evaluation of interproximal retention grooves in Class II amalgam cavity design. J. Prosthetic Dent. **17**:596-602, 1967.

Terkla, L.G., Mahler, D.B., and Mitchem, J.C.: Bond strength of repaired amalgam. J. Prosthet. Dent. **11**:942, 1961.

Voth, E.D., Phillips, R.W., and Swartz, M.L.: Thermal diffusion through amalgam and various liners. J. Dent. Res. **45**:1184, 1966.

Wagner, E. Beitvag zur Klarung des Corrosionverhalten der Siberzinn Amalgames. Deutsch Zahnaerztl Z. 17, 99, 1962.

Weaver, R.G., Johnson, B.E., McCune, R.J. and Cvar, J.F.: Three year clinical evaluation of spherical dental amalgam alloy. Int. Assoc. for Dent. Res. Abstracts, 48th General Meeting, p. 115.

Wilson, R.T., Phillips, R.W., and Norman, R.D.: Influence of certain condensation procedures upon the mercury content of amalgam restorations. J. Dent. Res., **36:**458-461, 1957.

Wilson, C.J., and Ryge, G.: Clinical study of dental amalgams. J.A.D.A. **66:**763, 1963.

Wing, G.: Clinical use of spherical particle amalgams. Aust. Dent. J. **15:**185-192, 1970.

Wing, G., and Ryge, G.: Setting reactions of spherical-particle amalgams. J. Dent. Res. **44:**1325, 1965.

Youdelis, W.V.: Dental amalgam. U.S. Patent 3, 305, 356, February, 1967.

Youdelis, W.V., and Innes, D.B.K.: Dispersion hardening of amalgam. IADR, 1962.

Zander, H.A., Glenn, J.F., and Nelson, C.A.: Pulp protection in restorative dentistry. J.A.D.A. **41:**563 Nov. 1950.

CHAPTER 5

Class I cavity preparation for amalgam

By definition, Class I cavity preparations are placed in pit and fissure lesions that occur in one or more of the following locations:

A. Occlusal surfaces of molars and premolars
B. Occlusal ⅔ of the buccal and lingual surfaces of molars
C. Lingual surfaces of the upper anterior teeth (usually the central and lateral incisors)
D. Any other unusually located pit or fissure involved with decay

Applications of the General Principles of Cavity Preparation in Class I Lesions:

I. Outline Form

The parameters of this cavity preparation should include all tooth enamel directly attacked by decay (either surface decalcification or actual penetration), all enamel undermined by backward decay, i.e., enamel not supported by sound dentin, all pits and fissures that come in contact with these margins, or grooves coming in contact with these margins if they are not readily cleansable after enameloplasty.

The width of any portion of the Class I cavity (mesio-distally or bucco-lingually) should be at least 1.5 mm. So, if after fulfilling all of the above mentioned parameters, there results a cavity width less than 1.5 mm, it is imperative to extend the cavity to that dimension.

Pulpally and axially, the preparation should be deep enough to accommodate at least a 1.5 mm bulk of amalgam in all locations. The pupal and/or axial surface of the restoration should seat on dentin in order to avoid sensitivity at the dentino-enamel junction. Usually, by having the cavity depth at 1.5 mm in cross-section, the restoration will be seated on dentin pupally and axially. However, occasions do arise when the enamel will be thicker than 1.5 mm. In these cases, if removal of all enamel substance directly attacked by the decay and the establishment of a 1.5 mm depth still results in sound enamel on the axial or pulpal floor, it may remain intact, provided it is not at the DEJ and is not undermined by backward decay (Fig. 1).

As the tip of the caries cone in dentin has a tendency to penetrate deeper than the sides and base of the cone, it is not unusual for the tip of this cone to extend deeper than the 1.5 mm required depth. In this case, prepare the pulpal floor and axial wall in *different* levels, i.e., one level at the tip of

the caries cone and another level at 1.5 mm from the surface. If there are several caries cones in the same cavity (multiple pits), each cone area will have a different pulpal or axial termination level within the preparation. In other words, there may be more than two levels for the pulpal floor and axial walls (Fig. 2).

The cavity margins, occlusally, should be located on smooth surfaces, inclined planes of cusps, marginal ridges, and crossing ridges. Sometimes, further occlusal extension including more of these inclined planes is necessary in order for the margins to be in more cleansable locations, e.g., closer to the cusp tips and ridge crests. This situation occurs when there are localized or generalized problems in plaque control, e.g., with third molars, or erupting teeth, or with a generally high caries index.

The margins of the facial and lingual Class I lesions must involve the entire facial or lingual groove in order to avoid feather-edged marginal amalgam. If the gingival margin can

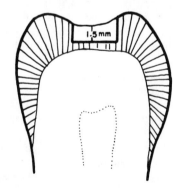

Fig. 5-1

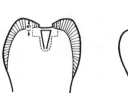 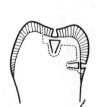

Fig. 5-2. As the caries cone in dentin deepens the cavity more than 1.5 mm pulpally or axially, different levelled-pulpal floors and axial walls are prepared.

be located at or occlusal to the height of contour, facially or lingually, that would be the ideal and desirable location. However, if these margins extend gingival to the height of contour, they should be handled as gingival margins are in Class II cavity preparations. The mesial and distal margins for the cavity preparation of the facial or lingual lesions may be located anywhere that fulfills the requirements for extension as mentioned previously.

Class I cavity preparations are seldom extended for convenience or retention reasons, as fulfilling the basic requirements for the outline form will sufficiently satisfy these purposes. However, if a facial or lingual cusp (or portion thereof) is badly thinned, or if the occlusal margin of the preparation reaches the tip of the cusp, reduce the height of part or all of cusp, thereby bringing some of the occlusal margins of the cavity preparation onto the facial or lingual surfaces. In so far as it is practically possible, the margins of the cavity preparations should not be in contact with opposing teeth in either centric or non-centric movements.

II. The Mechanical Problems in Class I Restorations and Their Solutions

A. All Class I cavity preparations will have a mortise shape, i.e., each wall and floor is in the form of a flat plane, meeting each other at definite line and point angles. This form is commonly applied in various mechanical structures, so its application here is understandable, and will contribute the following:

1. The seat of the restoration is placed at a distinct right angle to the direction of stresses, an ideal condition sought in all mechanical structures.

2. It is advantageous to have a mortise shape preparation in an inverted-cone shape to minimize shear stresses that tend to separate the buccal and lingual cuspal elements, i.e., to prevent the splitting of the tooth. The box-shaped mortise is less advantageous, and the cone-shaped is the least advantageous in this regard. So, whenever the anatomical and cariological factors allow, the cavity preparation should be an inverted cone shape.

3. Amalgam is readily adaptable against the smooth flat-planed surfaces of a mortise shape.

4. A mortise with two or more opposing walls will facilitate the gripping and frictional retention of amalgam in the cavity preparation.

5. A mortise shape is the most accessible type of cavity preparation for instrumentation.

B. When a caries cone penetrates deeply into dentin, removing undermined and decayed tooth structures can lead to a conical (hemispherical in cross-section) cavity preparation. Mechanically, two problems can occur if a restoration is inserted into such a cavity preparation (Fig. 3):

1. If the occlusal loading is applied centrically (Fig. 3A), the restoration may act as a wedge, concentrating forces at the pulpal floor, and leading to dentin bridge cracking, and an increased tendency for tooth splitting.

2. If the occlusal loading is applied eccentrically (Fig. 3C), the restoration will have tendency to rotate laterally, for there would be no lateral locking walls in definite angulation with a floor. Although these lateral movements are microscopic, they occur frequently enough to encourage microleakage

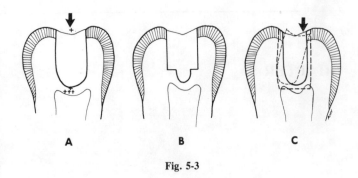

Fig. 5-3

around the restoration, predisposing to a recurrence of decay. These movements can also lead to fracture of marginal tooth structure, and even to splitting of lateral walls.

To solve these problems, *flatten the pulpal end* of the cavity preparation. However, if accomplishing this at a deep location (Fig. 3C) incurs increased risk of involving the pulp chamber, pulp horns, or recessional lines containing remnants of pulp tissues, make the pulpal floor at *more* than one level (Fig. 3B). One level will be the ideal depth level (1.5 mm) and the others will be the caries cone(s) level(s), dictated by the pulpal extent of the decay. The shallow level creates the flat portion of the pulpal floor at definite angles to the surrounding walls, adequately resisting occlusal forces and laterally locking the restoration, without impinging on pulp tissues. Reiterating, the other level(s) is (are) only necessitated by the caries extent, creating one or more concavities or cones in the pulpal floor. The first (ideal depth) level should be as pronounced and circumferentially continuous as possible. At least it should exist at two opposing locations in the cavity preparation in order to fulfill its objectives. This level is sometimes called "the ledge", and it can be circumferential (Fig. 4A), interrupted (Fig. 4B), or opposing (Fig. 4C).

C. When a cavity wall comes in contact with a marginal ridge, the wall should be divergent pulpo-occlusally, making an obtuse angle with the pulpal floor. This design allows for maximum bulk of tooth structure supporting the marginal ridge (Fig. 5), and avoids undermining of the marginal ridge, creating more mechanical and biological problems.

D. Whenever a cavity wall comes in contact with a crossing ridge, make the wall perpendicular to the pulpal floor, rather than diverging it. This is because there is more bulk of tooth structure in the crossing ridge than in the marginal ridge, yet, not enough to allow an acute angle with the pulpal floor (inverted truncated cone) without undermining the ridge (Fig. 5).

E. If cariogenic conditions do not dictate otherwise, the width of the cavity should be limited to ¼-⅓ the intercuspal distance (not less than 1.5 mm). This minimizes loss of tooth structure in this critical cross-section of the tooth. This width will also facilitate easy carving of the restoration, and minimize the possibilities of occlusal interferences.

F. The crossing ridges, whether they are oblique or transverse, should be preserved, i.e., no effort is made to include them in the cavity preparation, unless they are undermined by backward decay, crossed by a fissure, or their enamel is directly attacked by a penetrating lesion. Loss or involvement of such crossing ridges is often more detrimental for the tooth than loss or involvement of a marginal ridge.

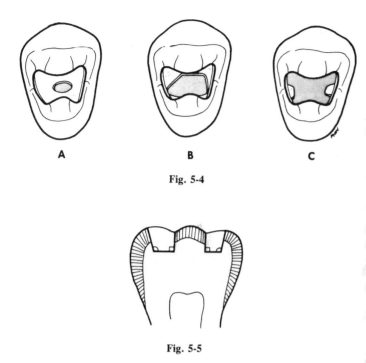

Fig. 5-4

Fig. 5-5

G. If the cariogenic and anatomical structures of the lesion and the tooth demand divergent walls around the cusps pulpo-occlusally, it is advisable to prepare at least the pulpal half of these walls perpendicular to the pulpal floor, creating a boxed-up relationship there, and to prepare the rest of the wall (the occlusal half or less) in the usual divergent configurations. This design modification will improve the resistance and retention forms.

H. Whenever the occlusal margins of the cavity preparation come very close to, or in contact with, the cusp tips, thinning them to the extent that they cannot be self-resistant, it is advisable to flatten these cusps creating a "table", with a minimum clearance of 1.5 mm from opposing teeth during centric and excursive occlusal contacts. This "table" does not have to involve the entire cusp; instead, it can be localized to the thinnest portion or portions of the cusp.

I. When it becomes necessary to cross a marginal ridge facially or lingually, the following rules should be observed:

1. Preserve the minimum mesio-distal width in the area being crossed, dictated either by the cariogenic factors or the ideal 1.5 mm, whichever is less.

2. If the crossing will isolate a small cusp from the rest of the tooth (e.g., the distal cusp in a facial extension of a lower first molar), an elevation in the pulpal floor at the crossing isthmus is advisable. This design modification will avoid isolating the small cusp from the rest of the tooth, and thereby preserve some of its self-resistance.

3. If possible, facial and lingual extensions should be in the form of a step, with a slanting axial wall, rounded axio-pulpal line angle, and retentive grooves at the expense of the mesial and/or distal dentinal walls.

J. In very deep occlusal lesions that also involve facial or lingual extensions, where the tip of the occlusal caries cone is more apical than the gingival periphery of the cavity prepa-

ration facially or lingually, we should not remove the intervening dentin wall. Instead, it is preserved between the occlusal and facial or lingual parts of the preparation, creating an occlusally stepped facial or lingual extension. Sometimes, leaving this wall will lead to a two-stepped extension, first occlusally, then gingivally, or it could lead to a no step facial or lingual extension (Fig. 19). These produce a more retentive and conservative cavity preparation.

K. Whenever cariogenic and anatomical factors dictate diverging the mesial, distal and gingival walls of the facial or lingual portions of the cavity preparation (e.g., when the mesial and distal margin are located on the convex part of the surface, and gingival margin is located in the gingival third of the surface), make two planes for each wall. The first plane is an internal "boxed-up" plane, i.e., perpendicular to the axial wall. The second, or external plane, is made with the ideal divergence. These two planes will avoid losing resistance and retention that would certainly occur with only divergence of the wall (see explanation with Fig. 6).

L. All cavosurface angles should be right-angled to create a butt-joint with the marginal amalgam. This configuration allows marginal amalgam to withstand stresses with the least possibility of failure (see explanation with Fig. 7). Generally speaking, when a cavity wall or its external plane follows the direction of the enamel rods, this right-angled configuration occurs, providing, of course, the amalgam restoration is not under- or overcarved.

M. All line and point angles, or any junction between different details in the cavity preparation, should be rounded but definite (Fig. 8B). This design has all the advantages of the mortise shape, while avoiding stress concentration in the tooth structure and restorative materials that may occur from sharp angulations (Fig. 8A).

N. If the general shape of the cavity preparation is not conducive to adequate retention of a restoration, it is necessary to resort to internal retentive modes, as described in Class I design 5.

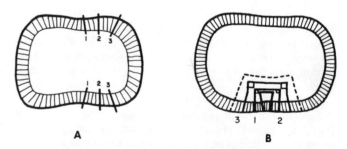

Fig. 5-6. If cariogenic conditions dictate putting the mesial and/or distal margins of a facial or lingual extension at position #1, following the direction of enamel rods, will create convergent walls axiofacially or lingually, which are self-resistant and retentive. If the same conditions dictate putting these margins at position #2, the mesial and distal walls there will be perpendicular to the axial wall, if prepared to conform with the direction of the enamel rods. In this case they will be self-resistant and fairly retentive. If the same cariogenic conditions dictate putting these margins at position #3, following the direction of the enamel rods in creating the mesial and distal walls will make a nonretentive preparation there (dotted lines). So the mesial and distal walls should be made in two planes, an internal boxed-up retaining portion and an outer plane going with the direction of the enamel rods.

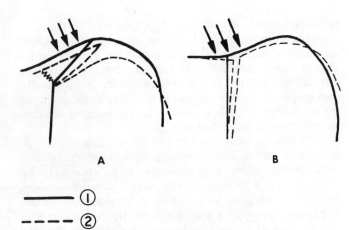

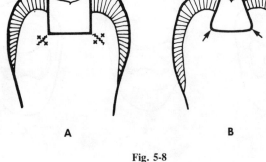

Fig. 5-8

Fig. 5-7. A, Occluding forces will tend to move marginal amalgam and tooth structures from position #1 to position #2. As vital tooth structures are more deformable than set amalgam, the displacement will not be equal thereby creating a gap between them. This places the marginal amalgam under intolerable tensile loading which may lead to amalgam failure if the amalgam is in thin cross-sections, i.e. acute-angled marginal amalgam will fracture. **B,** If marginal amalgam is right-angled, it can stand induced stresses from occlusal loading with less possibility of failure, even if the stresses are tensile in nature.

CLASS I AMALGAM
DESIGN I
lower right molar

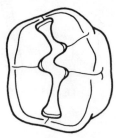

Fig. 5-9

Designs of Cavity Preparations

A. Class I, Design 1

Location: Occlusal surfaces of molars and premolars

1. Indications

a. The caries cone penetration into dentin does not exceed 0.5 mm-1 mm.

b. The involvement of both enamel directly attacked by decay or enamel undermined by backward decay, as well as all pits and fissures, will not widen the preparation more than one-fourth the intercuspal distance.

c. The patient has good oral hygiene and a low caries index.

d. This design is used in areas of the mouth with low cariogenic activity. For example, third molars and, occasionally, second molars, would be poor candidates for this design. Occasionally, however, this design is used as a prophylactic measure in defective pits and fissures in highly cariogenic situations.

2. General shape (Fig. 9)

The shape of this preparation varies from one tooth to another in accordance with specific occlusal anatomy, the application of aforementioned principles, and the extent of the lesion.

a. Premolars

In upper premolars these preparations are always "dumb-bell"-shaped with their ends somewhat triangular. In lower premolars, if they are confined to the pit only, the preparations are circular, resembling snake eyes. If, in lower premolars, they involve the entire occlusal surface, they will resemble the upper design, except that the mesial end of the dumb-bell in the lower first premolar will be more linear. In tricuspid lower premolars, the preparation will assume Y-shape with two of the arms of the Y ending in a triangular cavity.

b. Molars

Preparations in lower first molars (Fig. 9) and occasionally lower third molars will have an elongated shape mesio-distally, with three lateral extensions, two buccal and one lingual, corresponding to the primary grooves.

Preparations in the lower second molar and sometimes the lower third molars will have an elongated shape with two lateral projections, usually opposite one another, corresponding to the primary grooves. In upper molars, if the cavity involves all of the occlual surface, the preparation will be elongated, mesio-distally, with lateral projections not opposite one another. If the oblique ridge is not crossed, the mesial cavity preparation will assume a "kidney" shape, while the distal cavity preparation will assume a "heart" shape. In upper third molars with three cusps, the cavity will assume a T- or a Y-shape.

These above mentioned shapes are generalizations and no cavity preparations will assume these shapes exactly. They can be modified according to anatomical and cariogenic considerations.

3. Location of margins

a. Adjacent to ridges (marginal or crossing)

Whether located mesially or distally, buccally or lingually, any margin located next to a marginal or crossing ridge, should be placed on the inclined plane of that ridge, between the crest of the ridge and the adjacent pit or fossa (Fig. 10A).

b. Adjacent to cusps

Any margin near a cusp, whether is located mesially, distally, buccally, or lingually, should be placed on the inclined planes of that cusp between its tip and the nearby occlusal pit, fissure or groove. The mesio-distal and bucco-lingual widths of the isthmi between cusps will not exceed ¼ of the mesio-

CLASS I AMALGAM
DESIGN I
upper bicuspid

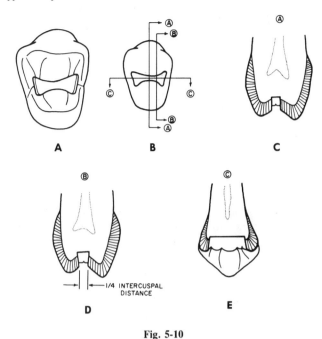

Fig. 5-10

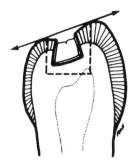

Fig. 5-11

distal or bucco-lingual intercuspal distance (Fig. 10A).

Margins should join each other in a very rounded fashion and should be in the form of sweeping curves at the base of the cusps and crossing ridges (Fig. 10A).

4. Internal anatomy (Fig. 10 C, D, and E)

a. Pulpal floor

This portion of the preparation is usually located in dentin, 0.2-0.5 mm from the dentino-enamel junction. It should be flat-planed and at a right angle to the long axis of the tooth. The only exception is the pulpal floor in the lower first premolar, where the lingual cusp is very small and the buccal cusp is very pronounced with a very large pulp horn. Creating a flat pulpal floor at a right angle to the long axis of this tooth would jeopardize both the minute lingual cusp and the buccal pulp horn (dotted outline, Fig. 11). So, in this case the floor is prepared in a flat plane, parallel to an imaginary line joining the tips of the buccal and the lingual cusp (continuous outline, Fig. 11).

b. Mesio-distal cross-section (Fig. 10E)

This cross-section should facilitate visualization of wall angulations in a mesial or distal direction. If the mesial and distal margins come in contact with a marginal ridge, the walls will be divergent, pulp-occlusally, forming a slightly obtuse angle with the pulpal floor. If any of these margins come in contact with a crossing ridge, the walls should be perpendicular, pulpo-occlusally, forming a right angle with the pulpal floor.

c. Bucco-lingual cross-section

This cross-section serves to facilitate visualization of wall angulations in a bucco-lingual direction. The area of the cavity preparation around each cusp will have its buccal and lingual walls in one of three angulations:

i. In the middle one-third of the cusp (Fig. 10C)

The buccal and lingual walls will be parallel to each other and perpendicular to the pulpal floor, to avoid encroaching on the pulp horn or recessional line without sacrificing resistance and retention form.

ii. In the mesial and distal one-third of the cusp (Fig. 10D).

Here, the buccal and lingual walls will be slightly convergent pulpo-occlusally, following the direction of the enamel rods, making a slightly acute angulation with the pulpal floor (75-85°). This cross-section constitutes the major parts of the cavity preparation walls, and it demonstrates the main retention feature of the preparation.

d. Buccal and lingual walls in contact with buccal or lingual marginal ridges

In molars, as the preparation extends buccally and lingually to incorporate the buccal and lingual primary grooves, the wall of the preparation frequently comes in contact with the buccal or lingual marginal ridge. If this occurs, the wall at the point should be diverged pulpoocclusally to support the marginal ridge in that area.

All walls should be devoid of any unsupported enamel rods marginally and of course all line and point angles should be rounded, but definite.

5. Cavity preparation instrumentation for Class I, Design 1

a. Prerequisites

The operator should be able to understand and visualize the general shape, location of margins and internal anatomy of this design in every tooth in the arch. A rubber dam must be applied properly. The proper tray set-up must be at the work area. Pain control measures should have been properly applied to the patient. The patient must be properly positioned, relative to the operator and the assistant.

b. Procedures

i. Gaining access

If the decay is backward, with a sizable dentinal caries cone, access to the lesion can be gained by cleaving the undermined enamel with direct cutting using a suitably sized hatchet, bin-angle chisel, or Wedelstaedt chisel (Fig. 12A). However, if the decay is still forward, access must be gained by preparing a "well", using a ¼ to a ½ round bur with pulpal pressure. The depth of the "well" should be less than the pulpal depth of the future cavity preparation (Fig. 12B and 12C).

ii. Gross removal (Fig. 12)

Using a 699 bur, loosely seated in the previously created "well", or access cavity (Fig. 12D), apply lateral pressure and occlusal dragging. Incorporate all pits and fissures and involve any indicated sound tooth structure in the cavity prep-

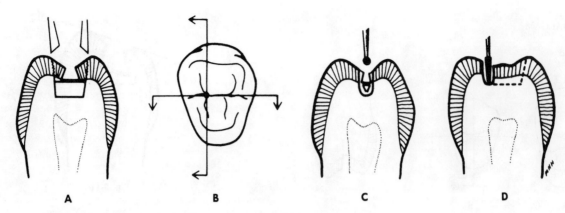

Fig. 5-12

aration at the established "well" depth. Always stop short of the previously determined location of the preparation peripheries.

iii. Removal of irreparably attacked dentin

Using the proper size spoon excavator, follow the procedures mentioned in Chapter I to remove the remainder of this type of dentin.

iv. Preliminary shaping

Using a 699 bur in lateral cutting strokes, establish the indicated angulation of the surrounding walls. The tip of the bur will grossly create point and line angles, pulpally.

v. Final shaping.

Using an 8-9 hatchet, a 10-11 hatchet or a binangle chisel, in a direct cutting action pulpally, plane all surrounding walls, establishing proper wall angulations and definite line and point angles.

Then, using an 8-9 hatchet or monangle hoe or chisel in lateral cutting actions scraping, flatten and smooth the pulpal floor, further defining the line and point angles.

vi. Cavity finish

With a Wedelstaedt chisel, using direct cutting actions parallel to the margins, trim away frail or undermined enamel, and establish a right-angled cavosurface.

vii. Intermediary basing

As indicated. See chapter on intermediary basing.

B. Class I, Design 2

Location: Occlusal surfaces of molars and premolars

1. Indications

a. The caries cones in dentin extend 1 mm or more from the dentino-enamel junction at one or more points.

b. The preparation involvement of the occlusal surface, due to cariogenic and anatomical considerations, and as a result of applying the principles of extension for prevention, is more than ¼ the intercuspal distance.

c. It is used as a preventive measure for lesions otherwise indicated for Design 1, but in patients with high plaque and caries indices.

d. It is used for teeth with intact cusps, i.e., cusps not undermined by backward decay.

2. General shape (Fig. 13)

The shapes of this preparation are similar to those of Design 1, except there are more deviations from the generalized shapes

previously mentioned. Also, there will be a less curved outline, and greater surface dimensions for these cavity preparations than for Design 1 preparations.

3. Location of margins (Fig. 14A)

Margin locations are also similar to those for Design 1; however, Design 2 margins are closer to cusp tips and crests of the ridges than Design 1 margins.

4. Internal anatomy (Fig. 14C)

In Design 2 preparations, the pulpal floor will probably have different levels: one (some) is (are) established by the penetration of the caries cones, and will have a concave shape; another, the main (ideal) level, which should be flat, is approximately 0.2-0.5 mm from the DEJ. As mentioned before, the latter level should consist of circumferential, interrupted, or opposing ledges.

a. Mesio-distal cross-section

This cross-section again serves to visualize wall angulations in the mesial-distal direction. In all instances the mesial and distal walls' angulations will be exactly as described for Design 1.

b. Bucco-lingual cross-section

This cross section serves to facilitate visualization and description of wall angulations in the bucco-lingual direction. At areas of the cavity preparation around the cusps, try to create the same anatomy for the buccal and lingual walls as described for Design 1. However, due to the lateral extent of these lesions, and in keeping with our effort to conform to the direction of the enamel rods, most of the buccal and lingual walls will be parallel to the long axis of the tooth crown making a right angle with the adjacent ledge portion of the pulpal floor (Fig. 14C). When the cavity margin is located in the occlusal third of the inclined planes of the cusps, the corresponding buccal or lingual cavity walls will have two planes—one perpendicular to the ledge portion of the pulpal floor and formed completely of dentin, and another plane following the direction of the enamel rods, i.e., diverging occlusally and formed of enamel supported by dentin (Fig. 15). By this design modification, it is possible to maintain the resistance and retention properties of the cavity walls while avoiding compromising the enamel and cavosurface integrity of those walls. The buccal and lingual walls adjacent to the facial and lingual marginal ridges should have the same divergent anatomy as described for Design 1.

5. Cavity preparation instrumentation

CLASS I AMALGAM
DESIGN 2
upper right molar

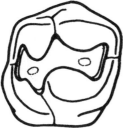

Fig. 5-13

CLASS I AMALGAM
DESIGN 2
upper bicuspid

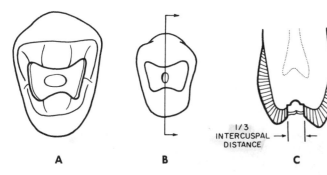

A   B   C

Fig. 5-14

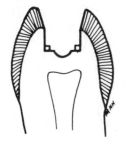

Fig. 5-15

Prerequisites and procedures are similar to those described for design 1, except that gaining access is usually done through removal of undermined enamel by hand instruments. The caries cone levels of the pulpal floor are usually created using excavators, and the ledge level is formed primarily with the 699 bur.

C. Class I, Design 3

Location: In the occlusal one- to two-thirds of the facial and lingual surfaces of molars and on the lingual surfaces of upper anterior teeth, usually the lateral incisors

  1. Indications

  a. A pit or fissure in the aforementioned location is decayed.

b. It is used to eradicate a pit or fissure in the aforementioned location as a prophylactic measure in decay-susceptible situations.

c. The involved pit in this location is not connected with other surface(s) or lesions in the tooth, either externally—via a fissure or enamel lesion, or internally—by backward decay or a dentinal cone.

d. It is used for invaginated teeth where the invagination does not reach the periapical region, periodontium or root canals. (Type one and two invaginations.)

  2. General shape (Fig. 16A)

The location in which this lesion occurs is usually self-cleansable. It is only necessary, therefore, to remove the decayed enamel and dentin and any undermined enamel. The resultant shape will be the cavity outline. Usually it is rounded, but it can also be triangular, oblong, etc.

  3. Location of margins (Fig. 16A)

Again, because the areas in which these lesions are located are naturally self-cleansable, the margin can occur anywhere that is dictated by removal of the affected tooth structure, i.e., extension for prevention need not be observed.

  4. Internal anatomy (Fig. 16C)

There will be no differentiation between the surrounding walls of this design; i.e., all walls are joined together in a seemingly continuous fashion. The axial wall should be flat and make a definite acute angle with this continuous surrounding wall. Usually this convergence of the surrounding walls from the axial wall (acute angulation at the junction between axial wall and surrounding wall) will be in the same direction as the enamel rods. If it is not, the surrounding wall, or the part of it that is not conforming to enamel rod direction, should be made in two planes—one making this retentive, acute-angulation relationship, and the other following the direction of the enamel rods. In any event, following the direction of the enamel rods will create the proper cavosurface angulation.

It is a good idea to carefully examine Class I carious lesions on the lingual surface of upper anterior teeth as 0.04% to 10% of these lesions are surface indications of an invaginated tooth (Dense-in-dent). Restoring the superficial lesion could leave a patent space within the tooth susceptible to leakage and decay recurrence. If discovered invaginations proved to be not continuous with the periapex, periodontal ligament or the root canal system, the invagination should be prepared to accommodate amalgam as an obturator and a restoration. The tooth

CLASS I AMALGAM
DESIGN 3
upper molar

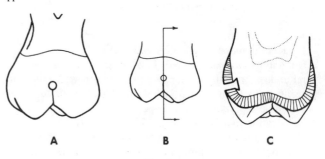

A   B   C

Fig. 5-16

preparation will have the same features as mentioned in the above description except the walls of the preparation could be more convergent and irregular according to the anatomy of the invagination. Also, the surrounding walls could be formed of enamel, if it is not attacked by decay. It should be clear that any invagination within a tooth should be obliterated to avoid eventual devitalization of the tooth.

5. Cavity Preparation Instrumentation

a. Prerequisites

These are the same as Design 1.

b. Procedures

i. Gaining access and gross removal is accomplished using a ¼-½ round bur placed in the involved pit, exerting pressure at a right angle to the tooth surface, and with lateral dragging, removing tooth structure within the proposed outline of the preparation.

ii. Removal of attacked irreparable dentin is accomplished with a spoon or discoid excavator. For invaginated lesion, excavators should have very long shanks.

ii. Preliminary shaping is completed using a 33¼ inverted cone bur with light lateral pressure. For preparations within invaginations one may use Gaites-Glidden or pesso-reamers.

iv. Final shaping is accomplished using an angle former, moving the blade point into the line angle and the side of the blade along the surrounding walls, thereby defining the line angles and smoothing the walls. Next, use an 8-9 hatchet, in lateral cutting strokes, to flatten and smooth the axial wall.

v. For deep and invaginated lesions, gingival margin trimmers can be used in this step.

vi. Cavity finish

Use a Wedelstaedt chisel, with direct cutting action, parallel to the margins to trim away frail or undermined enamel at the cavosurface area.

vii. Intermediary basing

Accomplished as indicated in a chapter on intermediary basing.

D. Class I, Design 4

Location: This design is applied in molars where in addition to involving their occlusal surfaces, the grooved part of the facial and/or lingual surfaces is also involved.

1. Indications

a. Caries lesions at the facial or lingual pits are connected to the occlusal surface or lesion through a fissure, enamel decay, or backward decay.

b. Decay undermines the facial or lingual marginal ridges, or thins them so they cannot be self-resistant.

c. Caries cones, facially or lingually, are confined to the concavity of their corresponding grooves.

d. Surrounding cusps are not undermined or thinned by backward decay.

2. General shape (Figs. 17A and 18A)

This cavity preparation will have an occlusal as well as a facial and/or lingual part; the occlusal portion will appear the same as in Designs 1 or 2, while the facial or lingual parts will assume a parallelogram shape.

3. Location of margins (Figs. 17A and 18A)

The margins of the occlusal part of the cavity preparation will be located at the same sites as described for Designs 1 or 2. The mesial and distal margins of the facial and lingual parts

CLASS I AMALGAM
DESIGN 4
lower right molar

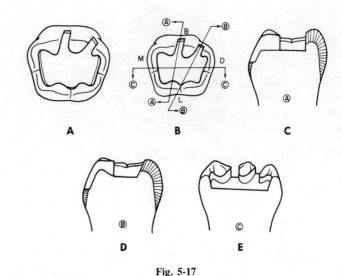

Fig. 5-17

CLASS I AMALGAM
DESIGN 4
upper right molar

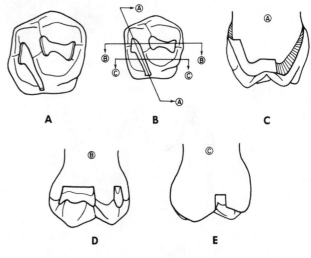

Fig. 5-18

of the preparation will be located on the corresponding surface. In these portions of the preparation, they must be separated from each other by at least 1.5 mm. In addition, they must involve all decayed tooth structure, as well as include all the respective pits, fissures and grooves. There would, of course, be no need for further extension since the surrounding area is self-cleansable.

The gingival margin should extend to include the involved pits, fissures and grooves, as well as the decayed tooth structure. If this puts the margin at, or occlusal to, the height of contour, no modification is indicated. If, on the other hand, the gingival margin ends up apical to the height of contour, it should be treated in the same way as the gingival margin of class II cavity preparation (next chapter).

4. Internal anatomy

a. Mesio-distal cross section

The cavity preparation anatomy in a mesio-distal cross-section through the occlusal part is very similar to the same section in Designs 1 or 2. The facial and lingual wall angulations of the occlusal part are the same as in Designs 1 or 2. Visualizing the cross-section through the facial and/or lingual extension, the axial wall will be flat mesio-distally. The mesial and distal walls of the extension are perpendicular to the axial wall. Each wall is always perfectly one-planed and flat.

If it is necessary to improve the self-retention of the facial or lingual part of this cavity preparation, cut a groove in the dentinal part of the mesial and/or distal wall, not exceeding ½ mm in depth, and not passing the pulpal floor occlusally. This groove should not undermine enamel occlusally, nor undermine or encroach on the axial angle of the tooth. Neither should this retention groove interfere with the pulp anatomy. In any of these situations, the mesial and distal walls, or part of them, should have two planes: one forming the wall proper of the groove, and another following the direction of the enamel rods.

b. Bucco-lingual cross-section passing through the facial and/or lingual extension of the cavity preparation (Figs. 17, 18)

This cross-sectional analysis should facilitate visualization of gingival and axial wall angulations. On the intact side of the tooth the buccal or lingual wall will have the same angulation as in Designs 1 or 2.

The pulpal floor may be flat or in different levels, except at an isthmus portion where the prepartion separates a small cusp from the rest of the tooth (e.g., the disto-lingual cusps of upper molars or the distal cusps in lower first molar). At this area, the pulpal floor will assume an occlusal elevation, which will act as a struss, connecting the small cusp with adjacent larger cusps (Figs. 17D and 18C). Also, this elevation in the pulpal floor will prevent this floor from encroaching on the small cusp's pulp horn which is usually mesio-buccally deviated. This is more important in the upper molar than in the lower molar. In addition, in molars where the apical ends of buccal or lingual grooves are frequently on the same level, or occlusal to, the prepared pulpal floor, the facial or lingual extension will have no steps (Fig. 19A) or a "reverse" step in the occlusal direction (Fig. 19B). In certain cases, the caries cone(s) occlusally may be very close to the facial or lingual marginal ridge, putting the deep part of the pulpal floor at the isthmus portion. Here again, a no-step or a "reverse" occlusal step facial or lingual extension is indicated. In many situations an occlusal and a gingival step facially or lingually is required. This produces a self-resistant, fairly pronounced stump of dentin between the occlusal and the facial or lingual portion of the cavity preparation (Fig. 19C).

5. Cavity preparation instrumentation

a. Prerequisites

These are the same as described for previous designs.

b. Procedures

i. Gaining access

This is always from the occlusal in the same manner as described for Design 1.

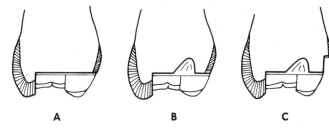

Fig. 5-19

ii. Gross removal

Occlusally, this is accomplished in similar fashion as described for Designs 1 and 2.

For the facial or lingual portion, use the side of #699 bur, while it is in the occlusal cavity preparation, adjacent to the facial (lingual) groove to be involved, and with lateral pressure and occlusal dragging through the surface, traverse the groove to be involved. Be sure to leave a gross elevation in the pulpal floor, if indicated. If the entire buccal or lingual groove is not involved by this cut, apply #699 bur on the groove, and using axial pressure and occlusal dragging, grossly create a facial (lingual) step with an axial wall.

iii. Removal of irreparably attacked dentin

This is accomplished in similar fashion described for Designs 1 and 2.

iv. Preparation of retention grooves

If a mesial retention groove is indicated in the facial or lingual extension, place a ¼ round bur at the mesio-gingivo-axial point angle, pressing mesially and dragging occluso-distally, disengaging the bur just short of the pulpal floor. If a distal retention groove is indicated, place a ¼ round bur at the disto-gingival-axial point angle, pressing distally and dragging occluso-mesially, disengaging the bur just short of the pulpal floor.

v. Preliminary shaping

For the occlusal portion this is accomplished utilizing the same instruments and technique described for Designs 1 or 2. For the facial or lingual portion in an upper tooth, the most efficient instrument is an off-set hatchet used in direct cutting acts apically. This will properly angulate and shape the mesial and distal walls. Then, using lateral cutting acts, shape the gingival and axial walls. For the facial and lingual parts in lower teeth, a hatchet or binangle chisel may be used to shape the mesial, distal, gingival, and axial walls.

vi. Final shaping

The occlusal portion is finished in similar fashion to that described for Designs 1 and 2. The mesial, distal and gingival walls of the facial or lingual extensions are finished with the same instruments used for preliminary shaping, but with more frequent and lighter strokes. The retentive grooves, if prepared, are finally shaped with gingival margin trimmers or pointed-edged off-set hatchets, using the movements as were used with the round bur, or by shaving strokes, occluso-gingivo-proximal. Line and point angles may now be rounded using a hatchet or binangle chisel in lateral cutting acts.

vii. Cavity finish

Internally, this is accomplished with the same instruments as final shaping. On the cavosurface, use a Wedelstaedt chisel in direct cutting actions parallel to the margins to trim away frail or undermined enamel, and to establish a right-angled cavosurface.

viii. Intermediary basing. As indicated. See chapter on intermediary basing.

E. Class I, Design 5

Location: This design is confined to molar teeth, where, in addition to involving part of the occlusal surface, most or all of the facial and/or lingual surfaces are also included in the cavity preparation.

1. Indications

a. Facial or lingual cusps are undermined by backward decay or directly attacked by forward decay, necessitating their total replacement by restorative materials.

b. The outline of the occlusal surface is not conducive to retention of the restoration.

c. The caries cones in dentin exceed 1 mm from the DEJ.

d. A foundation for cast restoration is needed.

2. General shape (Fig. 20A)

The occlusal part will be very similar in appearance to the Class I Design 2 preparations. The facial or lingual part will be parallelogram in shape, but larger than that described for Design 4.

3. Location of margins (Fig. 20A)

The occlusal margins will have locations similar to those described for Class I Design 2 preparations. On the facial or lingual surfaces, the mesial and distal margins will be located at, or near, the corresponding axial angles. The gingival margin will always be located in the gingival third of the facial or lingual surfaces, applying the same rules for gingival margins as for a Class II cavity preparation (next chapter).

4. Internal anatomy

The occlusal portion of these preparations will have similar anatomy to that of Class I, Design 2 (Fig. 20E). However, the pulpal floor will accommodate two internal boxes (Fig. 20E) at the mesial and distal thirds. These are, ideally, at least 2 mm in their width, depth, and length.

a. Mesio-distal cross-section in the facial or lingual extension

This cross-section will enable visualization of wall angulations in a mesial-distal direction (Fig. 20, A and B). At a depth of 0.5 mm from the DEJ, the axial wall should be convex or rounded, following the same curvature as the intact facial or lingual surface. There may be one or more depressions (concavities), corresponding to the tips of the dentinal caries cones, if they exceed the regular (ideal) depth, or any surface concavity on the involved facial or lingual surfaces (grooves, flutes, etc.).

The mesial or distal walls on the facial or lingual surfaces will have two planes: one plane is completely dentinal and makes a right angle with the tangent of the axial wall at the corresponding line angle. The other plane is an outer enamelo-dentin plane, following the direction of the enamel rods mesio- or disto-facially or lingually.

b. Facio-lingual cross-section (Fig. 20, C and D)

This cross-section facilitates visualization and understanding of design features of the axial and gingival walls. The gingival floor should be two-planed (Fig. 20C), i.e., an internal (dentinal) plane at a right angle to the long axis of the tooth, and

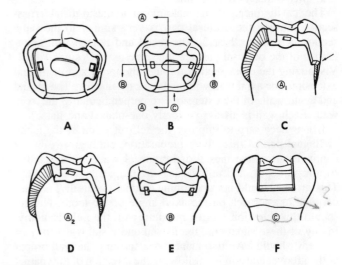

Fig. 5-20. Note in (A)₁ and (A)₂ that the gingival floor will be one- or two-planed depending on the direction of the enamel rods.

an outer (enamelo-dentinal) plane following the direction of the enamel rods. Rarely, it may be one-planed, e.g., (Fig. 20D), if the gingival margin is located at, or occlusal to, the height of contour or anatomical root surface.

The axial wall should slant gingivo-occlusally toward the pulpal floor (see Chapter 6) (Fig. 20, C and D). The axio-pulpal line angle should be very rounded (see Chapter 6) (Fig. 20, C and D). The configuration of the remainder of the cross-section will depend on where it crosses the occlusal part of the cavity preparation, e.g., the internal box area, the caries concavity area, etc.

5. Cavity preparation instrumentation

a. Prerequisites

These are as previously described for Design 1.

b. Procedures

i. Gaining access

This is accomplished in similar fashion to Designs 1 and 2.

ii. Gross removal

Occlusally, this is accomplished in similar fashion as in Designs 1 and 2, with the exception that we use 555 and 556 burs. For the facial or lingual portions, use 555 or 556 burs, in a buccal (lingual) pressure with lateral strokes, eliminating the cuspal elements involved in the preparation. Use the same bur with apical pressure and mesio-distal dragging to form the gingival floor stepping the extension apically. Both of these acts should be accomplished within the future designated outline of the cavity preparation.

iii. Removal of irreparably attacked dentin

This is accomplished in similar fashion as in Designs 1 and 2.

iv. Formation of internal boxes and retention grooves, using a 168 or 169 bur, at the predetermined location of the internal boxes in the pulpal floor, apply pulpal pressure and bucco-lingual dragging to grossly cut the two internal boxes at the expense of the pulpal floor. If mesial and/or distal grooves are indicated in the facial or lingual extensions, prepare them in exactly the same way as in Design 4.

v. Preliminary shaping

Using a 556 bur with lateral cutting, rough in the different planes and angulations for surrounding walls. Then, using a hatchet, with lateral cutting, create the different planes for the cavity floor.

vi. Final shaping

A hatchet, binangle chisel or Wedelstaedt chisel may be used in direct cutting acts to finally shape and make the different angulations or planes of the surrounding walls. Using the same instruments with lateral cutting, flatten, smooth, and shape the different planes of the floors. With a suitable hatchet (8-9) or hoe, with direct cutting, straighten the surrounding walls of the internal boxes. Then, with lateral cutting acts, smooth their floors. Use the hatchet or Wedelstaedt to round the junctions between the different cavity details, especially between the internal boxes and pulpal floor and the axio-pulpal line angles. If mesial or distal retention grooves buccally or lingually were prepared, these may be shaped as described for Design 4.

vii. Cavity finish

Internally, the same instrumentation as used in (vi), but with lighter, more frequent strokes. Externally, with a Wedelstaedt at right angle or parallel to the cavosurface margins, use direct cutting strokes to smooth and finish the cavity periphery, being sure to eliminate any remaining frail enamel.

F. Class I, Design 6

Location: This design of cavity preparation is used when it is necessary to include part of the occlusal surfaces of molars or premolars as well as a portion of the facial, proximal or lingual surface in the form of a "table" of an entire cusp (marginal ridge) or a section of a cusp (marginal ridge).

1. Indications

a. Portions or an entire cusp are undermined by backward decay, or badly thinned by direct decay, necessitating partial or total replacement of the cusp by a restorative material.

b. The cariogenic situation leaves a cusp or part of a cusp with a length to width ratio of 3:1 or more in a functional cusp, or 4:1 or more in a non-functional cusp, and there is no interruption in the continuity of the surrounding walls.

c. The cariogenic situation leaves a cusp or part of a cusp with a length to width ratio of 2 or more on the functional or 3 and more on the non-functional cusp and the continuity of the surrounding walls is interrupted at one part or another.

d. The marginal ridge adjacent to an occlusal preparation is crossed by a fissure to the facial or lingual embrasures (mesial marginal ridges of upper, first premolar, distal marginal ridge or upper second molars).

e. A foundation for a future cast restoration is needed.

f. A Class I occlusal lesion is continuous with a Class VI lesion on the cusp tips or their ridge crests.

2. General shape (Fig. 21)

The occlusal part of this design appears similar to Designs 1 or 2. The facial, proximal, or lingual part of these preparations will be box-shaped.

3. Location of margins (Fig. 21)

The occlusal part of this design resembles Class I, Designs 1 or 2. In the facial or lingual portions, the mesial and distal

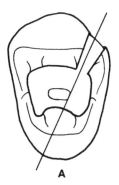
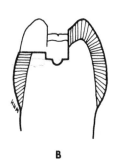

Fig. 5-21

margins are extensive enough to involve the thinned portion of a cusp or to include the adjacent groove if it is in proximity to the occlusal portion. In proximal preparations, the facial or lingual margins will extend sufficiently to involve the fissure crossing the marginal ridge.

The gingival margin should extend far enough to allow occlusal clearance of 1.5-3 mm from the opposing teeth. It should also serve to create a length to width ratio in the remaining part of the cusp or marginal ridge of 1:1. The gingival margin proximally should always be located within the occlusal and facial or lingual embrasures.

4. Internal anatomy (Fig. 21B)

The occlusal part of this design is very similar in appearance to Designs 1 or 2. The facial, proximal, or lingual parts should have a square, flat table in the mesio-distal and bucco-lingual direction. This table could be on the same level of the adjacent pulpal floor or at a different level, either occlusal or gingival to that of the pulpal floor. In the latter instances there will be an occlusal or gingival step from the pulpal floor to the table.

5. Cavity preparation instrumentation

a. Prerequisites

These are as described for previous designs.

b. Procedures

i. Gaining access is similar to that described for previous designs.

ii. Gross removal

The occlusal part is accomplished as in Design 1. The facial, proximal and lingual portions are done using a #555 or #556 bur with facial (lingual or proximal) pressure and dragging.

iii. Removal of irreparably attacked dentin

This is as described for previous designs.

iv. Preliminary shaping

The occlusal part is shaped using the instrumentation and techniques described for previous designs. Then, using a hatchet, binangle chisel or Wedelstaedt chisel in direct and lateral cutting, create the proper angulation and planes for the surrounding walls, the table, and floors.

v. Cavity finish

Internally, use the same instruments as previously used, but in more frequent, gentle strokes to abrade smaller increments of tooth structure. Cavosurface margins are prepared as in previous designs.

vi. Intermediary basing

Apply as in previous designs.

G. Class I, Design 7

Location: This design usually involves the occlusal, facial and/or lingual surfaces of molars and premolars.

Indications:

These are class I lesions with extensive carious involvement. Because of their substantial extent the resulting deficiency of surrounding walls, and, the placement of internal boxes in the floor of the preparation is impossible due to anatomical restrictions. Instead, pins and/or posts are indicated. This design is described in detail in the chapter on ''Pin- and Post-Retained Restorations''.

H. Class I, Design 8

Location: In molars and premolars, this design is used on the occlusal and sometimes on the occlusal and/or facial-lingual surfaces (Fig. 22). It also may be used on the lingual surfaces of anterior teeth (Fig. 23).

1. Indications

These preparations are designed specifically for endodontically treated teeth and they are confined to the occlusal and lingual or buccal surfaces of these teeth. Usually they are simply the access opening for the root canal therapy, or as preparation for final restoration of invaginated teeth, where the invagination has involved the periodontium, apical tissues, or the root canal system.

2. Location of margins (Fig. 22 and 23)

Depending on the extent of the endodontic access opening, and on the caries or invagination involvement, margins of these preparations should be lcoated in finishable, cleansable and supported areas as in the previous designs.

3. Design features of Class I cavity preparations for amalgam in endodontically treated teeth

For Design 8 cavities, the entire pulp chamber should be cleansed of any temporary cement or root canal filling material. The pulp chamber is the main retention form, especially if it is bulky as it usually is in molars (Figs. 22C and 23).

In these preparations, any pulpal floor not having a pulp chamber apical to it should be kept intact and as flat as possible (Fig. 22B). All thinned cusps should be tabled as described for design 6. Facial and/or lingual extensions of the preparation should have flat, pronounced gingival floors or tables. Bulky walls of the pulp chamber should accomodate a ledge, preferably a continuous one, but at least two opposing areas of ledging (Fig. 22C and D). All of these features serve to eliminate excessive loading to the subpulpal floor.

If these features are not present or if retention is insufficient for the magnitude of predictable forces, it will be necessary to intentionally extend the preparation buccally and/or lingually across the corresponding grooves, being sure to provide a gingival floor in these extensions. Also, in these situations, it is helpful to prepare ledges at the expense of the cusps, facially and lingually, or to intentionally cap portions of the facial or lingual cusps. Of course, marginal and crossing ridges should be preserved and protected as much as possible by avoiding placing ledges in walls in proximity to these areas. As usual,

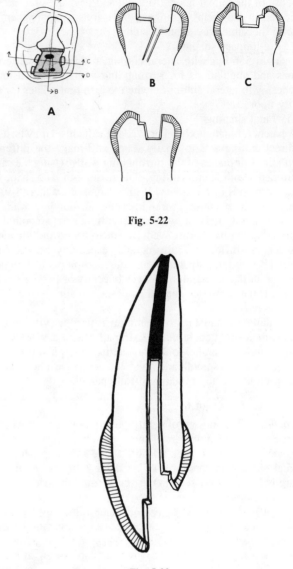

Fig. 5-22

Fig. 5-23

when margins come in contact with a facial or lingual groove, it is necessary to include the entire groove, preferably with a ''step'' in the cavity preparation.

4. Instrumentation for Class I, Design 8 cavity preparation for amalgam

Follow the same procedures in evacuating the pulp chamber and establishing the ledges as Class II, Design 8. Facial and lingual extensions can be done in the same steps as Class I, Designs 4 and 5. Capping the cusps or parts of the cusps can be accomplished using steps as described for Class I, Design 6.

See bibliography at the end of Chapter VII.

CHAPTER 6

Class II cavity preparation for amalgam

By definition, a Class II cavity preparation is the proximal, proximo-facial (lingual), proximo-occlusal (or combination thereof) tooth preparation. It is part of the mechano-therapy for a smooth surface lesion, involving the proximal surfaces of molars and premolars.

Applications of the General Principles of Cavity Preparations to Class II Lesions:

I. Outline Form

The following factors dictate the outline form of the Class II cavity preparations:

A. Proportional size of the caries cones in enamel to that in dentin, and their relative size to that of the uncleansable proximal areas

This may be exemplified by the following situations:

In a lesion of forward decay, in which the diameter of the caries cone in enamel is less than the size of the proximal uncleansable area, the governing factor for the cavity preparation outline is the extent of the uncleansable proximal area (Fig. 1A).

In a lesion of backward decay, in which the caries cone in dentin does not undermine all enamel of the uncleansable proximal surface, the governing factor for the cavity preparation outline form remains the extent of the uncleansable proximal area (Fig. 1B).

In a lesion of backward decay, in which the caries cone in dentin exceeds the size of both the uncleansable area and the undermined enamel in self-cleansable or protected areas, the governing factor for the proximal outline form of the cavity preparation is the extent of the dentinal caries cone (Fig. 1C).

Rarely, one encounters a situation in which the carious lesion is forward and the enamel decalcification is more extensive than the limit of the self-cleansable area. In such a case, the governing factor for the proximal outline of the cavity preparation will be the extent of the base of the cone in enamel (Fig. 1D). Seldom will the three possible governing factors coincide. In such a case a very limited extension of the cavity beyond its caries cone extent may be necessitated for proper finishing of the cavity preparation (Fig. 1E).

B. Extension for convenience or access

For most molars and premolars with proximal lesions, the occlusal surface or part of it should be included in the cavity preparation for access purposes. Seldom is there any other way to approach the lesion, or to formulate and locate the proximal cavity preparation walls and margins. However, there are a few cases in which the proximal lesion can be instrumented and the proximal cavity preparation can be prepared from the facial or lingual embrasures, e.g., a tooth with wide, accessible embrasures and intact marginal ridges (see design 5).

C. Location and condition of the gingiva

As mentioned in Chapter I, the most protected area in the gingival one-third of a proximal surface is that tooth surface

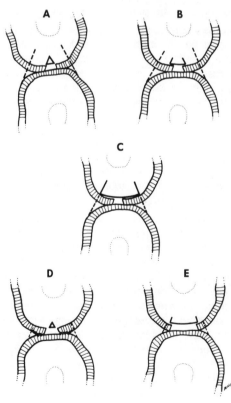

Fig. 6-1

which serves as one of the walls of the gingival crevice. Although placing the gingival margin in that location is difficult to achieve, (and sometimes contraindicated for periodontal reasons) one should try to locate the gingival margin there, especially in young teeth and in patients with high cariogenic activity (Fig. 2A). In other instances locating the margin even with the crest of the free gingiva is acceptable (Fig. 2B). In cases of gingival recession, the gingival margin should be located supragingivally, leaving intact a part of the proximal tooth surface apical to the gingival margin of the restoration. This exposes that margin to the cleaning mechanisms to be utilized by that patient (Fig. 2C). (See chapter on single tooth restoration and the periodontium).

When there is a very pronounced interdental col, it is imperative to avoid impinging on critical periodontal attachments. This is achieved by establishing a gingival floor at three planes in the bucco-lingual direction: a horizontal plane in the middle, corresponding to the bottom of the col, and two inclined planes connecting the flat portion of the gingival floor with the facial and lingual walls (following the same angulation as the descending parts of the col (Fig. 3).

D. Condition of the marginal ridge

If for any reason the proximal surface and carious lesion can be instrumented from the buccal or lingual embrasures, the integrity of the marginal ridge from the occlusal and proximal directions should be evaluated to ascertain whether or not it is undermined by caries. If the marginal ridge is not undermined or involved, a proximal cavity preparation, and even separate proximal and occlusal cavity preparations could be made, with the intact marginal ridge separating them.

E. Convexity of the proximal surfaces

As mentioned before, the more convex the proximal surfaces are, the wider are the embrasures, and the dimension of the contact area is smaller. Consequently, the less will be the required extension of the cavity preparation outline. So, if it is possible to increase the convexity of the contemplated restoration at its occlusal half, beyond the original convexity of the proximal surface, without compromising the periodontium, then one may minimize the extent of the cavity preparation outline.

F. Location and extent of the contact areas and their relation to the marginal ridges, embrasures and gingiva

The purpose of a Class II cavity preparation and restoration should be not only to replace diseased tissues with a suitable substitute, but also to correct local conditions which predisposed or initiated the carious lesion, in the first place. This might avoid a future recurrence of decay in that area. The proper relationship between four anatomical landmarks, i.e., the contact area (location and dimension), the marginal ridges, the embrasures, and the gingiva, is essential to achieve such a basic preventive measure. To establish this relationship in a restoration, the outline of the cavity preparation may need to be modified by overextension in some areas and underextension in others. Consequently, every lesion must be studied carefully and a restorative treatment planned specifically for it.

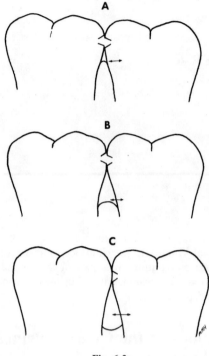

Fig. 6-2

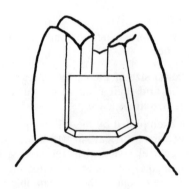

Fig. 6-3

G. Modifying factors influencing outline form

The following factors are to be considered modifying factors for the outline form.

1. Masticatory loads

Generally, the greater the masticatory loading, the less should be the extent of the cavity preparation facially and lingually. This is because a tooth subjected to a functionally physiologic high loading situation is *less* susceptible to decay than a tooth with less loading. In addition, this reduced extênsion should be done in order to decrease the surface area of the restoration that will be subjected to the high loading.

2. Generalized plaque index

The extent of the cavity preparation outline is directly proportional to the caries and plaque indices of the patient.

3. Localized cariogenic factors

Greater activity of local cariogenic factors (tooth location, partial denture attachment, etc.) indicates that a greater extent of cavity preparation into self-cleansable areas is necessary.

4. Esthetics

Esthetics can modify the outline form in a Class II cavity preparation by minimizing the facial extent of the cavity preparation, especially in the mesio-facial margins of premolars and first molars. Also, by making these margins curved, parallel to the curvature of the adjacent facial surface, the subsequent restorations are more acceptable esthetically.

5. Tooth position

Malalignment and rotation of teeth can impede or facilitate the access to proximal lesions and accordingly modify the outline form, e.g., a lesion on a clinical proximal surface of a rotated lower premolar may be instrumented from the facial embrasures without involving the occlusal surface, provided the occlusal surface together with the adjacent marginal ridge is intact.

Also, in some malaligned or rotated teeth the clinical contact area, which does not coincide with either the marginal ridge or occlusal surface adjacent to that ridge, may be involved in a lesion. In this situation, it is advisable not to cross onto the occlusal surface at the clinical contact area. This will avoid complications such as pulpal involvements.

II. Resistance Form

The fundamental concept of resistance form is based on the reaction within the restoration and the remaining tooth structure to occlusal loading. The nature of this reaction is the development of internal stresses. When these internal stresses exceed certain limits, structural failure will result. Such failure can be on atomic, microscopic or macroscopic levels. It is important to recognize that both the restoration and the remaining tooth structure must resist failure if the restorative effort is to succeed. At first, it will seem that providing bulk for the restoration can only be achieved at the expense of tooth structure; conversely, conservation of tooth structure can be accomplished only at the expense of the restoration bulk. The first, and basic, objective of a cavity preparation design is to establish the best possible configuration that can cope with the distribution and magnitude of the stresses in tooth structure and the restoration without failure. To design such a configuration, one must first comprehend the nature of loading and of resistance to such loading.

A. Occlusal Loading and Its Effects

During centric and excursive movements of the mandible, both the restoration and tooth structure are periodically loaded both separately and jointly. This brings about different stress patterns, depending upon the actual morphology of the occluding area of both the tooth in question and the opposing contacting cuspal elements. For the purpose of this discussion, one can classify these loading situations and their induced stress patterns in the following way:

1. A small cusp contacts the fossa away from the restored proximal surface, in a proximo-occlusal restoration at centric closure (Fig. 4).

As shown in a mesio-distal cross-section, due to the elasticity of the dentin, especially in young teeth, a restoration will bend at the axio-pulpal line angle (provided the proximal part of the restoration is self-retained). This creates tensile stresses at the

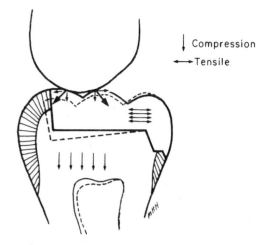

Compression

Tensile

Fig. 6-4

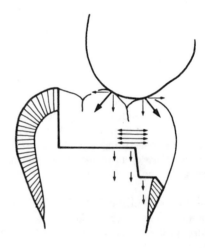

Fig. 6-5

isthmus portion of the restoration, shear stresses at the junction of the main bulk of the proximal part of the restoration and its self-retained parts, and compressive stresses in the underlying dentin.

2. A large cusp contacts the fossa adjacent to the restored proximal surface in a proximo-occlusal restoration at centric closure, either in the early stages of moving out of centric or at the late stages of moving toward it (Fig. 5).

As the diagram shows, the large cusps will tend to separate the proximal part of the restoration from the occlusal part. This creates tensile stresses at the isthmus portion of the restoration, even if the proximal portion is self-retained. This loading situation will deliver compressive forces in the remaining tooth structure, apical to the restoration.

3. Occluding cuspal elements contact facial and lingual tooth structure surrounding a proximo-occlusal or proximo-occluso-proximal restoration, during centric and excursion movements (Fig. 6).

As shown in this bucco-lingual cross-section, concentrated shear stresses will occur at the junction of the surrounding tooth structure and corresponding floors, with a tendency to-

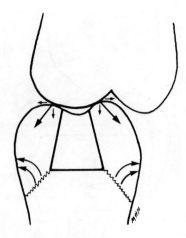

Fig. 6-6

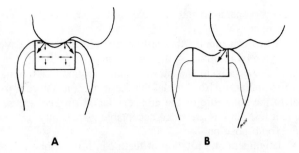

Fig. 6-7. **A,** Centric contact. **B,** Excursive movement contact.

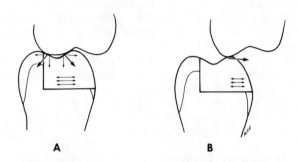

Fig. 6-8. **A,** Centric contact. **B,** Excursive movement contact.

ward fracture failure there. This loading situation can be unilateral or bilateral, depending on the direction of mandibular movement, occluding surfaces morphology, stage of the movement, and degree of intercuspation. It is the most deleterious to tooth structure, especially on the orbiting side if there is interference during lateral excursion.

4. Occluding cuspal elements contact facial and lingual parts of the restoration, surrounded by tooth structure during centric (Fig. 7A) and excursive movements (Fig. 7B).

As shown in this bucco-lingual cross-section, this arrangement will induce tensile and compressive stresses in the restoration which will be transmitted to the surrounding tooth structure.

5. Occluding cuspal elements contact facial or lingual parts of the restoration, completely replacing facial and/or lingual tooth structure during centric and excursive movements (Fig. 8, A and B).

As shown in the bucco-lingual cross-section, the stress pattern will be similar to #2 with tensile stresses induced at the junction of the occlusal and facial and/or lingual part of the restoration in both occluding situations.

6. Occluding cuspal elements contact a restoration's marginal ridge(s) or part of a marginal ridge during centric and excursive movements (Fig. 9).

As shown, in this mesio-distal cross-section (assuming the restoration is locked occlusally), there will be concentrated tensile stresses at the junction of the marginal ridge and the rest of the restoration. This will be especially true if it is an area of advance contact during mandibular closure.

7. Cuspal elements occlude or disclude via the facial or lingual groove of a restoration (Fig. 10).

As shown in the diagram, assuming that the restoration is locked occlusally, there will be tensile stresses at the junction of the occlusal and facial or lingual parts of the restoration at full intercuspation (Fig. 10A), and to and from that position (Fig. 10B).

8. Cusps (Fig. 11A) and crossing ridges (Fig. 11B) are part of the restoration in centric and excursive movement (Fig. 11).

Both will be subjected to compressive stresses during such positions and movements. Besides, tensile stresses could con-

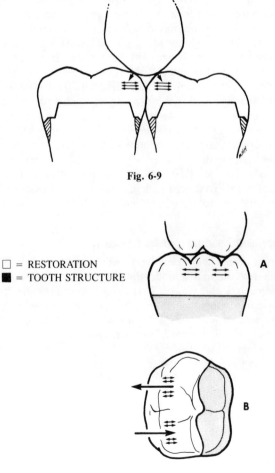

☐ = RESTORATION
■ = TOOTH STRUCTURE

Fig. 6-9

Fig. 6-10. **A,** At centric occlusion. **B,** To and from centric occlusion.

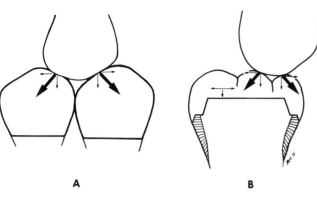

Fig. 6-11

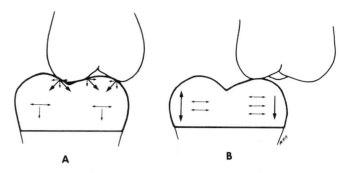

Fig. 6-12. A, Centric contact. **B,** Excursive movement contact.

centrate at their junction with the main restoration, especially during contacting excursive movement.

9. Axial portions of the restoration during centric occlusion and excursive movement contacts (Fig. 12).

As shown in the cross-section, whenever these portions are in contact with opposing occlusal surfaces, there will be induced compressive and shear (Fig. 12A) stresses. Whenever they are not reciprocating (one side not in contact with occluding surfaces, while the other axial part is), the axial surfaces will be stressed in a slight tensile and shear pattern at their junction with the main bulk of the restoration (Fig. 12B).

10. Remaining intact tooth structure will have the same stress pattern as described in Chapter I.

11. Marginal loading

Refer, again, to Chapter I for hazards of this type of loading on both the tooth structure and the restoration.

12. Restoration is not in occluding contact or is in premature contact during centric occlusion or excursive movement of the mandible.

The first situation is not conducive to function, insofar as the restoration will not be involved with direct loading from the opposing occluding teeth. After a period of time, however, the tooth will supraerupt, rotate, and/or tilt, establishing contact with the opposing cuspal elements. Usually, this newly acquired location will not be the most favorable position for the restoration, tooth, or the remainder of the gnatho-stomatic system, either mechanically or biologically. It is safer to build the restoration to predetermined contacting areas with opposing teeth which will lead to predictable physiologic stress patterns in the tooth structure and restoration. Conversely, any portion of the restoration occluding prematurely will tremendously exaggerate the same types of stresses normally induced in that area of the restoration. Besides, additional shear components of stress could be precipitated there. This, too, could lead to localized or generalized gnatho-stomatic disturbances, with eventual mechanical and biological failures.

Needless to say, pre-existing premature contacting areas should be eliminated before restorative treatment. This is done for many reasons (see chapter on single tooth restorations and the gnatho-stomatic system), but, primarily, because cavity preparation increases the susceptibility of remaining tooth structure to fracture failure. Besides, the restoration should be built to the predetermined occlusal position, even if the pre-existing tooth structures were not.

Several factors must be accommodated in designing Class II preparations for amalgam. Occlusal loading is dynamic and cyclic in nature, which is a far more destructive type of loading than static loading. Amalgam is least resistant to tensile stress and most resistant to compressive stress. Tooth structure, particularly when interrupted by a cavity preparation, is least resistant to shear stress. Therefore, Class II cavity preparations for amalgam restorations should be designed to resist cyclic loading while minimizing tensile loading in the amalgam and shear loading in the remaining tooth structure. The following discussion analyzes certain design features that will help achieve these goals.

B. Design features for the protection of the mechanical integrity of the restoration

1. Isthmus

In the isthmus, i.e., the junction between the occlusal part of a restoration and the proximal, facial or lingual parts, potentially deleterious tensile stresses occur under any type of loading. Most mathematical, mechanical and photoelastic analyses of these stresses reveal three things: (1) the fulcrum of bending occurs at the axio-pulpal line angle, (2) stresses increase closer to the surface of a restoration, away from that fulcrum, and (3) tensile stresses predominate at the marginal ridge area of a proximo-occlusal restoration. Materials tend to fail, therefore, starting from the surface, near the marginal ridge, and proceeding internally, toward the axio-pulpal line angle (Fig. 13).

These problems may be solved by applying common engineering principles. A theoretical solution might be to increase amalgam bulk at the axio-pulpal line angle, thereby placing the surface stresses away from the fulcrum (Fig. 14A). However, this actually results in increased stresses within the restorative material and a deepened cavity preparation, dangerously close to pulp anatomy. Therefore, such a solution, in and of itself, is wholly unacceptable.

Another solution might be to bring the axio-pulpal line angle closer to the surface (Fig. 14B), in an effort to reduce tensile stresses occuring near the marginal ridge. However, this, too, is unacceptable in that the consequent diminished bulk of amalgam would no longer adequately resist compressive forces.

A combination of the two solutions- i.e., increasing amalgam bulk near the marginal ridge, while bringing the axio-pulpal line angle away from that stress concentration area and closer to the surface, can be achieved simply by *slanting the axial wall toward the pulpal floor* (Fig. 14C). The obtuse axial-

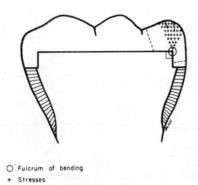

O Fulcrum of bending
+ Stresses

Fig. 6-13

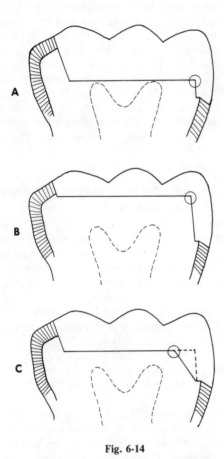

Fig. 6-14

Thirdly, by slanting the axial wall, bulk is improved by increased depth rather than increased width. Increasing the width at the isthmus portion only increases the surface area receiving deleterious occluding stresses.

As a fourth design feature, the pulpal and gingival floors at the isthmus should be perfectly flat in order to resist forces at the most advantageous angulation.

The fifth design feature is that every part of the preparation (occlusal, facial, lingual or proximal) should be self-retentive. If every part of the restoration is locked in tooth structure independently from other parts, there will be minimum stresses at the junction of one part with another, i.e., the isthmi. This can be achieved in amalgam preparations by retentive grooves, internal boxes, and undercuts.

Sixth, one should avoid, as much as possible, placing or leaving any surface discontinuities, such as carved developmental grooves, scratches, etc., at these critical areas in the restoration. These can precipitate and accentuate stresses leading to fatigue failure.

Finally, by checking occlusion to eliminate prematurities in the restoration, immediate overloading and failure can be avoided.

2. Margins

As discussed in the chapter on Class I amalgam preparations, amalgam has good compressive strength when it has sufficient bulk (1.5 mm minimum). However, frail, feather-edged margins of amalgam, which will occur when the cavosurface angles of preparations are bevelled, will fracture easily. Occluding forces will cause amalgam at the bevel to bend with maximum tensile stresses, occurring as a result of elastic deformation of the tooth structure beneath the bevel. Marginal excess of amalgam will similarly fracutre, leaving a ditch around the restoration that will enhance recurrence of decay. So, for the margins of these preparations, four design features should be observed: create butt joint amalgam-tooth structure at the margins, leave no frail enamel at the cavosurface margins, remove flashes of amalgam on tooth surface adjacent to amalgam margins, and, as practically as possible, the interface between amalgam and tooth structure should not be at an occluding contact area with opposing teeth either in centric or excursive mandibular movements.

3. Cusps and axial angles.

The following are the design features for these parts of a restoration.

a. Amalgam bulk in all three dimensions should be at least 1.5 mm.

b. Each portion of the amalgam should be completely immobilized with retention modes.

c. Amalgam should be seated on a flat floor or table in these areas.

d. Amalgam replacing cusps or axial angles should have a bulky connection to the main part of the restoration with similar design features as for the isthmus areas.

C. Design features for the protection of the physio-mechanical integrity of remaining tooth structure

In addition to design features in the restoration, there are also certain design features in the tooth structure, which enhance resistance of the restored tooth to deleterious stresses. The following discussion will analyze those features.

pulpal line angle thereby created not only provides greater amalgam bulk in the marginal ridge area of the restoration, but also reduces tensile stresses per unit area by bringing this critical area of the preparation closer to the surface of the restoration. Furthermore, this design feature improves accessibility to the proximal-facial and proximal-lingual parts of the cavity during preparation procedures. This is the first design feature.

Secondly, if the axio-pulpal line angle is rounded, structural projections or sharp junctions that may concentrate stresses at the isthmus would be avoided. This second feature will also improve the visibility for the facial and lingual gingivo-axial corners of the preparation proximally, as well as increase the amalgam bulk at the fulcrum.

1. Isthmus. Increasing the width of a cavity preparation, especially at its isthmus portion, will result in an increase in the internal stresses of the tooth (increased loading area and decreased tooth volume). This lowers the tooth's resistance to structural deformation and failure. It is necessary, therefore, to maintain the cavity width at one-fifth to one-fourth the intercuspal distance in order not to drastically affect the tooth strength. Knowing that one-fifth to one-fourth the intercuspal distance in the smallest premolar is still more than 1.5 mm, we nevertheless can still accommodate amalgam bulky enough to be self-resistant.

2. Occlusal Surface. If the Class II cavity preparation includes the occlusal surface, obviously all the design features of Class I cavity preparation must be present, namely, divergence of the walls toward the marginal ridges, perpendicularity of the walls toward the crossing ridges, preserving crossing ridges, where possible, three angulations for the walls around cusps (except at the isthmus portion), definite rounded line and point angles, and right-angled cavosurface angles. Facial and lingual walls at the isthmus should be perpendicular to the pulpal floor without any consideration to its location relative to the adjacent cusps. This feature will provide bulk for amalgam there. Occlusal ledging, as well as ledging on axial walls can be performed creating different levels axially. This minimizes tooth structure and pulp anatomy involvement.

3. Cusps and axial angles. As in Class I preparations, the ideal length to width ratio of a cuspal wall surrounding a Class II cavity preparation should be 1:1 or less in dimensions mesio-distally and bucco-lingually. If this ratio is more than 2:1 at any portion of the cuspal wall, this part of the cuspal wall should be shortened, until there is a maximum ratio of 1:1. This is done in the form of a flat table, to accommodate a minimum thickness of 1.5 mm of amalgam. If there are length to width ratios of between 1 and 2, the act of cuspal shortening and capping is considered according to loading and anticipated stresses. Usually, the partial replacement of a cusp and the shortening of a cuspal wall is indicated at the peripheral, proximal part of cuspal wall, which has been thinned by backward decay (see Class II Design 6).

In Class II preparations, every effort should be made to protect the axial angle of the tooth from proximal preparation involvement or undermining. As a design feature, the proximal cavity preparation should not include or encroach upon the axial angle; also, facial and lingual retentive grooves proximally should not be so deep as to undermine enamel at the axial angles of the tooth.

4. Margins. When the facial and lingual margins or walls on the occlusal surface approach the proximal surface, they should be prepared so as to meet the proximal surface at a right angle. Furthermore, these walls should terminate past the contact area, in the corresponding facial and lingual embrasures. If the occlusal and isthmus portion of these walls is narrow (facio-lingually), in order to make this right angle with the proximal surface they must be located either within the contact area (Fig. 15A, solid line) or past the axial angle through the cusp (Fig. 15B). Both of these situations are unacceptable. The first alternative would not include all uncleansable areas. The second unnecessarily involves sound tooth structure, impinging on pulp anatomy and weakening the remaining tooth structure. On the other hand, to continue the sweeping curves

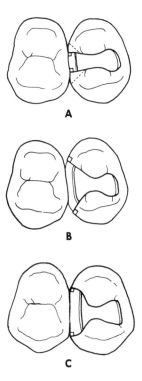

Fig. 6-15

of the occlusal outline proximally in an effort to include the whole contact area and end the facial and lingual margins in their corresponding embrasures, the facial and/or lingual cavosurface angles proximally would not be right angled (Fig. 15A, dotted line). This situation would lead to marginal failure of the amalgam.

To solve these problems, the normal direction of the sweeping curves of the outline in the occlusal portion of a proximo-occlusal cavity preparation must be reversed when it is necessary to include a broad contact area. This design feature enables involvement of the contact area as well as termination of proximal margins in the embrasures, with a right-angled cavosurface (Fig. 15C). This feature is almost always necessitated on the facial proximal walls of proximo-occlusal cavity preparation and occasionally on lingual proximal walls. With this design, it is possible to preserve tooth structures at this critical marginal area, to avoid impinging on the pulp anatomy, and to terminate margins in a right-angled cavosurface, including all of the uncleansable broad contacts.

Occluso-proximal cavity preparations are always made in a "stepped" form gingivally to avoid involving the pulpal anatomy, to improve retention, to assure proper resistance, and to facilitate access for the proximal portion of the cavity.

If the gingival margins are located at the gingival third of the involved axial surfaces, the gingival floors are always two-planed, i.e., an inner, horizontal dentinal plane for proper resistance against occlusal loading, and an outer enamelo-dentinal plane, inclined proximo-gingivally in the direction of the enamel rods.

In a proximal cavity preparation conserving the marginal ridge (direct access), the occlusal wall should be one-planed, i.e., divergent toward that marginal ridge, following the direction of the enamel rods. If retention is deficient, it may be made in two planes, i.e., a dentinal plane at right angles to the axial wall, and an outer plane divergent occluso-proximally following the direction of the enamel rods. There must be no undercuts for fear of undermining the intact marginal ridge.

III. Retention Form

In order to design a cavity preparation that will hold a restorative material, it is necessary to know the possible displacements that can happen to such a restoration, the forces that can cause them, and the fulcrum of these movements. There are four such displacements for a Class II proximo-occlusal restoration:

A. Proximal displacement of the entire restoration (Fig. 16)

In analyzing the obliquely applied force "A" into a vertical component "V" and a horizontal component "H" (Fig. 16A), it can be seen that "V" will try to seat the restoration further into the tooth, but "H" will tend to rotate the restoration proximally around axis "X" at the gingival cavosurface margin. To prevent such displacement, self-retaining facial and lingual grooves proximally are necessary, in addition to an occlusal dovetail (Fig. 16B).

B. Proximal displacement of the proximal portion

If one were to consider the restoration as being L-shaped, with the long arm of the L occlusally and the short arm proximally (Fig. 17), when the long arm is loaded by vertical force "V", it will seat the restoration more into the tooth. This is due to the elasticity of the dentin, especially in young teeth, wherein the pulpal floor will change location from position 1 to position 2. However, since metallic restorations are more rigid than the dentin, the short arm of the L will move proximally, as shown (interrupted line, Fig. 17A). The fulcrum of this rotation is the axio-pulpal line angle. In order to prevent such a displacement, proximal self-retention in the form of facial, lingual and/or gingival grooves are required (Fig. 17B). However, shear stresses will be induced at the junction between the amalgam of the main restoration and that in the grooves. Therefore, it is to be understood that these grooves are prepared *only* when there is complete assurance that there will be sufficient dentinal bulk to accommodate them, and that they will not impinge on the axial angle or on the pulp anatomy.

C. Lateral rotation of the restoration around hemispherical floors (pulpal and gingival) (Fig. 18)

As in Class I cavity preparations (Fig. 18A) this displacement can be prevented by definite point and line angles, and ledges where indicated (Fig. 18, B and C).

D. Occlusal displacement

This can be prevented by directing occlusal loading to seat the restoration and by inverted truncated cone shaping of key parts of the preparation.

Although the magnitude of these four displacements is minute, they are repeated thousands of times per day. This can definitely increase microleakage and initiate mechanical and biological failure of the restoration and surrounding tooth struc-

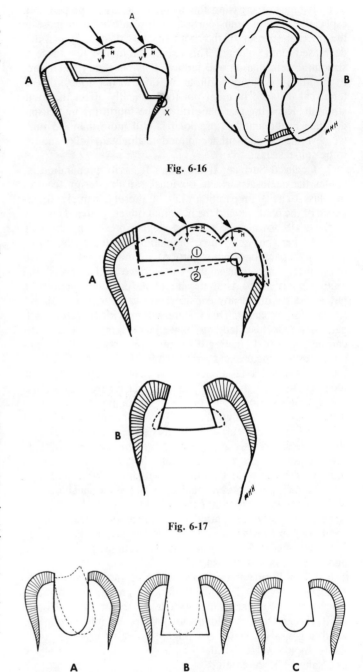

Fig. 6-16

Fig. 6-17

Fig. 6-18. A, A restoration seated on a hemispherical gingival floor will lead to rotation as the dotted line location. **B,** Flattening the gingival floor all the way bucco-lingually is detrimental to the remaining tooth structures. **C,** A two-levelled gingival floor provides the solution.

ture. Therefore, proper locking of the restoration into the tooth should be exercised to minimize these hazards.

To repeat every part of the cavity preparation should be self-retaining, if possible, i.e., independent in its retention from the rest of the cavity. This minimizes shear concentration areas at the junctions of different parts of the restoration, with less failure to be expected as a result.

IV. Convenience Form

Additional extension for the sake of access is seldom necessary in proximo-occlusal Class II cavity preparation. Actually, the occlusal involvement in many proximal lesions in molars and premolars is, in itself, a convenience form. However, when the Class II cavity preparation is confined to the proximal surface only, a limited facial or lingual extension may be needed to gain access.

Designs of Cavity Preparations

A. Class II, Design 1 (Conventional Design)

Involvement: Proximal(s) and occlusal surfaces

1. Indications

This design is indicated for:

a. A moderate to large size proximal lesion with the occlusal surface of the affected tooth involved in a lesion of similar size.

b. A proximal lesion undermining an adjacent marginal ridge(s) or not accessible through any other means but involvement of the occlusal surface.

c. The caries cones occlusally and/or proximally necessitate the cavity width to exceed one-fourth the intercuspal distance.

d. A Class II in stress concentration areas (i.e., a proximal lesion adjacent to a functional triangular fossa)

e. A patient with high caries and plaque indices.

f. An oral environment where local cariogenic conditions contraindicate a modern design.

2. General shape (Figs. 19, 20, 21, 22, 23, 24)

a. Occlusal portion

Occlusally, the outline of these preparations resembles Class I Designs 1 or 2, except they should have some dovetail form, which may be toward one side only.

b. Proximal portion

Proximally, these preparations assume an inverted truncated cone shape, with the occluso-apical inclination of the facial and lingual walls at the same occluso-apical inclinations of the adjacent facial and lingual surfaces (or at least the occlusal two-thirds of these surfaces). This shape will facilitate:

i. Improved retention.

ii. Improved resistance.

iii. Reduced chances of creating an acute-angled amalgam margin at the occluso-bucco-proximal and occluso-linguo-proximal point angles, compared to a boxed shape.

iv. Conservation of a portion of the marginal ridges with concomittant increased resistance to stresses; in addition, there will be more of a guideline for carving the proximal anatomy.

v. The placement of the gingivo-bucco-proximal and gingivo-linguo-proximal point angles at the proximal descending parts of the interdental col, i.e., areas of high relative immunity, if the adjacent periodontium is healthy.

vi. A less conspicuous outline, as it will follow the same inverted truncated cone outline of the tooth's proximal surface.

3. Location of margins (Figs. 19, 20, 21, 22, 23, 24)

a. Occlusal portion

Occlusally, margins in this preparation will assume locations similar to Class I Designs 1 or 2 cavity preparations.

b. Proximal portion

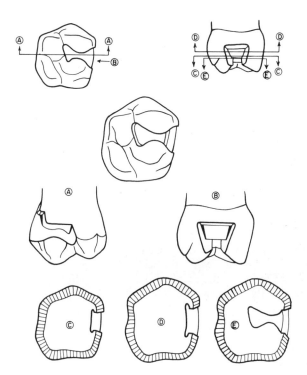

Fig. 6-19. Cross sections in a Class II conventional cavity preparation for amalgam showing internal anatomy.

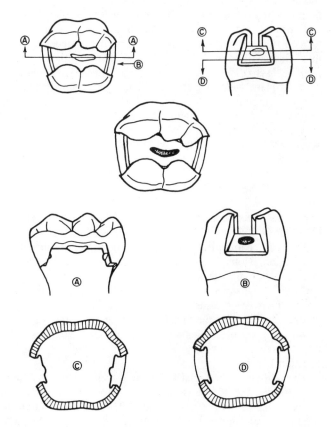

Fig. 6-20. Class II Amalgam conventional design (MOD) to accommodate intermediary base lower right molar

Proximally, facial and lingual margins are placed far enough facially and lingually to be located in the corresponding embrasures. As a rule of thumb, the tip of an explorer must pass freely occluso-gingivally between contacting proximal surfaces.

c. Gingival portion

Gingivally, margins are located ideally in the occlusal portion of the gingival sulcus space; otherwise, they are situated as indicated by the application of the general principles of cavity preparation.

d. Isthmus portion

Facial and lingual margins at the isthmus are located on the inclined planes of corresponding cusps and the remaining portion of the marginal ridge. These margins should be separated from each other by a distance not to exceed one-third the intercuspal distance. Usually, the facial margin and sometimes the lingual margin reverse the occlusal sweeping curve (in an S-shape) to create the required right angle with the proximal surface at the embrasure.

4. Internal Anatomy (Figs. 19, 20, 21, 22, 23, 24)

a. Occlusal portion

Internally, the anatomy of the Class II conventional preparation is similar to Class I Designs 1 or 2.

b. Proximal portion

i. Mesio-distal cross-section—this will facilitate visualization of the preparation details, especially gingivally and axially. If the gingival margin is located on cementum, cementum should be scraped from the cavosurface. Note that the gingival floor is perfectly flat, perpendicular to the long axis of the tooth and formed completely of dentin. If the gingival margin is located in the gingival third of the proximal surface, the gingival floor will be two-planed, i.e., an inner, dentinal plane at right angles to the long axis of the tooth, and an outer enamelo-dentinal plane following the direction of the enamel rods.

If the gingival margin is located at the middle third of the proximal surface, as in young, incompletely erupted teeth, the gingival floor will be formed of one plane made of enamel and dentin. Note, too, that the axial wall is slanted toward the pulpal floor, making an obtuse angle with the gingival floor. Its angle at the junction with the pulpal floor is very rounded. Occlusally, the anatomical features will be similar to Class I Designs 1 or 2.

ii. Cross-section at the apical third of the cavity preparation (Figs. 19D, 20D)

This will enable visualization of the proximal portion of the preparation. Note that the axial walls are rounded facio-lingually, following the same curvature as the proximal tooth surface. This insures a uniform thickness of the amalgam proximally, increases the surface area of the axial wall, and leaves an even thickness of the facial, lingual, and gingival walls. In addition, a uniform thickness of the dentin bridge, axially, results from this convexity, assuring even distribution of stresses against that wall.

The outline of the facial and lingual walls, from this view, may assume one of two variations. In situation (A), in which the proximal cavity preparations involve narrow contact areas, the facial and lingual walls may be perpendicular to the axial wall and at the same time follow the direction of the enamel rods. In this situation, the facial and lingual walls will be

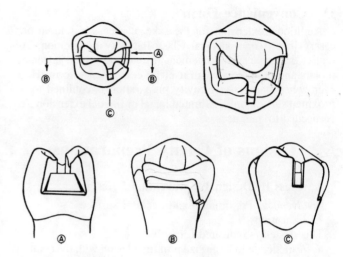

Fig. 6-21. Class II amalgam conventional design with groove extension (MOL) in a lower tricuspid premolar

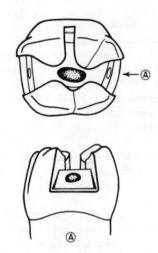

Fig. 6-22. Class II amalgam conventional design with groove extension and to accommodate intermediary base (MOD-B) lower right molar

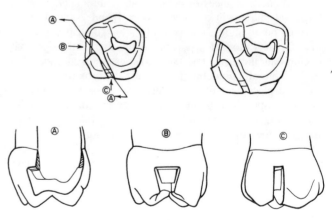

Fig. 6-23. Class II amalgam conventional design with groove extension (DO-L) upper left molar

composed of two planes, i.e., an internal plane in the form of a dentinal retention groove, and a straight external enamelo-dentinal plane, following the directions of the enamel rods and perpendicular to the tangent of the axial wall. (Fig. 33C)

In situation (B) the proximal cavity preparations involve wide contact areas. In this situation, if the facial and lingual walls follow the direction of the enamel rods, they will not be perpendicular to the axial wall. Therefore, it is necessary to prepare the facial and lingual walls in three planes (Fig. 19D, 20D); i.e., an inner dentinal plane, in the form of a retentive groove, a transitional plane, formed completely of dentin, perpendicular to the axial wall, and an outer enamelo-dentinal plane following the direction of the enamel rods.

Although situation (B) is almost always indicated for facial walls (because of the facial deviation of the contact areas and the usual location of their facial peripheries in the facial one-third of the proximal surfaces) it is not always necessary lingually. In other words, a combination of design features, utilizing situation (A) and situation (B), can be used in the same proximal cavity preparation.

iii. Cross-section at the middle third of the proximal portion (Figs. 19C, 20C)

This further facilitates visualization of proximal design features just apical to the pulpal floor. The axial, facial, and lingual walls will have the same general shape as they did at the apical third. The major difference is that the retention grooves will have a smaller dimension, due to the decrease of bulk of tooth structure facially and lingually.

iv. Cross-section at the level of the pulpal floor (Fig. 19E)

This view emphasizes one major feature: the retention grooves do not extend occlusal to the pulpal floor. This is to avoid undermining the axial angles and occlusal enamel. The axial wall configuration remains constant; the facial and ligual walls will be either one- or two-planed, depending upon the direction of the enamel rods at the margin.

It should be re-emphasized that the facial and lingual grooves have their greatest dimension at the gingival floor level, decreasing in depth going occlusally, and terminating at the pulpal floor level. These grooves may only be prepared if there is sufficient bulk of dentin to accommodate them. If there is any suspicion that these grooves will impinge on the axial angle or pulp anatomy, they should not be included in the internal design of the cavity preparation.

v. Wall configuration occlusal to the pulpal floor

Here, the facial and sometimes the lingual walls will have either the S-shaped configuration mentioned in the application of the general principles, or the universal sweeping curve coming from the occlusal walls.

5. Instrumentation for Class II, Design 1

a. Prerequisites

One should understand and be able to visualize the general shape, location of margins and internal anatomy of this design in every tooth in the arch, and the design modifications needed for this specific tooth to satisfy occlusal or esthetic requirements. The patient should be anesthetized and a rubber dam should be properly applied. Two wedges should be inserted adjacent to the proposed preparation site, ie., one from the buccal and one from the lingual, gingival to the contact area. These serve to apically displace and protect the gingival and

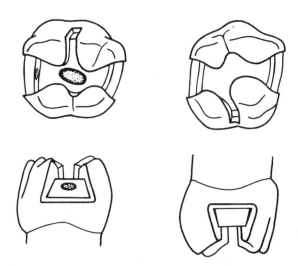

Fig. 6-24. MOB and MOL conventional Class II cavity preparations for amalgam.

rubber dam from proximal instrumentation. Also, they create a slight separation for better access.

b. Procedures

i. Gaining access

For occlusal access follow the same procedure described for Class I Designs 1 or 2 cavity preparations. For proximal access one of the following schemes may be used according to the degree of proximal involvement dictated by decay.

A. If the decay is confined to the part of the proximal surface apical to the contact area and the marginal ridge is still intact (Fig. 25):

With a 699 bur using the same movements as in preparing Class I, grossly rough in the occlusal portion of this design, being sure to keep the bucco-lingual width of the wall adjacent to the involved marginal ridge less than the bucco-lingual width of the future proximal cavity preparation. With a 699 bur thin the wall adjacent to the involved marginal ridge. This can be accomplished by pushing (pulling) the bur proximally and dragging it bucco-lingually. Proceed thinning until the proximal wall is formed only of enamel or has a thickness less than the anticipated axial depth of the proximal cavity preparation, whichever is less.

Mark the center of pulpal floor, adjacent to the thinned proximal wall. With a ¼ round bur, seated on this mark, use proximo-gingival pressure to create a tunnel (Fig. 25, A and B), from the occlusal (pulpal) floor to the proximal lesion, occlusal to the proposed location for the gingival floor.

With a 699 bur placed revolving in the tunnel, use bucco-lingual pressure to widen the tunnel in the bucco-lingual direction only (Fig. 25C). This should leave a thin, undermined proximal plate of enamel occlusal to the carious lesion and proximal to the future axial wall. Keeping this proximal plate of enamel is a very good protective measure against injuring the proximal surfaces of adjacent teeth. However, usually this enamel barrier breaks or shatters during working (Fig. 25D), especially when using snugly fitting burs or with any proximal pressure during this widening procedure.

B. If the proximal lesion caused the marginal ridge to be

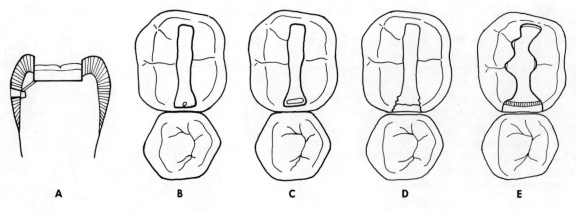

Fig. 6-25

partially lost (Fig. 26), the proximal access can be facilitated by continuing the occlusal cavity preparation in the form of two extensions: one buccally and another lingually, simulating the widened tunnel portion in this area as described in (i). Of course, it will be interrupted in the middle by the partial loss of the marginal ridge.

C. If the proximal lesion has caused loss of the marginal ridge to a degree coinciding with the uncleansable proximal area to be involved in the cavity preparation (or beyond it), there should not be any more preparation for access other than trimming undermined enamel facially and lingually, exposing the peripheries of the carious dentin.

ii. Gross removal

The occlusal portion of the Class II preparation is done in a similar manner to Class I Designs 1 or 2, or as described in Gaining Access for the proximal portion. For the proximal portion, however, it is done as follows:

Using a hatchet, binangle or Wedelstaedt chisel, cleave off the thinned overhanging proximal plate of enamel, if still present. Cleave all remaining undermined enamel in the rest of the cavity, preferably using a chisel of adequate size and shape. If this enamel is very thick, remove it with a proper size fissure bur. Sound tooth structure to be involved in the cavity preparation is removed using a 699 bur. In these three steps, be sure to stop short of the predetermined peripheries of the cavity preparation.

iii. Removal of irreparably attacked dentin

Most of this dentin will have been removed by now, except that located on the pulpal and axial walls. At either location it should be removed using the proper size spoon excavator, according to the rules mentioned in Chapter I and in the chapter on Management of Deep Carious Lesions. This step may create different levels of the pulpal floor and axial wall. At *no* instance should the uninvolved pulpal floor or axial wall be flattened to the depth of the caries cones.

iv. Formulation of facial and lingual retentive grooves

If, at this point, the preparation is seen to provide sufficient dentinal bulk facially and lingually in the proximal cavity preparation to accommodate retentive grooves without impinging on the axial angles or the pulp, the following steps in groove formation should be undertaken (Fig. 27).

Using a ½ round bur, the tip of a 699 bur, or a 33½ inverted cone bur in the slow speed handpiece (Fig. 27A), placed in

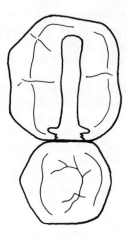

Fig. 6-26

the bucco-gingivo-axial point angle, use buccal pressure and occluso-lingual dragging to cut a shallow groove at the expense of the bucco-axial line angle. As previously described, this groove should ''fade out'' at the level of the pulpal floor.

Starting from the gingivo-linguo-axial point angle, use lingual pressure and occluso-buccal dragging. This creates a groove at the expense of the linguo-axial line angle. Again, the groove should ''fade out'' at the level of the pulpal floor.

With the tip of a gingival margin trimmer, starting at the gingival base of the retentive groove (Fig. 27B), use buccal pressure and occluso-lingual dragging to accentuate the buccal retention groove. Repeat this step for accentuation of the lingual retentive groove using lingual pressure and occluso-buccal dragging.

v. Preliminary shaping

The following steps are undertaken to accentuate design features of the preparation:

Angulations and different planes of the walls in the occlusal portion are created in the same way as their counterparts in Class I cavity preparation. Using a hatchet, Wedelstaedt chisel, or binangle chisel, in a direct cutting action, slant the axial wall toward the pulpal floor. As soon as the approximate location of the axio-pulpal line angle is established, the S-shaped curve, if indicated, should be cut at the expense of the buccal and/or lingual walls of the isthmus portion, placing the margins

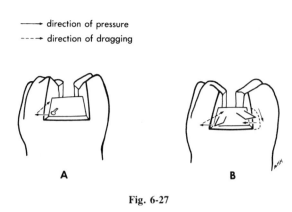

⟶ direction of pressure
---⟶ direction of dragging

Fig. 6-27

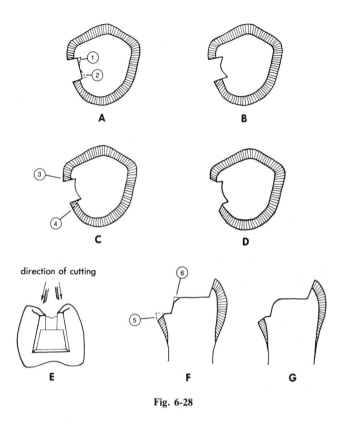

direction of cutting

Fig. 6-28

just short of opening the proximal cavosurface from its contact with the adjacent tooth.

The proximal preparation angulations and different planes are created by cutting a series of six triangles according to the following sequence (Fig. 28). Mentally, divide the axial wall into three equal portions in the bucco-lingual direction. Then, using a suitable size hatchet, binangle chisel, or Wedelstaedt chisel, in a direct cutting action, cut triangle #1 in the facial one-third and triangle #2 in the lingual one-third, leaving the middle third intact (Fig. 28A and B). Smooth the junction between the three portions. This process will round the axial wall in the bucco-lingual directions (Fig. 28C).

If it is indicated that the facial and/or lingual walls are to have three planes, cut triangle #3 and/or triangle #4, respectively (Fig. 28, C and D). These must include all enamel and part of the dentin, creating the outer plane of the wall that follows the direction of the enamel rods. A suitable size chisel, in a direct cutting action, will perform these cuts. The occluso-gingival cutting should follow the inverted truncated cone outline form of the proximal walls (Fig. 28E).

If a two-planed gingival floor is indicated, at the expense of the proximal one-third of the gingival floor, cut a triangle involving enamel and part of the dentin, to create an outer plane (formed of enamel and dentin). The instruments of choice here are either a gingival margin trimmer or a binangle hatchet. This is triangle #5 (Fig. 28, F and G). Of course, this step is not needed if the gingival margin is located either at the middle third of the proximal surface, or on the root surface. Using the same gingival margin trimmer or hatchet, cut triangle #6 at the expense of the axio-pulpal line angle. Use a lateral cutting action. This will round that line angle (Fig. 28, F and G).

vi. Final shaping

Use a hatchet, in a lateral cutting action, to ensure the flatness of the pulpal floor. With a hatchet or any other chisel, in a direct cutting action, plane all the surrounding walls, insuring proper angulation with the pulpal floor. All line and point angles may be defined, if necessary, using the same instruments that were used in creating them. Every junction between different portions of the cavity preparation should be rounded using either the same instrument that created them, or a round bur.

vii. Cavity finish

Using the same instruments used in final shaping, go over all cavity details in lighter, more rapid strokes to smooth these components. With the Wedelstaedt chisel in the occlusal and a hatchet on the proximal cavosurface margins, use a direct cutting action to eliminate frail enamel and to verify a smooth, right-angled cavosurface. (Fig. 25E)

viii Intermediary basing

Follow indicated procedures described in detail in the chapter on Intermediary Basing.

B. Class II, Design 2 (Modern Design)

Involvement: Proximal(s) and occlusal surfaces

1. Indications

This design is indicated for:

a. A moderate to small sized proximal lesion(s), i.e., not exceeding the area of near approach.

b. An occlusal lesion(s) undermining one or both marginal ridges and not exceeding a width of one-fourth the intercuspal distance.

c. A Class II in a stress concentration area (i.e., a proximal lesion adjacent to a functional triangular fossa).

d. Patients with good oral hygiene, low plaque and caries indices.

e. An oral environment where local conditions are conducive to low or remote potential cariogenic activities, e.g., not the last tooth in the arch or any tooth involved in abutting a partial denture, etc.

f. A lesion where after removal of the carious dentin and undermined tooth structure sufficient bulk in the buccal and lingual walls exits to accommodate retentive grooves, without impinging on important anatomy.

2. General shape (Figs. 29, 30, 31, 32, 33, 34)

a. Occlusal portion

Occlusally, the outline of these preparations appears very similar to Class I Design 1, and sometimes Design 2. However, there should be little if any dovetail shape on the occlusal outline.

b. Proximal portion

The modern design is characteristic in that proximally, there is only a unilateral inverted truncated cone (at the expense of one side only). In upper teeth there is a lingual inverted truncated cone only, and in lower teeth there is a buccal inverted truncated cone only, i.e., the linguo-gingival marginal angle in the upper will be acute, and the bucco-gingival marginal angle right-angled. In the lowers, the linguo-gingival marginal angle is right-angled and bucco-gingival marginal angle is acute-angled (Figs. 29B and 30P).

This inverted truncated cone on the functional side only is done to preserve tooth structure. Typically, there will be more tooth bulk on that side. Also, there is more axial convexity on the cusps on the functional side as compared to the non-functional side. This is partially due to the facial inclination of the upper posterior teeth and the lingual inclination of the lower ones.

3. Location of margins (Figs. 29, 30, 31, 32, 33)

a. Occlusal portion

In most cases the occlusal margins will resemble those seen in Class I Design 1.

b. Proximal portion

The gingival margin may be located anywhere on the proximal surface, provided (1) it is gingival to the contact area, and (2) the cavity preparation includes all carious and undermined tooth structures. It does not have to be located subgingivally.

Facial and lingual margins must be placed far enough facially and lingually to include all carious and undermined tooth structures and to include the contact area. However, the contact area need only be included to the extent of seeing light through the created space between the margin and the adjacent tooth. An explorer does not have to be able to pass interproximally.

c. Isthmus portion

The facial and lingual margins at the isthmus are placed on the corresponding surfaces of the inclined planes and the remaining areas of the marginal ridge, such that the width of the cavity will not exceed one-fourth the intercuspal distance. Because the cavity width is so limited, the universal sweeping curves of the facial and lingual margins occlusally will always reverse in the isthmus portion (in an S-shaped form) to include the contact area, while still ending with a right-angled cavosurface proximally.

4. Internal anatomy (Figs. 29, 30, 31, 32, 33)

a. Occlusal portion

Occlusally, the internal anatomy of the modern design is very similar to Class I Design 1 and, rarely, Design 2.

b. Proximal portion

Proximally, various cross-sectional analyses will facilitate visualization of internal anatomy.

i. Mesio-distal cross-section

Visualizing the modern design in this cross-section shows it to be very similar to the conventional design, except that very rarely the gingival margin may be located on cementum. Also, all line angles are rounded, especially the axio-pulpal one, with the exception of the gingivo-axial line angle, which should be kept sharp. This will help in stabilizing the restoration there.

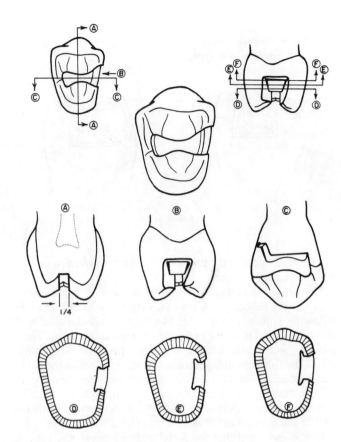

Fig. 6-29. Class II modern design cavity preparation for amalgam—upper premolar

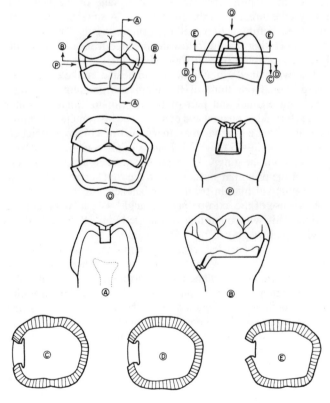

Fig. 6-30. Class II modern design cavity preparation for amalgam—in a lower first molar

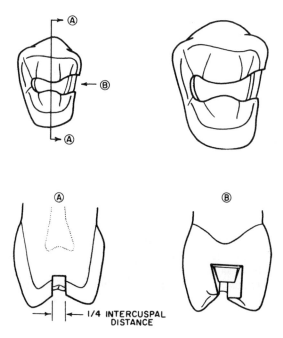

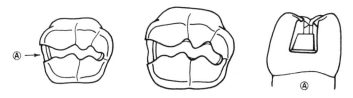

Fig. 6-32. Class II amalgam modern design lower right molar

Fig. 6-31. Class II amalgam modern design upper bicuspid

ii. Facio-lingual cross-sections at different levels of the proximal cavity preparation

These cross-sections show the modern design to be very similar to the conventional design, with the following variations. All details are on a smaller scale than in the conventional design. Buccal and lingual dentinal retention grooves will be present in every case, with no exception, in this design. With the facial and lingual walls, it is more common to encounter a two-planed configuration (situation A) rather than a three-planed configuration (situation B) because of the narrowness of the proximal cavity preparation in the modern design. Occlusal to the pulpal floor, the facial and lingual walls will almost always assume an S-shape, for reasons mentioned previously. The axial depth of the modern design cavity is much less than that of the conventional design, with more ledging possible axially. A regular depth of 0.2 mm from the DEJ is quite common. In fact, sometimes the axial wall and its peripheral parts are in enamel.

5. Preparation modifications

Occasionally we make one of the following two modifications for the modern design:

a. In tapered teeth (bell-shaped teeth) in which the gingival margin of the proximal portion of the preparation is located so far gingivally that preparing the regular facial and lingual retentive grooves will undermine tooth structure at the axial angle of the tooth, one of two types of facial and lingual grooves can be created.

In line with the axio-pulpal line angle facially and lingually a groove (Fig. 34A) is prepared on each of the facial and lingual walls, respectively. Each groove is started at the axio-pulpal line angle and continues occlusally to the occlusal surface. Of course, the groove will be formed of enamel and dentin and there should be enough tooth structure bulk there to accommodate them without seriously widening the occlusal portion. Or facial and lingual dentinal grooves may be prepared

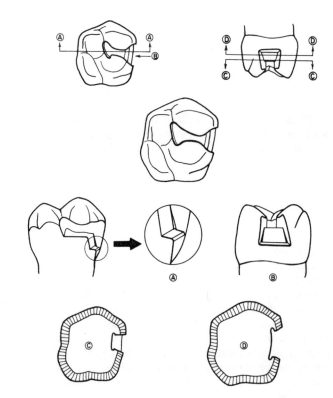

Fig. 6-33. Class II amalgam modern design (MO) upper molar

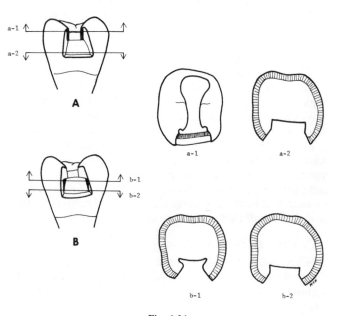

Fig. 6-34

at the expense of the facial and lingual walls of the proximal portion, respectively, but having their maximal dimension at the pulpal floor level, tapering to a point termination at the bucco-gingivo-axial and linguo-gingivo-axial point angles (Fig. 34B), i.e., the reverse arrangement of the regular retentive grooves. If sufficient dentinal bulk is available gingivally, a gingival groove could be prepared at the expense of the gingival dentinal floor via the axio-gingival line angle.

b. After preparing a Class II cavity preparation, if there presents an intact marginal ridge, crossed by a fissure, or carious groove (a situation usually encountered at the mesial marginal ridge of upper first premolar and sometimes the distal marginal ridge of second molars), it is not necessary to cross the ridge either in a conventional or a modern design fashion. All that is needed is a proximal extension in the form of a slit involving this fissure or groove. This "slit" may open proximally on the same level as the pulpal floor, or with an occlusal step, but never in a gingival step. Very often, the facial, lingual and gingival margins of the slit are located in the lingual (buccal) embrasures. Even if any or all of these margins are located in the contact area, this minimal opening does not necessitate the facio-lingual and occluso-apical involvement of the marginal ridge that is required for the conventional and modern design.

6. Instrumentation for Class II, Design 2.

a. Prerequisites

These are identical to Class II Design 1.

b. Procedures

Procedural steps are very similar to those described for Design 1, with the exception that smaller instruments are used, e.g., in gaining access and gross removal use a 168 bur, instead of a 699 bur. In preliminary and final shaping use the smallest sizes of chisels available. The proximal retention grooves, which are mandatory here, are created and accentuated with smaller gingival margin trimmers or angle formers.

c. Preparation of the Modifications

In preparing the modified facial and lingual grooves a tapered fissure bur is placed in line with the axio-pulpal line angle, with its tip at the level of the pulpal floor, and with buccal (lingual) pressure and occlusal dragging cut an enamelo-dentinal groove which will be symmetrical in dimensions from the level of the axio-pulpal line angle to the occlusal surface. Or, a small round bur is placed on the buccal wall at the axio-pulpal line angle. With purely buccal pressure, then apical and lingual dragging, cut deeper at the pulpal floor level and shallower proceeding apically. A groove will be formed having its maximal buccal depth at the pulpal floor level, while tapering to a point at the gingival floor level. A similar procedure is done to the lingual wall. To accentuate these grooves, a gingival margin trimmer (reverse of that used for regular grooves in same location) is used in the same way as the bur. To prepare a proximal slit extension simply use a tapered fissure bur, then box up the wall using a suitable size hatchet or chisel.

C. Class II, Design 3 (Conservative Design)

Involvement: This preparation is designed to involve primarily the proximal surface(s) and a very limited part of the occlusal surface, not extending beyond the adjacent triangular fossa.

1. Indications

This design is indicated when:

a. There are sound pronounced occlusal crossing ridges, and the inclined planes of the adjacent cusps are smooth and devoid of any crossing fissures.

b. The decay is restricted to the proximal surface only and the occlusal surface is completely sound.

c. The restoration is expected to be subjected to minimal loading, e.g., the mesial of premolars and the distal of second and third molars.

d. After removing decayed or undermined tooth structure and bringing the margins into their corresponding embrasures, there is sufficient bulk of remaining tooth structure to place substantial buccal, lingual and gingival retentive grooves without compromising important adjacent anatomy.

e. The patient exhibits good oral hygiene and low caries and plaque indices.

f. Local conditions, especially occlusally, are not conducive to unusual cariogenic activity.

2. General shape (Fig. 35)

These preparations appear proximally as a one-sided inverted truncated cone. The inverted truncated cone is located totally proximally, with the exception of its tip, which involves part of the adjacent occlusal triangular fossa (linear fossa in mesial of lower premolars) (Fig. 35).

3. Location of margins

a. Occlusal portion

The occlusal margin of Design 3 may be located on the occlusal inclined planes of the involved marginal ridge. If the entire adjacent triangular fossa (linear fossa) is included in the preparation, the occlusal margin will be located on the nearest inclined planes of the adjacent crossing ridge or ridge connecting adjacent facial and lingual cusps.

The facial and lingual margins occlusally are very limited in their extent, and they are always on the inclined plane of the involved ridge. Sometimes they are part of the inclined planes of the adjacent cusps.

b. Proximal portion

Proximally, Design 3 appears exactly like the modern design.

4. Internal anatomy (Fig. 35)

a. Mesio-distal cross-section

Visualizing the preparation in this cross-section, the gingival floor may assume one of two forms:

If the gingival margin is located at the gingival third of the proximal surface, the floor will be formed of three planes: an inner dentinal plane in the form of a groove; a middle, transitional, dentinal plane; and an outer enamelo-dentinal plane following the direction of the enamel rods and inclining gingivo-proximally. On the other hand, if the gingival margin is located at the middle third proximally, the gingival floor will be formed of two planes: an inner dentinal plane in the form of a groove, and another straight plane formed of enamel and dentin.

The axial wall, in this cross-section, can be seen to be formed of dentin and enamel, slanted pulpally to the occlusal surface (with more slanting angulation than in the modern design) so as to facilitate more bulk at the stress-receiving occlusal portion of the amalgam restoration, and to improve accessibility for the gingivo-axio-buccal and gingivo-axio-lingual corners. The axial wall will end in a butt joint with the occlusal surface.

b. A facio-lingual cross-section through the proximal part

This view shows the axial wall to be perfectly convex, as

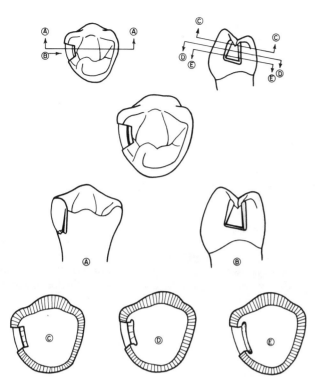

Fig. 6-35. Class II amalgam conservative design lower first bicuspid

in the modern design. The facial and lingual walls, if their margins are at the facial or lingual thirds of the proximal surface, will be formed of three planes: an inner dentinal plane in the form of a groove, which gradually decreases in depth going occlusally; a transitional dentinal plane; and an outer enamel-dentinal plane following the direction of the enamel rods proximo-buccally and lingually.

However, if either wall ends its margins at the middle third, it will be composed of two planes: an inner, dentinal groove plane, and an outer, straight enamel-dentinal plane, perpendicular to the tangent of the axial wall. These arrangements of the facial and lingual wall are followed to a point about 0.5-1 mm from the occlusal enamel. In other words, the facial and lingual grooves stop short of the occlusal enamel, as there should be sufficient dentin occlusal to their termination to support the enamel there.

5. Instrumentation for Class II, Design 3
a. Prerequisites
These are the same as previous designs.
b. Procedures
Gaining access

Usually, for this design to be indicated, the marginal ridge is still present. Using a ¼ round bur, start a tunnel on the occlusal inclined planes of the marginal ridge to be involved in the preparation, connecting this tunnel with the lesion, widening and breaking it in the same way as was done in preparation of the previous two designs. If part of the marginal ridge is lost, two lateral grooves may be prepared on the buccal and lingual behind the portion of the marginal ridge to be removed. In both situations, use a 168 bur to complete a rough-in of the outline form. The rest of the preparation is done similarly to the previous two designs, but using smaller sized instruments.

D. Class II, Design 4 (Simple Design)

Involvement: The proximal surfaces only

1. Indications

This design is indicated when:

a. The decay is restricted to contacting or proximal surfaces without undermining the corresponding marginal ridges.

b. There is a diastema or the adjacent tooth is missing facilitating direct access to the lesion.

c. The affected tooth is rotated or inclined, so that the contacting surface(s) is (are) not the anatomical proximal one(s), again facilitating access.

d. The proximal lesion is located very gingivally at, or apical to, the cemento-enamel junction, accompanied by gingival recession (senile decay), making accessibility to the lesion from the facial or lingual direction possible.

e. The proximal lesion occurs on tapered teeth with wide gingival embrasures facilitating facial or lingual access to the lesion.

f. The occlusal embrasures are pronounced in dimension so as to be cleansable enough to accommodate a margin.

2. General shape

There is no specific shape for this design of cavity preparation. Generally, it should follow the shape of the contact area and the proximal surface. Usually it will assume a trapozoidal or rhomboidal shape. (Fig. 36C)

3. Location of margins

If there is no proximally contacting tooth (diastema) (Fig. 36A), there is no specific location of margins, for the entire proximal surface is essentially self-cleansable. If the lesion is apical to the contact area (senile decay), the occlusal and gingival margins will be in the gingival embrasures (Fig. 36B), the facial and lingual margins will be located in the corresponding embrasures or their apical continuation, with more extension than otherwise necessitated for prevention on the access side.

If the lesion involves the contact area (clinical or anatomical), the occlusal margin will be located in the occlusal embrasure, the gingival margin in the gingival embrasure, both just clearing the contact area and involving the diseased tissues. The facial and lingual margins will be in the corresponding embrasures, with more extension on the access side.

4. Internal anatomy (Fig. 37)
a. Facio-lingual cross-section (Fig. 37A)

In this view, the axial wall is seen to be flat to slightly convex facio-lingually (interrupted line, Fig. 37A). If the axial wall, or part of it, occurs at a furcation area, or any concavity of the proximal surface of the tooth, that part of the axial wall should be prepared concave facio-lingually, paralleling the surface concavity (continuous line, Fig. 37A). This facilitates the preparation of a definite gingival floor in these concave areas of the proximal surface. It also accommodates amalgam bulk there without the possibility of creating overhangs proximally. In fact, this design feature may be applied to any proximal axial wall or part of a wall occurring adjacent to a surface concavity in any of the eight designs of Class II cavity preparations.

Also, as seen in this cross-section, the buccal or lingual wall (Fig. 37A), on the access side will be a one-planed enamel dentinal wall following the directions of the enamel rods. Because the margin of this wall is located at the facial or lingual one-third of the proximal surface, it will be slanting facio- or

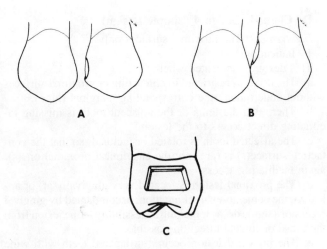

Fig. 6-36. A, Diastema enabling access proximally. **B,** Wide gingival embrasure enabling access proximally.

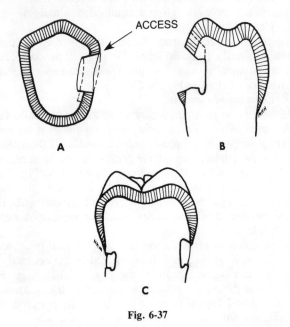

Fig. 6-37

linguo-proximally to facilitate access. On the non-access side, the facial or lingual wall may be formed in one of two ways. If its margin is located at the facial or lingual one-third of the proximal surface, it will be two-planed: i.e., a dentinal plane at a right angle to the axial wall, and an enamel-dentinal plane following the direction of the enamel rods (interrupted line, Fig. 37A). On the other hand, these walls will be one-planed, formed of enamel and dentin and perpendicular to the axial wall, if their margins are located in the middle third of the proximal surface (continuous line, Fig. 37A).

b. Occlusal-gingival cross-section (Fig. 37, B and C)

In this view, the gingival floor may be seen to occur in one of two ways. If the gingival margin is located on cementum, cementum should be removed, as it cannot be part of a cavity wall, and the gingival floor should be formed completely of dentin and in two planes: an inner one in the form of a groove and an outer one perfectly straight and flat (Fig. 37C). If the gingival margin is located on enamel, it will be formed of three

planes: an inner dentinal groove, a dentinal transitional plane, and an outer plane, formed of enamel and dentin and following the direction of the enamel rods (Fig. 37B).

If the gingival margin ends in a proximal surface concavity (e.g., furcation components), the part of the gingival floor involved in the concavity should be prepared in one plane without any grooves. Furthermore, it should form a right angle with the adjacent concave surface, which will usually create a divergent gingival floor proximo-gingivally. In fact, this design feature is to be applied to any gingival floor encountering a proximal surface concavity in any of the eight designs of Class II cavity preparations (see Class V, Design 5 for more details).

Also, in this cross-section, the occlusal wall can be analyzed. If sufficient bulk of tooth structure remains intact gingival to the marginal ridge, e.g., the lesion does not involve the contact area, prepare the occlusal wall in two planes: an inner dentinal plane at right angle to the axial wall and an outer enamelo-dentinal plane following the direction of the enamel rods (continuous line, Fig. 37B). If the occlusal margin is located at the middle third of the proximal surface, the enamel rods will be perpendicular to the axial wall, so there will be a straight one-planed occlusal wall. However, if the occlusal margin is located at the gingival third of the proximal surface and still on enamel, prepare the occlusal wall in one plane following the direction of enamel rods there (Fig. 38C), i.e., creating an undercut in the occlusal wall. If the occlusal margin is located on cementum, the wall is handled similar to the gingival wall at the same location, with the internal groove directed occlusally.

If, on the other hand, the tooth bulk apical to the marginal ridge is limited, it is advisable to prepare the occlusal wall in one plane following the direction of enamel rods there (interrupted line, Fig. 37B), i.e., divergent occlusally.

The axial wall in this cross-section can be seen to be almost flat. However, when it replaces a proximal surface concavity it, too, should be concave, for the same reasons as preparing it concave in the facio-lingual direction.

5. Instrumentation for Class II, Design 4

a. Prerequisites

These are similar to previous designs, with the exception that no wedges are used if they will interfere with access or if there is no contacting tooth.

b. Procedures

i. Gaining access and gross removal

From the access side, using a round bur (¼ the size of the proximal preparation) with axial pressure and lateral dragging, remove decayed and sound tooth structure within the contemplated outline.

ii. Removal of attacked irreparable dentin

This is accomplished in exactly the same fashion as described for other designs.

iii. Preliminary shaping

This is done using the base of an inverted cone bur. With buccal access, at the future location of the lingual wall, form the lingual wall in gingivo-occlusal movements. At the gingival floor location, use the same part of the bur moving it in a bucco-lingual direction to form the gingival floor. Then, using the side of the bur, in an occluso-apical direction, form the buccal wall. The occlusal wall could be formed with a tapered fissure bar, using bucco-lingual strokes.

If access is from the lingual, the exact reverse of the previous two steps can be done using the base of the inverted cone bur on the buccal and gingival, and the side of the bur on the lingual wall. Gingival retention grooves are prepared using a ¼ round bur, dragging it along the axio-gingival line angle with gingival pressure.

iv Final shaping is accomplished in several steps. The different planes for the buccal and lingual walls can be formed using a hatchet and Wedelstaedt chisel. Similarly, the different planes for the gingival and occlusal walls could be formed using a Wedelstaedt chisel from the buccal or a hatchet from the lingual. Slight rounding of the axial wall is accomplished with a hatchet as in Designs 1 and 2. Any necessary concavities can be created with the same instruments. Rounding the junction between the different parts of the cavity preparation is also done as in Designs 1 and 2.

v Cavity finish is accomplished with the same instruments utilized in the final shaping. Smooth all walls and internal details of the preparation using more frequent and lighter strokes of the instruments. A Wedelstaedt chisel and a gingival margin trimmer could be used to finish the cavosurface margins.

vi Intermediary basing is accomplished as described previously.

E. Class II, Design 5

Involvement: Part of the proximal surface, with a very limited access area on the facial or lingual surface.

1. Indications

There are two shapes for this design, each with certain indications. In *shape A* (Fig. 38A) the facial or lingual access will not have a dovetail form. The indications for this design are:

a. The cavity, when completed, will have four definite surrounding walls, with opposing retentive grooves in at least two of them.

b. Small to medium sized proximal lesions.

c. The restoration is expected to be subjected to normal displacing forces.

d. The marginal ridge is intact and adequately supported apically and occlusally with bulky tooth structure.

e. The lesion does not involve the contact area, nor does it undermine enamel in the contact area.

f. The patient has mastered or is expected to master interproximal plaque control.

g. The gingival embrasure is not accessible, exposed or pronounced enough to facilitate proximal instrumentation without cutting a facial or lingual access cavity.

h. Generally, it would be unrealistic from the biological, mechanical and conservative points to have an occlusal access to such an apically located proximal lesion.

In *shape B* (Fig. 38B), the facial or lingual access will have a locking feature in the form of a dovetail, unilaterally cut in the occlusal direction. The indications for the design are the same as shape A with these exceptions:

a. The final cavity preparation will not have four surrounding walls and either one wall or no wall is bulky enough to accommodate a groove.

b. For medium to large sized proximal lesion the self-retention proximally will not be compatible with the cavity size and the displacing forces.

2. General shape (Fig. 38)

The proximal part of this cavity will have no specific shape.

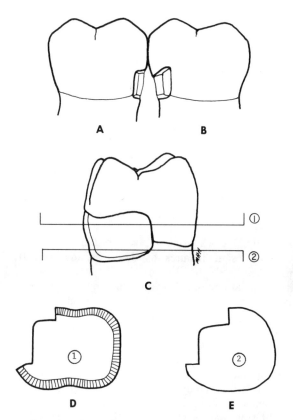

Fig. 6-38. C, Proximal view. **D-E,** Cross-section in preparation

Generally, however, it will appear either trapezoidal or elliptical. The facial or lingual part of this design will be either a box or rectangular shape (shape A) or it will be a one-sided dovetailed shape (shape B).

3. Location of margins

On the proximal part of this preparation, the gingival margin will be located in the gingival embrasure, even with the crest of the free gingiva, or it may be supragingival. The occlusal margin will also be in the gingival embrasure, just apical to the contact area. The facial or lingual margins, on the non-access side, will be located in the corresponding embrasure, short of the axial angle of the tooth. On the access side, the occlusal and gingival margins will be a continuation of the corresponding margins from the proximal portion. The proximal margins are far enough onto the facial or lingual surface (access) to include the axial angle and, maximally, one-fourth of the facial or lingual surface. When the access cavity is dovetailed, its dimension should be compatible with the size and displacement forces for the proximal restoration, but should not exceed one-fourth of the facial or lingual surface.

4. Internal anatomy (Fig. 38)

a. In an occluso-gingival cross section, the proximal and/or facial (lingual) access portion will present the same anatomy. The axial wall will appear flat occlusogingivally, except if replaces a surface concavity. Use the same design features as described for Class II Design 4.

The occlusal and gingival walls, if both are located on cementum or dentin, will be formed of two planes: an internal dentinal grooved plane, and an external dentinal plane which is perfectly flat and opening straight proximally. There is no place for cementum in any of these walls (see cross-section in Design 4, Fig. 37C).

If the occlusal margin is located on enamel, it is always at the gingival third of the surface, so the occlusal wall will be one-planed following the direction of the enamel rods. The resultant inclination axio-gingivally creates a needed undercut. If the occlusal or gingival margins are located in any other locations, refer to the simple design of Class II (Fig. 37, A and B) for a description of internal anatomy.

b. In a facio-lingual cross-section (Fig. 38, C, D, E), the axial wall will be, in essence, two distinct axial walls, i.e., one proximal, and another facial or lingual (access side). Both are perfectly flat, joining each other in a very rounded axio-axial line angle. The proximal axial wall may be slightly slanted toward the access side (isthmus). If any portion of the axial walls is adjacent to a proximal, facial or lingual concavity, use the same design features as described in Class II, Design 4.

If the facial or lingual wall on the non-access side has its margin on enamel, (located at the lateral one-third of the proximal surface), it will be composed of two planes: an inner dentinal plane at a right angle to the proximal axial wall, for resistance and retention; and an outer enamelo-dentin plane in the same direction as the enamel rods (Fig. 38D). However, if this wall has its margins at the middle third of the proximal surface, it will be composed of one straight plane which is at a right angle to the axial wall. Sometimes, in a very apically located lesion, part or all of this facial or lingual wall will be completely formed of dentin, always at a right angle to the axial wall (Fig. 38E). If the facial or lingual walls are bulky enough, cut a retention groove at the expense of the dentinal part of the wall as done in designs 1 and 2.

The mesial or distal wall on the access side is always one-planed. It is formed of enamel and dentin following the direction of the enamel rods. This makes it either convergent toward the proximal, creating an acute angle with the axial wall, or it makes it perpendicular to that axial wall, depending on the exact location of the margin. If it is convergent, it will add to the retention of the restoration.

The previous internal anatomy description fits shape A of Design 5. If shape B is necessitated, it will have less details according to the extent of the lesion, e.g., insufficient dentin bulk gingivally could prevent placing a gingival groove for fear of perforating the pulp chamber or the root canal. Occlusal margins very close to the contact area necessitate occlusal walls without grooves. Compensating for such a deficient retention form requires that the access cavity be ''dovetailed'' in form.

The decision to go from the facial or the lingual in this type of cavity preparation is mainly dictated by the extent of the decay and the condition of the axial angle, i.e., the more involved side is the side chosen for the access cavity. Also, the location of the access cavity is governed by the controllability of the surrounding tissues, muscular or non-muscular. Generally speaking, senile decay usually involves more facial than lingual tooth structure, because of the cleaning action of the tongue. Since tissues are more retractable facially than lingually, most of these cavity preparations have a facial approach.

5. Instrumentation for Class II, Design 5
a. Gaining access and gross removal

With a tapered fissure bur, using axial pressure and lateral dragging, on the access side cut the access window which usually will be in sound tooth structures. From this access preparation introduce the same tapered fissure bur proximally, using axial and lingual pressure (assuming it is a buccal access) and occluso-gingival dragging. Remove diseased and involved sound tissue within the future outline of the preparation.

b. Removal of attacked irreparable dentin

This is accomplished as in previous designs of Class II preparations.

c. Preliminary shaping

This is done using the tip and side of a 700 or a 169 bur to create definite surrounding walls, and to formulate the proximal axial wall. Retention grooves, if indicated, may be cut using a ¼ round bur, dragged along the axio-gingival and sometimes axio-occlusal line angle, with pressure gingivally and occlusally. The grooves are cut at the expense of the gingival and occlusal walls, involving both the facial (lingual) and the proximal part of these walls.

d. Final shaping occurs when the different planes of surrounding walls are formed using a hatchet for the access cavity and axial wall and a gingival margin trimmer for the non-access side walls and gingival walls. Defining and rounding of line and point angles is done using a Wedelstaedt or hatchet chisels.

e. Cavity finish is accomplished using the same instruments but with lighter and more frequent applications.

f. Intermediary basing is done as mentioned in a previous chapter.

F. Class II, Design 6

Involvement: The occlusal, proximal(s) and part of the facial and/or lingual surfaces

1. Indications

This design is indicated when:

a. The cusp length is double or more its width, either throughout or at certain portions of the cusp.

b. A cusp is completely missing or undermined.

c. A foundation for cast restoration is required.

d. Teeth have a doubtful prognosis endodontically and periodontally.

3. A badly broken down tooth needs to be prepared prior to endodontic or orthodontic treatment.

f. A cast restoration is not indicated.

2. General shape (Fig. 39)

The occlusal and proximal parts are similar in outline to Designs 1 or 2. The facial and/or lingual parts are rectangular in outline.

3. Location of margins

The occlusal and proximal portions have the same location of margins as in designs 1 or 2. In the facial or lingual portions of the cavity preparation the margins could be located in a variety of locations depending on several factors. In areas at or occlusal to the height of contour of the facial or lingual surfaces, margins could be placed anywhere provided it is a convex-surfaced area, e.g., do not place margins in grooves. In areas apical to the height of contour of the facial or lingual surfaces, apply the same principles as for locating margins in the gingival ⅓ of proximal surfaces.

With only partial mesio-distal replacement of a cusp, the

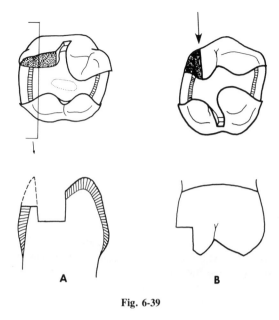

Fig. 6-39

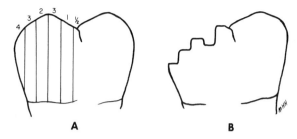

Fig. 6-40. Cusp reduction is directly proportional to the length:width ratio.

margin should not end at the tip of the cusp; rather it should be located mesial or distal to it. Similarly, if a margin comes near a groove, involve the groove in the cavity preparation, locating the margin past the groove in an effort to avoid feather-edged marginal amalgam.

4. Internal anatomy (Fig. 39)

In this design, the features of the occlusal and proximal parts are similar to those in Designs 1 or 2. However, in the cuspal replacement area (Fig. 39), a variety of internal features can be produced in replacing entire cusps (Fig. 40A) or parts of cusps (Fig. 40B), but there are certain rules which must be applied:

a. Cusps or parts of the cusps to be replaced or covered with amalgam should be reduced at least 1.5-2 mm from opposing cuspal elements in both static and dynamic contacts. This will accommodate sufficient amalgam bulk to resist loading. There should be more reduction on functional than on non-functional cusps. If the amalgam will serve as a foundation for a future cast restoration, more reduction is needed in order to leave the minimum of 1.5-2 mm of amalgam, after tooth preparation, as the foundation for the cast restoration.

b. Cuspal elements, or parts of them, which will accommodate amalgam must be cut flat, i.e., in the form of a table, with right-angled cavosurface margins.

c. Reduce cusps or parts of a cusp until there is a minimum length: width ratio of 1:1. If the length:width ratio is different at different cross-sectional locations of a cusp, tables can be prepared at these different levels. In addition to conserving tooth structure, this will add to the retention of the restoration (Fig. 40).

d. If the cusp or part of a cusp is formed of undermined or thinned enamel, it should be tabled until there is intact enamel supported by sound dentin.

e. The remaining part of the cavity preparation should have sufficient retention not only to be self-retentive, but also to help retain the amalgam replacing the cuspal portion(s).

f. It is always advisable to have a retention form, e.g., external box or groove, adjacent to the tabled cusp, especially

if it involves an axial angle. This will immobilize the amalgam cusp more efficiently.

g. Tables can be at any level, provided they fulfill the previous rules. They can be level with pulpal or gingival floors or there may be an occlusal or gingival step from the pulpal or gingival floors to the tabled area.

h. Never place pins on tables which will accommodate amalgam cusps or part of a cusp (see chapter on pin-retained amalgams).

i. In cavity preparations with multiple tables on the same cusp the junction between one table and another should be rounded.

5. Instrumentation for Class II, Design 6

Designs 1, 2, or 3 are partially prepared in the usual manner previously described. After evaluating the condition of the cusps and deciding whether or not a partial or complete cap is indicated, the following should be done during the preliminary and final shaping:

a. Using a 555 bur, reduce the cuspal area to be capped according to the previous rules.

b. Using a hatchet, Wedelstaedt or binangle chisel, flatten the cut area and round its junction with the adjacent walls and the main part of the cavity preparation.

c. The cavosurface is finished, along with the rest of the preparation, in the usual way.

G. Class II, Design 7 (Combination of Class II with Class V)

Shape A: The junction between the Class II and Class V via the proximal, crossing the axial angle(s) (Fig. 41).

Involvement: The occlusal, proximal, and part or all of the gingival third of the facial and/or lingual surfaces with the intervening part of the axial angle(s)

1. Indications

a. This design is indicated when at a location apical to the contact area, an occluso-proximal lesion joins a senile decay lesion via decalcification, or a defect that has spread laterally beyond the lateral limit of the original occluso-proximal lesion and the regular cavity preparation.

b. A Class V lesion undermines enamel or directly involves tooth structure of the adjacent axial angle(s), in a tooth having a proximo-occlusal lesion.

c. Surface defects or decalcifications at the axial angle(s) of the tooth are continuous with a proximo-occlusal cavity preparation or lesion apical to the contact area.

2. General shape (Fig. 41)

a. The occlusal portion of this design is similar in outline to Designs 1 or 2.

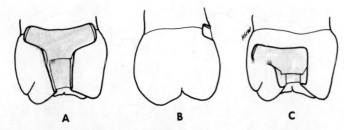

Fig. 6-41. A, Proximal view, bilateral extension preparation. **B,** Facial (lingual) view. **C,** Proximal view, unilateral extension preparation.

b. The proximo-facial and proximo-lingual portion, if the cavity extension will unilaterally involve the facial or lingual axial angle only, will be "L-shaped" (Fig. 41C). If the extension will be bilateral, i.e., involving both facial and lingual axial angles, it will be "inverted T-shaped" (Fig. 41A).

3. Location of margins

The occlusal margins and the main parts of the proximal margins will be exactly like those described for Designs 1 and 2. In the extensions, facially and/or lingually, the gingival margin will seldom be located subgingivally, but will be even with the free gingiva or supragingival.

The occlusal margin in the extension (Fig. 41, A and C) will be apical to the contact area, continuous with the facial or lingual margins of the main proximal cavity occlusally. The occlusal margin will be located mostly on the facial or lingual surface at the height of contour, crossing the axial angle there. In a unilateral "L-shaped" design, there is only one occlusal wall (Fig. 41C), but in the bilateral inverted T design there are two occlusal walls (Fig. 41A). The facial and/or lingual margins of the extensions (Fig. 41B) will be located past the axial angle on the facial or lingual surfaces.

4. Internal anatomy (Fig. 41)

The features of this design, in the occlusal and proximal portions proper, are very similar to those found in Designs 1 and 2. In the extensions, the internal anatomical features of the gingival and occlusal walls are very similar to those described for the design for senile decay. Facial and/or lingual walls, if their margins do not exceed the middle of the facial or lingual surface in the mesio-distal direction, will also have the same anatomy as the design for senile decay (Design 5). However, if they do exceed this width, the walls will be divergent toward the uninvolved axial angle.

Shape B (Fig. 42): The junction between the Class II and Class V is through the occlusal via the buccal and/or lingual grooves

Involvement: The proximal, occlusal, facial and/or lingual surfaces

1. Indications

This design is indicated when:

a. A Class V lesion connects with an occluso-proximal lesion via a facial or lingual fissured groove.

b. Surface defects or decalcifications on the facial or lingual surface connect a Class V lesion with an occluso-proximal lesion.

c. A Class V lesion is continuous with a Class I, Design 4, which, in turn, is continuous with an occluso-proximal lesion.

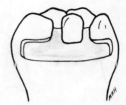

Fig. 6-42

2. General shape (Fig. 42)

The outline of the occlusal and proximal portions of this design are exactly as described for designs 1 and 2. The facial and/or lingual parts are "inverted T-shape".

3. Location of margins

The margins for the Class V portion are located as indicated in Chapter #7. Margins for the proximo-occlusal cavity are as described for Designs 1 or 2.

4. Internal anatomy (Fig. 42)

This may be described as three separate cavities, with the occlusal and proximal portions appearing exactly as previously described for Designs 1 or 2, and the facial and/or lingual portions as described in Chapter #5.

The connection between the occlusal and facial or lingual portion is in the form of the long arm of an inverted T. It will have the mesial and distal walls one-planed, formed of enamel and dentin. They are to be perfectly straight, perpendicular to a flat axial wall, which will slant toward the pulpal floor.

5. Cavity Preparation Instrumentation

a. The occluso-proximal cavity preparation proper is prepared in the conventional way as described for Design 1.

b. The facial and/or lingual extensions of the proximal part are prepared from the corresponding embrasure as described for Design 4. Here the instrumentation will be made easier by the possible formulation of part of the gingival floor from an occlusal access.

c. The Class V portion, if needed, is prepared as described in Class V cavity preparation, Chapter #7.

d. Using binangle chisel, hatchet or Wedelstaedt chisel, from a buccal, occlusal and lingual access, round and smooth the junctions between the different parts of the preparation.

H. Class II, Design 8

Involvement: Two or more surfaces of an endodontically treated tooth that does not require post retention

1. Indications

This design is indicated when:

a. The remaining tooth structure, after endodontics, can support and retain an amalgam restoration.

b. The tooth has a sufficient pulp chamber to accommodate retaining, self-resisting amalgam bulk, i.e., a minimum 2 mm thickness in three dimensions.

c. The post-endodontic pulp chamber has at least two opposing intact walls.

d. The tooth contains sufficiently large root canals to accommodate retaining, resisting amalgam bulk at its (their) occlusal one-thirds (i.e., minimum 1.5 mm thickness).

e. A foundation is needed for a reinforcing restoration (cast restoration).

f. There is sufficient remaining tooth structure to permit the preparation of flat planes at right angles to occluding forces.

g. There has been successful root canal therapy leaving an intact subpulpal floor.

h. The tooth does not show any signs of cracking or crazing.

2. General shape

The outline will appear exactly as described for Design 6.

3. Internal anatomy (Fig. 43)

An infinite number of shapes are possible for this design. It is necessary only to apply certain rules to arrive at the finished product:

a. Excavate from the entire pulp chamber any residual root canal filling materials or debris. Bare dentin should be exposed on the surrounding walls and subpulpal floor. (Fig. 43, A and E).

b. Large root canals that can accommodate an amalgam thickness of 1.5 mm should have the root canal filling removed to a 3-4 mm depth (Fig. 43B, C, D).

c. If possible, "square up" surrounding walls, provided this action will not perforate to the surface, furcation, or thin tooth structure to the extent of making these areas non-resistant.

d. In the bulky portion of the surrounding walls of the pulp chamber, cut flat ledges to receive most of the occlusal loading, thereby minimizing stresses on the subpulpal floor during such loading (Fig. 43, B, D, E, F).

e. Establish as pronounced gingival floors as possible. If they are in dentin, they will be one-planed; and if on enamel, they will be two-planed (Fig. 43, B and C).

f. Retain any residual pulpal floor, placing ledges in it and making it as flat as possible (Fig. 43, A and E)

g. Treat the cusps and cuspal elements as described for Design 6 (Fig. 43, D and F).

h. In preparing tables and ledges allow sufficient reduction depths to provide enough thickness of amalgam to serve as a foundation for a reinforcing cast restoration.

i. Any external boxes for retention should not perforate to the pulp chamber or cause thinning in the intervening walls.

j. Try to make every part of the preparation self-retaining.

k. Each flat portion of the preparation, e.g., tables or ledges, should be opposed by a similar flat component for proper reciprocation, to immobilize the restoration and evenly distribute stresses (Fig. 43, B, C, D, E, F).

l. Flat portions of the tooth preparation receiving forces at a right angle to their inclination should be strategically distributed, in order to be maximally concentrated in number and dimensions at locations of maximal loading.

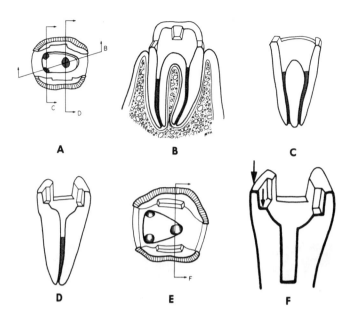

Fig. 6-43. A, Pulp chamber left no pulpal floor. **E,** Pulp chamber left pulpal floor distally.

4. Instrumentation for Class II, Design 8

The occluso-proximal cavity preparation and capping of cusps, short of pulp chamber and root canal preparation, is done in the same way as described for Designs 1 and 6. For intrapulpal and intraradicular preparation the following procedures may be done.

Ledges and shelves may be prepared using 555 and 556 burs in apical pressure and lateral dragging. Intraradicular preparation is started by removing the specified lengths of the indicated root canal material using hot gutta-percha pluggers, peaso reamers or bibevelled-sided reamers. Then, the specified length of the canal is widened and side-paralleled using large tapered, then cylindrical fissure burs (704, 558). Following this, the junction between pulp chamber and root canal preparations should be rounded using round burs. Finally, all junctional parts of the cavity preparations are rounded using a round bur or a very sharp gingival margin trimmer.

See bibliography at the end of Chapter VII.

CHAPTER 7

Class III, IV, and V cavity preparations for amalgam

Distal of the Cuspid Cavity Preparations for Amalgam

Amalgam is usually not indicated for anterior teeth due to its esthetic limitations, but the distal surface of the cuspid is a unique location that does necessitate a metallic restoration to replace lost tooth structure. Although the application of the general principles of Class III and IV cavity preparations will be described in detail in the chapter on direct tooth-colored restorations, sufficient information must be provided here to understand the purpose of design features for a cavity preparation on the distal of the cuspid.

Application of the General Principles:

I. Outline Form

General principles are applied to Class III amalgams in similar fashion to the Class II cavity preparation, with five areas of emphasis:

A. Esthetic concern

This makes it preferable to use a lingual access rather than a labial access to the cavity. Furthermore, any labial margin should be located just barely into the labial embrasure, unless there is need for further extension for other reasons. The labial margin of the Class III should also be convex, paralleling the labial contour of the canine. In addition, no undermined or thinned enamel, that would allow amalgam to show through, should remain.

B. Extension for access

To instrument a cavity preparation on the distal of a cuspid from a lingual approach, the lingual margin should not only be in the lingual embrasure, but sometimes must also have an incisal or gingival "turn", or overextension, on the adjacent lingual surface. This feature facilitates instrumentation of internal anatomy. The choice between the incisal or gingival "turn" is a clinical judgment, depending upon the width of the lingual embrasure incisally as compared to gingivally, the vault of the palate, tapering of the anterior segment of the upper arch, the degree of opening of the mouth, the location of the occluding contacts, and, most importantly, the extension

of the decay. From a mechanical point of view, it is preferable to have a gingival turn. An incisal turn may thin tooth structure in a critical area.

C. Stress considerations

Although the incisal margin of the cavity preparation is brought to the incisal embrasure, placing it in a self-cleansable and finishable area and making the contact area in alloy, it is not necessary to extend it too far incisally. This may undermine or involve the distal slope of the canine, an area of massive stress concentration during lateral disclusion of the mandible.

D. Enamel rod considerations

Whenever the lingual margin nears a lingual marginal ridge, it is necessary to include this section of the marginal ridge in the cavity preparation, as no rules exist for the direction of enamel rods there.

E. Incisal access

If a considerable part of the incisal slope is undermined or directly attacked by decay, necessitating involvement in the cavity preparation, access should be performed incisally, preserving as much of the labial and lingual walls as possible. This necessitates no "turns" and no extension for access, as these walls are needed to augment retention and resistance forms.

II. Mechanical Problems at the Distal of the Cuspid and How They Affect the Resistance-Retention Forms of a Restoration

The distal surface of the cuspid is an area of substantial stress concentration. It is one of the few areas in the mouth where the three types of stresses (i.e., compression, shear, tensile) are combined in substantial amounts. They are produced by the following:

A. The anterior component of forces (Fig. 1A) concentrates at the junction between the anterior segment of the arch and the premolar region. The cuspid stands at this corner, where these forces will first be received and resisted, especially on its distal surface.

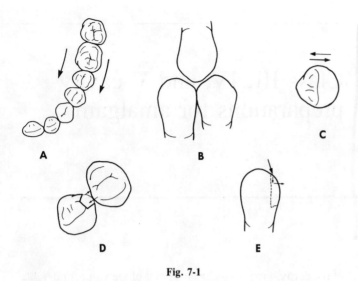

Fig. 7-1

B. The incisal slopes of the cuspid (i.e., the distal slope of the lower against the mesial slope of the upper, and the distal slope of the upper against the mesial inclined plane of the buccal cusp of the lower premolar (Fig. 1B), in a normal excursion mechanism, will be the last cuspal elements to disclude during lateral excursion. In other words, the canine carries the maximum occlusal load for the longest period of time. These lateral forces will subject the distal surface of the cuspid to a rubbing action, which, when combined with the anterior component of force, precipitates massive shear and abrading forces on that surface (Fig. 1C).

C. Because of the usual wide lingual embrasure on the distal of the cuspid and the very labial location of the contact area, these forces on the cuspid will tend to tip the restoration's lingual portion distolingually (Fig. 1D).

D. If the incisal margin of the cavity preparation is located far enough onto the distal slope, the restoration will be directly loaded vertically and horizontally (laterally) (Fig. 1E), a situation that necessitates tremendous strength and retention for the material placed there.

In addition to the previous four traumatizing factors at the distal of the cuspid, there are also the normal loading and displacing forces for anterior teeth which will be discussed in detail in a chapter for direct tooth-colored restorations. It is appropriate to at least enumerate some of these forces here.

For the upper teeth there is a linguo-labial force, and for the lower teeth there is a labio-lingual force. Both will try to rotate a restoration linguo-labially and labio-lingually, respectively. There is a vertical incisal force that will tend to displace the restoration proximally, as in Class II restorations. During protrusive excursion, there is a rubbing, vertical force trying to displace the restoration incisally. (All of this assumes that the occlusion is normal. For abnormal situations refer to a chapter on direct tooth-colored restorations). To counteract all these forces, the cavity preparation on the distal of the cuspid should have:

1. The bulkiest walls possible.

2. Minimal incisal extension, and if it involves parts of the incisal slope, additional retention or bulk for the restoration.

3. Retention placed in every available safe area of the cavity

preparation, e.g., point angles, grooves, gingival and incisal grooves, two-planed facial and/or lingual walls, etc.

4. Designs to accommodate only metallic restorations such as amalgam. Tooth-colored materials have no chance of withstanding the types of forces described above. If esthetics is of great concern here due to an extensive labial extension, an amalgam restoration can be built with a window-like cavity preparation placed in the labial portion of the amalgam, to be restored by a tooth-colored material. It is to be noted, however, that the entire contact area should remain in amalgam. An opacifier should be applied on any cavity floor made of amalgam so the amalgam will not show through the transparency of the direct tooth-colored materials. The retention for the tooth-colored material should have some tooth structure component, and should not be all in the amalgam material itself.

III. Convenience Form

The Class III cavity preparation should be designed with the following features of convenience form:

A. The access side wall, which is most often the lingual wall, is one-planed, divergent linguo-proximally. This lingual wall (the access side wall) is also shorter than the labial wall.

B. The convexity of the axial wall is always less than the convexity of the proximal surface to facilitate visualization of line and point angles.

C. There may be an incisal or gingival "turn" (i.e., extension) in the lingual margin.

Designs of Cavity Preparations to Accommodate Amalgam at the Distal of the Cuspid

A. Class III

This is the basic design for the distal of the cuspid.

Involvement: Distal surface of the cuspid and part of the lingual surface or, rarely, part of the labial surface

1. Indications

a. The lesion does not involve or undermine the distal slope of the cuspid.

b. Bulky walls will remain, especially incisally, after removal of diseased and undermined tissues.

c. The labial axial angle is intact.

d. The restoration will not be directly loaded by vertical forces and, preferably, not by horizontal forces either.

2. General shape (Fig. 3)

This design appears triangular with rounded corners. The labial side of the triangle conforms more to the proximal surface anatomy than the lingual side.

3. Location of margins

For a lingual approach preparation, the gingival margins will be located exactly as described for Class II, Designs 1, 2, 3. The labial margins will be situated barely into the labial embrasure. The lingual margins (Fig. 3) will be within the confines of the lingual embrasure, except for the incisal (Fig. 2B) or gingival (Fig. 2C) turn extension, if indicated. (The incisal or gingival turn is indicated when the lingual embrasure is not wide enough to facilitate instrumentation). Incisal margins should be placed in the incisal embrasure only enough to show

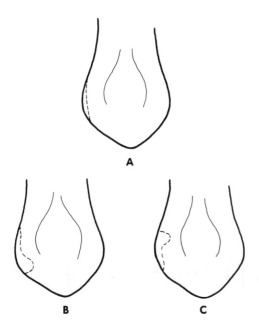

Fig. 7-2. A, No turn. **B,** Incisal turn. **C.** Gingival turn.

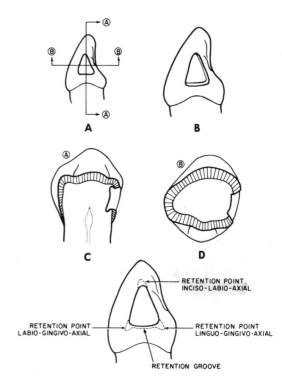

Fig. 7-3. Class III amalgam preparation (Distal) cuspid.

light passing between the margin and the adjacent proximal surface.

4. Internal anatomy (Fig. 3)

In a labio-lingual cross-section (Fig. 3D), the axial wall will appear slightly rounded (convex) labio-lingually, but not to the extent of that of the proximal surface of the tooth. It should be at a depth of 0.5 mm from the DEJ. Deeper portions, due to dental caries cones, may be at another level axially (i.e., the axial wall may have more than one plane).

As the labial margin will usually be located at the labial one-third of the distal surface, because of the labial deviation of the contact area, the labial wall in cross-section can be seen to be formed of two planes: one inner dentinal at a right angle to the tangent of the axial wall (resistance-retention) and an outer enamelo-dentinal plane following the direction of the enamel rods (usually diverging labio-distally). Rarely, the labial margin will be located at the middle third of the distal surface, which is usually due to labial rotation of the cuspid. In this case the cross-sectional analysis will show the labial wall to be a one-planed enamelo-dentinal wall, perpendicular to the axial wall.

The lingual wall (access) will be generally shorter than the labial wall, with the "turn" extension area, if present, showing as the shortest part. This emphasizes that in preparations with incisal or gingival turns, the lingual wall dimensions will not be symmetrical inciso-gingivally. In any event, the wall will be formed of one enamelo-dentinal plane, diverging linguo-distally.

In an inciso-gingival cross-section (Fig. 3C), if the gingival margin is located at the gingival third of the distal surface, the gingival wall will be formed of three planes: an internal retentive grooved area, a transition dentinal plane, and an outer enamelo-dentinal plane diverging disto-gingivally.

The axial wall will appear as almost flat, but it may accommodate one or more concavities corresponding to the axial extent of deep caries cones. Also, assuming the incisal margin is located at the incisal one-third of the distal surface, the incisal

wall will be seen to be formed of three planes. The first is an inner dentinal plane, 1.5 mm deep, corresponding to the grooved area. This parallels the adjacent slope, but with a slight labial inclination. Next is a transitional plane, formed of dentin. Finally, there is an outer enamelo-dentinal plane following the enamel rods and inclining inciso-distally so as to leave sufficient bulk of enamel supported by dentin to protect the distal slope and angle.

Retention points also will appear in this cross-section, starting at the gingivo-labio-axial and gingivo-linguo-axial point angle, in a direction trisecting each point angle to a depth of 1 to 2 mm in dentin. The labial groove should be bulkier than the lingual (due to pulp chamber deviation). However, each groove should have at least 1 to 1.5 mm dimensions in three directions, and they should join the gingival groove and the rest of the preparation anatomy in rounded, bulk-accommodating, junctions. Also, these retention points should end bluntly in dentin.

5. Modifications

a. The decay extent may dictate a labial approach, in which case the wall anatomy of the labial and lingual walls, as described, will be reversed. However, there will be no turns for either the labial or lingual margins, as access can be gained easily from the labial without these extensions.

b. If the incisal wall is not bulky enough to accommodate a retentive groove without undermining the distal slope, it may be replaced by a labial and, to a lesser extent, lingual groove.

c. If the horizontal gingival groove cannot be located without perforation to a surface concavity or without coming close to one, it can be replaced by deepening the point angle retention grooves.

d. If the labial or lingual wall is lost (Fig. 4), it is essential to at least create a very short wall to try to lock the restoration.

This can be accomplished by deepening the axial wall at its labial or lingual periphery and by establishing a very pronounced axio-labial or axio-lingual line angle (Fig. 4).

e. If the gingival margin is at the middle third of the distal surface, the gingival wall will be two-planed: an inner grooved plane, and an outer, straight (flat) plane following the direction of the enamel rods. If the gingival margin is on cementum, there will be a two-planed gingival wall: an inner grooved plane, and an outer flat plane. Both are in dentin. Cementum should be removed if it is close to the margins (Fig. 5D).

f. If the incisal margin is at the middle third of the distal surface, the incisal wall will be formed of two planes: an inner grooved dentinal part, and an outer enamelo-dentin plane opening straight, proximally, at a right angle to the long axis of the crown (Fig. 5D).

g. In senile decay, where the incisal margin of the lesion is apical to the contact area, the incisal wall will be one-planed, inclining gingivally-distally, making an acute angle with the axial wall (undercut) (Fig. 6). The gingival margin here will definitely be on cementum, with the same arrangement as mentioned before (Fig. 6).

h. If the entire preparation can be confined to the gingival embrasure (Fig. 5A), either due to senile decay or decay affecting periodontally exposed root surface, the preparation will not need any turns in its outline (Fig. 5A), nor point retention grooves, nor the divergent one-planed lingual or labial walls (Fig. 5, B and C). If the margins of the later walls are on cementum or at the middle third of the surface, the walls will be one-planed (Fig. 5C). Otherwise they will be two-planed as usual. This is because of the accessibility of the gingival embrasures and the non-proximal loading for the restoration there.

6. Instrumentation for Class III

a. Prerequisites

Understand and visualize the general shape, location of margins and internal anatomy of this design in all cuspid teeth. A rubber dam must be properly applied. Wedges are introduced from both the labial and the lingual, gingival to the contact area, to protect the interceptal dam and gingiva and to create slight separation.

b. Procedure

i. With a ¼, ½, or 1 round bur, introduced at the lesion from the lingual, use axial pressure and lateral dragging to remove tooth structure within the anticipated depth and outline form of the preparation. It may help to increase the length of the bur shanks or to use burs with lengthy shanks to facilitate this operation.

ii. Removal of undesirable attacked dentin is accomplished using instruments and procedures previously described.

iii. Preliminary shaping (Fig. 7, B, C, D)

With the base of a 33½ or 33¼ inverted cone bur seated at the location of the future labial wall, use labial pressure and incisal gingival dragging to preliminarily shape the labial wall (Fig. 7B). Next use the side of the same inverted cone bur seated on the future lingual wall location and apply lingual pressure and inciso-gingival dragging to create a roughed-in lingual wall (Fig. 7C). Then, with the base of a 33½ inverted cone bur seated on the future gingival wall location, apply gingival pressure and labio-lingual dragging to rough-in gingival floor (Fig. 7D).

iv. Preparation of point angle and line angle grooves

With a ¼ or ½ round bur seated at the gingivo-labio-axial

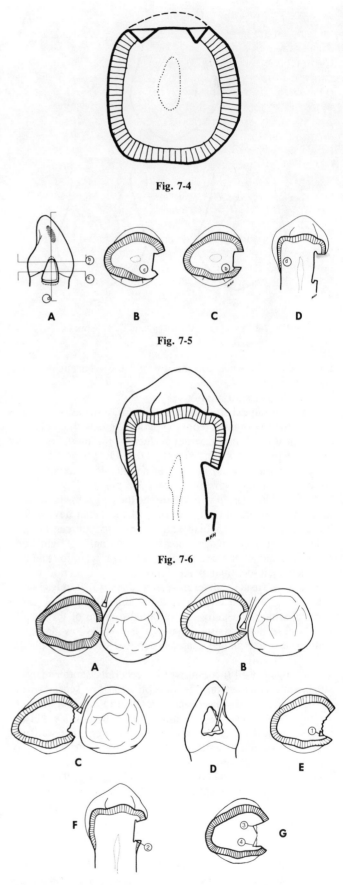

Fig. 7-4

Fig. 7-5

Fig. 7-6

Fig. 7-7

point angle, use direct cutting pressure to drill a retention point in dentin (2 mm deep and directed gingivo-labio-axially). Then, pull the bur out slightly and drag it lingually, along the axio-gingival line angle, to create a retention groove at the expense of the gingival floor, at a depth shallower than the point angle groove. Next, with the ¼ or ½ round bur seated in the linguo-gingivo-axial point angle, use lateral cutting pressure to slowly drill the other retention point in dentin (2 mm deep and directed gingivo-linguo-axially). With the same bur seated at the inciso-labio-axial point angle, slowly drill a retention point in dentin, slightly directed inciso-labio-axially and paralleling the distal slope of the cuspid.

v. Final shaping (Fig. 7E, F, G)

Use the flat blade of the angle former, hatchet, or gingival margin trimmer to cut triangles #1 and #2 (Fig. 7E, F), making two planes for the labial and gingival walls. Also, cut triangles #3 and #4 (Fig. 7G) to round the axial wall in the labio-lingual direction. Then, with a properly angulated bi-bevelled hatchet that fits the incisal groove, use shaving actions to widen and deepen this groove. With the tip of the gingival margin trimmer or angle former, widen and deepen the gingival grooves.

vi. Cavity finish

Use a suitably sized gingival margin trimmer or angle former to round the junctions between the different retention grooves, and between these grooves and the rest of the wall details. Next, with a suitable size Wedelstaedt chisel, hatchet, hoe or gingival margin trimmer, use lateral cutting motions to smooth all walls and floors and to define all line angles. Finally, with a Wedelstaedt chisel, trim all cavosurface margins to make them right angled. (Application of intermediary basing will follow the principles described in that chapter.)

B. Class IV

Involvement: This design encompasses not only the distal surface, but also part or all of the distal incisal slope of the cuspid.

1. Indications

This preparation is indicated when:

a. The incisal angle is undermined or involved by the lesion.

b. The labial and lingual walls are intact and bulky.

c. There is a pronounced intact gingival floor.

d. A restoration that replaces the distal slope or part of it will be subjected to that slope's mechanical problems.

2. The general shape (Fig. 8A) of this cavity preparation is an inverted truncated cone.

3. Location of margins

Gingival and labial margins are exactly as described for Class III. The lingual margin is located in the lingual embrasure, just clearing the contact area. The incisal margin is located on the slope of the incisal edge.

4. Internal anatomy (Fig. 8A, B, C)

Overall, the internal anatomy of this design bears a great resemblance to the Class II conservative design. In labio-lingual cross-section, the axial wall appears almost flat, although it may have different levels dictated by the depth of caries cones.

The labial and lingual walls, assuming the labial and lingual margins are located at the labial and lingual one-third, respectively, of the distal surface, will each appear in cross-section

as being formed of three planes. First is an inner (dentinal) plane in the form of a groove that has its maximum divergence and dimension at the gingival floor level. This dimension decreases gradually, going incisally, until it ends just short of undermining the labial and lingual enamel plates. Next will occur a transitional (dentinal) plane, and finally there will be an outer (enamelo-dentinal) plane diverging disto-labially and lingually. If any margins must be located elsewhere, refer back to Class II design 3 for descriptive details of the cross-section analysis.

In an inciso-gingival cross-section, the gingival wall appears exactly as in Class III. The axial wall will be flat, with a slight slant to the enamel surface of the slope. This wall may have different levels (as Class III), depending on carious invasion.

Point retention grooves are evident in this cross-section, located exactly as in Class III.

5. Modifications

a. Modifications c, d, e, as described for Class III, may be applied here also.

b. In addition, if the labial or lingual walls are not bulky enough to accommodate retention grooves, it is advisable to make these walls in two planes: i.e., an inner (dentinal) plane at a right angle to the axial wall, and an outer (enamelo-dentinal) plane following the direction of the enamel rods. To further compensate for the absence of retention grooves, it is necessary to accentuate the rest of the retention modes.

c. Sometimes, the entire cavity preparation may be inclined inciso-lingually, especially in the upper cuspid, resulting in the preparation opening partially at its incisal end onto the lingual surface (Fig. 8D). In such cases, the lingual wall must be more slanted in an inciso-gingival direction than the labial wall. This should not be an intentional preparation modification, rather, it should be dictated by tooth inclinations and the extent of incisal involvement.

d. If retention forms are deficient, and some walls are either partially or totally lost, pins should be used to help retain the

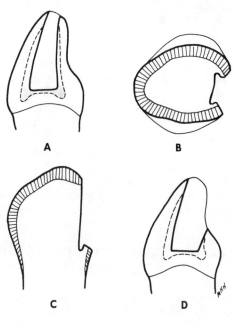

Fig. 7-8

amalgam in this design. This modification will be discussed in detail in the chapter dealing with pin- and post-retained restorations.

e. Two other designs of cavity preparations for the distal of the cuspid are not used now, as they have proved to be too detrimental. One involves a dovetail at the incisal two-thirds of the lingual surface. This is contraindicated except to replace a restoration into the same cavity preparation. A dovetail in this location will further thin already thinned tooth structure and will bring the metallic restoration close to the lingually deviated pulp. Furthermore, such a design does not lock the restoration completely in all directions. The other abandoned design has no lingual wall at all, and retention is achieved through a gingival, labial and incisal groove at the junction of each of the gingival, labial and incisal walls with the axial wall. The absence of the lingual wall, although it facilitates access, deprives the restoration from a most needed locking mechanism. In addition, such retentive grooves are not strategically located relative to the displacing forces. However, if replacing a restoration in such a cavity preparation, it is acceptable to follow the same design of tooth preparation.

6. Instrumentation for Class IV

a. Prerequisites

These are the same as those mentioned for Class III.

b. Procedures

i. Gaining access is usually accomplished through the incisal or inciso-lingual direction. Access is facilitated by removing undermined enamel there, using a chisel. In addition, access is made easier by utilizing wedges.

ii. Gross removal of carious tooth structure is performed exactly as in Class III preparations. Similarly, the removal of undesirable attacked dentin is accomplished as described previously.

iii. Preliminary shaping of the preparation may be done with a 168 or 169 bur. Using apical pressure and facio-lingual dragging, roughly prepare the gingival, labial, lingual, and axial walls.

iv. Final shaping is done using the same instruments as in Class III. Five triangles are cut, one on each of the proximal peripheries of the labial or lingual wall, making two planes out of each wall: one on each of the labial and lingual one-thirds of the axial wall, rounding that wall, and another on the proximal periphery of the gingival floor, creating two planes for that wall.

v. The gingival grooves are prepared in the same way as described in Class III, but with direct cutting action facilitated by the incisal access.

vi. Facial and lingual grooves are prepared as the facial and lingual grooves of the conservative design of a Class II cavity preparation, using a ¼ round, 168, or 33¼ burs.

viii. The cavity is finished as described for Class III, using the same instruments.

Class V Cavity Preparations for Amalgam

By definition, Class V lesions involve smooth surfaces apical to the height of contour on the facial and lingual surfaces of all teeth. Amalgam will usually be used in class V cavity preparations in molars and premolars. This area of the facial and lingual surfaces, apical to the height of contour, is a location for many destructive activities, e.g., erosion, abrasion, attrition, hypoplasia, hypocalcification and aplasia, in addition to caries. The restorative treatment for defects created by such activities is usually a Class V cavity preparation and restoration.

Application of the general principles

I. Outline form

1. In addition to the rules mentioned in the general principles and in the discussion of Class II cavity preparations concerning gingival margins, for Class V preparations it is also important to have adequate dimensions of attached gingivae, apical to the gingival margin and separating this margin from the adjacent fornix. If this type of gingivae is limited or not present at all, decay will recur around these margins and gingival sulcular problems will be initiated. It is not always advisable to locate margins of amalgam subgingivally in Class V cavity preparations, except in those situations enumerated in the chapter on single tooth restorations and the periodontium.

2. Occlusal margins of Class V preparations, especially in the most posterior molar teeth, should be located at, but not including the height of contour. Although this location is not mandatory in premolars and in prominent, easily cleansable molar tooth surfaces, locating the margins apical to the height of contour should be decided upon only after carefully considering the cleansing ability and plaque control technique of the patient as well as the natural pattern of cleansing these teeth.

3. Similarly, the cleansability of the facial or lingual surfaces apical to the height of contour should be carefully evaluated before deciding on locations for mesial and distal margins. Generally speaking, when the vestibule (fornix) is deep, there is a greater occluso-apical dimension of attached gingivae, and less static adjacent musculature. In this situation, the mesio-distal dimension of the cavity may be more restricted, locating margins further from the adjacent axial angles. In fact, in the extreme, it is only necessary to include the tooth structure directly attacked or undermined by decay. On the other hand, if a tooth is the last molar tooth in the arch, with very limited attached gingivae, and with very tight, static cheek musculature, it is advisable to include the entire facial surface apical to the height of contour in the Class V preparation, bringing the margins nearby, but not involving, the axial angles.

4. If the caries extends past the height of contour or the axial angle of a tooth, it is necessary to extend only part of the cavity preparation to include this area. This is done in a very limited manner, i.e., without extending the entire occlusal or proximal margin to include the area of decay.

II. Resistance and retention form

1. Class V restorations confined to one surface and not subjected to direct loading may be thought of as free of any mechanical problems. However, as the mandible moves in lateral excursion, the lingual slopes of the buccal and lingual cusps of maxillary teeth load the buccal slopes of the buccal and lingual cusp of mandibular teeth. Assume that we have a facial

Class V restoration in the lower molar tooth (Fig. 9). As the tooth is firmly seated in bone, the tooth structure of the crown can move from position #1 to position #2, making a V-shape opening at the margin (usually the occlusal one), together with a facial component of force driving the restoration facially. Although this opening and the facial component of force are very minute and may not displace the restoration completely, their repetition, thousands of times per day, can create marginal failures and, eventually, facial protrusion of the restoration. The same thing can happen for a lingual restoration in lower teeth and a facial or lingual one in upper teeth. The amount of force as well as dimensions of this V-shaped space are increased with increasing steepness of the cusps, the width and depth of the cavity preparation, the length of the clinical crown, the occluso-apical taper of the tooth, the less bulk of the tooth at the level of the cavity preparation, and the frequency of lateral excursion forces. To minimize the effects of these displacing forces, grooved occlusal and gingival walls are essential for any Class V cavity preparation for amalgam, in addition to definite surrounding walls, line and point angles.

2. In many instances, the gingival margin of a Class V preparation is located on cementum. However, there is no place for cementum in any cavity wall or floor because it lacks self-resistance. Therefore, cementum on a gingival wall as well as on the gingival portion of the mesial and distal walls should be eliminated, so that the wall will be formed completely of dentin.

3. In some situations, caries and erosion lesions involve the bifurcation or its flutes, especially facially in the upper and lower molars. In these cases, special attention should be given to the gingival margins and walls. The gingival margins should follow the curvature of the furcation and they should be as external in the furcation flute as possible. This is because as more of the furcation is involved, the possibility of creating a definite gingival floor and a cleansable gingival margin becomes remote. The gingival floor in these situations should be flat, one-planed, and with no retentive grooves. This allows more tooth bulk to support the furcation. Furthermore, the occlusal walls should carry a more pronounced retention groove than usual to compensate for the absence of a corresponding gingival groove.

4. To protect the critical axial angle of the tooth, the mesial and distal walls of the Class V preparation should diverge axio-facially or lingually when they come close to this critical anatomy. This allows maximum tooth structure bulk when com-

pared to a boxed-up or convergent wall in this location.

5. If the occlusal margins approximate the facial or lingual cusps or marginal ridges, it is advisable to make the occlusal walls devoid of any occlusal grooves as this may undermine the structure of these cusps or marginal ridges. Occlusal walls should be divergent axio-facially or lingually toward the occlusal. If retention is drastically decreased by the divergence of the occlusal wall, this wall could be made in two planes: an inner (dentinal) one at a right angle to the axial wall and an outer plane following the direction of the enamel rods, formed of enamel and dentin.

Designs of Cavity Preparation

A. Class V, Design 1 (Conventional Design)

1. Indications

a. The lesion is large to medium-sized, confined to the gingival third of the facial or lingual surface.

b. The axial angles are intact.

c. There is no furcation or root involvement.

d. Facial or lingual lesions facilitate definite occlusal and gingival walls.

2. The general shape (Fig. 10) of this design may be described as trapezoidal with rounded corners, with the short side of the trapezoid being the gingival arm.

3. Location of margins

The gingival margin for Class V design 1 is located similar to the gingival margin described for Class II cavity preparations. The mesial and distal margins should be located far enough mesially and distally to include all decayed and undermined tooth structures, yet not encroaching on the axial angles of the tooth. Furthermore, there should be sufficient tooth structure bulk between these margins and critical angles and proximal anatomy. However, the mesial and distal margins must be far enough from each other to facilitate a 1.5 to 2 mm amalgam bulk within the preparation. The occlusal margin in this design must be located far enough occlusally to include all decayed and undermined enamel, while preserving the

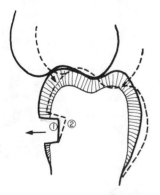

Fig. 7-9

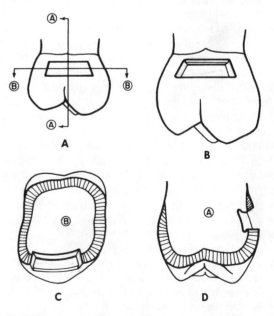

Fig. 7-10. Class V amalgam preparation. Upper molar (facial).

height of contour. There should be a minimum cavity width between the occlusal margin and the gingival floor to accommodate 1.5 to 2 mm amalgam bulk.

4. Internal anatomy (Fig. 10)

In a mesio-distal cross-section (Fig. 10), the axial wall (Fig. 10C) occurs 0.5 mm from the dentino-enamel junction. The wall is rounded, following the curvature of the facial or lingual surfaces. It may have different levels if caries cones exceeded the 0.5 mm limit from DEJ at one or more points.

The mesial and distal walls (Fig. 10C) will appear divergent facio- or linguo-mesially or distally, allowing maximum tooth bulk for protection of the axial angles. In an occluso-gingival cross-section (Fig. 10D), the axial wall will be seen as flat to slightly convex. Again, it may have one or more levels as dictated by caries extent.

The occlusal wall can appear in one of two ways in this cross-section. If the occlusal margin is located at the middle third of the facial or lingual surfaces, it will be formed of two planes: a grooved internal plane and an outer enamelo-dentinal plane following the direction of the enamel rods. However, if the occlusal margin is located in the occlusal one-third of this surface, the wall will be formed of three planes: an inner grooved dentinal plane, a transition plane, then an outer enamel-dentinal plane following the direction of the enamel rods occluso-facially or lingually.

The gingival wall can also vary in appearance, depending on its location. In this cross-section, if the gingival margin is located on enamel at the gingival third, the wall will appear with three planes: a grooved dentinal plane, a transition plane, and an enamel-dentinal plane, going axio-facially or lingually. However, if the gingival margin is located on dentin, the wall will appear with two planes: an internal grooved plane and an outer flat plane, both made of dentin.

5. Modifications

a. If most of the facial or lingual surface is involved in a Class V lesion, and they are to be part of the cavity preparation, since the occlusal margin will be very close to a cusp tip or marginal ridge crest, it is necessary to diverge the occlusal wall axio-facially or lingually in the occlusal direction. Because such a wall angulation will decrease the retentive capability of the preparation, it is advisable to make this divergence only at the areas where the margin approximates the occlusal surface. At other areas, prepare a two-planed occlusal wall: i.e., a dentinal plane perpendicular to the axial wall, and an enamelo-dentinal plane diverging facially or lingually. In this situation, the gingival retention grooves should at least be doubled in size, and the mesio-axial and disto-axial line angles should be accentuated considerably.

b. In the event the mesial or distal wall is lost, it is advisable to reduce the curvature of the axial wall. If it is at all feasible, the loss of these walls should be confined to only a portion of them. This can sometimes be accomplished by extending the cavity slightly occlusally and/or gingivally, so as to be able to create a portion of a mesial or distal wall occlusally and/or gingivally. Also, more retention can be obtained by deepening the axial wall near the lost mesial or distal wall. This creates and/or accentuates the mesial-axial and distal-axial line angle. (If the mesial or distal wall is shortened rather than lost entirely, the same remedy can be followed, with the goal of improving the maximum height of these walls.)

In both of the above mentioned situations, retention form in the rest of the cavity preparation should be exaggerated to compensate for the loss or decrease in the retention and resistance features that resulted from the shortening or loss of walls.

6. Instrumentation for Class V, Design 1

a. Prerequisites

i. The operator should be able to visualize the general shape, location of margins, and internal anatomy of this design in every tooth in the arch.

ii. A rubber dam must be properly applied with a 212 clamp.

iii. A tray set-up with the necessary instruments should be ready.

b. Procedures

i. Gaining access is simple for this design. Usually, simple retraction of adjacent soft tissues and removal of undermined enamel using a suitable size hatchet or a Wedelstaedt chisel is all that is required.

ii. Gross removal of carious tooth structure can be accomplished with a #2 or #3 round bur, preferably in a straight handpiece. Apply axial pressure and lateral dragging to remove tooth structure within the anticipated cavity preparation outline form. Removal of undesirable attacked dentin is accomplished, using the previously mentioned procedures and instruments.

iii. Preliminary shaping of the cavity can be done with the base of a 33½ inverted cone bur, in a straight handpiece. Seating the bur distally, apply distal pressure to primarily formulate the distal wall using occluso-gingival dragging. Then, with the base of the same bur seated gingivally, apply gingival pressure and use mesio-distal dragging to primarily formulate the gingival floor. With the side of the same bur seated mesially, apply mesial pressure, and use occluso-gingival dragging to create the mesial wall. Again, with the side of the same bur seated occlusally, apply slight occlusal pressure, and use mesio-distal dragging to establish the occlusal wall.

iv. Final shaping (Fig. 11) can be done with a Wedelstaedt

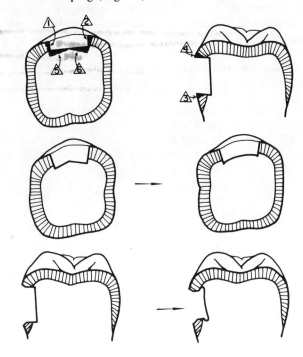

Fig. 7-11. Triangles involved in preparation of Class V cavity preparation for amalgam.

chisel, a hatchet, margin trimmer or a hoe. Use lateral cutting action to cut triangles #1, 2, 3 and 4. This will flare the mesial and distal walls and will make two planes for occlusal and gingival walls. With the flat cutting edge of an angle former or a gingival margin trimmer, in lateral cutting action, cut triangles #5 and #6. This will round the axial wall in a mesio-distal direction.

v. Line angle and groove preparation is done with a ¼ round bur. Seating this bur at the gingivo-disto-axial point angle, use gingival pressure and mesial dragging to cut a groove at the expense of the gingival floor between the two gingival point angles and via the axio-gingival line angle. Then, with a ¼ round bur repeat step 1 in the occluso-axial line angle, starting at the occluso-disto-axial point angle using occlusal pressure.

vi. Finally, this cavity is finished with a Wedelstaedt chisel, hatchet or gingival margin trimmer. With lateral scraping action, smooth all walls and floors, and define all line angles. Using a Wedelstaedt chisel in direct cutting action, smooth all cavosurface margins and make them right-angled.

B. Class V, Design 2

This design may be described as a typical facial or lingual preparation, except with a proximal "handle" extension.

1. Indications

a. Lesions on the facial or lingual gingival third have concomitant encroachment on the axial angle.

b. Lesions on the facial or lingual gingival third are continuous with a proximal lesion apical to the contact area.

c. The contact area proximally is not involved or encroached upon by any lesion.

d. Moderate to severe gingival recession facially places the margin of the proximal extension solely in the gingival embrasure.

2. The general shape (Fig. 12A) of this design, as mentioned, consists of a facial or lingual preparation similar to Design 1, as well as a proximal portion which is parallelogram or rectangular in shape, with rounded corners.

3. Location of margins

The facial or lingual portion of this design will have its margins in the same location as in Design 1. The proximal part (Fig. 12C) will have its margin in the adjacent facial (lingual) and/or gingival embrasures. The occlusal and gingival margins are a continuation of the same margins facially or lingually, but with some occlusal deviation. The lingual or facial margins will be located either in the adjacent embrasure or past the contact area in the opposite embrasure.

4. The internal anatomy (Fig. 12, B and D) of the facial or lingual part is exactly as described for Design 1. The proximal part will have the same appearance in occluso-gingival cross-section as the facial or lingual parts (Fig. 12D), with the exception that sometimes, if the occlusal margin is very close to the contact area, there will be no groove there.

In mesio-distal cross-section (Fig. 12B), the axial walls will appear flat, and the intact lingual or facial walls proximally seem to be inclined with the direction of enamel rods there, i.e., toward the adjacent proximal surface from the axial wall.

5. Modification

This design can occur with two proximal extensions. Some-

times, the two proximal extensions are continuous with another Class V preparation on the opposite facial or lingual surface, i.e., creating band type cavity preparations with two proximals, facial and lingual portions. The general shape and the location of margins and internal anatomy of each portion is exactly as mentioned above.

6. Instrumentation for Class V, Design 2

a. Gaining access is accomplished exactly as in Design 1. The facial or lingual portions will facilitate access to the proximal portion.

b. Gross removal of carious tooth structure is also accomplished exactly as described for Design 1, as is removal of irreparably attacked dentin.

c. Preliminary shaping follows procedures enumerated for Design 1, except the facial or lingual walls proximally are created as in Class II designs. The occlusal and gingival walls proximally may not be preparable by inverted cone burs, especially if they pass the contact area facio-lingually. In this case, a 169 or 700 bur can be used in lateral cutting action to preliminarily shape both walls.

d. Final shaping is done as for Design 1, cutting one or two triangles fewer according to the number of the lost walls, and cutting a triangle at the axio-axial line angle to (round it).

e. Retention grooves are placed and the cavity is finished using procedures and instruments described for design 1. The axio-axial line angle is rounded to follow the contour of the adjacent facial- or lingual-axial surface.

Class V, Design 3

This preparation may be described as Class V with an occlusal "moustache" extension.

1. Indications

a. A lesion on the gingival third facially or lingually is continuous with isolated decalcifications or lesions occlusal to the height of contour.

b. The height of contour is very gingivally curved in the mesio-distal direction.

2. General shape (Fig. 13)

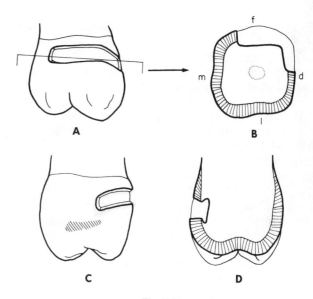

Fig. 7-12

This design consists of trapezoidal gingival third portion, with a unilateral (Fig. 13A) or bilateral (Fig. 13B) "moustache" extension at the very mesial and/or distal part of the central cavity, passing the height of contour.

3. Location of margins

In the center of the "basic cavity", margins are located as in Design 1. In the extension, margins will be located anywhere, as long as all decayed and undermined tooth structure is involved, since the area occlusal to the height of contour is self-cleansable.

4. Internal anatomy

The basic cavity has the same anatomy as Class V Design 1, but the extension will have its mesial and distal walls perpendicular to a flat axial wall. The mesial and distal walls of the extension will meet occlusally at a rounded junction with no undercuts.

5. Instrumentation for Class V, Design 3

Instrumentation and technique are very similar to Design 1, except smaller instruments are used in preparing the moustache extension and in blunting (rounding) the junctional components at the tip of the occlusal extensions.

D. Class V, Design 4

This is known as the "multiple isolated boxes" cavity preparation.

1. Indications

a. There are multiple lesions or defects in the gingival third which are very limited in size, with sound tooth structure separating them from each other.

b. Cariogenic factors justify placing vertical margins within the facial and/or lingual surface, apical to the height of contour.

2. The general shape (Fig. 14) of this design, is of several (2 or more) preparations which are small, box-shaped, and with rounded corners.

3. Location of margins

Margins, in this design, may be situated anywhere on the enamel or dentinal surface after removal of decayed and undermined tooth structures.

4. Internal anatomy (Fig. 14)

Internally, this design appears as a small scale copy of Design 1, except that the mesial or distal walls may be perpendicular to the axial wall if they are located in the middle third of the facial or lingual surfaces in the mesio-distal direction. There should be sufficient sound tooth structure between one part and another, in order for them to be self-resistant.

5. Instrumentation for Class V, Design 4

This is very similar to that described for Design 1, using smaller size instruments and with little or no triangle cutting in the final shaping.

E. Class V, Design 5

1. Indications:

The lesion involves a bifurcation or part of it. Due to advancement in periodontal therapy, especially in handling furcation involvements, carious or erosion lesions involving the furcation are seen more often, necessitating this design of cavity preparation.

2. The general shape (Fig. 15) of this design is basically trapezoidal, with a gingival wall curved occlusally following the furcation outline, and sometimes with an extension on one or both surrounding roots (Fig. 16).

3. Location of margins (Fig. 15 and 16)

The occlusal, mesial and distal margins are located similar to Class V Design 1. The gingival margin should be located as superficially as possible, within the furcation and root surfaces. The deeper the location in the furca, the more difficult it is to keep its interface clean.

4. The internal anatomy (Fig. 15B and C) of this design resembles Class V, Design 1, with the following additions:

a. The curved portion of the gingival wall, surrounding and following the furcation outline, should be formed of one flat dentinal plane (Fig. 15B).

b. The remainder of the gingival wall (flat portion) may

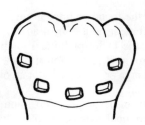

Fig. 7-14

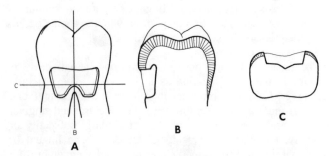

Fig. 7-15

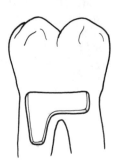

Fig. 7-16

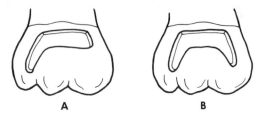

Fig. 7-13

accommodate a gingival groove if it is situated occlusally enough in the anatomical crown. (It is very hazardous to place a groove in the gingival wall if it is located on the root surface (Fig. 16).

c. The axial wall, especially in the flutes of the furcation, will have the same concavity as the furcation anatomy (Fig. 15C). This is to facilitate creating a pronounced gingival wall and to provide adequate bulk of amalgam there.

d. It is very critical that the maximum possible bulk of tooth structure be left between the gingival margin and the furcation proper (Fig. 15B).

e. Because of minimal or no gingival retentive grooves, the occlusal retention groove should be exaggerated to compensate for this deficiency (Fig. 15B).

f. The junction of walls around the furcation should be as rounded as possible to minimize stress concentration at this critical area.

5. Instrumentation for Class V, Design 5

The same procedure as described for Design 1 should be followed, except a wedge is placed in the involved furcation, if possible. This serves to retract the gingival tissues there and to maintain the dimensions of the furcation and the surrounding tooth structure during the procedure. Furthermore, it is advisable to use hand instruments as much as possible. Rotary instruments should be used with smaller burs than in Design 1. The axial concavity, corresponding to the furcation concavity should be created with a round bur.

BIBLIOGRAPHY

Almquist, T.C., Cowan, R.D., and Lambert, R.L.: Conservative amalgam restorations, J. Prosthet. Dent. May 73; **29**(5):524-528.

Amorim, A., de Lima Navarro, M.F., Mondelli, J., and Lopes, M.S.: Influence of axiopulpal line angle and proximal retention on fracture strength of amalgam restorations, J. Prosthet. Dent. 1978 Aug. **40**(2):169-173.

Barkmeier, W.W., Murrin, J.R., and Anderson, R.W.: Amalgam restoration of posterior teeth before endodontic treatment, J. Endod. 1980 Feb. **6**(2):446-449.

Baum et al.: Operative Dentistry, Philadelphia, 1981, Saunders.

Bhat, K.S., and Murthy, K.S.: Marginal microleakage at cementum-amalgam interface; an in vitro study, J. Indian Dent. Assoc. Nov. 74; **46**(11):421-426.

Black, G.V., and Black, A.P.: A work on operative dentistry. Vol. I and II, 6th ed. Medico-Dental Publ, 1924.

Bouschor, C.F., and Martin, J.R.: A review of concepts of silver amalgam retention, J. Prosthet. Dent. Nov. 76; **36**(5):532-537.

Chan, K.C., Edie, J.W., and Svare, C.W.: Scanning electron microscope study of marginal adaptation of amalgam in restoration finishing techniques, J. Prosthet. Dent. 1977 Aug. **38**(2):165-168.

Charbeneau et al.: Principles and practice of operative dentistry. Philadelphia, 1980, Lea and Febiger.

Craig, R.G., and Farah, J.W.: Stress analysis and design of single restorations and fixed bridges, Oral Sci. Rev. 1977; **10**:45-74.

Crockett, W.D., Shepard, F.E., Moon, P.C., and Creal, A.F.: The influence of proximal retention grooves on the retention and resistance of Class II preparations for amalgams, J. Am. Dent. Assn. Nov. ●● **91**(5):1053-1056.

D'erand, T.: Marginal failure of amalgam Class II restoration. J. Dent. Res. 1977 May. **56**(5):481-5.

Farah, J.W., Hood, J.A., and Craig, R.G.: Effects of cement bases on the stresses in amalgam restorations. J. Dent. Res. Jan-Feb 75; **54**(1):10-5.

Galan, J., Gilmore, H.W., and Lund, M.R.: Retention for the proximal portion of the Class II amalgam restoration. J. Indiana Dent. Assoc. Nov-Dec 75; **54**(6):16-9.

Gilmore, H.W., et al.: Operative Dentistry. 3rd ed. St. Louis, The C.V. Mosby Co., 1977.

Leidal, T.I., and Dahl, J.E.: Marginal integrity of amalgam restorations. Acta Odontol. Scand. 1980; **38**(2):81-8.

Mondelli, J., Ishikiriama, A., de Lima Navarro, M.F., Galan, J., Jr., and Coradazzi, J.L.: Fracture strength of amalgam restorations in modern Class II preparations with proximal retentive grooves. J. Prosthet. Dent. Nov. 74; **32**(5):564-71.

Mondelli, J., and Vieira, D.F.: The strength of Class II amalgam restorations with and without pins. J. Prosthet. Dent. Aug 72; **28**(2):179-88.

Mount, G.J.: The use of amalgam to protect remaining tooth structure. NZ Dent. J. 1977 Jan. **73**(331):15-20.

Oilo, G.: Adaptation of amalgams to cavity walls. J. Oral Rehabil. Jul 76; **3**(3):227-36.

Osborne, J.W., and Gale, E.N.: Failure at the margin of amalgams as affected by cavity width, tooth position, and alloy selection. J. Dent. Res. 1981 Mar. **60**(3):681-5.

Sturdevant et al.: The art and science of operative dentistry. New York, McGraw-Hill Book Co., 1968.

Terkla, L.G., Mahler, D.B., and Van Eysden: Analysis of amalgam cavity design. J. Prosthet. Dent. Feb. 73; **29**(21):204-9.

Wilson, R.A., and Fiocca, V.L.: Current concepts in cavity design for amalgam restorations. Ill. Dent. J. May 75; **44**(5):275-8.

CHAPTER 8

Direct tooth-colored restorations

One of the basic requirements of esthetics in dentistry is to restore anterior teeth and any extraorally conspicuous aspects of posterior teeth, with a restorative material that has the same color, shade and all visual perceptions as that of the adjacent tooth structure while keeping them unchanged in function. Since the birth of dentistry there have been continuous attempts to formulate a material and technique with such esthetic requirements, besides having the expected physical, mechanical and biological properties to behave favorably in the oral environment. Unfortunately, all attempts to this point in time fall short of that ideal goal. This chapter will attempt to elucidate the present status of the everchanging subject, "direct tooth-colored restorations".

Presently, there are five types of tooth-colored materials that can be made directly into restorations inside the mouth. In chronological order of development, these are silicate cement, unfilled resin, filled resin, composite resin, and alumino-silicate-polyacrylate cements (ASPA). Also, there are other types that are fabricated outside the mouth and then cemented into or onto the tooth: porcelain, cast moldable ceramic, and porcelain fused to metal restorations.

Composition and Setting Reactions

I. Silicate Cements

Silicate is the oldest of the direct tooth-colored materials and although it is rarely used nowadays, knowledge of its chemical composition and behavior is an important prerequisite to the understanding of newer materials.

Silicate is composed of a powder and a liquid which are mixed together into a workable consistency, then introduced and allowed to set in a retentive cavity preparation. The powder consists mainly of silicone dioxide and alumina (aluminum trioxide), with small amounts of trisodium phosphate and calcium oxide. It also contains a large percentage (up to 25%) of fluorides in the form of calcium fluoride and sodium aluminum fluoridate, which act as fluxes during the processing of the powder and subsequently remain. Some inert coloring additives are incorporated into the powder to produce multiple shades for the material. The liquid is a 35%-50% phosphoric acid solution, with some buffers in the form of sodium and aluminum phosphate.

The setting reaction of silicate is an ordinary acid-base reaction, producing a reaction type composite material, of which the interrupted phase is the unattacked portions of the original powder particles. The attacked peripheral portions of these powder particles will be replaced with a gel-structure almost depleted of cations. The product of the acid-base reaction, mostly phosphates and silicic acid, will serve as the continuous phase, joining the unreacted portion of the original particles. There are four things in the silicate cement structure that affect its clinical behavior. First, the phosphate matrix is an irreversible gel with a specific amount of liquid in it. Any loss or reduction of that liquid will drastically affect the properties of the material, especially its optical properties. Second, the matrix and gel peripheries of the original powder particles contain large amounts of fluoride ions that may be available to surrounding enamel. Third, the Ph of the mass can stay as low as "3" for two days to a week. Fourth, the bonding between the matrix ingredients themselves, and that between the matrix and the gel peripheries of the original particles, is mainly ionic and in some areas physical. The latter is easily liberated by many agents, especially acids.

II. Unfilled Resins

This material is the result of addition polymerization, and it can be supplied in three forms:

A. Powder-liquid form

The powder is mainly methyl-methacrylate polymer particles, refined to smooth surfaced, small diameter particles; it also contains the accelerator (activator) for the polymerization reaction. The accelerator is usually a tertiary amine. Pigments and inert coloring agents are added to the powder to create different shades of the material. The liquid is a monomer methyl-methacrylate, with traces of polymerization inhibitors (hydroquinone) to prolong its shelf life. It also contains the initiator, which is always benzoyl peroxide. Mixing the powder with the liquid decomposes the initiator and starts a chain reaction of addition-polymerization. The final product is a mass of polymethyl-methacrylate acccommodating residual unreacted monomer, coloring agents, voids, and traces of original additives. The intramolecular bonding in unfilled resin is mainly strong covalent. The intermolecular bonding in the material is a weak physical one.

B. Liquid form

This form contains the monomer and initiator (benzoyl-peroxide) and a visible or ultraviolet light energy transformer, like benzoin-methyl-ether. The polymerization in this form is started by applying light rays. These are transformed by benzoin-methyl-ether to usable energy, decomposing the benzoyl-peroxide and starting the chain reaction addition-polymerization. The resin in this form is not always methyl-methacrylate; sometimes it is either bisphenol-A-glycidyle-methacrylate (BIS-GMA) or urethane.

C. Three part form

In this form, the powder and liquid are supplied separately, and they do not contain either an accelerator or an initiator. These, too, are supplied separately, to be incorporated just before use.

Certain problems exist in the final products of all these forms that drastically influence the clinical behavior of this material:

1. The volumetric shrinkage during polymerization may be up to 7%.

2. The residual monomer enhances solubility and weakens the material.

3. The coefficient of thermal expansion is 10-12 times that of the tooth structure.

4. Decomposition of the tertiary amine accelerator occurs by natural ultraviolet light, creating discolorations. In an attempt to counteract this, resin systems with different accelerators, e.g., sulfinic acid derivatives, are used. Also, ultraviolet light absorbers have been added to some of these materials.

5. Bonding between the material components is mainly covalent and physical. The greater the percentage of covalent bonding (large macromolecules), the less will be the solubility, and the better the mechanical properties of the material.

III. Filled Resins

Filled resin is mainly methyl-methacrylate containing up to 25% inorganic fillers incorporated within. These fillers are not chemically bonded to the resin phase. This resin can come in one of the three forms mentioned with the unfilled resins. The liquid form of the filled resin, however, is better described as a "semi-liquid", because of the increased viscosity caused by the fillers in the filled resins. The intramolecular bonding is mainly covalent, the intermolecular bonding is physical, and the bonding between the filler particles and the resins is physical with a high percentage of voids.

IV. Composite Resins

Presently, these composites are the most universally used direct tooth-colored materials. Although there are now different types of composite resins available to the profession, they are all dependent on the original ideas and research of Raphael Bowen. Composites are all reinforced materials with a continuous (dispersion or reinforced) phase and an interrupted (dispersed or reinforcing) phase.

The continuous phase usually consists of synthetic resin macromolecules, with a skeleton of epoxy and reactive radicals of methacrylate. It is, in fact, a product of the reaction between bisphenol-A and glycidyle methacrylate (BIS-GMA). There are several other resins that are presently being used as the continuous phase, e.g., modified BIS-GMA from elimination of the hydroxy group, urethane diacrylate, and TEG-DMA (triethylene-glyco-dimethacrylate). Polymerization of the continuous phase will bring about the setting (hardening) of the

material. This occurs through a set of activators (catalysts or accelerators), and initiators (reactors) which may be thermochemical, photochemical, or chemico-chemical. In other words, polymerization can occur through heat-curing, light-curing, or chemical-curing. In all three methods, benzoyl-peroxide is the usual initiator (reactor). The activator differs in each of the three methods of polymerization. In heat-curing, no activator is needed, as the applied heat, itself, is capable of deteriorating the benzoyl-peroxide to start polymerization. In light-curing, benzoin-methyl-ether is a typical chemical capable of serving as a photon absorber that converts photon energy to polymerization energy. In chemical curing, a tertiary amine deteriorates the benzoyl peroxide on contact, starting the process of polymerization. In all of these situations, the "HO" group of the deteriorated benzoyl peroxide will collide with the continuous phase molecules, starting a chain reaction that leads to the creation of giant macromolecules and/or to the lengthening and cross-linking of these macromolecules. The degree of polymerization that occurs is understandably crucial to the clinical behavior of the material. Generally speaking, maximum polymerization is achieved best by heat curing, followed by light curing, and finally by chemical curing. In actual practice, light and chemical curing are the only feasible clinical procedures.

The interrupted (reinforcing or dispersed) phase may consist of either one or a combination of the following:

A. Macro-ceramics

This is the reinforcing phase of the first generation composite resins, and consists of slica-silicate (SiO_4) based materials. Examples of these in use are quartz, fused silica, silicate glasses, crystalline lithium aluminum silicate, barium aluminum-boro-silicate, etc. Those that contain heavy metals (barium) will be radiopaque. Although original particle diameters were between 5 and 75 micrometers, today they are reduced to between 1 to 5 micrometers. They are produced from large particles by crushing and grinding, which produces irregularly shaped particles. To improve the surface texture and packing factor of the final materials, a decrease in the surface irregularity through more sophisticated grinding techniques, and use of different size particles, mathematically calculated to occupy the maximum available space, as well as use of softer ceramics have all been incorporated into today's conventional composites. With these more refined particles, it is possible to create systems that are 50% by weight and 80% by volume of these reinforcing silica-silicate ceramics.

B. Colloidal and micro-ceramics

These comprise the reinforcing phases for the second generation of composite resins. Originally, these fillers were colloidal silica in the form of silicic acid, formulated by a chemical process of hydrolysis followed by precipitation. To be in the colloidal state, the diameter of these particles cannot exceed 0.04 micrometers. Recently, part of these particles have been replaced with larger particles of pyrogenic silica, with an average diameter of 0.05 to 0.1 micrometer. In either of these dimensions, the particles are smaller than the wave length of visible light; consequently, they give the final product an extremely smooth surface. Because of the large surface area resulting from such dispersed phases, the viscosity of systems utilizing them will be very high. Therefore, there is a limit to the dispersion of these types of particles if a workable system is to result. The maximum percentage of such dispersion, to maintain reasonable workability, is 50% dispersed phase by volume and 30% by weight.

C. Fabricated macro-reinforcing phases with colloidal-micro-ceramic component bases

In an attempt to reinforce composite systems more with colloidal or micro-ceramics, without interfering with the workability of the material, several procedures are indicated:

Pyrogenic silica and silicic acid (colloidal state) are dispersed in a resin system as the continuous phase. This will cause viscosity to be very high, as the system is loaded to its maximum capacity with the dispersed micro-colloidal particles. The system is then heat-cured. The created mass is then ground into small, irregularly shaped particles, ranging in size from 1-200 micrometers. These highly filled particles could then be used as a dispersed phase in a continuous resin phase that may be cured photo-chemically or chemico-chemically.

Colloidal or microceramics are introduced into partially thermo-chemically polymerized spherical particles of a resin system. The diameter of these spheres may range from 20-30 micrometers. The highly reinforced spherical resin particles are then used as reinforcers for a continuous phase resin, forming a composite resin.

In both of the aforementioned situations, intelligent distribution of particle diameters to be used in dispersion (reinforcement) is essential to attain the maximum packing factor in the final mass.

Using a sintering process of heat and pressure, the colloidal microceramic particles are agglomerated to form irregularly shaped and sized, highly porous particles. These range in size between 1-25 micrometers. Dispersing these agglomerated particles into a suitable continuous phase resin, to be photochemically or chemico-chemically cured, will create the most highly reinforced composite resin presently available. A minimum amount of the continuous phase is needed to bind the reinforcing particles together, because the porous nature of the reinforcing particles allows mechanical locking-in of the continuous phase. This enhances the physico-chemical bonding between the two phases. A composite resin with such reinforcement, could even be condensable.

The interface between the interrupted and the continuous phase is the most crucial in determining the final behavior of these systems. Usually, the interface is enhanced by a coupling agent in the form of a bi-polar molecule (usually organo-silanes and their derivatives). These agents are ionically and physically bonded to the inorganic parts of the reinforcing particles, and chemically and physically bonded to the inorganic and organic parts of both the continuous and interrupted phases. On the other hand, this interface may be a co-polymeric or homopolymeric bonds (covalent and physical) between the organic matrix and the partially organic dispersed phases.

The continuity, chemical stability, and minimum thickness of these interfaces is essential to the overall integrity of the final composite resin. The better the bonding at these interfaces, the more the reinforcing phases that may be added, enhancing the physical and mechanical properties of the composite.

Modifiers are added to the mass to create certain effects or characteristics. For example, hydroquinone 0.008% (mono-methyl ether) stabilizes the resin, preventing undue polymerization (polymerization retarder); coloring agents, usually in the form of inorganic oxides, or sulfides, establish certain visual effects in the material; ultraviolet light absorbers prevent discoloration of the resin due to ultraviolet rays.

V. Types of Composite Resin

It should be obvious from the previous description of the different possible phases, that a variety of composite resin formulations are possible. The following is a brief description of the types that have become available to the profession, in order of their chronological development:

A. First generation composites consist of macroceramic reinforcing phases in an appropriate resin matrix. This type enjoys the broadest clinical experience, has the highest mechanical properties in lab testing, and the highest proportion of destructive wear clinically due to the dislodging of the large ceramic particles. The first generation composites have the highest surface roughness. Newer versions of these materials, with smaller, softer, more rounded particles of variable dimensions have reduced these drawbacks tremendously.

B. Second generation composites, with colloidal and micro-ceramic phases in a continuous resin phase, exhibit the best surface texture of all composite resins. However, the properties of strength and coefficient of thermal expansion are unfavorable because of the limited percentage of reinforcers that can be added without increasing viscosity beyond the limits of workability. Despite the difficulty in fully wetting the reinforcing particles with the coupling agents, wear resistance is better than that of first generation composites due to the dimension proximity of dispersed particles to dispersion matrix macromolecules, and difficulty of engaging these minute ceramic particles in the abrading element.

C. Third generation composite is a hybrid composite in which there is a combination of macro- and micro(colloidal) ceramics as reinforcers. They exist in a ratio of 75:25 in a suitable continuous phase resin. The percentage of ceramic reinforcement approaches that of the first generation materials. As may be expected, the properties are somewhat of a compromise between the first and second generation materials.

D. Fourth generation composites are also hybrid types, but instead of macroceramic fillers, these contain heat-cured, irregularly shaped, highly reinforced composite macro-particles with a reinforcing phase of micro(colloidal) ceramics. Although these materials do produce superior restorations, they are very technique sensitive. There are, in fact, two prerequisites for their successful use:

1. The concentration of the dispersed microceramics must be equal in the pre-polymerized particles and in the polymerizable organic matrix to ensure their uniform distribution throughout the mass. In other words, the non-polymerized resin matrix is highly reinforced with the microceramics and will have a very high viscosity. However, because of the limited percentage of this resin matrix, workability is not affected.

2. The bonding between the continuous organic matrix and the partially organic, complex reinforcing particles should be a strong cohesive bond. Sensitivity to technique variables play a major role here, as regards insertion, finishing and polishing. In addition to their technique sensitivity, these fourth genera-

tion materials exhibit the maximum shrinkage of all composite resins. Nevertheless, they are able to most permanently preserve a created surface, which has a texture and esthetic capacity only slightly less satisfactory than second generation materials. They exhibit physical and mechanical properties between those of the first and third generation systems.

E. Fifth generation composites are a hybrid system in which the continuous resin phase is reinforced with microceramics (colloidal) and macro, spherical, highly reinforced, heat cured composite particles. The continuous phase of these particles is the same as (chemically bondable with) the final composite continuous phase. The spherical shape of the macrocomposite particles will improve their wettability, and consequently, their chemical bonding to the continuous phase of the final composite. Using many different sizes of these spheres, in a mathematically calculated manner, will improve the packing factor of the final composite. Furthermore, because of the specific shape of the macromolecules, the workability is improved. This results from the easy ''slip'' that occurs among the particles, in spite of the high viscosity of the highly reinforced matrix.

From this micro-structural description, it should be apparent that the surface texture and wear of these materials would be comparable to that of the second generation composite systems. Physical and mechanical properties are similar to those of the fourth generation materials.

F. Sixth generation composites are hybrid types in which the continuous phase is reinforced with a combination of micro (colloidal)-ceramics and agglomerates of sintered micro (colloidal)-ceramics. This type of composite exhibits the highest percentage of reinforcing particles. Of all composites, it has the best mechanical properties. Its wear and surface texture characteristics are very similar to fourth generation systems. Also, it exhibits the least shrinkage, due to the minimum amount of continuous phase present, and also due to the condensable nature of these systems.

Composite resins may be supplied in one of six systems:

1. Chemically cured paste-paste system

Each paste contains the monomer of the continuous phase as well as the dispersed phase treated particles. Only one paste contains the initiator. The other contains the activator (accelerator) and coloring agents.

2. Chemically cured or photocured liquid-powder system

The liquid in this system contains the monomer of the dispersion phase resins, with the accelerator (activator) and photon energy absorber and convertor. The powder contains the polymer of the dispersion phase, the particles of the dispersed phase, the initiator and the coloring agents.

3. Chemically cured or photocured paste-liquid system

The paste in this system contains the monomer of the dispersion phase, the particles of the dispersed phase, the initiator, and coloring agents. The liquid contains the monomer of the dispersion phase, the activator (accelerator), or ultraviolet visible light energy absorbers, and a convertor to activate decomposition of the initiator. When the paste is mixed with the liquid, the benzoyl peroxide will be decomposed chemically or by the application of the visible or ultraviolet light rays and this will precipitate the polymerization of the continuous phase. Liquid is added to paste, in this system, in an effort to vary the viscosity of the mix, as required by different restorative situations.

4. Photocured one paste system

The paste in this system is provided in varying viscosities and contains the monomer of the dispersion phase, treated particles of the dispersed phase, the initiator, coloring agents, and energy absorber of ultraviolet or visible light rays. This last chemical will direct the energy to decompose the initiator and start polymerization of the dispersion phase.

5. Photo-cured one liquid system

This consists of a highly viscous liquid that contains all the ingredients found in the one-paste system, but with a lower percentage of reinforcing phase. It is usually used in intricate areas of a cavity preparation where high wettability is needed.

6. Chemically cured three- or four-part system

The main powder part contains the polymer of the dispersion phase, the dispersed phase particles, and coloring agents. The main liquid part is the monomer of the dispersion phase. A third part, consisting of the initiator, and a fourth part consisting of the accelerator, are supplied separately. Sometimes the second and third parts are supplied together, and are to be incorporated with the fourth and first parts just before the mixing.

The final structure of composite resin produced by anyone of the above mentioned systems is a classical, reinforced composite material with the following features influencing its clinical behavior:

a. Although the bonding between the different components of the matrix, and between the matrix components with the treated silica-silicate dispersed particles is physical and covalent, the weakest link in the entire structure is still that between the matrix and the reinforcing silica-silicate phases.

b. Because of the high viscosity of most of the mixes, voids are inherent in these materials, especially if they are two component systems which are to be mixed together in an open atmosphere. This allows incorporation of air in the matrix.

c. As in unfilled resins, residual monomers in the final mix are very influential in shaping the physical and biological behavior of the material.

d. If macrosize silico-silicate dispersed phase particles are on the restoration's surface in the final structure, finishing and polishing to a smooth surface is impossible.

e. The set structure of all the systems has great affinity for water filling its pores and being adsorbed via its polar groups.

f. If reinforcing silico-silicate particles are not in sufficient concentration and/or dimension to prevent kinking and unkinking of the continuous phase macromolecules, due to thermal energy, the material will exhibit increases in th coefficient of thermal expansion.

g. Because the silica-silicate particles are the strongest phase in all systems, the closer together these particles are brought, the better will be the transmission of stresses from one particle to another, rather than being absorbed by the weaker reinforced phases.

h. The higher that the molecular weight (maximum polymerization) of the continuous phase macromolecules is, the closer will be the mechanical properties to those of the interrupted phase. This creates a more evenly strained system, one that is more durable and stable.

V. Alumino-Silicate Polyacrylate Cement

It is the newest addition to tooth-colored restorations. It was introduced in the mid-seventies by McLain, Wilson and Kent. As they stated in their introduction, ''It is a trial to combine the advantages of silicate, composite resin and polycarboxilate cement.''

The material is supplied in the form of a powder and liquid. The powder is a special ion-leachable silicate glass, similar to that of silicate cement. Alumina and calcium fluorides are the major ingredients, besides silica. It is cold-fritted, and ground to small particles averaging 20 microns in diameter. The liquid is an aqueous solution of polymer copolymer of polyacrylic acid.

The final product is a classical polymer-cemented composite structure. During mixing of the powder with the liquid, the polyacrylic acid attacks the surface of the powder particles, depleting them of their cations, and leaving a siliceous gel. The metal ions migrate to the liquid, connecting the macromolecules of the polyacrylic acid in three dimensions to form metallic salts. This combination may be intramolecular (through chelation) or intermolecular, producing a highly cross-linked matrix. This matrix itself is chemically bonded to the original powder particles through their peripheral cation-depleted siliceous gel-layers. Calcium ions are the first to react with the liquid acid, creating one or two dimensional linking of the polymer molecules. Aluminum ions react later, as soon as certain criteria are fulfilled, establishing a more rigid three-dimensional cross-linked bridging between the polymer molecules. So the material sets in two stages. After the first stage (calcium ion reaction), carving is still possible. However, after the second stage (aluminum ion reaction), the material is un-carvable.

The set structure has the following features that influence its clinical behavior:

1. It contains a sizable percentage of fluoride that is available to the surrounding environment.

2. Bonding between the matrix molecules, and between the matrix components and the original ceramic particles, is mainly strong covalent. Such bonds are almost inseparable by acid action, especially plaque acids.

3. Although the PH of the liquid may be less than that of the silicate cement, the size of the polymer molecules of the polyacrylic acid and its entangled attachment to the main mass decreases its mobility and, consequently, its penetrability into the dentin.

4. The polymeric matrix of the material can chelate some of the calcium ions of the hydroxy-apatite crystals of the enamel and dentin, binding the material to tooth structures.

Comparison of Tooth-Colored Materials

I. Strength Properties

Observing the accompanying table, it is obvious that composite resin (excluding second generation types) possesses the highest tensile and compressive strengths. Filled resin has the lowest compressive strengths, and silicate cements and ASPA have the lowest tensile strengths.

The modulus of elasticity, which is a measure of rigidity of the material, is high in silicate and composite resins. The modulus of resilience is very low in composite resin, which may explain some of the crazing, cracking and wear failures of this resin. Compared to tooth structures, composite resin will have the closest strength properties of all the direct tooth-colored materials.

Material	Compressive Strength P.S.I.	Tensile Strength P.S.I.	Flexure Strength P.S.I.	Modulus of Elasticity P.S.I.	Setting Shrink. %	Kt P.P.M.	Hardness Knoop	Abrasive Resist. mgm/hr 1500 PPM	Water Sorption	Solubility % in Water and Plaque Acid	Surface Roughness Scratches and Irregularities per Square Meter: Microinches	Refractive Index Degree	Opacity % Relative to Opaque Glass
Enamel	40-56,000		—	2.3			300				25-250 0.1-0.2	1.60°	21-67%
Dentin	30-50,000	7500	—	12 millions		8-11 PPM	65	1.46 1.90		—	—	1.56°	50-90%
Silicate	24,000-31,000	700	—	3.1 millions	L-0.03% V-0.25%	8	65	1.5	0	Water 1.4-2% A(5%)	100,000	1.47°-1.60°	55%
ASPA	23,100 28,000	650	—	1.9 millions	0.2%	20	60	2.13	0.01	Water 0.4 A(1.390)	100,000 11-24	2°	73%
Unfilled Resin	10-11,000	4,000	—	260,000	L-2-3% V-7%	127	16	1.5	7%	Water & acid 0.1	50,000	1.9°	60%
Filled Resin	8,000	1500	1	100,000	L-1-2% V-5%	90	80		5%	Water & acid 0.7	90-120,000 10-50	1.7°	59%
Composite Resin	2nd 25,000 1st 45,000 Hybrid 55,000	6400 7000 9000	10-14,000 14,000 16,000	1.7-2 million 2.2 millon	L-0.2% V-0.5%	56-65 30-50 23-33	30-100	0.57-1.46	1.5	Water & acid 0.3	30-60,000 250,100 14-100 100-120,000	1.8°	58%

Strength properties are drastically decreased by the amount of residual monomer in the resinous materials. Voids and a decrease in the powder:liquid ratio drop these properties in the silicate and ASPA cements. Discontinuity in the bonding between the dispersed and dispersion phase of composite materials (silicate, ASPA and composite resins) discourages attainment of maximal strength properties in these materials. Surface roughness and cracks or crazing in the set product of a composite material enhance mechanical failures, and also drop the strength properties of these materials. Incomplete polymerization or gelling of the matrix components in composite materials will prevent the attainment of the highest possible strength properties. On the other hand, excessive powder:liquid ratio in silicate ASPA and powder-liquid systems of resinous materials could lead to the same results as incomplete polymerization or gellation.

Compared to the strength properties of the tooth structure, it is clear that these materials fall drastically behind enamel in the different strength properties. Although composite resin can have comparable strength properties to that of dentin, both silicate and ASPA have a low modulus of toughness compared to that of dentin. All resinous materials have a considerable modulus of toughness, but not to the level of dentin. The modulus of elasticity of silicate cement is considerably high, denoting a very rigid material. Those for ASPA, composite resin, enamel and dentin are fairly close to each other, denoting a moderately rigid material. All in all, it is obvious that none of these materials can replace tooth structure and satisfy all its mechanical properties. Thus, restorations made from any of these materials are to be considered provisional, or semi-permanent at best.

II. Dimensional Stability

A. (Shrinkage During Setting)

Using the bulk pack technique in inserting these materials, as shown in the table, the unfilled resin exhibits the maximum shrinkage during polymerization. The least shrinkage is exhibited by silicate cement. The shrinkage for composite and ASPA is of no clinical significance. When using the brush bead or laminated techniques for inserting unfilled and some composite resins into cavity preparations, shrinkage can be directed away from cavity walls and details, i.e., toward the surface of the restoration, and compensated for by further additions of material.

B. Coefficient of Thermal Expansion

The closest coefficient of thermal expansion to that of the tooth structure is exhibited by silicate cement (8 PPM/1° C). As mentioned before, the coefficient of thermal expansion of unfilled resin is from 10 to more than 12 times that of the tooth structures (127-150 PPM/1° C) and the highest of all restorative materials. This situation will lead to percolation, increased microleakage, recurrence of decay, marginal discoloration, etc.

The coefficient of thermal expansion of composite resin (with the exception of second generation types) is close to that for amalgam (25-35 PPM/1° C). Second generation composite resins have a high coefficient of thermal expansion (close to that for unfilled resins) 65 PPM/1° C. Therefore, these materials should not be used either for large restorations or at lo-cations of extreme temperature fluctuations. They are best utilized as veneers for other generation of composites because of their excellent surface characteristics.

C. Abrasive Resistance

Material abrasion in the oral environment is a complex phenomenon controlled by known factors (e.g., fatigue, adhesion, abrasion, and chemical disintegration) and many unknown factors. There is no reliable lab test for the abrasion resistance of dental materials that will simulate problems in the oral environment, and that is why the abrasive resistance lab figures are not consistent with the clinical behavior of some tooth-colored materials. This is very clear in comparing amalgam and first generation composite resin. Although both show very similar abrasive resistance figures in lab experiments, the composite resin wears faster and more dramatically in Class I and II restorations, as compared to the same types of amalgam restorations. It has been well documented that the main mechanism for wear of composites starts at the interface, leading to a debonding of the attachments of the reinforcing particles from the resin matrix. Consequently, abrading forces dislodge the particles. This interfacial failure is precipitated, first, by its exposure through abrasion of the matrix resin and, second, through deterioration of the coupling agents by environmental factors.

On the accompanying table, the lab figures show that the direct tooth-colored materials most resistant to abrasion are still the composite resins; the least resistant are the unfilled resins. Silicate cement and ASPA rank very close by. Recent available data indicate that the newer generations of composite resins show higher abrasive resistance than conventional first generation materials. This may be explained by the reduction of the exposed surface area of the resin matrix, and the resulting difficulty in dislodging the microceramic particles reinforcing most of the newer generation materials. The same factors that decrease the hardness of these materials, also decrease their strength properties and reduce their resistance to abrasion.

D. Solubility

In water and plaque acids like acetic, citric and pyruvic acid, silicate cements are the most soluble tooth-colored materials. Solubility of ASPA is much less than that of silicate cement, which can be explained by the difference in the type of bonding between the matrix ingredients and between the matrix and the reinforcing original particles. Nevertheless, ASPA's solubility is still higher than that of other resinous materials. Although resinous materials and organic components of composite resins have low solubility in water and plaque acids, they are soluble (or at least softened) in organic solvents which may be introduced orally (e.g., ethanol). If softened by these solvents, their wear resistance could be drastically reduced. The inorganic ceramic components of composites and silicate cements could be soluble in acidulated fluorides topically applied during certain clinical procedures. However, ASPA's solubility is still higher than that of resinous materials which are close to each other.

Solubility of resinous restorative materials can be drastically increased by an increase in the residual monomer and discontinuity or weakness in the bond between the dispersed and dispersion phase in composite and filled resins.

Solubility of silicate cements and ASPA is increased by any change in the water balance of its liquid, and by decreasing the powder:liquid ratio. Also, increasing the aforementioned ratio more than certain limits or changing the liquid percentage in the gel matrix due to evaporation, can drastically increase their solubility.

E. Water Sorption

This combines both water absorption within the material and water adsorption, both of which are characteristics of polymeric resinous materials with polar radicals in their macromolecules. This phenomenon is enhanced by increasing the number and dimensions of pores within the material, and also by increasing the surface area of the final mass. Absorption and adsorption are most pronounced in unfilled and filled resins and significant in composite resins. They are present to some extent in ASPA and silicate cements. These phenomena can increase the dimensions of the restoration with a lot of favorable and unfavorable results, including compensation for polymerization shrinkage, adhesive bond disruptions, susceptibility to dislocation, increased plasticity, etc.

F. Synersis

By this process, a loss of water or liquid contents of the material matrix occurs when it is gel-structured. The phenomenon is very much observed in silicate cements and, to a lesser extent, in ASPA. It may lead to a minimum decrease in dimension; but, most importantly, it will deleteriously affect the mechanical and optical properties of the material.

G. Plasticity

Although most of these materials fall under the category of brittle materials, i.e., they fracture, rather than change shape. Composite resins and unfilled resins have some limited plasticity and are viscoelastic in nature. This may lead to change in their shape under loading, if it does not exceed their breaking point. This is determined not only by the amount of loading, but also by the rate of loading. Resinous materials can withstand high rates of loading better than low rates. Even loading under the proportional limits of these materials might permanently strain them, if these loads are cyclic (e.g., occlusal loads).

H. Disintegration

This process involves gross loss of material and it can be a combination of solubility, abrasion, erosion, and low strength properties. Disintegration is an inherent property of reinforced composite materials, in general, due to failure at the interface between the dispersed and dispersion phases. Disintegration is most obvious in silicate cements and composite resins and leads to variable features of failure, such as surface roughness, leakage, and a partial or complete loss of the material.

III. Hardness

As shown in the table, the Knoop hardness number of these materials is much less than that of enamel. Silicate and ASPA cements have close figures; the lowest is that for unfilled resins. The figure for composite resins depends on where the indenter was applied in the material specimens. If it occurred on the dispersed phase, a reasonably high figure will result. However,

if it occurred on the continuous resinous phase, a very low figure will be recorded. Hardness is affected by the same factors that control the strength properties of all these materials.

IV. Surface Roughness

This feature is measured by the average number of scratches per square inch (meter), the average depth of irregularities in microinches (meters) and surface profile of the material specimens after proper finishing and polishing. From the accompanying table it is apparent that composite resins in general have the highest number and deepest scratches of all restorative materials after all finishing and polishing procedures. Comparatively, the best surface, at least after polishing and before subjecting it to the oral environment, is that of unfilled resin followed by second generation composite resins, ASPA, silicate cements. It is a well established fact that the best surface that can be obtained from these materials, with the least number and smallest depth of scratches, is that produced by the matrix strip, when the material sets against it during fabrication of the restoration. Any further manipulation of the surface will worsen the surface textures.

Attempts are being made to improve this surface impediment of composite resins. One method is to use a glaze, usually the monomer for the matrix resin polymerized onto the surface. The immediate effect is very adequate and can create a surface very similar to that produced by the matrix. Unfortunately, it is a very temporary layer because of its low abrasive resistance.

Surface roughness of restorative materials is responsible for many possible problems, ranging from plaque adhesion and its harmful effects on the tooth and the periodontium, to surface discoloration of the restoration, fatigue failure of the restoration, and patient consciousness of the restoration, with possible mechanical irritation to the tongue, lips and cheeks.

V. Microleakage

Comparison of the circumferential dimensions and the extent of leakage space around restorations made of these materials reveals that the maximum size and extent of leakage space is that under and around unfilled resins and second generation composites, especially if inserted with a bulk-pack technique. Enamel etching and the use of coupling agents prior to insertion of the resin restoration (especially composite resin), decreases the leakage space to almost none, at least for a period. The leakage picture around and under silicate restorations is clinically acceptable in a newly placed restoration, but it is worsened by solubility and disintegration of the material, and can be very advanced in an aged restoration. In the case of ASPA, leakage is greatly minimized by the physico-ionic adhesion between the material and tooth structure. Leakage around any restorative material is an extremely complex phenomenon controlled by multiple factors, e.g., coefficient of thermal expansion, solubility, disintegration, strength properties, wettability toward tooth structures, viscosity at the time of insertion, abrasive resistance, adhesiveness to tooth structure, polarity toward tooth structure compounds, etc. From the previous discussion, it is very clear that none of these materials will completely seal a cavity preparation without a leakage space between it and the surrounding tooth structures at some period in the lifespan of the restoration. Leakage cannot be prevented, except if there is true adhesion between the tooth structure and the restorative material. Such adhesion is not exhibited by any of these materials, except partially so in ASPA restorations.

VI. Anticariogenicity

Imparting resistance to decay recurrence in the tooth structures, surrounding and underlying the restoration is mainly accomplished by three factors:

A. The restorative material's sealability of the prepared cavity in the tooth, which is the reverse of microleakage discussed in the previous section

B. The inability of the material's surface to retain cariogenic plaque, which is the result of its surface texture previously described

C. The leachable fluorides from the restorative material which can be taken in by the surrounding tooth structure, reducing its solubility and susceptibility to decay.

Only two tooth-colored restorative materials have fluoride available for the surrounding enamel and dentin, i.e., silicate and ASPA cements; ASPA has much more available fluorides than silicate cements (2200 PPM compared to 700 PPM for silicate cement). Investigators have verified that the uptake of fluoride ions from these restorations by the surrounding enamel is substantial during the first week, and is continuous on a lesser scale for the life of the restoration. Also, decay recurrence around these restorations was shown to be the least of all restorative materials. In addition, the bacterial activities of plaque attached to these materials were shown to be the least of any other restorative materials. Many attempts are being made to incorporate fluoride in resinous restorative materials, but with no apparent success.

VII. Optical Properties

Although the visual perception of a restorative material and the closeness of its shade to that of the tooth structure is subjective, it can be evaluated and predicted by objective testing, namely tests for refractive index, opacity, transparency, translucency, reflectiveness, hue, value, chroma and metamerism. The figures for the refractive index of silicate cement is the closest to that of enamel and the dentin. The other materials rank very close to each other, with ASPA having the highest figures. It should be remembered that saliva on tooth or restorative material surface can modify a refractive index. Although opacity of enamel and dentin varies between one tooth and another and from one individual to another, it does not come close to that of the present ASPA material, which has the highest opacity figures of all tooth-colored materials. The other materials are very close in their opacity figures.

Transparency is chiefly controlled by the absence of, presence of, and type of fillers in the material. That is why unfilled resin has the highest transparency figures. Translucency depends mainly on the type and nature of unreacted particles of the original powder material or its fillers. Silicate cement and composite resin have the most approximate translucency to that of tooth enamel.

Reflectiveness is mainly the product of surface texture. The smoother the surface, the more rays will be reflected, giving a shiny bright surface impression visually. The reflectiveness is a major modifying factor for any shade. It should be emphasized that saliva will impart a certain reflectiveness on the surface of the tooth and restorative material; that is why in choosing a shade the tooth should be covered with saliva.

The hue, value, and chroma are products of the inherent coloration of the material and the nature of incorporated pigments. Inorganic pigments seem to produce the most stable and predictable coloration and shading of tooth-colored restorative material. The more stable the interface between the component phases of a material, the more permanent will be the effect of pigmentation. To imitate the shade of a tooth, several pigments should be added by the manufacturer and/or by the dentist via tinting kits. To formulate the appropriate shade at chair side requires a thorough understanding of the factors that affect the hue, value, and chroma of materials, and the proper use of different colors, e.g., red, yellow and blue, to formulate the exact tooth color.

This discussion would not be complete without mentioning that the shade of a material can be different under different illuminating sources, a phenomenon called metamerism. The best medium to choose and formulate a shade of a restoration is the sunlight of midday.

VIII. Color Stability

None of these materials are as color stable as tooth enamel. Discoloration can be brought about either intrinsically or extrinsically.

A. Intrinsic discoloration can be due to chemical changes or deterioration of one or more of the component phases of the material with coloring byproduct(s), e.g., the effect of ultraviolet light (sunlight) on the benzoyl peroxide–tertiary amine combination in polymeric resins, loss of some of the components of the gel-matrix of some materials, or brown (black) discoloration in restorative material or tooth structures around pins resulting from the corrosion of pin material due to leakage.

B. Extrinsic discoloration is the most common type. It can occur marginally or surfacewise. Marginally, it is always due to leakage and recurrent decay, and sometimes to dissolution of varnish, if it is used under resinous materials. Surface discoloration is mainly due to surface roughness that increases the stainability and possibility of plaque adhesion to material's surface. Also, it can be as a surface continuation of intrinsic discoloration. It should be mentioned here that enamel and dentin surfaces etched by acids and not covered subsequently by restorative materials will be more stainable than untreated surfaces.

IX. Rate of Hardening

Resinous materials, namely unfilled resin, filled resin, and composite resin, can gain most of their mechanical properties within 15 minutes, and can be usually finished and polished after 5-8 minutes. Silicate cements will not gain such a state until after 48 hours. ASPA, as mentioned before, hardens initially in two stages, with a 10-15 minute interval between them. ASPA attains its final mechanical properties only after 48 hours. That is why silicate cement and ASPA restorations should be covered with a non-soluble protective agent for the first 48 hours, at which time finishing and polishing can be performed.

X. Biologic form

As with all restorative materials and techniques the first biologic inquiry about these materials should be: ''Are the materials irritant to the P-D organ?'' The answer is ''Yes.''

The next inquiry should be: ''What will be the irritating characteristics and ingredients?'' The answers are—

A. For silicate cements:

1. The original acidity of the cement which remains high up to one week in some cases
2. Microleakage around and through the disintegrated restoration, which increases with age
3. Acidity of the matrix phase and part of the interphase between the original particle and the matrix
4. Traces of arsenic in the original powder from natural origin

B. For unfilled and filled resins:

1. Residual monomer
2. The exothermic heat of polymerization
3. Leakage, especially when accompanied by marginal percolation
4. High coefficient of thermal expansion
5. Enamel etching acids accidentally applied on dentin

C. For composite resins:

1. Residual monomer
2. The exothermic heat of polymerization
3. Leakage
4. Surface roughness allowing plaque accumulation, especially around gingival margins
5. Acids used for enamel etching, if it comes in contact with any part of the pulp-dentin organ

D. For ASPA:

1. Acidity of the original liquid and non-set matrix, i.e., that of the restoration undergoing hardening
2. Surface roughness that leads to plaque accumulation
3. The cleaning acid for the dentin surface

All materials share the factor of heat production due to the acts of finishing and polishing, especially for a cervical lesion or any other location close to the pulp chamber and root canal system.

The third biologic inquiry is: ''What will be the material's effect at different effective depth?'' The following effects and average figures brought to the closest rounded number are the answers, assuming that there is no other modification for the P-D organ reaction to these materials.

A. For silicate cements:

1. Usually there is no healthy reparative reaction in the P-D organ of teeth restored with these materials.
2. If the effective depth is 3.5 mm or more, expect an unhealthy reparative reaction in the P-D organ.
3. At an effective depth less than 2-2.5 mm, expect destruction in the P-D organ.

B. For filled and unfilled resins:

Assuming that etching acids did not come in contact with dentin:
1. A P-D organ with effective depths of 3 mm or more in teeth restored with this material will usually show a healthy reparative reaction.
2. Teeth having cavities with effective depths from 2-3 mm

and restored with this material will have their P-D organ exhibiting an unhealthy reparative reaction.
3. If any of these materials restored a tooth having a cavity preparation with an effective depth less than 2 mm, expect destruction in the P-D organ.

C. For composite resins:

Also, assuming that the acid etching the enamel did not come in contact with the underlying dentin of the involved P-D organ:
1. As with unfilled and filled resins, if the effective depth of the involved P-D organ is 3 mm and more, expect a healthy reparative reaction.
2. If the effective depth of the P-D organ is 1.5-3 mm and the tooth is restored with composite resin, expect an unhealthy reparative reaction and sometimes destruction, especially if it is in the lower level of these measurements.
3. In teeth with P-D organs having an effective depth less than 1.5 mm and restored with this material, always expect destruction.

D. For ASPA:

In general, the pulp-dentin organ reaction will be very similar to that of polycarboxylate cement.
1. In teeth restored with this material, expect a healthy reparative reaction in the P-D organ up to as low as 1.5 mm effective depth.
2. An unhealthy reparative reaction has been reported in the P-D organ of teeth restored with this material having an effective depth as low as 0.5-1 mm.
3. Destruction can be expected if the effective depth is less than 0.5 mm, especially when the material comes in direct contact with the pulp or root canal tissues.

The fourth biologic inquiry is: ''What will be the indicated protective intermediary basing procedure for the P-D organ of teeth to be restored with each of these materials?''

A. For silicate cement:

1. Varnish should be used routinely whenever the effective depth is 3.5 mm or more, whether it is formed of dentin or brought up to that thickness by a subbase-base combination or a base. Varnish should be removed from enamel surfaces, so as not to hinder the fluoride exchange between the restoration and surrounding enamel.
2. At the safe depth for zinc phosphate cement (2.5 mm with varnish) or polycarboxylate cement (1-1.5 mm), use a base of either material under the silicate cement.
3. With less than the safe depth of zinc phosphate cement and PCC, use a subbase of calcium hydroxide or unmodified ZOE (according to the condition of the P-D organ) and a base of either zinc phosphate cement or polycarboxylate cement. It should be emphasized again here that ZOE cannot be used under or in conjunction with polycarboxylate cement.

B. For all resinous or resin-based materials:

Before enamel etching, the proper intermediary basing should be applied in the following indications:
1. If the effective depth of the P-D organ is 3 mm or more, no protection is needed for the P-D organ, except for etching acids which not only drastically affect the P-D organ, but also

increase the permeability of the underlying dentin and make the area more susceptible for decay recurrence.

2. In cavity preparations with effective depths from 2 mm to 3 mm one could use cavity liners on all dentinal walls and floors only. Usually, the varnish carrier in these liners is dissolved by the composite resin monomer, creating a halo discoloration effect, so, preferably, a base of polycarboxylate is used.

3. In cavity preparations with effective depths of 1-2 mm, use a base of PCC.

4. In cavity preparations with effective depths less than 1 mm, if calcium hydroxide will not interfere with the normal physiology of the P-D organ (according to the condition of the P-D organ and location of the lesion), use a carried calcium hydroxide or chelated calcium hydroxide cement as a base, or use any other form of calcium hydroxide as a subbase, then apply varnish and a base of ZPC, or use the calcium hydroxide as a subbase to be covered by a PCC base. If calcium hydroxide is contraindicated, use a subbase of unmodified ZOE, varnish, then a base of zinc phosphate cement. This is because ZOE is a depolymerizer to resinous polymeric materials.

After applying the indicated intermediary basing and before etching the enamel surface or walls, all dentinal surrounding walls plus dentinal and/or based floor should be covered with a carried calcium hydroxide. After enamel etching, this calcium hydroxide should be removed (it neutralizes etching acids inadvertently arriving to the dentin).

If this type of calcium hydroxide is the indicated base, it should be applied over all surrounding dentinal walls and floors before etching. Then, after etching, all surrounding walls of the cavity preparation, if present, should be cleaned from the calcium hydroxide, before insertion of the restoration.

C. For ASPA:

As this type of the restorative material does not usually necessitate a point line angle cavity preparation, it is very difficult to apply bases.

1. It is advisable to protect the P-D organ in the deepest part of the lesion before applying the acid cleaners, by applying a bead of calcium hydroxide chelated cement. Remove the cement after acid-conditioning.

2. Usually, no intermediary base is needed for this material because of its previously discussed effect on the P-D organ, and because of the barrier effect of any intermediary base on the adhesion of the material to tooth substance and the fluoride leaching to the dentin and enamel.

3. In extremely deep lesions, with less than 1 mm effective depth, it is advisable to apply a base of calcium hydroxide

chelated cement to the deep area only, if it will not interfere with the circulation and metabolism of the P-D organ, or a subbase of unmodified ZOE, varnish, and a base of zinc phosphate cement, if calcium hydroxide is contraindicated. In the latter case, any traces of varnish or ZOE external or peripheral to the ZPC base should be eliminated as they will interfere with the adhesion and setting of the ASPA.

BIBLIOGRAPHY

Bassiouny, M.A., and Grant, A.A.: The surface finish of a visible light-cured composite. J. Prosthet. Dent. 1980 Aug.; **44**(2):175-182.

Bassiouny, M.A., and Grant, A.A.: Physical properties of a visible light-cured composite resin. J. Prosthet. Dent. 1980 May; **43**(5):536-541.

Bowen, R.L.: Adhesive bonding of various materials to hard tooth tissues. II. Bonding to dentin promoted by a surface-active comonomer. J. Dent. Res. **44**:895 Sept.-Oct. 1965.

Bowen, R.L.: Effect or particle shape and size distribution in a reinforced polymer. JADA **69**:481 Oct. 1964.

Bowen, R.L.: Properties of a silica reinforced polymer for dental restorations. JADA **66**:57 Jan. 1963.

Bowen, R.L., and Reed, L.E.: Semiporous reinforcing fillers for composite resins: I. Preparation of provisional glass formulations. J. Dent. Res. Sept.-Oct. 76; **55**(5):738-747.

Charbeneau, G.T.: Appraisal of finishing and polishing procedures for dental amalgam. J. Mich. Dent. Assn. **46**:135 May 1964.

Fan, P.L., Powers, M., and Craig, R.G.: In vitro wear of microfilled and visible light-cured composites. J. Dent. Res. 1979 Nov. **58**(11):2116-2119.

Hamilton, A.I., et al.: Special report: report of the Committee on Scientific Investigation of the American Academy of Restorative Dentistry. J. Prosthet. Dent. 1980 June; **43**(6):663-686.

Lutz, F., Setcos, J.C., Phillips, R.W., and Roulet, J.F.: Dental restorative resins, types and characteristics. The Dental Clinics of North America, 1983 October; **27**(4):697-712.

McLean, J.W.: Status report on the glass ionomer cements. Council on dental materials and devices. J. Am. Dent. Assoc. 1979 Aug.; **99**(2):221-226.

Numm, W.R., Hembree, J.H. Jr., and McKnight, J.P.: The color stability of composite restorative materials. ASDC J. Dent. Child 1979 May-June; **46**(3):210-213.

Peterson, E.A., Phillips, R.W., and Swartz, M.L.: A comparison of the physical properties of four restorative resins. JADA **74**:1324 Dec. 1966.

Phillips, R.W.: Restorative resins. Dent. Clinics of North America. Vol 19, No. 2, April 1975, p. 223.

Phillips, R.W.: Skinner's Science of Dental Materials, 3d ed. Philadelphia, W.B. Saunders Co., 1973.

Phillips, R.W., Avery, D.R., Mehra, R., Swartz, and McCune, R.J.: Observations on a composite resin for Class II restorations: Three-year report. J. Prosthet. Dent. **30**:891-897 Dec. 1973.

Qvist, V.: Correlation between marginal adaptation of composite resin restorations and bacterial growth in cavities. Scand. J. Dent. Res. 1980 Aug.; **88**(4):296-300.

Raptis, C.N., et al.: Properties of microfilled and visible light-cured composite resins. JADA **99**:631, 1979.

Reinhardt, K.J., and Vahl, J.: A comparison of light-hardened and UV-polymerizable sealants and composites. Disch Zahnaerztl Z 1979 March; **34**(3):245-250.

CHAPTER 9

Cavity and tooth preparations for direct tooth-colored materials

Direct tooth-colored materials described in the previous chapter are usually used to restore anterior teeth affected with Class III, IV (with the exception of the distal surfaces of the cuspids), or V lesions. Under certain conditions these materials may also be used for Class I and II lesions, as well as for Class III lesions on the distal of a cuspid. Designs of tooth preparation have been subjected to many changes in the past few years, due to the introduction of new materials and to the advancements in available materials. This chapter is an attempt to give the bases for designing cavity and tooth preparations for direct tooth-colored materials. The actual designs are a compromise between the restorative requirements, especially the esthetic ones, the material's deficiencies and the tooth's limitations.

Application of the General Principles

I. Outline Form

There is no other area in operative dentistry where the general principles advocated by G.V. Black are violated as much as in restoring teeth with direct tooth-colored material. In fact, the only inviolabe principle is that "the cavity preparation should include tooth structures directly attacked by the lesion." The following are some features of the outline form for the tooth preparation to accommodate the direct tooth-colored materials which were discussed in the previous chapter.

1. Gaining access to the lesion, especially in Class III and some Class II cavities, will necessitate the choice between a facial and a lingual approach for tooth preparation. In the final analysis, the choice is dictated by the extent of the decay and the esthetic requirements, even though the latter makes lingual approach preferable. The problem of extension for access is not found in Class I, IV and V and most Class II preparations.

2. There is seldom a need for a cavity extension for prevention utilizing direct tooth-colored restorative materials. This should be obvious and after studying the physical, mechanical, and biological properties of these materials, from which we can conclude that none of these materials can come close to efficiently replacing tooth structures during function. Moreover, some of the materials have variable degrees of anticariogenecity.

3. In proximal surface lesions, the operator should try to prepare cavities so as to leave contact areas or parts of the contact areas in tooth structure, and not in the restoration. These restorative materials cannot maintain the integrity of the contact or the mesio-distal dimension of the tooth for a long time. This will necessitate placing one or more margins of the cavity preparation within the contact area.

4. Cavity preparations to receive any of these materials can accommodate undermined enamel in their surrounding walls, as even this is better attached and mechanically stronger than any of these materials that would replace it. Undermined enamel that is left, however, should have the following specification:

a. It should not be badly thinned by backward decay such that it becomes non-self-resistant or creates a prisming effect.

b. It should not be discolored by the lesion or such discoloration should not be conspicuous facially.

c. It should not be directly loaded at centric and eccentric contacts of upper and lower teeth. Also, the same situation should be exhibited during the movements from centric to eccentric locations.

d. If the tooth is to be restored in composite resin, remaining undermined enamel should be etched internally and externally, enabling the restorative material to embrace it.

e. Remaining undermined enamel should not be carious itself, and should not interfere with removal of all irreparable carious dentin from the cavity preparation.

f. Ragged peripheries of this undermined enamel should be smoothed to improve its own resistance and prevent a prisming effect.

g. Undermined enamel to be retained should not show any signs of cracks or crazing.

5. The gingival margin of any preparation to receive one of these materials should be located supragingivally, as any proximity of these materials to the gingiva will initiate periodontal problems. This results from the rough surfaces of these materials allowing plaque adhesion.

6. The outline of the cavity preparations should be in definite lines with rounded junctions between these lines. If possible, the conspicuous margins should parallel certain landmarks on the tooth surface or the parameters of the tooth, to partially mask the differentiating line between the tooth structure and the restorative material. This line will be the first to show up from any discoloration of the restorative material.

II. Retention and Resistance Form

The mechanical problems of Class I, II, and V restorations are fully described in the chapters on Class I, II, and, V cavity preparations for amalgam. Therefore, the mechanical problems of proximal restorations in anterior teeth (Class III and IV), with the exception of the distal of the cuspid, will be described here.

For any proximal restoration in anterior teeth, there are two possible displacing forces. The first (H in Fig. 1) is a horizontal force displacing or rotating the restoration in a labio-proximo-lingual or linguo-proximo-labial direction. It has its fulcrum almost parallel to the long axis of the tooth being loaded. The second (V in Fig. 1) is a vertical force displacing or rotating the restoration proximally (sometimes facially or lingually), and having a fulcrum at the gingival margin of the preparation. The latter has a loading arrangement similar to occluso-proximal (occluso-facial or occluso-lingual) restorations in posterior teeth. The amount of each depends upon the location, extent, and type of occluding contacts between the upper and lower teeth during function.

The mechanical picture can be summarized as follows:

1. In anterior teeth with normal overbite and overjet during centric closure of the mandible (from centric relation to centric occlusion), mainly the horizontal forces will be in action. Those forces, if loading the proximal restoration directly, would try to move it linguo-proximo-labially (for the upper restoration) and labio-proximo-lingually (for the lower one). The magnitude of the horizontal force component at this stage of mandibular movement is not very substantial, and the vertical one is almost nil.

In protrusive and lateral protrusive movements of the mandible, directly loaded proximal restorations in anterior teeth will be subjected to substantial horizontal as well as vertical displacing forces, especially in restorations replacing the incisal angle. The results of this loading are rotational forces (previously described), as well as forces rotating the restoration labially and proximally (for the upper) or lingually and proximally (for the lower).

2. If anterior teeth meet in edge-to-edge fashion at centric occlusion, loading of the proximal restoration, involving incisal angles (Class IV) will be similar to any Class II proximo-occlusal restorations, i.e., vertical displacing forces with very limited horizontal components. This loading will continue during all centric closures and excursion movements of the mandible. However, if the incisal angle is intact (Class III), these displacing forces will be minimal.

3. If the upper and lower anterior teeth meet such that the lowers are labial to the uppers in centric occlusion (Angle's Class III), there will be the same type of loading conditions mentioned in (1) except the horizontal loading will tend to rotate or displace restorations labio-proximo-lingually (for uppers) and linguo-proximo-labially (for lowers). During excursive movements, if teeth are in contact and there is a possibility of retrusive mandibular movements, the loading will be much less than that described in (1), with its horizontal displacement capability exactly the reverse to that described in (1).

4. In occlusions with deep anterior overbite and normal or no overjet, the horizontal type of loading will be greatly exaggerated. The vertical displacement, although present, will be minimal by comparison.

5. In occlusions with anterior open bite or severe overjet, or any other condition that creates a no-contact situation between upper and lower anterior teeth during centric occlusion and excursive movements of the mandible, proximal restorations will not be loaded directly either vertically or horizontally. The situations just described should be examined carefully, for

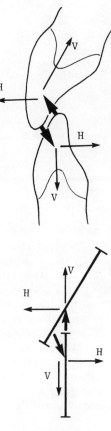

Fig. 9-1

in many cases where there is no apparent contact either in centric or in border positions, there may be momentary contact during excursions from one location to another.

6. In cases when the proximal restoration of an anterior tooth is a part of a mutually protective occlusion, i.e., an incisor and the adjacent cuspid are involved in an anterior lateral disclusion mechanism, the teeth and restoration will be part of that disclusion mechanism with excessive horizontal and vertical loading forces. This situation should be properly diagnosed, so that the tooth preparation can be designed and prepared accordingly. It should be understood that none of these loading forces work separately. They work together and simultaneously. However, they may differ in magnitude at different stages of mandibular movement. It should be mentioned here that a restoration replacing part or all of the incisal ridges of an anterior tooth will have the same pattern of loading as mentioned in (1)-(6), but with increased intensity. Loss of the incisal angle of a tooth, i.e., conversion from a Class III to a Class IV represents a major complication in the mechanical problems of anterior tooth restorations. This loss will lead to definite direct loading of the restoration, loss of the incisal wall which would normally accommodate one of the two possible main internal retentive modes for the restoration, definite vertical loading with its sequelae, and the placement of margins on the incisal ridge. This further exposes the restoration to the maximal loading possible in anterior teeth, and it is with the minimal tooth structure to be used for resistance and/or retention against such loading.

The structure of anterior teeth themselves, have a comparatively different stress pattern, as a result of occlusal loading, from that of posterior teeth. The unique shape as well as the mechanical structure and function of these teeth is very important to comprehend before designing a cavity and/or tooth preparation for a direct tooth-colored restoration. The following is a summary of these unique features:

a. Anterior teeth have their maximal bulk gingivally. They taper incisally with the least bulk at the incisal ridge. So resistance to stress fractures will be maximum at the gingival end and decrease incisally.

b. Forces are directed horizontally and vertically on anterior teeth as mentioned with the force analyses on restorations for these teeth. These forces accumulate maximal shear stresses at the junction of the clinical root with the clinical crown and maximum tensile stresses at the incisal ridges, especially their corners (incisal angles).

c. The labial enamel plate is much thicker than the lingual or proximal ones, with maximal thickness of enamel usually at the incisal ridge.

d. The incisors may be involved in a disclusion mechanism of the mandible with loading similar to that of the cuspid, but to a much lesser extent.

e. Occluding surfaces of anterior teeth, especially the lingual surfaces of the upper teeth and incisal ridges of the lowers, are the most important anterior determinant of mandibular movements. The extent and degree of concavities on these upper teeth lingually and the inclination and roundness of the incisal ridges of the lower ones, determine to a great extent the amount of loading, their directions, and the pattern of mandibular movements anteriorly and latero-anteriorly.

f. Cervical portions of anterior teeth when they are affected with a Class V lesion or cavity preparation will have a stress pattern similar to posterior teeth, and the stress pattern is governed by the same factors as in posterior teeth. In addition, the deeper the overbite is, the more induced the stresses are at these cervical areas.

g. As mentioned previously, loss of an axial angle, incisal angle, or tooth structure at the neck of the tooth will dramatically reduce that tooth's ability to resist loading without fracture failure.

Ideally, a restoration made of tooth-colored materials should not be loaded directly, i.e., there should be intervening tooth structure between the occluding tooth and the restoration. This situation can only be achieved by four intact walls surrounding the restoration. Unfortunately, this is usually not the case. That is why the clinical performance of tooth-colored materials differs from one situation to another, sometimes dramatically.

Composite resins used with acid etching and/or bonding techniques are the only non-cast restorative materials that can combine undermined enamel and cuspal elements to sound tooth structure, thereby improving their resistance form. They are reinforcers, similar to cast restorations, but in a much more conservative way.

There are four methods to accommodate and properly retain a restoration of these materials within tooth structure. They are:

i. Acid conditioning of surface enamel
ii. Retentive cavity preparation with internal details
iii. Physico-chemical adhesion to some components of the tooth structure

iv. Pins and posts (to be discussed in a separate chapter)
v. Combination of 1 to 4

i. Acid Conditioning of Surface Enamel

In 1959, Bounocore reported on the effects of 85% phosphoric acid application to enamel on the retention of acrylic resin restorations. There was little use of the idea until 1969 when the methodology was further explored. Now it is becoming an integral part of any direct tooth-colored resin restorative technique. At the present time, a 35-50% aqueous solution of phosphoric acid is used as a conditioning agent to enamel before inserting tooth-colored resin. Recent reports, however, state that much lesser concentrations (e.g., as low as 15%) produce sufficient enhancement of retention.

A. Effects of acid conditioning on surface enamel

It has been agreed upon by many authorities that 35-50% phosphoric acid applied on tooth enamel for 60 seconds will render the following effects and changes in the treated enamel.

1. It will etch the enamel substance, with preferential dissolution of the interprismatic enamel first, followed by the tops (surfaces) of the prisms themselves. The least dissolvable are the sides of the prisms (Fig. 2A).

2. From the preferential dissolution pattern mentioned in (1), the surface area of the enamel will increase up to 2000 times that of its original unetched surface area.

3. Also, from the actions mentioned in (1) the enamel surface will be very irregular, accommodating valleys in place of the interprismatic enamel, which sometimes will be undercut in shape (Fig. 2B). The top (surface) of the enamel prisms will have circumscribed depressions which also may have some undercuts (Fig. 2C). Both valleys and depressions will have irregular surfaces (Fig. 2d) and an average depth of 25 microns (Fig. 2E).

It is obvious from (2) and (3) that the retention of the restorative material which can wet all or most of the details of these irregularities (right side of Fig. 2A) will be several fold that of a restorative material wetting and adhering only to an unetched enamel surface (left side of Fig. 2A).

4. Acid etching will expose proteinaceous organic matrix substance of enamel, which can add to the restoration's retention if it becomes adequately embedded within the restorative material (Fig. 2F).

5. Mechanical cleaning and acid etching of enamel will assure removal of substrates, enamel cuticles, salivary deposits, plaque components and any possible adhesives to the enamel surface, thus exposing a cleaner, less contaminated, and more wettable enamel surface for adhesion with a restorative material (Fig. 2G).

6. Acid can, to some extent, completely remove surface enamel (Fig. 2G) which has been subjected to the surrounding environment for varying periods of time. Such long standing exposure will make this enamel fully reacted, with minimal or no surface energy left to be able to react with and adhere to a new adhesive, e.g., a restorative material. The freshly exposed enamel might have sufficient surface energy to facilitate a reaction with and adhesion to the restorative material to be applied (compare left side of Fig. 2A with right side). Mechanical removal of a fraction of 1 mm of the surface enamel can greatly improve the action of acid in this respect.

7. It has been suggested by several authorities that, by phos-

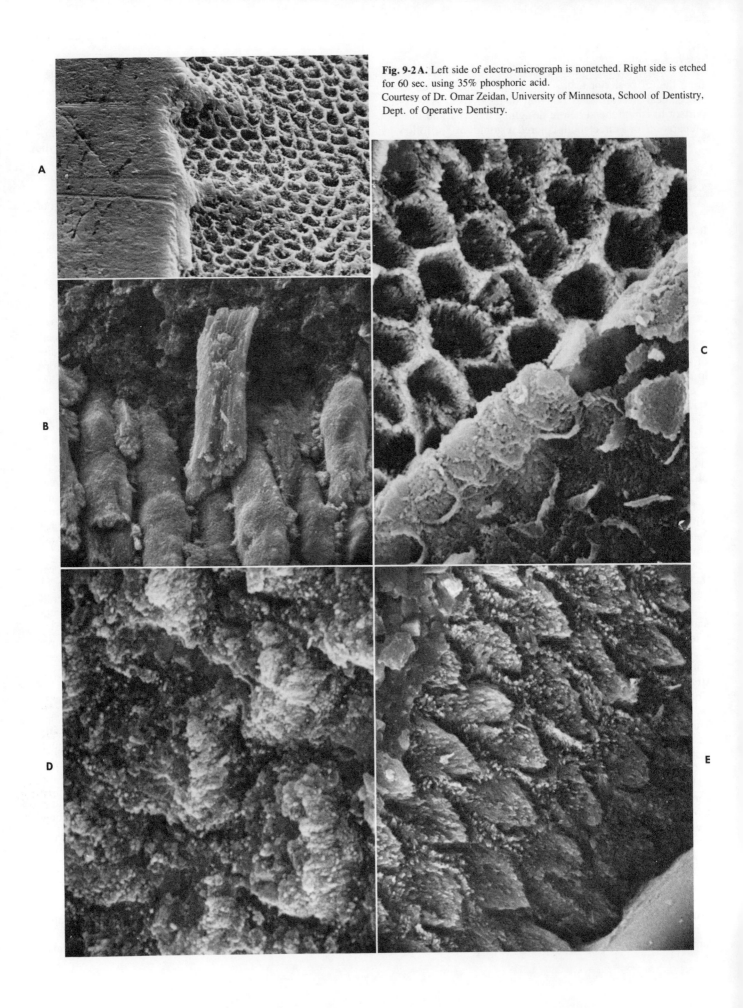

Fig. 9-2 A. Left side of electro-micrograph is nonetched. Right side is etched for 60 sec. using 35% phosphoric acid.
Courtesy of Dr. Omar Zeidan, University of Minnesota, School of Dentistry, Dept. of Operative Dentistry.

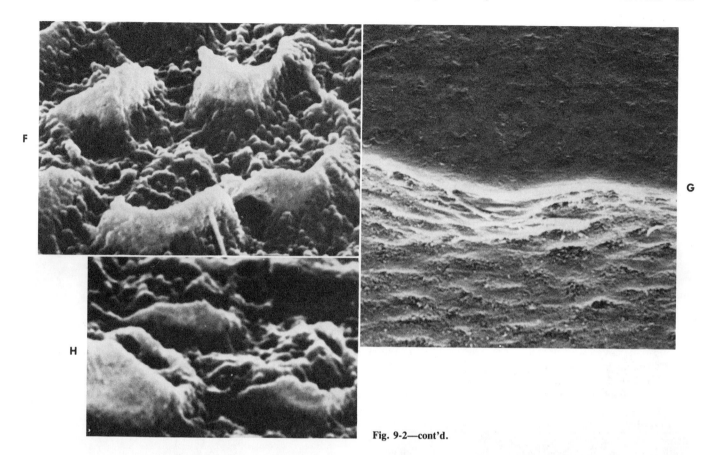

Fig. 9-2—cont'd.

phoric acid treatment, a newly precipitated phase of calcium oxalate and organic tungstate complexes could be created in isolated surface areas which can adhere both to enamel and to resinous substances (Fig. 2H).

8. It has been verified that enamel treatment with phosphoric acid will add to the enamel surface a highly polar phosphate group, which will increase the adhesive ability of the enamel surface.

From the above mentioned possible changes in human enamel, as a result of acid treatment, it is obvious that etching is not the only possible change. At any rate, with such type of treatment, the enamel surface will have an adhesive capability toward a wetting resinous material, a mechanical locking capability for a restorative material that can fill the created microscopic cavities, and the capability to create a fairly lasting joint with a wetting restorative material exhibiting minimum or no leakage (Fig. 3, A and B).

B. Requirements and principles of acid conditioning of surface enamel

First and foremost, the enamel surface should be mechanically cleansed from adhesive deposits and stains using a nongreasy non-fluoridated abrasive carried on a revolving rubber cup. If conditioned enamel is to be the only retentive mode for the restoration, it is necessary to involve an enamel surface that is at least double the surface area of the defect to be restored or minimally 1 mm in width. Conditioned enamel should be strategically distributed around the defect, taking into consideration the type, amount and directions of displacing forces, as mentioned before.

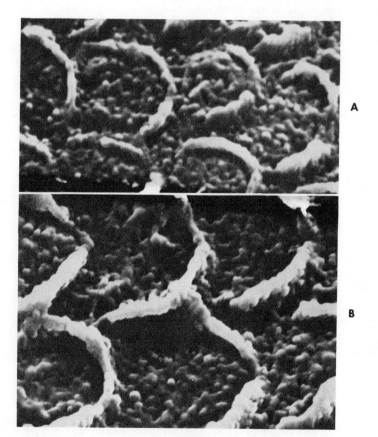

Fig. 9-3

There is no sense in etching enamel from the sides of the prisms (parallel to enamel surface), as the resulting effect will not be conducive to any retention of the restorative material. Rather, etching should be performed at a right angle to the enamel surface (prisms heads), so as to produce the retentive valleys and honey-combs as described. Any indicated intermediary basing should be applied to the tooth preparation, and all its exposed dentin surfaces should be covered with calcium hydroxide before applying the phosphoric acid on adjacent enamel.

If acid conditioning is to be used in conjunction with a cavity preparation to retain a resinous restoration in a tooth, the enamel walls should be prepared in one of the following fashions:

1. Partial bevel (Fig. 4)

This should involve about ⅓ to ½ of the enamel wall at 45-70° to the cavity walls. It is always used when the cavity preparation's internal anatomy and walls can adequately retain the restoration, and acid conditioning is used only to reduce marginal leakage. It is also to be used with restorative resins exhibiting minimal setting shrinkage.

2. Long bevel (Fig. 5)

In this design feature, the entire enamel wall is bevelled at 45-70° to the cavity wall. It is used when the cavity preparation details are not retaining enough for the resinous restoration, or when the resinous material used exhibits considerable shrinkage during polymerization. Of course, this design feature will also decrease microleakage.

Both shapes have the distinct disadvantage of having no definite marginal termination, especially after acid treatment. As a result, marginal overhangs (flash) of resinous material peripheral to the restoration will usually be present at the cavosurface margins treated in (1) or (2) fashion. Also, this marginal flash will occur in a weak acute-angled cross-section. Accordingly, do not use design features (1) or (2) in uncleansable areas, stress concentration areas (direct loading), inaccessible areas, and/or next to the periodontium. To increase the extent of the above mentioned bevels, increasing their angulation, relative to the adjacent cavity wall could be attempted. This will not only enhance the advantages of these bevels, but it will also increase the bulk of the composite next to the wall proper of the preparation.

3. Hollow ground bevel (Fig. 6)

In this design feature, about two-thirds of the enamel wall thickness is ground in a concave manner so the cavity margin will have a right angled cavosurface angle, with butt joint between the restorative material and the marginal enamel. This combines the advantages of the retaining, sealing, and acid conditioning of the enamel with the strong butt-joint and definite junction of tooth structure and restorative material. The hollow ground bevel is indicated for inaccessible areas, e.g., gingival walls to avoid possible overhangs which could occur with either (1) or (2) finish lines. It is also indicated for areas of direct loading, to accommodate the maximum bulk of restorative material.

4. Scalloping the margins (Fig. 7)

This feature can be used in conjunction with a partial or long bevel, in order to further increase the surface area and irregularities of the enamel that is to be conditioned. It is used when conditioned enamel will play a major role in the retention of the restoration. Scalloping has the disadvantage of greater pos-

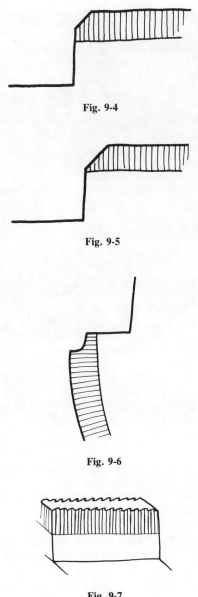

Fig. 9-4

Fig. 9-5

Fig. 9-6

Fig. 9-7

sibilities of flash and overhangs. Under no circumstances should scalloping be used for gingival walls or inaccessible portions of any wall margin.

5. Skirting (Fig. 8)

This feature is used if conditioned enamel will be the main retentive mode for resinous material. In restoring a wide and shallow defect (e.g., Class II, III or IV traumas, or Class III and IV proximal lesions having short or no surrounding wall), it is essential to involve enamel from the surrounding surfaces of the tooth. In these cases, mechanically remove a fraction of 1 mm from the surface enamel (0.1 mm) adjacent to the defect. As mentioned before, any such surface involvement should be double the surface area of the defect. Also, the involved enamel surface should be distributed around the defect so that principal, auxillary, and reciprocating retaining areas are in accordance with the magnitude, location and direction of loading forces, both in static and dynamic occluding con-

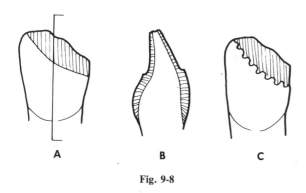

Fig. 9-8

tacts. Such surface involvement is called a skirt. It should have a definite termination (mini-chamfer, Fig. 8B, or scalloping, Fig. 8C) to improve retention and finishing. The skirt can also be used to circumscribe undermined enamel or thinned cuspal elements. In these situations, the weakened tooth structure is covered with restorative material and connected to more self-retained tooth structure.

A single cavity-tooth preparation can have more than one of the previously mentioned enamel preparations for acid conditioning. For example, a Class III cavity preparation may have a partial bevel on its incisal wall, a skirt labially (because of loss of the labial wall), a long bevel lingually (to reciprocate with the labial skirt) and a hollow ground bevel gingivally. Any of these, with the exception of the latter, could be scalloped.

If acid conditioning of the enamel is the only mode of retention for the restoration, it is advisable to mechanically remove the superficial, fully reacted, and sometimes prismless (in deciduous teeth) enamel layer using a fine diamond stone. Also, if the margins will be away from the gingiva, scalloping the peripheries of the enamel surface to be conditioned improves retention.

Acids should be applied on enamel with a soft sponge or cotton pellet, using light patting touches with *no rubbing at all*. Rubbing may fracture the thinned enamel rods, thereby reducing the depths of the created valleys and irregularities and obliterating what is left of them with the fractured enamel pieces. Leave acid on enamel for 60 seconds.

Acid conditioned enamel should be washed for one minute, using a copious stream of water. It should then be air dried before applying the components of the restoration. After drying, a characteristic whitish or chalky appearance is the sign for proper enamel conditioning.

In older teeth, and in areas with substantial flouride precipitation the signs for proper enamel conditioning may not appear after one minute of acid treatment. In this case a second and maybe a third application could be needed. It is advisable to resort to other means of retention, if three applications of acid do not produce the signs indicative of proper conditioning.

Absolutely no saliva should come in contact with the etched enamel surface. It has been shown that with only momentary exposure to saliva a proteinaceous film (biofilm) of salivary glycoproteins will instantaneously adhere to the etched enamel. This will prevent any other adhesives from wetting this enamel. Any further exposure to saliva will initiate remineralization of the area. This, of course, encourages the use of rubber dam

isolation. Enamel may be reconditioned after saliva contamination occurs, however.

Inadvertently etched areas of enamel surface that are not to be used to retain the restoration should be left for such salivary remineralization, a process which may take from a few hours to a few days. Most importantly, this untreated etched enamel should always be kept free from plaque accumulation, which is easily attached to such surfaces, until that enamel regains its prior mineral contents.

ii. Cavity Preparations

All direct tooth-colored materials, with the exception of ASPA and other materials that have a physico-chemical adhesion potential, need a mechanical cavity and/or tooth preparation. The following general features should be evident in these cavity preparations:

A. As many walls as possible should be established around the lesion. These walls should have rounded but definite angles between them and the involved floor or axial wall (mortise form). The roundness of the line angles should be far more exaggerated than in amalgam preparations, because of the brittle nature of direct tooth-colored restorative materials.

B. Surrounding walls should make right angles or preferably acute angles with floors or axial wall. In any event, try to avoid an obtuse angulation relationship.

C. Walls directly loaded, i.e., in contact with opposing teeth in centric and non-centric occlusion, should be formed of enamel supported by dentin.

D. Any unattacked enamel (directly or indirectly), pulpally or axially, should be maintained if etching is to be part of the restorative technique.

E. If bonding or acid-etching is to be part of the restorative technique, the preparation dimensions (width, length, depth) may be kept minimal (as low as 0.5 mm).

F. Any surface defects (e.g., pits, fissures, cracks, etc.) which are in contact with the preparation margins, should be included in the tooth preparation after eliminating their diseased parts.

G. In extensive Class I or II lesions, where the width of the preparation exceeds one-third of the intercuspal distance, substantially angulated long bevels should be prepared peripheral to the wall proper, and should be etched prior to insertion of composite resin.

H. In extensive Class I or II lesions which have areas of cusp with a length:width ratio of 3 or more, it is advisable to skirt all or part of the elongated cusp. This skirt must be prepared distant to the occluding contacts (both centric and excursive). It should be prepared only if:

1. The cusp has sound, bulky enamel that will accommodate a minimum skirt of 0.5 mm depth.

2. Reciprocating cusp or tooth structure is self-retaining (i.e., length:width ratio is 1 or less), and has sufficient sound enamel to accommodate a reciprocating skirt or long bevel.

Such skirting of elongated cusp elements should be applied more stringently on functional rather than non-functional cusps.

I. If a Class I or II lesions is extensive and backward in nature, creating severe undermining of cuspal enamel, occlusally overhanging (unsupported) enamel should be eradicated. However, any facial, lingual, or proximal unsupported enamel may be left, provided it will be skirted and etched externally as well as internally. Any knife-edged enamel should be trimmed to a blunted or flat-tabled form before skirting. Also, the reciprocating cusp or tooth structure should be self-resistant and treated with a skirt or long bevel as described in H.

j. When confronted with a situation as described in H and I, but with reciprocating tooth or cusp structure also thinned or formed of unsupported enamel, one or both reciprocating areas should be reduced to be self-resistant (length: width ratio of 1). Then, skirting of both could be accomplished prior to etching.

K. In highly stressed areas during centric and excursive contacts, it is essential to create in the tooth preparation sufficient reduction and depth for bulk of composite resin.

L. When bevelling of enamel walls is indicated prior to conditioning, and it is cariogenically and anatomically feasible, it is preferable to bevel supported enamel in walls or planes following the direction of the enamel rods.

M. Internal auxiliary retention should always be in the form of bulky dentinal grooves. The most efficient grooves are gingival and incisal (occlusal) for Class II, III, and V, and gingival, facial, and lingual for Class II and IV cavity preparations.

N. Extension for retention in the form of a dovetail should absolutely be avoided in anterior teeth for the following reasons:

1. Dovetails may expose more restoration surface to occlusal loading.

2. Dovetails thin the labio-lingual bulk of tooth structure in an already thinned tooth. This minimizes its resistance ability.

3. In upper teeth, for the dovetail to be effective, it should be cut on the lingual surface, a location precariously close to the pulp chamber.

4. Dovetails do not ''lock'' restorations in all directions. There are always one or two directions in which the restoration will be free to move if the dovetail is the only means of retention. *Therefore, the hazards (compared with the possible benefits of the dovetail) do not warrant using it in Class III and IV cavity preparations for direct tooth-colored materials.*

O. When cavity margins come close to important anatomy, e.g., the incisal angle, marginal ridge or axial angle, where their loss means more complicated mechanical problems for the tooth and the restorative material, it is advisable to diverge the adjacent wall inward-outward and to avoid placing any retentive forms in the adjacent walls. This will leave tooth bulk, especially dentinal, to support these critical anatomies.

P. Involvement of the incisal angle or a cusp in a defect always varies. The extent of this involvement should be evaluated facio-lingually, mesio-distally and occluso-gingivally, to try to maintain as much of it as possible (see chapter on Restoration of Badly Broken Down Teeth). Similarly, involvement of the facial and lingual axial angle or marginal ridges can also vary. Only the involved part needs to be restored, so the facial and/or lingual walls of the tooth preparation may be interrupted, if necessary, to avoid losing them completely. Bear in mind that *any* small portion of a wall can help with resistance and retention.

Q. Of all the surrounding walls in Class II, III and IV cavity preparation, the gingival wall is the most critical in shaping the resistance and retention form of the restoration. That is why it should be present in any Class II, III and IV cavity preparation for tooth-colored materials. This gingival wall should be as pronounced as anatomically and cariogenically possible, both facio-lingually and proximo-axially. It should be as close to the contact area with occluding teeth (center of loading) as anatomically and cariogenically possible. As mentioned previously, this wall should accommodate one of the main internal retention modes (grooves). Furthermore, it should be flat or have a flat component if formed of different planes, and should meet a facial and a lingual wall, even if very short in definite angles to help lock the restoration. Finally, the gingival wall should accommodate a hollow ground bevel if it has an enamel component.

iii. Physico-Chemical Adhesion to Some Components of Tooth Structure

A restorative material that can adhere and chemically combine with tooth structures will be a solution for many restorative problems, especially retention and microleakage. This goal is rapidly becoming a dream come true for restorative dentistry. Nevertheless, despite considerable progress in this field in the past few years, it is still in its infant stage.

Rather than discuss the details of these modes of retention, the reader is referred to the everchanging literature in this field. It deserves mention, however, that for any adhesive bond to be effective and serviceable there must be close proximity between the adhesive and adherend, complete wettability of the adhesive to the adherend, physical and/or primary bonding between the adhesive to the adherend, and most importantly, permanency of the bond under environmental changes and functional stresses. The tooth as an adherend leaves much to be resolved to make it amenable to an adequate adhesive restorative material. Its heterogeneous structure, especially that of dentin, its water components, the impossibility of removing all debris from its surface by present techniques and instruments, and the difference in tooth composition in different individuals and various geographical areas are just a few of the problems that need to be overcome.

Although there have been several breakthroughs in the past few years, the present status of adhesive dental restoratives still leaves much to improve upon. There are adhesive systems available that can bond with one or more components of tooth structure but not with all of them. These systems may be classified as follows:

A. Adhesives to the inorganic phase of the tooth (hydroxyapatite-$Ca_{10}(PO_4)_6(OH)_2$) through complexation of calcium or a reaction with its PO_4^{+++} and OH^- group

Examples of these are the polycartoxylates (PCC and ASPA). The macromolecules having multiple carboxyl and hydroxyl groups in certain spatial combinations can complex $Ca++$ from the apatite crystal of enamel and to a lesser degree from dentin. Such chelation is severely inhibited, both by improper debridement of the tooth surface and by the non-availability of polyacrylic acid macromolecules.

Also included in this group are solutions which improve the wetting of acid-etched enamel with composite resin. Carboxy monomer and polymer, such as 4-methacryloxyethyl trimelletic acid anhydride, and a solution of butyle-acrylate acrylic acid copolymer in isoprorananol are examples of such wetting agents.

In addition, amino carboxy monomer (like that developed by Bowen) which is a condensation product of n-phenyl glycine, and glycidyle methacrylate, have been shown to adsorb effectively to calcium and were used commercially as a primer to adhere composite resin to cervical erosions.

Recently, Bowen reported a more sophisticated and complex adhesive procedure using amino-carboxy and amino-hydroxy polymers as surface active copolymers, on, a mordanted tooth surface (enamel and dentin). Basically, the procedural steps were as follows:

The mechanically prepared teeth were treated with 5.3% aqueous solution of ferric oxalate ($Fe_2(C_2O_4)_3$) (mordant solution) for 60 seconds. This precipitates ferric ions, that could be a more stable chelate with the surface active copolymer than calcium ions. This is due to the Fe_3 being more electronegative than the tooth calcium, thereby decreasing the possibility of water ionization at the interface and diminishing hydrolysis of the chelate. The treated surfaces were then washed with water for 10 seconds. A 10% acetone solution of N (p-tolyl) glycine and glydidyl methacrylate (NTG-GMA) aminohydroxy was then applied for 60 seconds, during which time most of the solvent evaporated. Next, a drop of clear acetone was applied for 10 seconds and then removed. This eliminated any free NTG-GMA. After drying the surface with air, a 5% acetone solution of pyromelletic dianhydride and 2-hydroxyethyl methacrylate (PMDM) amino-carboxyl was applied for 60 seconds. After the surface was again dried, a suitable composite resin was applied. Bonding strength was reported to be up to 1 ton/sq. inch. to dentin and even more to properly etched enamel.

Silanes, such as those used to create bonding between ceramic particles and resin matrix in composite resins, can also be used on etched enamel. Although silanes do not create strong bonds with enamel apatite, they do improve the wettability of enamel to composite resin.

Polyphosphates (e.g., glycerophosphoric acid dimethacrylate) and phosphonates (e.g., vinylbenzene phosphonates) show a great capacity for chelating calcium, although phosphate chelates are readily hydrolyzed in the oral environment, phosphonate chelations better withstand such deterioration. They bond similarly to both enamel and dentin.

B. Adhesion to organic phases (mainly collagen)

Many possibilities of reacting with side-chain groups of the amino-acids of tooth collagen, namely NH_2, OH, and COOH groups, do exist. However, dentinal collagen is not very reactive, so a vigorous chemical reactant must be used. Many such attempts have been made, e.g., grafting of methylmethacrylate to dentin collagen induced by an agent containing the polymerization initiator tributyl boron. However, this procedure resulted in dentin degradation and ultimate loss of the bond.

C. Crystal growth bonding

This is a new concept in which a clean tooth surface is treated with a solution of polyacrylic acid containing SO_4^- ions. The liberated Ca^{++} will react with these SO_4^- ions forming $CaSO_4^- 2H_2O$ (gypsum) in one to two minutes. As these crystals are nucleated within the tooth and grow outwardly with irregular, rough surfaces, they are similar to an etched enamel without loss of tooth structure. To this surface, primers

and appropriate resins may be applied, creating an adhesive restoration.

Despite all of these aforementioned advances in adhesive dentistry, using presently available materials and techniques for bonding we can expect to have islands of attachment surrounded by areas of non-attachment between the adherend (tooth) and the adhesive (restorative material). Indeed, this situation is conducive to increased retention; but, by all measures, this retention is incomplete. The areas of non-attachment invite microleakage, stress concentration, and eventually failure (detachment) at the interface.

III. Convenience Form

The very nature of access to Class III and IV lesions necessitates some modifications in outline form, internal anatomy of cavity preparation, and instrumentation for convenience of preparation. Examples include:

i. Separation, using different devices, helps to gain access proximally in anterior teeth.

ii. Convenience form is facilitated by making the wall of the access side shorter and divergent compared to the wall on the non-access side.

iii. In order to reach all the cavity preparation details, it is necessary to reduce or eliminate convexity of the axial wall.

iv. Specific instruments are used which are designed with multiple and different angulations in their shanks.

IV. Removal or Carious Dentin

This procedure is performed as described in the general principles; however, in these preparations there will be the challenge of removing carious dentin without removing all overlying enamel. As described above, some will be left as part of the cavity walls.

After grossly removing the softened dentin, small bi- or triple-angled discoid excavators are introduced into the cavity preparation under the undermined enamel and moved laterally while in contact with this enamel. Finally, the tip of a blunt explorer is used in the same way to be sure that there are no remnants of that softened irreparably decayed dentin.

V. Biologic Form

This procedure follows the general principles previously outlined, with special emphasis on creating different levels of pulpal and axial walls.

VI. Finishing of Enamel Walls

The unique situation in these preparations of leaving undermined enamel and conditioning of enamel surfaces before restoration, make the finishing of enamel walls completely different from that described in the general principles. Both situations have been explained in detail above, and the procedure for handling the enamel will be mentioned later.

VII. Preparation Debridement

This procedure, too, follows the general principles. Bear in mind, however, that there is no other place in restorative dentistry where debris-free preparation details are as vitally important as in these preparations. In addition to reagents and techniques described for debridement in the general principles, several additional reagents are used here (e.g., 0.5% EDTA, citric or acetic acids for enamel and dentin, and phosphoric acid for enamel).

Designs of Tooth Preparation for Direct Tooth Colored Restorations

The following is a description of basic designs of tooth preparations for direct tooth-colored materials, or modified designs for these materials. The most varied modifications involve the handling of enamel walls or enamel margins prior to acid conditioning.

I. Class I and Class II Cavity Preparations
(Figs. 9, 10)

Of all direct tooth-colored materials, only composite resin could be used for Class I and Class II restorations, and even then, only in the following situations:

A. Minimal incipient involvement

B. Removal of undermined tooth structure leaves sound, etchable enamel as circumferentially as possible

C. Areas in the dentition with low cariogenic activity

D. Areas of minimal masticatory loading, especially those with abrasive components

E. As a provisional restoration in teeth with doubtful prognoses

F. In badly broken down teeth prior to endodontics, orthodontics, or periodontics

G. As a treatment restoration to create a tooth or occlusal pattern of specific configurations, to test its compatibility with surrounding tissues and to allow correction of any discrepancies (either by addition or elimination of material) before replicating them in a permanent restoration

H. Only used for supragingival lesions

I. When esthetics is the major objective of the restoration

J. For prophylactic purposes in fissures and grooves that are apparently highly caries susceptible

K. For provisional splinting of teeth

L. As provisional veneering for unsightly amalgam restorations

There are some similarities, at least in the general outline form, between Class I and II tooth preparations for amalgam and composite resin. However, the differences between these preparations for both materials may be enumerated as follows:

1. The intercuspal width of the preparation of direct tooth-colored materials may be as small as one-fifth the intercuspal distance (Fig. 9).

2. In preparations for direct tooth-colored materials, internal line and point angles are extremely rounded, especially if they are in enamel.

3. If anatomically, cariogenically, and mechanically possible (described in the General Principles) surrounding walls and/or pulpal and gingival floors could all be in enamel in preparations for direct tooth-colored materials.

4. Surrounding walls or floors having dentinal components may accommodate dentinal grooves as reciprocating and auxiliary means of retention (Fig. 10).

5. In direct tooth-colored preparations, undermined enamel may be retained, subject to the provisions enumerated earlier in this chapter.

6. Unlike preparations for amalgam, these preparations do not require a reverse curve at the occluso-proximal juncture (Fig. 10).

7. For thinned cuspal elements circumferential skirting is indicated. Of course, this is not the case for amalgam preparations.

8. Dentinal portions of preparations for direct tooth-colored materials should always be mortise shaped.

9. Peripheral portions of enamel walls to be etched should be beveled, as described earlier in the chapter.

10. Saucer-shaped Class II preparations for tooth-colored

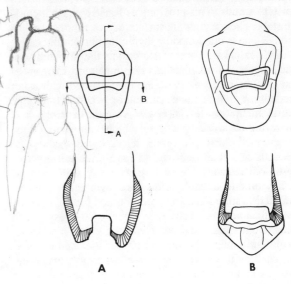

A   **B**

Fig. 9-9

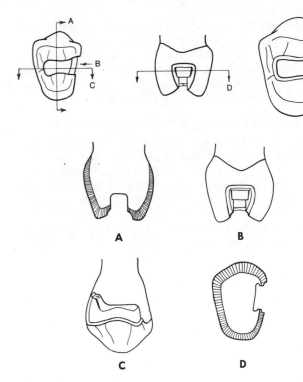

A   **B**

C   **D**

Fig. 9-10

materials could be used if the lesion is confined to enamel with minimal, forward dental involvement at its center.

11. When restoring with direct tooth-colored materials, the preparations should allow for contact areas to remain totally or partially in tooth structure.

II. Class III Tooth Preparations

A. Class III, Design 1 (conventional labial approach)

Involvement: Part of the proximal surface of anterior teeth

1. Indications

a. Proximal surface lesions in anterior teeth, except the distal of the cuspid, where decay is extending more labially than lingually, and involving part of the labial embrasure.

b. Class III lesions in labio-verted rotated teeth where lingual access would involve excessive sound tooth structure on the lingual surface.

c. In situations wherein direct loading of the restoration cannot be avoided with any possible location of the lingual margin if trying to prepare the cavity with a lingual access, but such deleterious loading can be avoided by a labial access.

d. For the distal of the cuspid, if part of the contact area remains in tooth structure.

e. For any type of direct tooth-colored material except unfilled resin and first generation composite resin.

2. General shape (Fig. 11, A and B)

This should be triangular with rounded corners.

3. Location of margins

a. The labial margin is located in the labial embrasure, between the labial axial angle and the contact area.

b. The lingual margin is located mostly in the contact area, just past the lingual extremity of the carious lesion.

c. The gingival margin is located in the gingival embrasure, just apical to the gingival limit of the lesion, sometimes in the contact area.

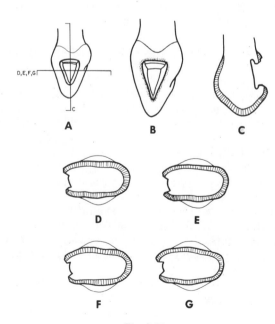

Fig. 9-11

d. The incisal margin is located always in the contact area, just past tooth structure directly attacked by decay.

4. Internal anatomy (Fig. 11, C, D and E)

The internal anatomy details described in the following section represent the ideal situation, i.e., assuming that no undermined enamel will be left as a part of the preparation components. Unfortunately, this situation is not true in most cases. Undermined enamel can be part of the remaining tooth structure to accommodate the restorative material provided it satisfies the criteria mentioned previously. That is why, in addition to the details to be described next, the retainable undermined enamel component(s) should be added as described elsewhere in the chapter.

a. Inciso-gingival cross-section (Fig. 11, C)

This cross-section enables visualization of the axial wall, which is flat to slightly rounded, and which may have different levels. The peripheries and various levels should maximally be 0.5 mm from the dentino-enamel junction.

The incisal wall, in this cross-section, will vary in appearance, depending on the location of the incisal margins. It is seen to have two or three planes. If the incisal margin is located at the middle third, there will be two planes—one in the form of a dentinal groove at the expense of the incisal wall, and another following the direction of the enamel rods formed of enamel and dentin. If the incisal margin is located in the incisal third of the proximal surface, there will be three planes—a dentinal plane to form a groove incisally, a transitional plane, and a third plane following the direction of the enamel rods inciso-proximally and formed of enamel and dentin.

The gingival wall will appear very similar to the incisal wall in this cross-section. If the gingival margin is located at the middle third of the proximal surface, there will be two planes, with the inner dentinal plane creating a gingival groove at the expense of the gingival floor. If the gingival margin is located at the gingival third of the proximal surface, there will be three planes, but directed in the reverse direction of the incisal situation. If the gingival margin is located on cementum, it should be handled the same way amalgam gingival floors are handled, but with an inner dentinal groove. As mentioned before, the gingival groove is required for *any* Class III cavity preparation. The incisal groove will be reduced in dimensions the closer the incisal margin is to the incisal angle. The incisal groove may be eliminated altogether, if it jeopardizes the support for the incisal angle. Of course, for resinous material, it is necessary to place a partial bevel incisally and a hollow ground bevel gingivally before etching, if they are not contraindicated.

b. In the labio-lingual section (Fig. 11, D and E), the axial wall is seen to be flat to slightly rounded, but not to the extent of the proximal surface. The labial wall appears to be a one-planed, enamelo-dentinal wall, divergent proximo-labially. It is usually shorter than the lingual wall, at least at one location of its inciso-gingival extent. Prior to acid etching it is necessary to place a partial or long enamel bevel labially (Fig. 11, D and E), if not contraindicated.

The lingual wall, in this cross-section, due to the extent of the decay or narrowness of the proximal surface, is located at the lingual third of the proximal surface. It will have two planes: an inner dentinal plane at right angle to the axial wall, and an outer plane following the direction of the enamel rods diverging proximo-lingually (Fig. 11D). However, if the decay extent is limited lingually and/or the proximal surface is wide so that the lingual margin is located in the middle third of the proximal surface, the lingual wall will be formed of one plane (straight) proximally, following the direction of the enamel rods, and at a right angle to the axial wall (Fig. 11E). Each of these two possible wall configurations can be formed at different levels of the wall according to each specific area's marginal location. If not contraindicated, peripheral parts of these walls could contain a partial or long enamel bevel for acid etching (Fig. 11, D and E).

B. Class III, Design 2. (conventional lingual approach)

Involvement: Proximal or part of the proximal surface of anterior teeth

1. Indications

a. This design is preferred for all Class III lesions if anatomical, cariogenic, and loading situations will allow a lingual approach.

b. This design is indicated for all direct tooth-colored materials except unfilled resins and second generation composites.

2. General shape (Fig. 11)

This is similar to the labial approach.

3. Location of margins

The incisal and gingival margins are located similar to the labial approach.

The labial margin is almost always in the contact area, just past the labial limit of the lesion. It may also be located at the very lingual limit of the labial embrasure.

The lingual margin is in the lingual embrasure. At one point or another it may be located on the lingual surface proper, if decay involves part of the marginal ridge, or if required to improve access.

4. Internal Anatomy (Fig. 11, C, F, and G)

In the inciso-gingival cross-section, the features of the internal anatomy are similar to those seen in the labial approach. In the labio-lingual cross-section (Fig. 11, F and G), however, features that are the exact reverse of the labial approach are seen. Compared to the labial wall, the lingual wall (excluding any enamel beveling) is always one-planed and shorter either as a whole or at one location. Due to the limited bulk of lingual tooth structure in some anterior teeth, skirting all or part of the lingual enamel wall may be necessary (Fig. 11F). The labial wall, as seen in this cross-section, may consist of one (Fig. 11G) or two (Fig. 11F) planes (excluding any bevelling). This will depend on the marginal location.

In these designs, if the enamel walls are to be bevelled (partially or completely) or skirted, prior to conditioning them for resinous restorative material, the anatomy of each wall will be modified marginally to accommodate the indicated bevel described in the previous section (Fig. 11, F and G).

5. Instrumentation for Class III, Designs 1 and 2

a. Gaining access

Wedge separation will create some space for instrument introduction. The removal of undesirable undermined enamel overhanging the proximal lesions can also facilitate the access.

b. Gross removal

With a ½ or 1 round bur introduced through the labial embrasure use axial pressure and lateral dragging to grossly remove tooth structure within the contemplated preparation outline. This should not exceed 0.5 mm from the DEJ.

c. Removal of irreparable carious dentin

Follow the same procedures described in application of the general principles.

d. Preliminary shaping

Use a smaller round bur than the one used for gross removal. First place it on the future location of the gingival floor. Then, with very light gingival pressure and with facio-lingual dragging and intermittent strokes that have proximal withdrawal, primarily shape the gingival floor.

Then repeat the same actions with the same bur on the future location of the labial, and then the lingual walls in inciso-gingival strokes. This will preliminarily formulate these walls and join them with the gingival floor in very rounded fashion. During the preliminary shaping, it is necessary not to remove any retainable undermined enamel.

e. Retention grooves formulation

With a ¼ round bur placed into the incisal point angle, use incisal pressure and *slight* labial dragging to create a short retention groove at the expense of the incisal wall. Placing the same bur into the gingivo-linguo-axial point angle, use gingival pressure and labial dragging to create a retention groove at the expense of the gingival floor.

f. Final shaping

With a Wedelstaedt chisel, use direct cutting strokes in an inciso-gingival direction to create the plane(s) for the labial and lingual walls. Be careful not to remove any retainable undermined enamel that can remain as part of the preparation walls. With an angle former or small gingival marginal trimmer, round the axial wall in a labio-lingual direction by cutting two triangles (mentioned in Chapters 6 and 7). A suitable size round bur may now be used on all point and line angles to further round out any sharpness that might have occurred from hand instrument cutting.

g. Cavity finishing

With an angle former or gingival margin trimmer, remove loose, thinned, and ragged enamel from cavosurface margins. Then with an angle former and Wedelstaedt, go over all walls, avoiding point and line angles (which should be kept very rounded), using light strokes to smooth them, in order to enhance material adaptability.

h. Intermediary basing and dentin protection from conditioning acids

Intermediary basing should be done as planned in the chapter on intermediary basing and according to the indications mentioned in the section on biologic form. If acid is to be used on the preparation or the surrounding enamel, all exposed dentin should be covered with a methyl cellulose carried or chelated cement form calcium hydroxide, whether or not the cavity received intermediary basing. If, in fact, the preparation did receive an intermediary basing, this calcium hydroxide will be in addition to that base.

i. Enamel wall preparation and conditioning

First, decide about the type of enamel wall for each part of the preparation. Then, using a fine diamond stone, prepare the partial or long bevels or the skirt at the indicated angulations, using fluent strokes.

A very small ball-shaped stone or a ¼ round bur may be used to prepare a hollow ground enamel bevel gingivally. Care must be taken here not to thin or penetrate the enamel at this location. Next, polish the surface enamel surrounding cavity margins with pumice mixed with water, then wash and dry the tooth thoroughly. Be sure the calcium hydroxide covering the dentin was not disturbed by these procedures. If it was, more should be applied.

Apply acid conditioning solution on prepared enamel using a very small cotton pellet with a *gentle tapping* movement. Allow the acid solution to remain in place for 60 seconds, then wash the tooth for one full minute with a gentle water spray. Then dry with a strong blast of oil free air. At this point, the enamel margins should appear as chalky white. If this characteristic appearance is absent, repeat the acid conditioning steps. Apply the available primer (usually monomer or coupling agent) on etched areas, using a camel(sable)-hair brush. All of these procedures should be done just before insertion of the restorative material.

Instrumentation for Class III Design 2 cavity preparation to accommodate a direct tooth-colored material is exactly the same as Design 1, except that access is gained from the lingual embrasures instead of from the labial.

C. Class III, Design 3. (without a lingual or labial wall)

Involvement: The proximal and part of the lingual or labial surface of anterior teeth

1. Indications

  a. All labial and lingual approach indications are included.

  b. The entire labial or lingual wall is lost during access, or for cariogenic reasons.

  c. The incisal angle is approached too closely by the incisal margin in a Design 1 or 2 cavity preparation, making it impossible to place a bulky retention form incisally.

  d. The remaining labial or lingual wall should be bulky enough to accommodate a retentive groove.

  e. This is used for the distal of cuspids, if the contact area will remain in tooth structure.

  f. This is used for all direct tooth-colored restorative materials except unfilled resin or second generation composite resins.

2. General shape (Fig. 12)

This design is almost parallelogram in shape except for the tendency of the incisal portion to be triangular. Both areas have very rounded corners.

3. Location of margins

Labial, lingual, incisal, and gingival margins can be similar to those described for the second design. If the lingual wall is lost, the lingual margin is located on the lingual surface, past the marginal ridge or the proximo-lingual axial angle. If the labial wall is lost, the labial margin is located on the labial surface, past the axial angle.

4. Internal anatomy (Fig. 12)

In the inciso-gingival cross-section (Fig. 12C), the internal anatomy appears very similar to the previously described designs. However, the incisal groove may not be present in most cases. In the labio-lingual cross-section (Fig. 12D), the axial wall may be seen to be perfectly flat, opening directly to the lingual (or labial) surface, and formed of dentin and enamel. It may have different levels, depending on the caries extent.

The labial wall, for preparations with lingual access, excluding any enamel bevelling, will usually be in the labial embrasure, i.e., labial one-third of the proximal surface, and it will be formed of three planes: an inner plane in the form of a groove at the expense of the labial wall, a dentinal tran-

sition, and an enamelo-dentinal plane that will follow the direction of the enamel rods labio-proximally. However, if the labial margin is located in the contact area, i.e., middle third of the proximal surface, the labial wall will only be formed of two planes, i.e., a grooved dentinal area and a dentino-enamel plane opening straight proximally at a right angle to the axial wall (Fig. 12D). When this design is applied to a labial approach, the same planes mentioned previously for the labial wall will be found on the lingual wall, instead. The only exception will be the grooved plane (Fig. 12D), which should be omitted in the labial approach due to the relative flatness or convexity of the lingual surface, and to the narrowness of the lingual embrasure as compared to the labial embrasure. Both of these situations increase the possibility of undermining tooth structure lingually or of perforation to the lingual surface if a groove was attempted.

Therefore, when confronted with a cavity preparation involving a lost labial wall, to use Design 3, the tooth must have sufficient bulk of tooth structure to accommodate deeper incisal and gingival retention grooves, and/or a labial enamel skirt. If these are not possible, it will be necessary to resort to another design of cavity preparation.

If enamel bevels are indicated, they should change the wall anatomy as previously described (Designs 1 and 2). Here, also, a lingual or labial surface enamel skirt may be indicated as a reciprocating retention means. In this case the cavity will have a lingual or labial surface enamel extension as described before.

5. Instrumentation for Class III, Design 3

  a. Gaining access

Wedge separation, as well as the fact that the lingual (or labial) axial angle (marginal ridge) will be involved in the preparation, will definitely facilitate access.

  b. Gross removal

With a 699 tapered fissure bur at the lingual (labial) embrasure, use lateral pressure and inciso-gingival movements with proximal dragging strokes to remove tooth structure to a 0.5 mm depth, short of the predetermined location of the margins.

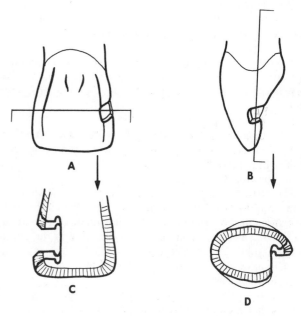

Fig. 9-12

c. Removal of irreparable carious dentin

This is accomplished exactly as discussed for Designs 1 and 2.

d. Preliminary shaping

Following the same scheme as described for the previous design, tentatively formulate labial (lingual), gingival, and incisal walls. This step will be much easier in this design, as the tapered fissure bur used in the gross removal should, to some extent, have partially created these walls.

e. Groove preparations

The gingival and incisal grooves should be prepared as in the previous design. Using the same size round bur, start at the gingivo-labio-axial point angle, with lateral pressure and incisal dragging cut a groove at the expense of the labial wall via the labio-axial line angle. Access for preparing this groove is generally facilitated by loss of the lingual wall.

Final shaping, cavity finish and intermediary basing for the preparation are done exactly as described for the previous two designs.

f. Preparing enamel walls for surface conditioning

This is done as in the previous two designs with the exception that the lingual (labial) surface enamel next to the margin may be skirted and sometimes also scalloped, using tapered diamond stones.

D. Class III, Design 4, (both labial and lingual approach)

Involvement: Anterior teeth, always involves the proximal surface and sometimes very limited parts of the labial and/or lingual surfaces

1. Indications

a. Decay extent labially and lingually brings the margins to corresponding embrasures.

b. There has been partial or complete loss of labial and/or lingual walls.

c. There are pronounced labial and/or lingual embrasures facilitating two-way access.

d. There is a diastema or spacing between teeth facilitating the two-way access.

e. There is a very limited size lesion in the gingival embrasure proximally, with noticeable sound tooth structure between it and the contact area.

f. In its limited form, any direct tooth-colored restorative material except unfilled resin. In its extended form only composite resin with the exception of second generation composites.

2. General shape (Fig. 13, A and B)

This design is similar to the first two designs with either of two extremes, a limited width (Fig. 13A) or an exaggerated width (Fig. 13B) triangle.

3. Location of margins

The gingival margin will be located in the gingival embrasure. Lingual and labial margins may be in the corresponding embrasure or the proximal surface, depending on the extent of the lesion. The incisal margin will be either in the gingival embrasure, in the contact area, or in the incisal embrasure, depending on the extent and location of the lesion.

4. Internal anatomy

a. In the inciso-gingival cross-section (Fig. 11 and 12C), the internal anatomy will appear very similar to the first two designs. However, if the gingival margin is located on cementum, the gingival wall will be formed of two planes, both in dentin, i.e., an inner plane in the form of a groove, and an outer plane going straight proximally, perpendicular to the axial wall. Residual cementum should be scraped off the tooth surface at that location.

b. In the labio-lingual cross-section, the axial wall will appear to be perfectly flat labio-lingually, although it may have different levels depending on the extent of the decay.

The labial and lingual walls (Fig. 13, C, D, E, F, and G), excluding any bevels, each will be formed fo two planes, if their margins are located on the labial and lingual one-third of the proximal surface. One plane will be at a right angle to the axial wall, and the other diverging proximo-labially or lingually, following the direction of the enamel rods. Other than that, the outer inclination will be just enough to acquire access to the cavity. The major parts of the labial and lingual walls will have a right angulation relationship with the axial wall (Fig. 13 E). If the labial and/or lingual margins are located on cementum or the middle third of the anatomical crown axial surface, the labial and lingual walls will open straight proximally, at a right angle to the axial wall (Fig. 13, C and D).

When this design of cavity preparation is used for extensively wide lesions labio-lingually, each of the labial and/or lingual walls may not have the same height (depth) in all locations inciso-gingivally (Fig. 13). In fact, at some locations, there may not be any labial or lingual wall at all (Fig. 13F). In the extreme, this design may be used when both lingual and labial walls are lost completely. In such situations, in order to create at least partial walls, the gingival and/or incisal walls should be intentionally extended gingivally and/or incisally. This is done to involve some sound tooth structure labially and lingually around the preparation, that can be used to establish short labial and lingual walls, even though they may be interrupted in the middle. In addition, part of the enamel surface, labially and lingually, that is adjacent to the area where walls are absent, should be skirted. On the other hand, if this design is used for a limited size cemento-enamel junction gingival embrasure lesion or a lesion approached through a diastema (Fig. 13A), the labial and lingual walls will be consistent in height inciso-gingivally (Fig. 13, C and D).

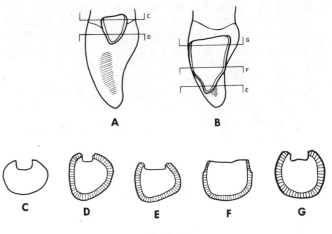

Fig. 9-13

5. Instrumentation for Class III, Design 4

This design, in its different configurations, can be prepared in the same way and with the same instruments as Designs 1 and 2. There will be a distinct advantage, with this design, of the availability of labial and lingual access, facilitated by the location and/or extent of the lesion.

In any one of the four previously described designs of cavity preparation, some walls can be formed partially or completely of enamel only (i.e., unsupported enamel). These walls, or parts of walls, if their presence is justified, will have no specific configuration or angulation with the surrounding or adjacent walls. Most probably, if unsupported enamel is the whole or part of the labial or lingual wall, it will make a definite acute degree of angulation with the axial wall. These enamel walls devoid of dentin should not be smoothed internally (Fig. 14).

In the previous designs, if undermined enamel is to be left, the configuration of the surrounding walls formed by such enamel will be completely different in the following ways:

a. Dentinal portions of these walls should make from an acute to a right angulation with the adjacent axial wall.

b. The enamel portion of these walls, follows the angulation of the dentinal walls (or has a lesser degree of angulation). Such angulation, in any event, should not be less than half of that angulation which the dentinal wall makes with the axial wall.

c. If the whole wall is formed of undermined enamel, it should meet an axial wall formed of enamel, at least at their junction.

d. Although retained undermined enamel will not be mechanically prepared internally, its periphery should accommodate at least a partial bevel away from the cavity preparation.

E. Class III, Design 5 ("saucer-shaped")

1. Indications

a. Conditioned enamel and sometimes treated dentin will be the principal means of retention.

b. The restorative material to be used should possess some physico-chemical adhesive ability to tooth structure or to part of it.

c. Systemic and local conditions contraindicate mortise-shaped cavity preparation.

d. It is used as a caries control measure, preparatory to permanent restorative treatment.

e. It is used in deciduous or young permanent teeth.

f. It is used for rampant lesions with extensive surface decalcification, where there is no definite demarcation between the affected and sound enamel.

2. General shape (Fig. 15)

The outline of this design is saucer-shaped, not perfectly rounded, but oblong in the inciso-gingival and labio-lingual directions (Fig. 15B).

3. Location of margins (Fig. 15)

There is no specific location for the labial or lingual margins, as they will gradually blend with sound enamel on the lingual or labial surfaces. There should, however, be definite margins incisally, mostly in contact areas, and gingivally, where they should be in the gingival embrasure.

4. Internal anatomy (Fig. 15, C and D)

Cross-section analysis shows no definite walls or floors, nor line and point angles. However, there should be an attempt to create definite cavosurface margins preferably in enamel. The preparations will be dishshaped in any cross-section (Fig. 15, C and D) with the deepest part at the center of the lesion proximally. The only detail would be at the enamel part of the preparation, which should terminate in a hollow-ground bevel (Fig. 15D) gingivally and incisally, and in the form of an enamel skirt facially and lingually (Fig. 15C), which could also be scalloped. Both termination arrangements are preparatory to acid conditioning.

5. Instrumentation for Class III, Design 5

The actual tooth structure removal is very limited in this design, as the preparation details are mostly accomplished by the lesion itself. Yet, the first step is to shave off the undesirable attacked dentin, i.e., that which cannot be used for retentive purposes. For this action, use a Wedelstaedt chisel.

The second step is to remove the irreparable carious dentin, as described for the previous designs. Third, prepare the labial and lingual skirts, then the incisal and gingival hollow-ground bevels, as described for the previous designs.

The rest of the procedures consists of preparing enamel walls for surface conditioning and the enamel conditioning itself are as described for the previous designs.

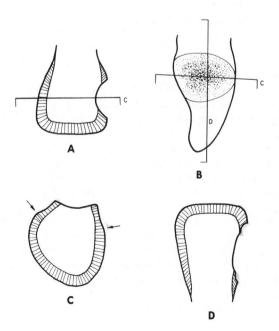

Fig. 9-15

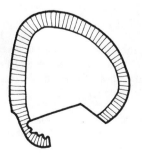

Fig. 9-14

III. Class IV Tooth Preparations

A. Class IV, Design 1 (conventional design)

1. Indications

a. After the removal of diseased tooth structure, bulky labial and lingual walls should connect with a gingival floor.

b. Incisal angle involvement in the preparation is very limited, i.e., almost to the corner only.

c. Teeth have normal occlusal contacts during centric and excursive relation of the mandible.

d. The tooth is fairly thick labio-lingually.

e. This design is used for Class II trauma.

f. Any composite resin is used for this design, excluding second generation composites.

2. General shape (Fig. 16A)

The outline of this design is triangular, with rounded corners, or an exaggerated bilateral inverted truncated cone shape.

3. Location of margins

Because this design of cavity preparation involves almost an incisal approach, the margins can have very minimal labial and lingual extensions. The labial and lingual margins, if the extent of the decay will allow, can be put in the contact areas, or barely within the corresponding embrasures. The gingival margin will be in the same location as those described for Class III Design 1 or 2. The incisal margin will be located on the incisal ridge, just past the location of the incisal angle (Fig. 16B).

4. Internal anatomy (Fig. 16)

In the inciso-gingival cross-section (Fig. 16B), the axial wall will appear flat, slanting toward the incisal ridge, and making a butt enamel joint with the incisal ridge. The gingival wall will appear the same as the gingival walls in Design 3 of Class II for amalgam, i.e., containing a groove. Its anatomy depends on the location of the gingival margin, e.g., if the margin is on enamel, prepare a hollow-ground bevel before conditioning the enamel.

In the labio-lingual cross-section, at the very gingival end of the preparation, excluding any bevels, the labial and lingual walls may have two or three planes, according to the location of the corresponding margins on the proximal surface. Each wall will have its innermost dentinal plane making a pronounced rounded acute angle with the axial wall (part of the dentinal groove) (Fig. 16C).

Viewing the cross-section at the middle third of the preparation, excluding any bevels, the labial and lingual walls will have the same details, but the inner, dentinal, grooved plane makes a less acute angle with the axial wall (Fig. 16C).

Viewed close to the incisal periphery of the preparation (Fig. 16D), each of the labial and lingual walls are seen to be formed of one or two planes, just like the wall anatomy of the non-access side of Class III Designs 1 or 2, and with the same factors dictating the choice between one or two planes. In other words, each of the labial and lingual walls accommodates a groove, which will have its maximum depth at the gingival end of the preparation (bulkiest part of the tooth relative to the preparation). This groove tapers incisally, with the point of termination depending on how close it will be to the labial, lingual, and incisal plates of enamel. This situation differs from one tooth to another. At no location should the groove undermine or involve any of these enamel plates.

Prior to enamel etching, each of the labial, lingual and/or

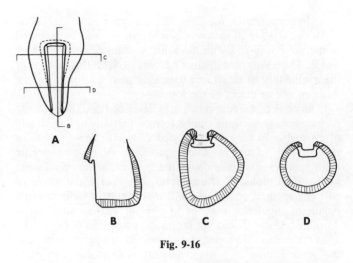

Fig. 9-16

incisal enamel walls should accommodate the indicated bevel as previously described in this chapter. The handling of retained unsupported enamel is similar to that described for Class III preparations.

5. Instrumentation for Class IV, Design 1

a. Gaining access

Of course, access is facilitated by the loss of the incisal angle. This is further improved by wedge separation.

b. Gross removal

With a tapered fissure bur (#699) use apical pressure and proximal dragging, to grossly remove tooth structure within the limits of the predetermined outline.

c. Removal of irreparable attacked dentin

This, too, is accomplished as previously described for other designs.

d. Preliminary shaping

Use a 168 bur to box up the labial, lingual, axial and gingival walls.

e. Groove formation

This is accomplished as in Class II Design 3, i.e., using a ¼ round bur, stopping short of undermining enamel labially, lingually, or incisally.

f. Final shaping

Using a gingival margin trimmer, angle former, and/or Wedelstaedt, formulate surrounding walls, according to the indicated configuration and the anatomical and mechanical needs. It may be necessary to cut a triangle or two at the expense of each of the labial, lingual, and gingival walls. Then, using an angle former, cut the two triangles on the axial wall to round it up. Finally, accentuate retention grooves using gingival margin trimmers as described for Class II Design 3.

g. Cavity finishing

The same instrumentation is used here as in the final shaping stage, except that it may be necessary to go over all preparation angles with a round bur to further round them out. Also, the cavosurface margins should be finished using a gingival margin trimmer and a Wedelstaedt chisel.

B. Class IV, Design 2 (labial and/or lingual approach, conditioned surface enamel skirts and at least one surrounding wall)

1. Indications

a. Incisal angle loss is substantial, i.e., the defect not only involves part of the incisal corner, but also more than one-fourth of the incisal ridge in the mesio-distal direction.

b. The entire labial and/or lingual walls are lost.

c. The labial and/or lingual walls are formed completely of unsupported enamel, or the supporting dentin is too thin to accommodate a groove.

d. The contemplated Class IV restoration will be directly loaded.

e. This design is used for Class II or Class III trauma.

f. The defect to be restored has one or more of the aforementioned features, but still has a proximal involvement larger than its incisal involvement.

g. Not to be used for the distal of cuspids unless a sizable portion of the contact area remains in sound tooth structure.

h. Only composite resins, excluding second generation types, should be used in this design.

2. General shape (Fig. 17)

The outline of this design of preparation will have two parts: a cavity proper which is inverted truncated cone in shape, and surface extensions labially and lingually in the form of skirts over the corresponding axial angles. These skirts may also be scalloped.

3. Location of margins

For the cavity proper margin locations are very similar to those described for Design 1. For the skirted part, however, margins will be located past the corresponding axial angle on the labial and/or lingual surfaces. The extent of the skirt is directly proportional to:

a. The amount of occlusal loading.

b. The extent of wall loss labially and lingually.

c. The absence or shallowness of grooves labially, lingually and gingivally.

d. The need for reciprocation in retaining the restoration.

e. The size of the defect.

f. The inability to properly etch the enamel.

g. The degree of permanency of the restoration.

Very seldom is it necessary to skirt part of the incisal ridge. If this is done, it should be very minimal, as the material bulk and the loading environment at that location can be incompatible.

4. Internal anatomy (Fig. 17)

Because this design is used in many lesions with varying tooth involvement and occlusal loading, the internal anatomy will differ from one case to another. The following description will be just an example for a Class IV Design 2 tooth preparation where the tooth has lost its lingual marginal ridge, and consequently there will be no lingual wall.

a. In the inciso-gingival cross-section (Fig. 17B), the internal anatomy will appear similar to Design 1, except that the incisal involvement is greater. In the labio-lingual cross-section, the axial wall will appear perfectly flat. Usually it will have deeper concavities at different levels.

b. Lingual cavity anatomy (Fig. 17C)

Because the lingual wall is almost absent, the axial wall will be continuous with the enamel surface, reduced to 0.1 mm in depth. This reduction will end in a definite finishing line on the lingual surface, short of the gingival and incisal ridge. The skirt extension to the other proximal surface is governed by the factors mentioned in the discussion of the location of the margins. If there is a bilateral Class IV, it will be continuous with the cavity anatomy on the other proximal surface.

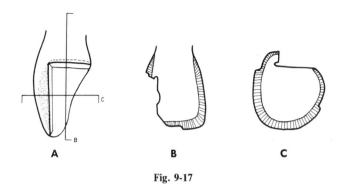

Fig. 9-17

c. Labial wall cavity anatomy (Fig. 17C)

If the labial wall is intact, it will appear exactly as in Design 1. The outer enamelo-dentinal plane (if present) will be continuous with an enamel surface similar to that on the lingual, i.e., reduced to 0.1 mm depth. Because this conditioned enamel area is for reciprocal retention, it will be extended less than the lingual one. If the labial wall is formed solely of enamel, the labial surface reduction should be even less than on the lingual. At its thinned portion, there should be at least 1 mm thickness of enamel to be encased by the restorative material. Bear in mind that the lingual cavity anatomy may replace the labial one if the labial wall is the lost one, and tooth structure remains to create a lingual wall. If both walls are lost, badly shortened, thinned, or formed only of enamel, the lingual anatomical details just described will be used for both labial and lingual sides of the preparation.

If the skirt is to be extended over the incisal ridge for the purpose of retention, enamel reduction there should be deeper than either labially or lingually. The reduced conditioned enamel area incisally should connect with similar areas labially and lingually by means of bulky junctions, and the incisal retention area should be reciprocated with pronounced gingival retention modes.

Very seldom is it necessary to resort to cutting an incisal dentinal groove to accommodate material to help immobilize the restoration at that area. It should be apparent from this discussion that there can be infinite shapes for this design, as it is the most universally used.

7. Instrumentation for Class IV, Design 2

Preparing this design involves the same instrumentation as used for Design 1 preparation. Usually, there will be shortened one-planed wall preparations and labial and lingual skirts. The gingival hollow-ground bevel and sometimes the incisal skirt are prepared in the same way as in Class III, Designs 3 and 4.

C. Class IV, Design 3 (unilateral angle involvement)

1. Indications

a. The defect involves more of the incisal ridge than the proximal surface.

b. This design is used for Class II or Class III trauma.

c. It is used for young teeth with large pulp chambers.

d. Only composite resin, excluding second generation composites should be used for this design.

e. This design is not indicated for the distal of cuspids if contact in tooth structure is lost.

2. General shape (Fig. 18)

The outline of this preparation, proximally, appears either parallelogram or inverted cone shape, while the incisal part has a non-specific outline form.

3. Location of margins

Proximally, all margins, even the gingival, will be in the contact area. Incisally, margins may be anywhere on the incisal ridge, lingual, or labial surfaces, just so far as they involve adequate extent of conditioned enamel according to the rules mentioned in the section on enamel conditioning.

4. Internal anatomy (Fig. 18)

The proximal part (Fig. 18B) of this preparation is a very short extension from the defect, designed merely to improve the restoration's retention and resistance. In the inciso-gingival cross section (Fig. 18D), axial wall appears flat, continuous with the incisal defect. The gingival wall also appears flat and one-planed, ending with a concave enamel bevel. Its margin is always at the incisal or middle third of proximal surface. In the labio-lingual cross-section (Fig. 18E) the axial wall again appears perfectly flat. The labial and lingual walls are seen to be one-planed enamel-dentinal walls perpendicular to the axial wall, and ending proximally with a partial bevel. In the incisal part (Fig. 18C), any cross-section shows the center part to be saucer-shaped with variable dimensions and extent according to the nature of the defect. The peripheral part (Fig. 18, A, C, and E) is seen to be prepared in the form of a reduced enamel surface (to a depth of 0.1-0.2 mm) ending in definite finishing lines. Surface enamel reduction will be greater on incisal ridges and less on lingual surfaces, especially on the lower teeth. Avoid placing enamel reduction margins either in proximal contact areas or subgingivally.

5. Instrumentation for Class IV, Design 3

The procedures and instruments for this design are not too different from Design 2. In this design, the extent of the skirts is less, and the internal walls have no retention grooves.

D. Class IV, Design 4 (bilateral angle involvement)

1. Indications

a. Include all indications for Design 3.

b. The incisal defect is larger than the proximal defect.

c. This design is used for bilateral Class IV lesions.

d. Only composite resin, excluding second generation composites, should be used for this design.

2. General shape

The outline for this design is very non-specific.

3. Location of margins

Margins are located as described for the incisal portion of Design 3, except that in Design 4 there is a greater possibility of bringing the margins of the reduced enamel closer to the gingival and the contact areas. Every effort should be made not to place the margins under the gingiva or into the contact areas, as marginating and finishing restorative material in such bulk at those locations is almost impossible.

4. Internal anatomy (Fig. 19)

In a mesio-distal cross-section (Fig. 19A) an irregular pulpal floor is seen ending mesially and distally in an enamel portion that is hollow-ground for acid conditioning. There appears no skirting, either mesially or distally.

In a labio-lingual cross-section (Fig. 19B), an irregular pulpal floor continuous with variant extents of the reduced enamel

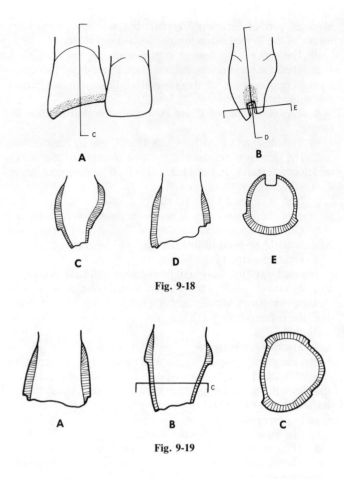

Fig. 9-18

Fig. 9-19

surface area is seen. This reduced enamel is of approximate depth of 0.1-0.2 mm. The peripheries of this area might be scalloped, but they must end in definite finishing lines. The facial and lingual skirts should not have any proximal extensions. Also, they should have vertical (Fig. 19C) as well as horizontal (Fig. 19B) definite terminations on the corresponding surfaces.

5. Instrumentation for Class IV, Design 4

Preparing this design involves procedures and instrumentation similar to those described for the previous designs of Class IV, except no intracoronal preparation will be required.

IV. Class V Tooth Preparations

A. Class V, Design 1 (mortise-shaped preparation)

1. Indications

This is a conventionally indicated design, where it is anatomically and cariogenically possible to create distinctly walled, mortise-shaped preparations.

2. General shape

The outline of this design is very similar to that described for amalgam restoration (five designs). In addition, all or part of the preparation's enamel walls and the adjacent surface enamel may be prepared in one or more of the different ways described earlier in this chapter (Fig. 20). In addition, the line and point angles must be more rounded than for the amalgam preparation.

Figure 20 shows the usual marginal enamel modification for

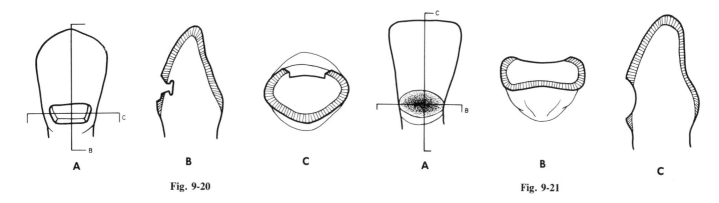

Fig. 9-20   Fig. 9-21

a Class V Design 1 cavity preparation to accommodate a resinous restorative material. Other designs can be modified in the same way.

B. Class V, Design 2 (non-mortise saucer-shaped design)

1. Indications

a. The same indications as for saucer-shaped Class III are included.

b. It is used for erosion and abrasion lesions where the teeth are very sensitive and cavity preparation may increase that sensitivity.

2. General shape (Fig. 21)

The outline of this design is similar to that described for the saucer-shaped Class III.

3. Location of margins

Margin locations are non-specific. However, they should avoid the proximal contact area, as well as the sub-gingival and incisal (occlusal) surfaces (ridges).

4. Internal anatomy (Fig. 21)

This design has no definite wall. It is dish-shaped in any cross-section (Fig. 21, B and C). Its center is in dentin and all peripheries are made of enamel, except the gingival peripheries which may sometimes be on dentin.

BIBLIOGRAPHY

Abe, J.L.: Chemical changes in human enamel demineralization by etching agent. Nippon Kyosei Shika Gakkai Zasshi, 1977; 36(4):286-301.

Alexieva, C.: Character of the hard tooth tissue-polymer bond. II. Study of the interaction of human tooth enamel and dentin with N-phenyl-glycine-glycidyl methacrylate adduct. J. Dent. Res. 1979 Sept. 58(9):1884-1886.

Asmussen, E.: Penetration of restorative resins into acid etched enamel. I. Viscosity, surface tension and contact angle of restorative resin monomers. Acta Odontol Scand. 1977; 35(4):175-182.

Asmussen, E., Dreyer, and Jorgensen, K.: The stability of water in the pores of acid etched human enamel. Acta Odontol. Scand. 1978; 36(1):43-44.

Beech, D.R., and Jalaly, T.: Bonding of polymers to enamel: influence of deposits formed during etching, etching time and period of water immersion. J. Dent. Res. 1980 July 59(7):1156-162.

Bowen, R.L.: Investigations of the surface of hard tooth tissues by a surface activity test. In adhesive restorative dental materials, Phillipa, R.W., and Ryge, G. (ed.). Spencer, Ind., Owen Litho Service, 1961, p. 177.

Bounocore, M.: Adhesive retention and adhesive restorative materials. JADA, vol. 67, Sept. 1963, 382.

Bounocore, M.G.: Simple method of increasing the adhesion of acrylic filling materials to enamel surface. J.D. Res. 34:849 Dec. 1955.

Dennison, J.B., and Craig, R.G.: Characterization of enamel surfaces prepared with commercial and experimental etchants. J. Am. Dent. Assoc. 1978 Nov. 97(5):799-805.

Dogan, L.: Acid etching. 3 M Co. 1977.

Gilmore, H.W.: Textbook of operative dentistry. St. Louis, C.V. Mosby Co., 1967, p. 380.

Glantz, P.O.: Adhesion to teeth. Int. Dent. J. 1977 Dec. 27(4):324-332.

Grajower, R., Glick, A., Gedalia, I., and Kochavi, D.: Tensile strength of the bond between resin to enamel etched with phosphoric acid containing fluoride. J. Oral Rehabil. 1979 July 6(3):267-272.

Hembree, J.H. Jr.: Microleakage of composite resin restorations with different cavosurface designs. J. Prosthet. Dent. 1980 Aug. 44(2):171-174.

Leidal, T.I., and Eriksen, H.M.: Microleakage along composite restorations in human premolars after treatment with different cleansing agents. Scand. J. Dent. Res. 1979 Dec. 87(6):470-474.

McCabe, J.F., and Storer, R.: Adaptation of resin restorative materials to etched enamel and the interfacial work of fracture. Br. Dent. J. 1980 Mar. 18; 148(6):155-159.

Nation, W., Jedrychowski, J.R., and Caputo, A.A.: Effects of surface treatments on the retention of restorative materials to dentin. J. Prosthet. Dent. 1980 Dec. 44(6):638-641.

Nordenvall, K.J., Brannstrom, M., and Malmgren, O.: Etching of deciduous teeth and young and old permanent teeth. A comparison between 15 and 60 sec. of etching. Am. J. Orthod. 1980 Jul. 78(1):99-108.

O'Keefe, T.J., and Christie, R.D.: Electroless and chemical metal deposition on human tooth enamel. J. Dent. Res. 1977 Jun. 56(6):595-602.

Prevost, A.P., and Fuller, J.L.: Consequences of the acid etchant drying on the enamel surface. J. Dent. Que. 1981 Feb. 18:33-36.

Restorative dental materials. Graig et al. St. Louis, C.V. Mosby Co., 1981.

Schneider, P.M., Messer, L.B., and Douglas, W.H.: The effect of enamel surface reduction in vitro on the bonding of composite resin to permanent human enamel. J. Dent. Res. 1981 May; 60(5):895-900.

Smith, D.C.: A milestone in dentistry. Journal of Operative Dentistry, 1982 Winter.; 7(1):14-25.

Sturdevant, C.M., Barton, R.E., and Brauer, J.C.: The art and science of operative dentistry. New York, McGraw Hill Book Co., 1968, p. 457.

Zidan, O., Asmussen, E., and Jorgensen, K.D.: Correlation between tensile and bond strength of composite resins. Scand. J. Dent. Res. 1980 Aug. 88(4):348-351.

CHAPTER 10

Principles for fabricating direct tooth-colored restorations

After completing mechanical and/or chemical preparation of an affected tooth, which, in many cases, may include conditioning its enamel and its dentin, the tooth will be ready to receive the tooth-colored material. Hopefully, this material will restore the functional, esthetic, phonetic, and stabilizing capacities of the tooth. The restorative process usually is performed in the following 10-step sequence:

    I. Choice of direct filling material
   II. Shade determination
  III. Matricing
  IV. Dispensing of restorative material
   V. Priming tooth structure surfaces involved in the restoration
  VI. Formation of appropriate mix or mixes
 VII. Insertion and curing
VIII. Margination and contouring
  IX. Finishing and polishing
   X. Glazing

I. Choice of Material

Actually, the choice of direct filling material should be made before starting the preparation of the tooth, as the material can dictate the design of tooth and cavity preparation. With an understanding of the information presented in the two previous chapters, the clinician should now be able to diagnose the restorative needs of the tooth, the mouth, the stomato-gnathic system, and patient as a whole (mentioned in sequence of their importance).

An evaluation should be made of each of the five direct tooth-colored materials, to determine what quality(ies) each can offer that will satisfy these needs and the appropriate selection can be made.

It should be emphasized that every material has an indicated use in restorative dentistry; therefore, the following points should be kept in mind during this search for the appropriate material:

A. Unfilled resins should be used as provisional, or temporary, restorations, e.g., between visits for a cast restoration or as a diagnostic, preparatory restoration preceding a more permanent type of procedure. Also, it can be utilized as a primer or glaze for composite or filled resin restorations due to its high wetting ability.

B. Silicate cement is only used as a therapeutic restorative material in cases of rampant decay and uncontrolled lesions.

ASPA is becoming even more popular for these therapeutic restorations due to its high fluoride content.

C. Before deciding which brand of a material to choose, it might be helpful to try several, provided they are accredited by the ADA and/or the FDA.

D. It would behoove the operator to use only those materials which have been proven clinically acceptable after reliable, convincing research data. As the field of direct tooth-colored materials is an ever-changing one, new and modified materials are introduced to clinicians every day, some without sufficient clinical evaluation.

E. The choice of the different composite resins should be dictated by the following factors:

1. First generation composites have the longest history of clinical use, even though it has been substantially modified over the years. Nevertheless, it should not be used in locations of heavy loading, especially from lateral (abrading) movements, or in highly conspicuous areas due to its susceptibility to staining. Furthermore, because of its adhesiveness to plaque, it should be kept away from the periodontium.

2. Second generation composites are indicated for conspicuous areas, where esthetics is of major concern. However, its lesser strength precludes its use in stress concentration areas. These composites could be used to veneer over generations 3, 4, and 5 (sometimes generation one) in order to realize the advantages of each type of material.

3. Generations 3, 4, and 5 should be the most universally used composites for most uncomplicated situations.

4. Generation six composites are indicated specifically for highly loaded areas, and in situations wherein the contact area is to be completely restored by composite. This is due, of course, to its condensability.

5. Light-cured resins should be the material of choice, except for those areas where light cannot be delivered in curing amounts to the inserted composite, or in situations necessitating that a large bulk of composite be inserted and cured non-incrementally (e.g., post build-ups). The light-cured resins will generally have more complete polymerization than auto-curing resins.

The clinician should be well informed about the material's component, makeup, and to which class it belongs. Bear in mind that the clinician who builds the restoration establishes, to a great extent, its clinical behavior by his understanding of the material's weaknesses and strengths. Accordingly, he should master manipulation of materials as well as tooth preparations, in order to mask the weaknesses and fully realize the strengths.

II. Shade Determination and Formulation

Every direct tooth-colored material is supplied with a shade guide in the form of sample teeth, each with a different shade and identification number or letter. The identification corresponds to the items in the containers for the material (powder or paste). Shade varieties differ among manufacturers. They may range from three shades for one material, to 33 shades for another, and there is no standardized numbering for shades.

The procedures to determine the proper shade are as follows:

A. Tooth shade should preferably be determined before applying the rubber dam, i.e., before preparing the tooth, while the saliva is covering the tooth. If this is not feasible, the tooth whose shade is being taken should be wetted with water, or preferably, the patient's saliva prior to determining its shade.

B. The shade guide should match a well scaled and polished intact tooth surface, adjacent to the contemplated restoration, as well as the adjacent tooth and opposing teeth.

C. Shade selection should be made twice, while the patient is in an upright position, under two illuminating lights, one of which is preferably a full spectrum light. The closest shade that matches under each of the two light sources should be the one selected.

D. For areas of the tooth not receiving direct lighting, a lighter shade (lower value) than that of the adjacent directly lighted area should be chosen, e.g., proximal areas should have lighter shade value than the labial areas, especially incisally.

E. After looking at the tooth, pick out at least two shades closely matching that of the tooth. Soak them in water, and hold them, one at a time, next to the tooth to be restored. Then start comparisons in the sequence mentioned previously, until it is possible to select the closest match.

F. Always consider the stainability of each material with age. In other words, the more stainable the material is, the lighter the chosen shade value should be, compared to an exact match.

G. Some large restorations may need two or more shades for their different parts. In this case, mix or choose different mixes, each for a specific location.

H. When choosing a shade, always look from different position and angles. Involve the assistant and even the patient in making the correct decision.

I. Some transparent materials may need an opacifier on discolored but healthy tooth structures, metal pins, or metallic backings (substructures) before being covered with these materials. These opacifiers are supplied with certain materials and should be chemically combined with the restorative material.

J. During shade selection, it is best not to observe the shade guide or tooth for more than five second intervals. The eyes may be rested between these intervals by looking at a light blue hue background.

K. The procedure for choosing a shade is a very empirical, trial and error process. The paste(s) or powder is supplied in a preset hue, value and chroma. Although the hue can be easily matched, the tooth value and chroma are extremely difficult to simulate with such a system. In spite of the procedure's primitiveness and inadequacies, it does usually produce surprisingly acceptable results.

L. If it is impossible to find a close shade match, it is necessary to formulate a shade for this restoration in one of two ways:

1. Add powder or paste of the two closest shades and use them as a shade guide. One can even make a trial mix to facilitate the proper match. The added parts might be unequal, according to the emphasis or deemphasis needed from each shade, in formulating the restoration's overall shade.

2. Use the tinting kit supplied with some material. (It should be used for the material for which it is manufactured.) The tinting pastes or powders contain more coloring agents than those identified by the shade guide for the material, i.e., they have deeper chroma. Usually they come in four colors—brown, yellow, white, and gray. The paste or powder with the closest shade to the desired one is chosen. (Sometimes a universal one is supplied and the operator will tint it according to his or her desire.) The appropriate tint is added and mixed thoroughly to the universal part. The resulting mix is carried close to the tooth, and the shade is checked. Other tinting components may be added, until the paste or powder with the exact shade is formulated.

III. Matricing

The principles and procedures for matricing will be presented in detail in the chapter on contact and contour. Needless to say, a properly contoured, adapted, and confining matrix is the most important factor in creating a biologically and esthetically acceptable restoration surface. For Class I and II restorations, in order to build occlusal, facial, or lingual surfaces out of composite resin, it is essential to fabricate a clear, non-adhering, plastic matrix which will form those surfaces. A study model may be taken before restoration to ensure that any defect in the tooth is corrected to the most appropriate anatomy. A clear plastic sheet is then molded to this corrected configuration by thermoplastically softening it and subjecting it to vacuum molding. The created template should then be perforated in several locations (cusp tips) and used as a matrix to hold and form the inserted composite while it polymerizes. Such a matrix will shape occlusal, facial, and lingual surfaces. So, for composites in premolars and molars involving proximal extensions, the regular matrix technique for proximal surfaces (described in Chapter 6), as well as this thermoplastically formed matrix, is used. Because of the polymerization shrinkage of composite resins, double (heavy) wedging should be used with these matrices.

IV. Dispensing

As mentioned before, there are numerous ways these resin materials are supplied; therefore, the dispensing procedure will vary. The main objective of dispensing is to supply the exact amount of the material component(s) to be incorporated to produce not only an adequately workable mix but also the expected physical characteristics of the set materials. Of all the components of the direct tooth-colored materials, the liquid of silicate cement and ASPA are the most sensitive because of their water contents. Dispensing this liquid should be done without exposing the rest of the unused liquid to the surrounding atmosphere, which may increase or decrease its water content. Also, the dispensed liquid should be exposed to the surrounding environment for a minimal time. This can be done by using squeeze bottles or calibrated hypodermic syringes to aspirate and dispense the liquid from rubber stopped sealed bottles. Sometimes the liquid is supplied in a large calibrated syringe which injects the desired amount when needed. The amount of liquid is better measured with such a calibrated syringe than with a squeeze bottle.

Before the dispensing step in a two-paste system of filled and composite resins, it is advisable to stir the contents of the jar. When they have not been used for a long time, the fillings and reinforcing particles tend to settle to the bottom of the containers.

The most appropriate way of dispensing chemically setting materials is by preweighed capsules, each containing the different components of the material system, separated from each other by a thin, breakable diaphragm. The capsule can be activated before mixing by rupturing these diaphragms.

Chemically curing cavity primers could be activated before insertion. They should not be dispensed before the tooth is made ready to receive them, as they have a very short maturation time. When dispensing different components of one material system, do not use the same tool tip in more than one component, as this may lead to premature setting or contamination of the unused materials.

Although the liquids of silicate and ASPA are the most sensitive, all these material components can be affected by the surrounding atmosphere, especially in urban areas. As soon as the material components are dispensed, seal their containers immediately. Also, use clean instruments for dispensing and discard any unused material component that has been dispensed out of its container. Most importantly, follow manufacturers' instructions.

V. Priming Tooth Structure Surface Involved in the Restoration

With today's understanding, priming can mean the application of coupling agents on unconditioned or acid-conditioned tooth structure. These di-functional agents will adhere to parts of the tooth substance in a physico-chemical way, and they will bind to the applied resinous material in a chemico-physical way, thus assuring the cavity seal. Most of the present coupling agents are silane or silane derivatives. Priming may also mean painting the monomer of a composite resin polymeric matrix on an acid conditioned enamel surface. This monomer has a lower viscosity and, consequently, a high wettability. It can wet more details of the conditioned enamel surface than its companion composite resin. The monomer can be polymerized in one of three ways. The first is to add to it its initiator and/ or accelerator just before painting. The second is to apply it, then photocure it, in which case it should contain an appropriate photon energy absorber and initiator (Fig. 3). The third way is to apply it and then insert the composite resin mix. Some of the mix initiators and accelerators will diffuse to polymerize the monomer in the conditioned enamel or dentin.

VII. Formulation of the Appropriate Mix or Mixes

Because there are four ways or procedures to insert direct tooth-colored material and its components into a prepared tooth, each will necessitate a specific consistency, ranging from complete fluidity to "buttery" pastes. To formulate such consistencies, utilize the following techniques and principles:

A. Most of the powder and paste parts of these materials contain very abrasive particles that can abrade metallic instruments, incorporating metal filings in the mix, thereby discoloring it. Therefore, to mix these materials, always use wood, non-reacting plastic, or ivorine instruments.

B. For silicate and ASPA cements, a cool glass slab should be used in order to incorporate as much powder in the liquid as practically possible. But, be sure the slab is not cooled to the dew point, as this can accumulate atmospheric water that may change the properties of the material if incorporated into the mix.

C. For chemically cured composite resin, mixing on non-absorbent paper pads is most practical if using a two-paste system.

D. To chemically activate a liquid to be painted on the tooth as a primer, by adding the catalyst and initiator to it, use a microdish, preferably a disposable plastic one, as these materials could adhere to glass dishes causing great difficulty in cleaning the dish for further use.

E. Formulating bead mixes is best done using three dappen dishes, as will be described in the brush-bead technique.

F. For non-trituration mixing of silicate and ASPA cement, spatula movements should be in "padding-folding" acts, using the minimum surface area of the glass slab. This is done to minimally expose the material to the atmosphere. Addition of the powder and mixing should be continued until arriving to a creamy mix that will stick to the spatula but not be stringy when moving the spatula away from the slab.

G. For the non-trituration mixing procedure of two-paste composite resin, rapid incorporation of the two pastes into each other in folding actions will be sufficient until arriving to a homogeneously colored mix.

H. For the non-trituration mixing of powder-liquid system resinous material, it is advisable to dispense the recommended amount of liquid into a dappen dish, then add the recommended amount of powder slowly, in a circular action. Then, leave it to set until the late part of its sandy stage. It may be inserted into the cavity while in its rubbery stage.

I. Any of the previously formulated mixes in (F), (G), or (H) or paste of light-cured resin can and should be loaded into a syringe with the appropriate attachment for injection into the tooth (Fig. 2).

J. The most efficient way of mixing is to have the material in preweighed injectable capsules. Capsules for chemically cured materials can be activated by rupturing the internal diaphragm, separating the reacting components. It should then be triturated in an amalgam triturator for 5-15 seconds, according to the manufacturer's suggestion. Capsules for light cured resin do not need activation or trituration. These capsules can then be accommodated into a special gun to inject the mix directly into the preparation without manipulating it outside of the tooth preparation with any instruments (Fig. 1).

Some capsules are not directly injectable. Therefore, after trituration mixing, the mix is taken from the capsule with a plastic instrument to the cavity, or it may be loaded into a syringe for injection into the cavity preparation.

Preweighed capsules can be used with silicate cement, ASPA, and composite resins, but not with unfilled resins. The

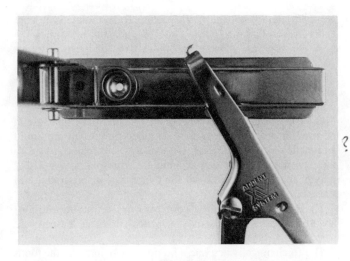

Fig. 10-1

latter do not have a sufficient weight to effect their trituration mixing. The capsule should be refrigerated before use to partially neutralize the heat of trituration energy which may accelerate the setting and make the mix unworkable. For a light-cured resin, this step is not always used, except to formulate a mix out of powder and liquid components, or to thin viscous pastes with the addition of resin monomer, or to mix two pastes in an effort to arrive at a more suitable shade.

VII. Insertion and Curing

There are four ways to insert direct tooth-colored materials or their components onto or into a tooth preparation. For a single restoration, in many cases, more than one way is used to incrementally build up the restoration.

A. Painting technique

This is used mainly for the priming parts of the restoration build-up. Whatever the primer is, unactivated or activated in the microdish, the tip of a sable-hair brush is dipped into it and carried to the designated parts of the tooth preparation. With light painting actions, apply the liquid, avoiding the pooling of any excess. If the brush is soaked with the liquid, it should be partially blotted, with a dry piece of gauze.

Try to make one application only. Excessive amounts of the primer will not completely polymerize, if it is to be chemico-chemically activated in the tooth by initiators or catalysts within the main bulk of the restoration. This will lead to a weak link between the tooth and the bulk of the restoration. A weak link can still occur, if the painted resin is excessive and completely polymerized, as it is not reinforced. Also, the excessive primer may weaken the main bulk of the restoration by diluting its dispersion phase.

B. Brush bead technique

This is mainly used with unfilled resins and should never be used with silicate and ASPA cements. Three dappen dishes, two containing the liquid and one containing the powder, are utilized. A sable or camel-hair brush is dipped in the first dish containing a liquid. Then it is carried to the cavity to wet its surfaces. The brush is dried, and only its tip is immersed in the liquid dish. Then, with the monomer soaked tip, a bead of powder is taken and carried to the wetted cavity. The bead will

flow into the preparation details. The brush is then washed in the second liquid dish and dried. The brush tip is again dipped in the first liquid dish, a bead is taken from the powder dish to the preparation, and so on, until the restoration is built up. Light should be applied to cure each bead, if using a photo-curing resin. In this way any setting shrinkage will be directed toward the walls and can be compensated for by the subsequent bead. Also, the low viscosity of the bead mix will assure wetting all the details of the cavity and previously introduced materials. This method can be used in the powder-liquid system or the paste-liquid system, of composite and filled resins, preferably, if the resin is to be cured with light (Fig. 3).

C. Bulk pack technique

The preferred way to utilize this technique is to load the material into a syringe (Fig. 2) and inject it immediately into the cavity preparation. The internal details are obliterated first, withdraw the syringe as the cavity is filled, keeping the syringe tip always buried in the material to prevent voids. A less preferred method is to carry the material to the cavity preparation in two parts, using suitably sized plastic instruments. The first, small part will fill the internal details of the preparation, and the other part will fill the rest of the cavity preparation. In either method, after filling the cavity, the matrix is applied under pressure and held for the prescribed time. The bulk pack technique is the most universally used technique for small-sized composite resin restorations that do not require multi-shade characterization. It is the only technique to be used in silicate and ASPA cements. The applied pressure can be used, to some extent, to compensate for the setting shrinkage of the material, for wetting and filling all the details of the preparation, to reduce voids, and to bring enough matrix material to the surface to make the restoration smoothly surfaced.

D. Laminated technique

This is a combination of the principles of the brush-bead and the bulk-pack techniques. In this technique, several mixes are used: a first mix with low viscosity to wet minute details, a second mix with medium viscosity to fill up larger details and partially obliterate the cavity preparation, and a third mix with higher viscosity to complete filling of the cavity and to be pressed upon with the matrix. The first one or two mixes can be applied by brush bead, the last mix or two may be injected or carried with a plastic instrument. More than three consistency mixes could be necessary for very large restorations (e.g., foundations). Also, the different mixes can be of the same consistency, but introduced and cured separately to minimize voids and compensate for setting shrinkages. Also, this technique can be used for several mixes with the same consistency but with different value and chroma to simulate dentin (body) and enamel (veneering) layers or to cover an underlying opacifier mix. Furthermore, this technique can be used to obliterate one segment of a tooth preparation in a specific shade, followed by other parts filled to the surface, in differing shades. In this way, the laminated technique is ideal for medium to large sized cavities with torturous details, and for restorations with multiple shades. Light-cured resins inserted with this technique should be cured layer by layer. Silicate cements and ASPA should never be inserted by the laminating technique.

Sixth generation composite restorations can be inserted in-

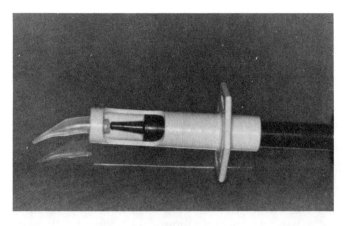

Fig. 10-2

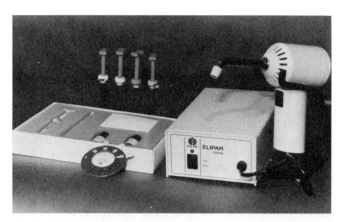

Fig. 10-3

crementally, with each portion condensed before inserting another. Condensing instruments are very similar to amalgam condensers in both shape and dimension, but their nibs are made of a rubbery, non-adhering material.

The number and intensity of photons to be delivered to resinous materials for curing will vary according to:

1. The thickness of the increment—the greater the thickness, the more the needed photons and the greater the speed in which they are delivered.

2. The shade of the resinous material—the darker the material (high value or chroma) the more photons necessary and the faster their required delivery pace.

3. The type and thickness of tooth structure through which photons must pass—enamel is more penetrable by photons than dentin, and the thicker either of them are, the less the penetrability.

4. The reflectiveness of the resin surface—fluidy resin will not allow complete absorption of photons.

5. The number of photons supplied—this is a product of the intensity of the producing source and time. Both factors may be under the control of the operator.

Although the use of photo-curing resins permits an extended working time, it should be pointed out that these materials are setting (albeit slowly), as long as it is exposed to any source of light energy.

VIII. Margination and Contouring

These procedures can be accomplished in many different ways, but the following scheme is well tested and easy to use with excellent results.

After the prescribed time for their initial setting, the matrix is removed, and flashes on tooth surfaces peripheral to preparation margins are shaved off using a sharp scalpel or knife. The movements for flash removal should always be from the tooth surface to the restoration surface, or placing the instrument edge partly on the material, partly on the tooth surface and moving parallel to the preparation margin. Either of these ways is essential to avoid "shelving" or "ditching" the restoration margins. Most flashes will be removed by these acts.

Gross overhang removal, contouring, finishing and polishing can be done immediately in the case of composite, filled and unfilled resins, but only after 48 hours for silicate and ASPA. ASPA and silicate cements should, therefore, be covered with a non-soluble grease or varnish for 48 hours after insertion, in

order to complete their setting undisturbed. To remove gross overhangs a flame-shaped 12-fluted carbide bur with copious water coolant is very efficient in thinning the excess material so it may then be easily shaved off with a sharp scalpel.

For proper contouring of the restoration, there is nothing that can replace an adequate matrix. Ideally, the restoration surface should be created by the matrix, so that no further instrumentation is needed. Most of the time, however, this is not practically feasible, and overcontoured restorations result. In these cases, 12-fluted carbide burs and diamond stones with abrasive particles averaging between 15-40 microns, in different shapes (preferably, flame taper and pear shape) are used with moderate speed and a lot of cooling water. Contouring should be done in intermittent strokes and with the least possible pressure in the least time possible.

Final margination should be done using a 40-fluted, flame finishing carbide burs, with the maximum amount of cooling water possible. These types of burs do not actually cut, but rather abrade in a very superficial manner, causing a lot of friction and heat.

A word of caution here—there is no place for coarse diamond stones in marginating or contouring of any tooth-colored materials. There are good possibilities of injuring surrounding enamel or dentin, overheating, or roughening the restoration surface beyond any possible finishing and polishing procedure's abilities.

If during or prior to this procedure a discrepancy is discovered in the restoration, due to a void, underfilling, or overinstrumentation, it can be corrected in one of three ways:

A. Prepare a locking preparation within the restoration, or partly in the restoration and partly in the tooth, and restore the area locally.

B. Etch the material with proper etchant (hydrofluoric acid), copiously wash it, and then restore the defective area.

C. If the restoration is resinous and the defect is close to the enamel, etch that enamel and clean the restoration surface prior to adding more material for contour adjustment.

IX. Finishing and Polishing

There is no ideal way for finishing and polishing of tooth-colored materials. It should be emphasized again that the best surface possible for any of these materials is that produced by the matrix. Any instrumentation of the material surface that had set in contact with the matrix surface will roughen it even more. But after instrumentally contouring the surface it definitely needs some finishing and polishing, even though the resulting surface is not as smooth as that produced by the matrix. There are numerous ways for finishing and polishing. The most affected material by this process is the unfilled resin, and the least affected is the composite resin. Polishing can be summarized in the following sequential steps:

A. For delineated, concave, and non-accessible areas use finishing burs, mainly 40-fluted carbide burs or extremely fine diamond stones with a maximum particle diameter of 15 microns (no stainless steel as it will be abraded by the silica containing materials) or alumina stones. Do not try to remove too much from the surface. Use a lot of water and do not touch the margins with these instruments. Do not exert a lot of pressure when the tool does not appear to be cutting. This could loosen or dislodge the filler particles from the surface, causing it to become even rougher.

B. For accessible, convex, and conspicuous areas use descending grades of abrasive paper, preferably Al_2O_3, cuttle, and/or silicone dioxide soft discs and strips according to the available access. Discs should be used in slow speed, and strips in "shoe-polishing" hand actions. Vaseline or petrolatum should be used as a lubricant during these actions, especially with silicate and ASPA.

C. Abrasive polishing pastes with glycerin or water as a carrier can be rubbed against the restoration using wheel or cone-shaped brushes, rubber cups, linen strips, or dental tapes. Their effect varies according to the type, particle size, particle shape, hardness and abrasive resistance of the abrasive particles. These pastes can contain pumice, tin oxide, alumina, silicone carbide, zirconium silicate, etc. Many believe that silicone carbide can produce the smoothest of all the surfaces in composite resins. Some believe that a paste (or a stone) formed of the reinforcing particles of the composite resins or Al_2O_3 particles are the best polishing agent for that specific resin. There are some composite resins that have their polishing pastes (stones) made of their own reinforcing ingredient particles. For silicate cement, ASPA and unfilled resin, pumice is usually relatively efficient for polishing. Because of the tooth-abrading properties of these materials, there is a good chance of injuring adjacent enamel and dentin surface by these finishing acts. Therefore it is advisable to apply some non-staining fluoride solutions on adjacent tooth surfaces after the restoration is finished and polished.

X. Glazing

It is a well established fact that the smooth surface created next to the matrix-band surface of most of the direct tooth-colored materials is due to a surface layer of the continuous phase of the resin material devoid of any filling, reinforcing or original powder particles of the material. So if a material can allow the adhesion of a thin layer of its own continuous phase (dispersion phase) after it is contoured, finished, and polished, it will be possible to simulate the matrix set smoothness of the surface. This idea has been applied to composite resin, but with only limited success. After finishing and polishing, the composite resin surface is cleaned, dried, and then painted with an activated continuous phase monomer or unactivated monomer, to be photo-cured. The produced surface is initially very smooth, but only for a short period. Eventually it is abraded away during function, a process that may take a day to three months, depending on such factors as occlusal contact, habits, type of ingested food, nature of plaque control measures used, etc. It can be obvious from the structure and the prescribed way of applying this glaze material that it lacks abrasive resistance and complete adhesion to the restoration. Besides, it is located in the most exposed area for the surrounding environment. In order to improve the adhesion of these glazes to resinous restorations, careful etching of the restoration surface, using low concentrations of hydrofluoric acid, should be used prior to glazing. In any event, applying a fluid form of the continuous phase of the composite, preceded by thorough drying of the restoration and its interface with the tooth structure, will allow the microleakage space at the interfaces, created by the setting shrinkage of the composite resin, to be at least partially filled and obliterated. Glazing cannot be used in silicate cements and ASPA, and it is not necessary in unfilled resin. For composite resin glazing is, as mentioned, only considered a transient smoothing of the surface, and for successful results it should be periodically reapplied.

BIBLIOGRAPHY

Fontana, U.F., Dinelli, W., and Gabrielli, F.: Comparative study of translucence of composite resins and silicate cement. Effects of immersion medium and time. Rev. Assoc. Paul Cir Dent. Mar.-Apr. **33**(2):162-168, 1979.

Garberoglio, R., and Cozzani, G.: In vivo effect of oral environment on etched enamel: a scanning electron microscopic study. J. Dent. Res., 1979, Sept. **58**(9):1859-1865.

Hayashibara, H., Goto, Y., Shintani, H., and Indue, T.: Clinical use of a new, visible-light-cured composite resin. Shikai Tenbo, 1980 Aug. 15; **56**(2): 222-226.

Hormati, A.A., Fuller, J.L., and Denehy, G.E. Effects of contamination and mechanical disturbance on the quality of acid-etched enamel. J. Am. Dent. Assoc., 1980 Jan. **100**(1):34-38.

Itoh, K., Iwaku, M., and Fusayama, T.: Effectiveness of glazing composite resin restorations, J. Prosthet. Dent. 1981 Jun. **45**(6):606-613.

Jedrychowski, J.R., Caputo, A.A., and Foliart, R.: Effects of adhesion promoters on resin-enamel retention. J. Dent. Res., 1979 Apr. **58**(4): 1371-1376.

Miyagawa, Y., Powers, J.M., and O'Brien, W.J.: Optical properties of direct restorative materials. J. Dent. Res. 1981 May **60**(5):890-894.

Powers, J.M., Dennison, J.B., and Lepeak, P.J.: Parameters that affect the color of direct restorative resins. J. Dent. Res. 1978 Sept.-Oct. **57** (9-10):876-880.

Ortiz, R.F., Phillips, R.W., Swartz, M.L., Osborne, J.M.: Effect of composite resin bond agent on microleakage and bond strength. J. Prosthet. Dent. 1979 Jan. **41**(1):51-57.

Sproull, R.C.: Color matching in dentistry. Part I. The three-dimensional nature of color. J. Pros. Dent. **29**:416, 1973.

Sproull, R.C.: Color matching in dentistry. Part II. Practical applications of the organization of color. J. Prosthet. Dent. **29**:560, 1973.

Sproull, R.C.: Color matching in dentistry. Part III. Color control. J. Prosthet. Dent. **31**:146, 1974.

CHAPTER 11

Pin- and post-retained non-cast restorations and foundations

Pins and posts are used as retentive means for restorations. It is a misconception that they serve to reinforce or improve either the mechanical or the physical properties of restorative materials. On the contrary, they may reduce these properties.

Pin-Retained Amalgam and Direct Tooth-Colored Restoration

I. Indications

Auxillary retentive means, in the form of pins are often required for restoration of mutilated and badly broken down teeth, especially in young patient's teeth, in which the pulp chamber is relatively large, the dentinal tubules are comparatively immature, and the gingival lines are still high. These same features contraindicate the massive tooth preparations necessitated by cast restorations. Frequently, it is necessary to place a transitional restoration in badly broken down teeth prior to endodontic or orthodontic treatment. Here, pin-retained restorations act as build-ups for rubber dam application or band attachment.

Also, pin retention may be required in foundations for partial or full veneer cast restoration or metalo-ceramic restorations. This procedure will save a considerable amount of tooth structure by eliminating the need to remove undercuts for the cast fabrication.

In teeth with questionable prognosis endodontically or periodontically, pin-retained restorations may be used as an economic provisional restoration until definitive prognosis is established after a specific waiting period.

Pins are also indicated for use as a cross-linkage mode between two bulky, sound parts of the remaining tooth structure which are discontinued by abnormal tooth involvement or cracks. These pins and their restorations reinforce the tooth only by the act of joining the two discontinued portions together.

As an auxillary or reciprocal retention mode for preparation containing principal retention modes which are insufficient to prevent restoration displacement in a given direction, and as an adjunct retentive mode with a post in endodontically treated teeth to prevent rotation of the restoration around the post in the root canal, placing pins are the indicated procedure. Finally, pin retained build-ups in amalgam or composite may serve as an economical restoration. This is the least desirable indication, especially when the time involved in the procedure is considered.

II. Types of Retaining Pins for Amalgam and Direct Tooth-Colored Materials

A. Cemented pins (Fig. 1A)

For this type, the pin channel is larger in diameter than the pin. These come in two sizes:

Pin channel diameter	Pin diameter
0.027″	0.025″
0.021″	0.020″

B. Frictional grip, or friction lock, pins (Fig. 1B)

In this type, the pin channel is slightly narrower in diameter than the pin. These come in one size only:

Pin channel diameter	Pin diameter
0.021″	.022″

C. Threaded pins

In this type, the pin channel diameter is narrower than that of the pin. These come in four sizes (Fig. 1C):

Pin channel diameter	Pin diameter
0.027″	0.031″
0.021″	0.023″
0.018″	0.020″
0.013″	0.015″

III. Mechanical Aspects of Pin-Retained Restorations

Pins and Tooth Structures

A. Stressing capabilities of pins:

Stresses are always induced in dentin substance as a result of pin insertion. If these stresses exceed the elastic limit of the dentin, permanent (plastic) deformation will occur. These stresses might concentrate to a point exceeding the dentin's plastic limit, resulting in microscopic and/or macroscopic dentinal cracks, i.e., interrupted and/or continuous fractures of the dentin substance. Either can lead to pulpal, suface, and/or periodontal involvement with their sequelae (cracked tooth syn-

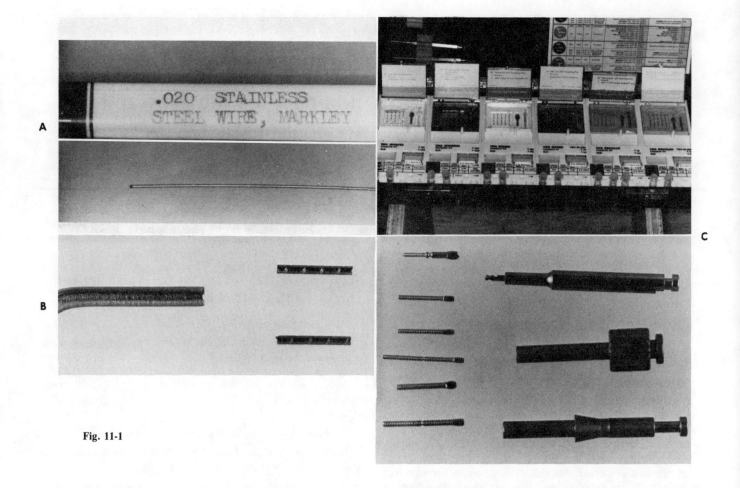

Fig. 11-1

drome, gross fracture of the tooth or part of the tooth, loose restorations, etc.) The same results occur if these stresses are applied in such a way to immediately arrive at the breaking point of the dentin substance. There are many factors in pin techniques and materials that can increase or decrease these stresses:

1. Type of pins (Fig. 2)

The smaller that the diameter of the pin is relative to that of the pin channel, the less will be the amount and concentration of stresses in dentin during insertion of the pin. Thus, in cemented pin techniques, there are little or no stresses. Maximum stresses are associated with the friction grip technique, where, in addition to the relative diameter of the pin and pin channel, the impact forces introduced during insertion can magnify these stresses.

The threaded pin technique introduces stresses intermediate to the other techniques. The threading acts dissipate and consume some of the insertion energy by cutting part of the pin channel in dentin walls. The greater the difference between the pin diameter and pin channel diameter, the greater will be the stresses. Also, the blunter that the threads are on these pins, the greater will be the induced stresses.

Furthermore, the less that the distance is between the threads of the pin, the more concentrated will be the induced stresses. This is because the intervening dentin will be of lesser dimensions, while the number of shearing threads per pin increases.

2. Diameter of pins

The greater that the diameter of a pin is, the greater will be the induced stresses.

3. Pin depth and dentinal engagement (Fig. 3)

The greater that the depth of a pin channel is, the greater will be the stresses. This situation is most marked in threaded and friction grip pin techniques, which is due to the greater dentinal involvement. With threaded pins, the deeper that the engagement of the pin is into surrounding dentin, the more will be the stresses.

Because of the factors mentioned in items 1, 2, and 3, manufacturers have seen to it that modern pins have a lesser number of threads with a greater distance between these threads. Threads are designed to be self-tapping and sharp, extending very short distances laterally. Pin diameters, themselves, have been scaled down. All of these features represent an effort to minimize possible induced stresses without a drastic decrease in their retaining capabilities.

4. Bulk of dentin (Fig. 4)

The greater that bulk of dentin pulpally or toward the surface from the pins is, the less will be the amount of stresses per unit volume of dentin.

5. Type of dentin

Regular, primary dentin of young teeth is the least affected by stresses induced by pin techniques because of its high elastic and plastic limit, i.e., the modulus of resilience and toughness. The greater that the mineralization and dehydration of the den-

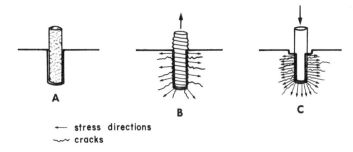

— stress directions
〜 cracks

Fig. 11-2. A, Pin channel diameter greater than the pin diameter. **B,** Pin channel diameter is smaller than pin diameter. Pin is to be inserted by threading. **C,** Pin channel diameter smaller than pin diameter. Pin is to be inserted by impact energy.

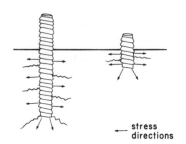

— stress directions

Fig. 11-3. Stresses are directly proportional to pin-dentin engagement.

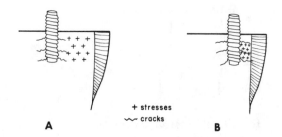

+ stresses
〜 cracks

Fig. 11-4. Same stress units induced by the two placements A and B; more stress concentration in B than in A. The only difference is dentinal bulk.

tin is, and the greater that the obliteration of the dentinal tubules is, the less the dentin will be able to tolerate stresses without some eventual failure. Accordingly, the sequence of stress tolerance of different types of dentin in decreasing order is: secondary dentin, sclerosed dentin, tertiary dentin and calcific barrier. When the dentin loses its vitality, its stress tolerance drops drastically, with non-vitality being exemplified by endodontically treated teeth and dead tract areas. Therefore, it is a basic principle in pin technique to *not* use threaded or frictional grip pins in endodontically treated teeth and areas of dead tract formation in the dentin. Rather, cemented pins should be used routinely in these situations. Also, it is advisable that friction grip and threaded pins should be avoided in tertiary dentin, sclerosed dentin and calcific barrier areas. Cemented pins are most preferred in these situations.

6. The inter-pin distance (Fig. 5)

The closer that the pins are inserted to each other, the greater will be the possibility of stress concentration beyond the tolerable limits of the dentin. It is advisable to not insert pins

closer than 4 mm from each other when using small threaded pins. This distance should be increased for larger threaded pins and for all friction grip pins. The distance can be decreased for the cemented pin technique.

7. Non-coinciding eccentricity in pins or pin channel circumferences (Fig. 6)

Eccentricity is usually due to non-centrically running drills causing elliptical or irregularly shaped pin channels to occur that are not in conformance with the pin shape. The pin will contact the surrounding dentin at only one or two points, thereby concentrating stresses that should be distributed evenly over all surrounding dentin.

8. Loose pins

A loose pin within its pin channel could result in a pin-retained restoration that is partially or completely mobile. Consequently, the pin will definitely move inside its pin channel with every movement of the restoration. The energy created by this movement will be precipitated as induced stresses within the dentin. These stresses will be directly proportional to the amount and the degree of pin movement within the dentin.

9. Wedge, chisel, or irregularly shaped dentinal end of pins (Fig. 7)

Irregularly shaped pin-ends can happen during pin manufacturing or pin adjustment prior to the insertion procedure. This situation can invite concentration of stresses at small cross-sections of dentin which may result in stresses beyond its tolerance.

10. Ratio of depth of the pin in dentin to that protruding into the cavity preparation (Fig. 8)

The ideal ratio of dentinal engagement: pin protrusion is 2:1. Although a ratio of 1:1 is tolerable, a lower ratio will make the dentinal portion of the pin the short side of a type one lever. This will put the dentin around the pin at a distinct disadvantage when the cavity end of the pin is moved during loading of the restoration.

11. Number of pins in one tooth

It is not only the number of pins per tooth that will dictate the type and amount of induced stresses, but also the number of pins per unit volume of dentin. Generally speaking, the fewest pins needed that will help retain a restoration should be the number used.

12. Twist drill variability

Blunt-edged drills, vibrating drills, or a twist drill used with laterally applied forces can magnify the induced stresses in the dentin to a greater level than will be consumed in the pin-channel cutting. It will also introduce different types of stresses that are not used for cutting dentin. Both situations can invite crack formation in the involved dentin.

13. Overthreading or overdriving of pins into the pin channel

These situations can magnify and induce unnecessary stresses in the underlying and involved dentin.

14. Stresses induced during shortening pins inside the cavity preparation

After dentinal engagement, any energy not consumed in cutting the pin can induce intolerable stresses in the involved dentin.

15. Bending or aligning pins after their dentinal engagement

Trying to bend pins inside preparations after engaging them

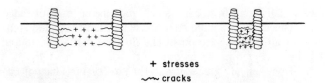

Fig. 11-5. Induced stress concentration in holding dentin is reversely proportional to the interpin distance

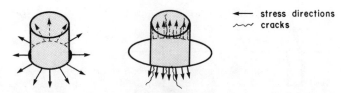

Fig. 11-6. The more the pin peripheries are coinciding with the pin channel circumference, the more evenly distributed are the induced stresses, and the more the retention of the pin in dentin will be.

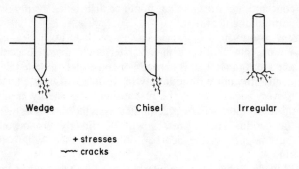

Fig. 11-7

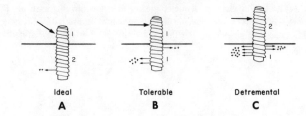

Fig. 11-8. Stresses in dentin induced from lateral loading are least when the cavity arm (receiving arm) of a Class I lever (pin) is shorter than its dentinal arm (resisting arm) as in A. Stresses can be tolerable, if both arms are equal as in B. However, they are intolerable when the reverse of A occurs as in C.

within dentin can also introduce intolerable stresses in the investing dentin.

16. Retentive features in the remaining portion of the cavity preparation

The greater that the number and extent of these features are, especially if they are of the principal type, the less will be the displacing forces that will filter through to the pins. Consequently, stresses on investing dentin are lessened. To repeat a general rule, *"pins should be used only as an auxillary means of retention."*

17. Inserting pins in a stress concentration area of a tooth (Fig. 9)

In stress concentration areas, (e.g.: the axial angle or incisal angle or the junction between clinical crown and clinical root), inserting pins will complicate pre-existing stress patterns, especially if the bulk of tooth structure has already been reduced.

B. Retention of pins in dentin

The main objective of using pins in a restoration is to acquire or improve retention of the restoration in dentin. Such retention of pins in dentin is dictated by the following factors:

1. Type of pins

Provided pins are of equal diameter and depth of dentinal engagement, self-threading pins will be 5-6 times more retentive than cemented pins. Friction grip pins will have 2-3 times the retention of a cemented pin.

2. Depth of pin engagement in dentin

According to Moffa, a graph which plots the depth of pin engagement in dentin against tensile forces needed to create failure at the pin-cement-dentin complex will illustrate the following:

a. A linear relationship without a plateau exists in case of cemented pins. Failure usually occurs at the cement-dentin interface.

b. The plotting for friction grip pins shows no increase in the resistance to failure after 2 mm of dentinal engagement. Failure always occurs at the pin-dentin interface.

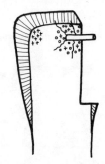

+ functional customary stresses
∘ additional stresses due to pin placement

Fig. 11-9

c. In the case of small threaded pins, there is no increase in the resistance to failure after 2 mm of dentinal engagement. Failures usually occur within pins themselves.

d. A plateau is formed after 1.5-2.0 mm of dentinal engagement in case of large threaded pins (regular). The failure usually occurs in the dentin itself.

3. Pin channel circumferential shape relative to that of the pin (Fig. 6)

It stands to reason that the greater that the coincidence of these two shapes is, the better will be the retention. The ideal arrangement is to have a truly (centrically) revolving drill creating a perfectly rounded pin channel circumference to accommodate a pin with a circular cross-section. This will make for continuous contact between the pin and the dentin (cement), thereby increasing the frictional retention.

4. Number of pins

Pin proximity and location relative to displacing forces (not the total number of pins per tooth) affects the retention. Pins placed closer than 2 mm to each other in one tooth will result in a loss of pin retention in dentin. This may be caused by microcracks occuring during placement of the pins, which then become continuous with each other prior to or as a result of functioning (see Fig. 5).

5. Type of cement

In the case of cemented pins, copper-phosphate cement (which is only to be used in non-vital teeth) is the most retaining cement. This is followed by zinc phosphate cement, polycarboxylate cement, and ZOE, in that order. Using varnish with zinc phosphate cement will decrease its retaining power by almost 40%.

6. Type of involved dentin

Young, resilient, primary dentin is the most retaining type of dentin, followed by tubular secondary dentin. Hypermineralization (sclerosis and calcification) and dehydration (non-vitality) of dentin will drastically decrease its pin-retaining power.

7. Surface roughness of the pins

Pins with surface serrations or threading will have increased retention in dentin, especially in the case of the cemented pin technique.

8. The ratio of dentinal engagement of the pins to their protruding lengths in the cavity preparation

The ideal ratio for the pin retention in dentin during function is 2:1. A higher ratio will increase the pin retention, while a lower ratio will definitely decrease the retention (see Fig. 8).

9. Mode of shortening the pins after insertion

Ideally, pins should not be manipulated after insertion, but frequently it is necessary to shorten them after they are engaged within the dentin. The least disturbing method to the retention of the pin is to clip the excess with a cutting plier. In many cases, access will prevent using pliers, and rotary instrument cutting is the only available way. The following techniques will minimize the disturbance of pin retention in dentin when shortening pins with rotary instruments:

a. Use the smallest carbide bur applicable, preferably a ¼ round or 699 bur.

b. Apply pressure in a clockwise direction in the case of threaded pins, i.e., the direction of threading the pins.

c. Hold the pin with a hemostat (plier or holding instrument) while applying the lateral cutting pressure.

d. During all these acts use light intermittent pressure at the highest speed possible to minimize vibration that may disengage the pin from the dentin.

e. Nick the pin at the designated level of shortening. Then bend the excess to fracture using a hemostat or pliers.

10. Bulk of dentin around the pin

The greater that the cross-section of dentin separating the pins from the pulp, tooth, and root surface is, the greater will be its retention. This is probably due to the lesser number of interconnecting cracks per unit volume of dentin (see Fig. 4).

C. Microcracking and crazing

Microcracking or mechanical separation of enamel components from each other can start at the surface or at the DEJ. The most common crazing, and the least detrimental to the tooth, is that originating at the surface. This type will encounter the gnarled enamel, decreasing the possibility of its propagation, and usually occurs due to age (enamel hypermineralization) and externally applied trauma. Crazing starting from the DEJ and appearing on the surface must penetrate the gnarled

Fig. 11-10

enamel, implying that it is driven by much stronger and more destructive forces. Unfortunately, this type of crazing is being seen more frequently, which can generally be attributed to improper and indiscriminate use of high speed rotary instrumentation, highly calcifying intermediary basing, and the frequent use of pins and posts in restorative dentistry. It is a well documented fact that crazing can predispose to "cracked tooth syndrome," partial or complete fracture of parts of the tooth, and flaking of enamel veneers with or without tooth instrumentation. Unfortunately, pins can cause the second type of crazing mentioned, and the following factors can dictate its occurrence, type, extent and number:

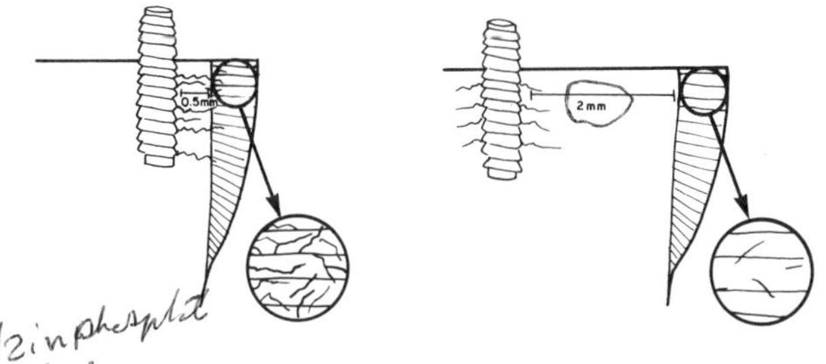

1. Type of pins

According to Moffa, cemented pins, even if they are located at the DEJ, do not create any crazing in the adjacent enamel. Friction lock pins create the maximum number and extent of crazings even at 1.5 mm from the DEJ. Threaded pins are intermediate etiologic agents especially when smaller sizes are used.

2. Proximity of pins to the DEJ (Fig. 10)

More crazing can be expected the closer a pin is inserted to the DEJ. It is considered that areas 0.5-1.0 mm from the DEJ are a safe location for cemented pins, 1.5-2.0 mm from the DEJ is safe for threaded pins, and there is *no* practical safe location for friction grip pins.

3. Induced stresses in involved dentin

One of the products of stress concentration in dentin is microcracks that will propagate to the DEJ, where it will encounter a "snag" (gnarled enamel). If the stress inducing forces are strong enough and frequent enough, the cracks can overcome this "snag" and appear on the enamel surface. Therefore, any factor that will enhance stress induction in the dentin can definitely increase the possibility of enamel crazing.

4. Thickness of adjacent enamel

The thinner that the adjacent enamel is, the greater will be the possibility of crazing within it.

5. Type of dentin between the pin and adjacent enamel

The greater that dehydration or mineralization in the intervening dentin is, the faster a crack will travel from the pin site to the enamel, and the greater will be the possibility of crazing.

Pins and Restorative Materials

A. Effect of pins on the strength of amalgam and composite resins

1. Pins will *not* increase the compressive strength of the restorative material. They only help in retaining it mechani-

cally. In fact, there will be a drop in the compressive strength of these restorations if:

a. The cavity end of the pin is chisel- or wedge-shaped or irregular in shape. These situations will lead to creation of shear lines, enhancing fatigue failure of the restoration under compression (Fig. 11).

b. Pins are closer than 2 mm to each other. This situation will drastically affect the restorative material strength, possibly due to increased incidence of voids and decreased bulk of the material. The pins will actually segment the restorative material (Fig. 12).

c. Pins protrude through or approximate the surface of the restoration. This situation leads to segmentation and separation of the restorative material with less bulk and more interfaces. In the final analysis there will be complete negation of the retentive property of the pin (Fig. 13).

d. Less than 1.5-2.0 mm exists between the pin surface and the restoration surface. In this circumstance, the restorative material bulk will be less than the minimum bulk for amalgam or composite resin to successfully resist mechanical failure under compression (Fig. 13).

e. There is non-adapatability of the restorative material to the pin (see Fig. 12) due to improper wettability or voids. This will lead to movement of the restorative material independent of the pin, a situation which will induce unnecessary, intolerable stresses within the restorative material. For this reason, the failure rate of composite resin restorations retained by pins is higher than the amalgam restoration retained in the same way. As can be expected, amalgam offers less voids and more adaptability around pins than composite resins do.

2. Tensile strength

The same pin factors that affect the compressive strength of amalgam and composite resins also affect their tensile strengths. In addition:

a. There will be severe reduction (30-40%) in the tensile strength of the restorative material if the pins are placed at right angles to the direction of the tensile stresses induced during function.

b. A moderate reduction (10%) in tensile strength can be expected if the pins are placed at 45° to the direction of the induced stresses in the restoration during function.

c. No reduction of tensile strength will occur if the pins are placed parallel to the direction of tensile stresses in the restoration.

These three factors dictate the necessity to avoid the insertion of a gingival pin in isthmus portion of a cavity preparation, especially in cavities with shallow gingival floors.

B. Retention of pins to restorative materials

The following factors control pin retention to the restorative material:

1. Type of pins

Friction grip pins are the least retentive for amalgam and composite resins due to their smooth surfaces. Cemented pins and threaded pins are four times more retentive than the friction grip, mainly due to the gnarled and threaded roughness of their surfaces.

2. Pin length in restorative material

For friction grip pins, retention is directly proportional to the length of pin in the restorative material, without any plateau. Failure will almost always occur in the pin-restorative

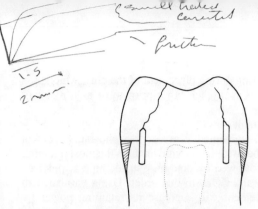

Fig. 11-11. Shear line in a pin-retained restoration resulting from wedge, chisel, or irregular shape cavity end of the pin.

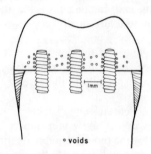

Fig. 11-12. Too many or too close pins lead to less adaptability of restorative materials, voids, and segmentation of the restoration.

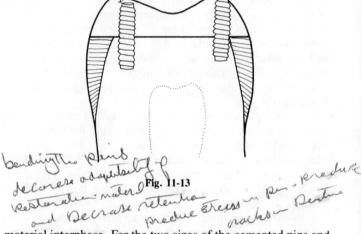

Fig. 11-13

material interphase. For the two sizes of the cemented pins and the small threaded pins, the retention in the restorative material is directly proportional to the length of the pin in the material up to a length of 2 mm where a plateau is reached. Usually, failure will occur in the pins themselves. For large threading pins, the plateau for retention in the restorative material will occur at a pin length of 1.5 mm within the restorative material. Failure will always occur in the restorative material itself. There is no evidence that bending pins will increase retention of restorative materials to the pins.

3. Pin diameter

There is a gradual increase in pin retention to restorative material with increasing pin diameter up to 0.035″. Any diameter larger than this will have no significant increase in retention, up to diameters not practical for pin use.

4. Interpin distance

Bringing pins closer to each other will increase retention up to a distance of 2 mm. Interpin distances closer than this will cause a definite reduction in the pin retention within the restorative material.

5. Proximity of the restorative material to the pin surface

The greater that the wetting ability of a restorative material to the pin surface is, the greater will be the adaptability and consequently the frictional retention components. It is a well documented fact that the proximity of the restorative material to the pin is the most influential factor in pin retention to the restorative material.

6. Surface material of the pins

If the surface layer of the pin can chemically combine with the restorative material or one of its phases (mercury), and still be of sufficient thickness to leave a considerable part of it still adhering (cohering) to the pin bulk, an ideal retention mode will exist at this interphase. Unfortunately, gold or silver plating of SS pins is not as effective as would be expected. Amalgam mercury will combine with the silver veneering layer found in some pins, dissolving it and reacting with it completely. If pins are gold plated, gold must be pure and cleansed of any surface impurities for the mercury to react with it, a condition that cannot be attained inside a tooth preparation without endangering the tooth itself. All-silver pins are not effective retaining means because of their plasticity and affinity to mercury.

As mentioned, there is no advantage of bending pins into teeth preparation. It will not improve retention and it can interfere with the proper adaptation of the restorative material to the pin surface, the single most important factor for retention. A bent pin could also complicate the stress pattern, i.e., pin parallelism to induced stresses compared to perpendicularity to these stresses. Bending the pin while it is in the cavity induces stresses in the tooth and may fracture tooth structure superficial to the pin itself and/or weaken the pin at its bending point.

IV. Anatomical Aspects of Pin-Retained Restorations

To preserve the anatomical integrity of a tooth to receive a pin-retained restoration, one should confine the tooth retained part of the pin to dentin only. Of course, it is undesirable to approximate or perforate to the tooth surface (Fig. 14), pulp chamber, root canal system, furcation (Fig. 15) or the cementum. The following factors will assist the operator in acquiring the appropriate instrumentation for pin placement:

A. Knowledge of anatomy

Full comprehension of the tooth anatomy, its invested and investing tissues, particularly in a spatial three-dimensional pattern, is basic to the drilling of pin channels without perforation or encroaching on that essential anatomy.

B. Radiographs

Although x-rays only illustrate the tooth in one plane, they are helpful in getting a basic idea about the dimensions of the dentin in this plane.

C. Outer surface of the tooth (Fig. 16)

The outer surface of the tooth next to the contemplated location of the pin in the dentin is the ideal guiding landmark

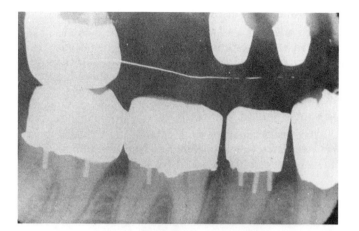

Fig. 11-14

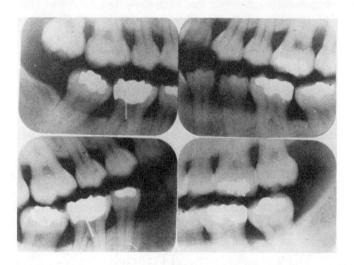

Fig. 11-15

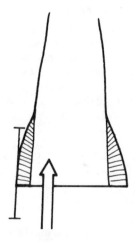

Fig. 11-16

for the drilling location and angulation. It is a good habit to apply the drill on that adjacent surface, then move it with the established inclination to the drilling location, so the resulting pin channel will be parallel to the adjacent surface.

D. Amount of dentin

Factors which lead to obliteration of the pulp chamber or root canal spaces will increase the dimension of dentin. On the contrary, previous pathology or instrumentation (during endodontic therapy) may enlarge the aforementioned space, decreasing the dimension of dentin.

E. Anatomical features

Abnormal anatomy on tooth surfaces, in the form of grooves or concavities, approximating the planned pin location (Fig. 17) will increase the possibility of surface perforation.

F. Tooth alignment

Malalignment of teeth in the form of rotation or inclination, etc., necessitates individual evaluation of the tooth involved to determine the best access, location, and angulation of pin channel. One of the most difficult teeth in which to insert a pin is an inclined tooth which has completely lost its crown (Fig. 18). Usually, a surface perforation occurs toward the inclination, or a pulp chamber (root canal system) perforation occurs away from the direction of the inclination.

G. Cavity extent

The more apically located that a gingival floor is, the higher will be the possibility of surface and pulp-root canal perforation (Fig. 19) in trying to prepare a pin channel. This is due to decrease in dentin bulk, root surface concavities and grooves, and the taper of the tooth as one proceeds apically.

H. Age or relative age

Aging decreases the size of the pulp chamber and root canal system and increases the dentin dimension. e.g., first molars are always older and have bulkier dentin than third molars.

V. Mechano-Anatomical Principles for Pin-Placement

A. Maxillary central incisor

This tooth has four pulp horns—three in the mesio-distal direction and one in the labio-lingual direction (cingulum). The cingulum pulp horn is the most pronounced. The lateral horns are close to the incisal angles and the whole pulp chamber is deviated lingually. In a cross-section at the cervical margin, there is an average of 1.5-1.8 mm of dentin circumferentially gingivally, with more dentin labially than lingually.

1. Pin locations (Fig. 20, A, B, C)

The ideal location is gingival, close to the proximo-labial and proximo-lingual corners. The second choice is the middle of a proximal gingival floor or the middle of a labial gingival floor and the third choice is incisal, where there is at least 2 mm or more of dentin between the labial and lingual enamel plates.

Areas to be avoided include the middle of a lingual gingival floor, incisal when the dentin between the labial and lingual enamel plates is not bulky enough to stand pin insertion without possible failure, and incisal near a proximal pulp horn.

2. Pin angulation

Proximal and labial pins always should have a slight labial angulation in the labio-lingual direction. All gingival pins

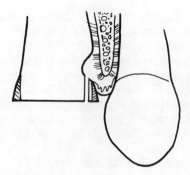

Fig. 11-17

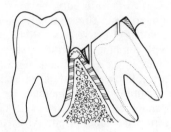

Fig. 11-18. Mesially inclined lower molar, with very limited crown landmarks available for pin channel guidance. Mesial perforation to root surface and distal perforation to pulp chamber are imminent.

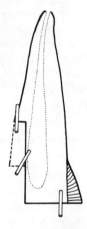

Fig. 11-19. The more apical the pin location, the greater the possibility of perforation to the surface, pulp chamber, and root canal system.

should have a very limited angulation (10-20%) with the longitudinal axis of the tooth in the mesio-distal direction. Incisal pins should be parallel to the incisal ridge.

B. Maxillary lateral incisor

These teeth have the same general anatomy of the pulp horn and chamber as central incisors. Circumferentially gingivally at the cervical line, there is an average of 1.2-1.5 mm of dentin.

1. Pin location (Fig. 20, D and E)

The ideal location and second choices are the same as for the central incisors. The areas to be avoided are the middle of a lingual gingival floor and incisally.

2. Pin angulation

MAXILLARY TEETH

- ● ideal location
- △ areas to be avoided
- □ second choice
- ○ third choice

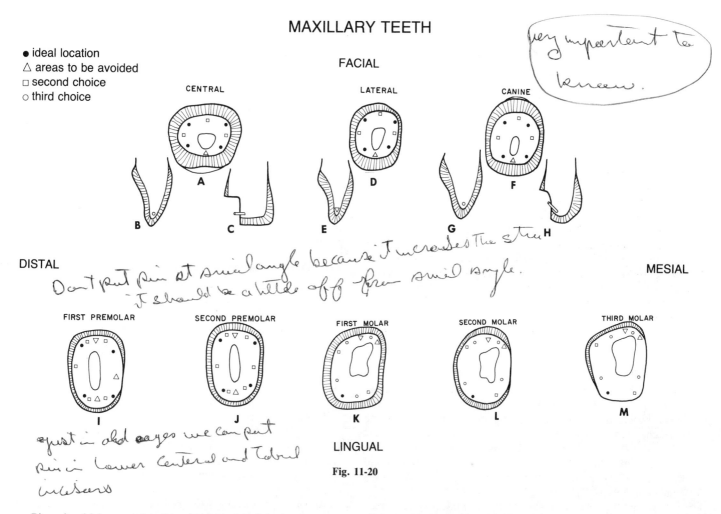

very important to know.

Don't put pin at axial angle because it increases the stress. It should be a little off from axial angle.

just in old ages we can put pin in lower Central and Labial incisors

LINGUAL

Fig. 11-20

Pins should be angulated as in the central incisor, except that all gingival pins should have slightly more angulation (15-20%) with the longitudinal axis of the tooth in the mesio-distal direction.

C. Maxillary cuspid

In this tooth, the pulp chamber has only two pronounced surfacewise projections, incisally in the middle of the tooth and lingually (cingulum). The pulp chamber is lingually deviated. At a cervical line cross-section, on the average there is from 2.5-3.5 mm of dentin circumferentially gingivally. There is more dentin labially than lingually.

1. Pin location (Fig. 20, F, G, and H)

This tooth ranks second only to the upper first molar in freedom of pin insertion. The ideal location is at or close to the facio- and linguo-proximal corners of the tooth. The second choice is the middle of a proximal gingival floor and middle of a labial gingival floor. The third choice is incisal, close to the incisal angle. Areas to be avoided include the middle of the lingual gingival floor, and gingival pins close to surface concavities or grooves, which can occur proximally.

2. Pin angulation

Gingival pins proximally and labially should have a slight labial angulation in the labio-lingual direction. All gingival pins should form an angle with the long axis of the tooth in the mesio-distal direction, coinciding with the taper of the root.

This angle can be between 20-35°. Incisal pins should be parallel to the adjacent proximal slope of the tooth.

D. Maxillary first bicuspid

The pulp chamber in this tooth is narrower mesio-distally than bucco-lingually. The mesial and distal walls of the pulp chamber are flat, and the buccal and lingual walls are concave from inside. There are two pulp horns, of which the buccal is the most pronounced. Always there is a pronounced concavity on the mesial surface of the tooth (canine fossa). The tooth may be birooted, having a mesial and a distal furcation. It may also be trirooted in which case there is an additional facial or lingual furcation. Circumferentially gingivally at the cervical line, there is an average of 2 mm of dentin bucally and lingually, 1 mm mesially and 1.5 mm distally. There is more dentin lingually than bucally.

1. Pin location (Fig. 20I)

The ideal location is at or close to the proximo-facial and lingual corners of the tooth gingivally. The second choice is gingival between the corners of the tooth and the middle of the axial surfaces with the exception of the mesial surface. Areas to be avoided include the mesial gingival floor (canine fossa), the middle of the gingival floors bucally and lingually (because of the concavity of the pulp chamber, especially bucally), and the gingival floors, occlusal to furcations.

2. Pin angulation

All gingival pins should be parallel to the longitudinal axis of the tooth.

E. Maxillary second premolar

This tooth resembles the first premolar in its pulp anatomy, with more dentin circumferentially gingivally (on the average mesially and distally 1.5 mm, bucally and lingually 2.5 mm). There is no mesial surface concavity. Very infrequently the tooth may have three roots, and sometimes it has two roots with possible mesial and distal furcations. There is more dentin lingually than bucally.

1. Pin location (Fig. 20 J)

There is more freedom in using pins in the second bicuspid than in the first bicuspid. The ideal location is the same as for first premolars. The second choice is at gingival floors between the corner and their middle proximally, facially, and lingually. Areas to be avoided include the middle of the gingival floor facially and lingually (concavity of the pulp chamber), and areas of the gingival floor occlusal to furcation, if present.

2. Pin angulation

The same angulations apply to both first and second premolars.

F. Maxillary first molar

The whole pulp chamber of the upper first molar is mesio-buccally deviated. Although there are four pulp horns, the mesio-buccal one is the most pronounced. The walls of the pulp chamber are almost convex inwardly. Circumferentially gingivally at the cervical line, the dentin measures an average of 2-2.5 mm mesially and distally and 2.5-3.5 mm bucally and lingually. There is more dentin distally, especially disto-lingually, than mesially, especially mesio-buccaly.

There are three furcations; one is located buccally, and each of the other two are located proximally. The proximal furcations are deviated lingually and inwards. The closest furcation to the surface is the buccal, followed by the distal and the deepest furcation apically and inwardly is the mesial furcation.

1. Pin location (Fig. 20K)

The ideal location is the gingival floor at or close to the disto-lingual corner. The second choice is the gingival floor at or close to the disto-buccal and mesio-lingual corner of the tooth. The third choice is the gingival floor lingually, mesially and distally if you can avoid the furcation and the isthmus portion of the future restoration. Areas to be avoided include the gingival floor or tables at the mesio-buccal corner of the tooth, any part of the gingival floor occlusal to a furcation (facially and proximally), its flutes, or a root concavity, and areas mesio-buccal to the cusp tips (pulp horns).

2. Pin angulation

Gingival pins facially and lingually should be approximately parallel to the occlusal two-thirds of the lingual surface. Gingival pins mesially and distally should be parallel to the longitudinal axis of the tooth.

G. Maxillary second molar (Fig. 20 L)

This tooth is very similar to the first molar in all aspects, except there may be less dentin circumferentially gingivally and the pulp horns are less pronounced.

H. Maxillary third molar (Fig. 20M)

This is the youngest upper tooth and, unfortunately, there are numerous varieties in its morphology and pulp anatomy. If quadri-tubercular, it can be similar to the first molar. If tri-tubercular, the anatomy will be very peculiar for each tooth. Generally speaking, the pulp chamber can be expected to be more occlusally located, and its walls can be expected to converge more toward the cervical line following the slope of the tooth crown. There is always a disto-buccal inclination of the crown, which can invite distal and buccal surface perforation, as well as mesial and lingual pulpal perforation. To avoid unwanted perforation or encroachment during pin channel preparation in these teeth, they should be studied carefully and pin placement decided upon and executed carefully. To say the least, upper third molars are very poor candidates for pin-retained restorations.

I. Mandibular central incisor

This tooth has a very peculiar pulp chamber, which is wider mesio-distally at its incisal half than labio-lingually; yet its gingival half or less is wider labio-lingually than mesio-distally. There are three pulp horns: two in the mesio-distal direction and one in the lingual direction (the most pronounced of the three). The pulp chamber is generally lingually deviated. Circumferentially gingivally the tooth has the least amount of dentin in a cross section, 0.8-1.7 mm on the average. There is more dentin labially than proximally or lingually.

1. Pin location (Fig. 21, A and B)

There is no ideal place for pin location in this tooth. In fact, pins are to be avoided as retention means for restorations in this tooth. Pins may be used at the gingival floor proximally in an aged tooth where the pulp has receded appreciably.

2. Pin angulation

As in the maxillary incisors, all gingival pins should be angulated slightly labially in the linguo-labial direction. Mesio-distally, to prevent perforation to the rooth surface or involving the mesio-distal widening of the pulp chamber in its incisal half, pins could have an angulation of 30-40° to the longitudinal axis of the tooth. Understandably, there is no place for incisal pins in this tooth.

J. Mandibular lateral incisor

The morphology and pulp chamber anatomy of this tooth are very similar to those of central incisors. The tooth and pulp chamber are more fan-shaped inciso-apically. Circumferentially gingivally in cross-section, the tooth has an average of 1-2 mm dentin.

1. Pin location (Fig. 21, C and D)

Pins should be located exactly as in the central incisors, with similar advice not to use pins except in aged teeth.

2. Pin angulation

This tooth is similar to the central incisors, except in the mesio-distal direction, the angulation relative to the long axis of the tooth could be up to 50° to avoid perforation and encroachment.

K. Mandibular cuspid

Surface, pulp chamber, and root canal system anatomy are very similar to those features of the upper cuspid. Aside from the fact that the pulp chamber is slightly compressed mesio-

MANDIBULAR TEETH

● ideal location
△ areas to be avoided
□ second choice
○ third choice

FACIAL

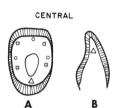

CENTRAL

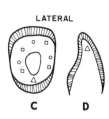

LATERAL

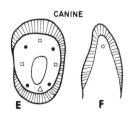

CANINE

A   B   C   D   E   F

MESIAL

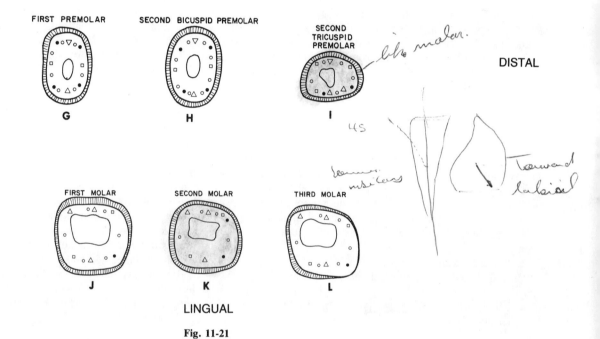

FIRST PREMOLAR

SECOND BICUSPID PREMOLAR

SECOND TRICUSPID PREMOLAR

DISTAL

G   H   I

FIRST MOLAR

SECOND MOLAR

THIRD MOLAR

J   K   L

LINGUAL

Fig. 11-21

distally, the pulp horns are a little bit blunt in this tooth and there is a distant possibility of two root canals. Circumferentially gingivally, the average amount of dentin in a cross-section is 2.2-3 mm, with more dentin labially than mesially, distally, and lingually. Pin location (Fig. 21 E and F) and angulation are very similar to those of the upper cuspid.

L. Mandibular first bicuspid

This tooth has the most predictable pulp chamber and root canal system anatomy. It has a very pronounced buccal pulp horn and, infrequently, a blunt lingual pulp horn (usually there are no lingual pulp horns). The pulp chamber and most of the cervical half of the root canals is oval in shape. The pulp chamber is wider bucco-lingually than mesio-distally. The average thickness of dentin circumferentially gingivally at the CEJ is 2-2.5 mm. There is more dentin bucally and lingually than mesially and distally.

Pin location (Fig. 21G) and angulation

The ideal location is close to or at the proximo-facial and proximo-lingual corners of a gingival floor or table. The second

choice is on the gingival floor between the mesial or distal corners and their centers, facially and lingually. The third choice is gingivally, anywhere between the two distal or mesial corners, avoiding the isthmus part of the restoration. The areas to be avoided are the middle of the gingival floor, bucally and lingually. Pin angulation should always be parallel to the long axis of the tooth.

M. Mandibular second premolar

If this is a bicuspid premolar, its anatomy will be very similar to the first premolar, with the exception that it always has a lingual pulp horn and the pulp chamber is more rounded. If it is a tricuspid premolar, its pulp anatomy will be different, in that the pulp chamber will be mesio-bucally deviated, with three pulp horns. Circumferentially gingivally, the average thickness of dentin at the CEJ is 2-3 mm bucally and lingually, 2.3-2.6 mm mesially and distally.

1. Pin location (Fig. 21 H and I)

In a bicuspid premolar pin location is exactly like the first premolar (Fig. 21 H). In a tricuspid premolar, the ideal location

(Fig. 21 I) is the disto-lingual corner on the gingival floor. The second choice is gingival floor of the other corners, except the mesio-buccal one. The third choice is the mesio-buccal corner gingival floor and in-between the four corners except areas to be avoided. The latter include the area under the lingual groove (pulp horn), and the middle of the buccal gingival floor (maximum concavity of pulp chamber and pulp horn).

2. Pin angulation

In bicuspid second premolars, angulation is exactly like first premolars. In tricuspid premolars, it should be like first lower molars.

N. Mandibular first molar

This tooth usually has five pulp horns, the mesio-buccal being the most pronounced and closest to the surface. The whole pulp chamber is mesio-bucally deviated with more dentin distally, especially disto-lingually, than mesially, especially mesio-buccally. The floor of the pulp chamber is smaller than its roof. The side walls of the pulp chambers are flat to concave inwardly. Circumferentially gingivally, the average thickness of dentin is 2-3 mm at the cervical line. There are two furcations between the mesial and distal roots: one in the buccal and another in the lingual.

1. Pin locations (Fig. 21J)

The ideal location is the disto-lingual corner gingival floor. The second choice is the disto-buccal and mesio-lingual corner gingival floor, and the third choice is the gingival floor mesially or distally avoiding the isthmus portion of the future restoration. Areas to be avoided include the mesio-buccal corner gingival floor, the middle of the buccal and lingual gingival floors (furcation), and mesio-buccal to any cusp tip (pulp horn).

2. Pin angulation

Mesially and distally, gingival pins should be parallel to the long axis of the tooth. Bucally and lingually, gingival pins should be approximately parallel to the occlusal two-thirds of the buccal surface.

O. Mandibular second molar (Fig. 21K)

This tooth is very similar to the first molar, except that the pulp chamber has four pulp horns only, and less surrounding dentin bulk.

P. Mandibular third molar (Fig. 21L)

As in the upper third molars, there are infinite anatomical variations in these teeth. They can have some similarities to first molars if they have five cusps, yet, they can be similar to the second molar if they have four cusps. As in the upper third molars the pulp chamber in the lower is very much deviated occlusally, with severe flaring of the pulp chamber apically. There is a great tendency for a mesio-lingual angulation of the tooth as a whole, which increases the probability of mesial and lingual surface perforation, together with distal and buccal pulpal perforation in attempting to prepare pin channels there. As in the upper, every lower third molar should be studied carefully as an individual case. Whatever approach is used, it should be executed very cautiously, with an understanding that pins are the last resort for retaining restorations in these teeth because of the unpredictability of their anatomy.

Post-Retained Amalgam and Direct Tooth-Colored Restorations

It should be emphasized again that posts are only used for retaining the restorative material in the remaining tooth structures, and by no means will they reinforce or improve the strengths of these tooth structures. On the contrary, they may decrease their strengths.

I. Indications

A. Foundations for reinforcing cast restorations, allowing a two-part restoration for the endodontically treated tooth. This has the following advantages:

1. It prevents further intracanalicular instrumentation if the surface restoration fails marginally.

2. It obliterates undercuts in the remaining tooth, so as to save tooth structure that must be removed if a cast restoration have to be done without a foundation.

3. A post retained foundation minimizes the amount of cast alloy necessary for fabricating the surface restoration.

4. It improves retention of the future cast restoration by increasing the surface area.

B. Posts are used for provisional restoration during orthodontic or periodontic therapy for the endodontically treated tooth and its supporting structures.

C. Posts are used as a cross-linking mechanism between an intact crown and root (except for the instrumental opening to the root canal(s)), if the teeth have relatively large crowns and masticatory forces are applied laterally.

D. Posts should be the last resort for retention form. They should be considered only when confronted with remaining tooth structures that cannot accommodate retentive modes compatible in dimension and location to the size of the restoration and the magnitude of the displacing forces. The most prominent indication for a post is where the pulp chamber walls are lost, deficient, or what is left of them are not reciprocally opposing each other.

II. Types of Retentive Root Canal Posts for Amalgam, Direct Tooth Colored, and Resin-Based Materials

This section will be devoted to prefabricated retentive root canal posts. These are usually made of stainless steel, although some are made of chromium cobalt or chromium nickel alloys. There are numerous post systems currently available to practitioners, and all of them use the principle of preparing part of the root canals to a specific dimension to fit a premade post. Each system has its armamentarium, i.e., different types and sizes of drills, measuring devices, root canal posts, etc.

All prefabricated posts are wrought metals, a product of cold working. Therefore, they are much more resistant to torsion and tensile loading than cast types of cores and dowels. Premade root canal posts can be classified into three main types, according to the general shape of their root portion:

A. Parallel-sided (Fig. 22)

This type is cylindrical in shape, with rounded corners and have the same diameter from one end to another.

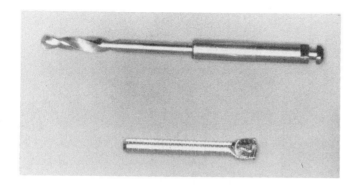

Fig. 11-22

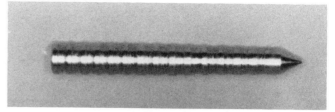

Fig. 11-23

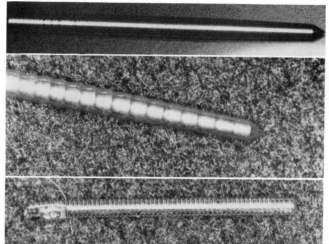

Fig. 11-24

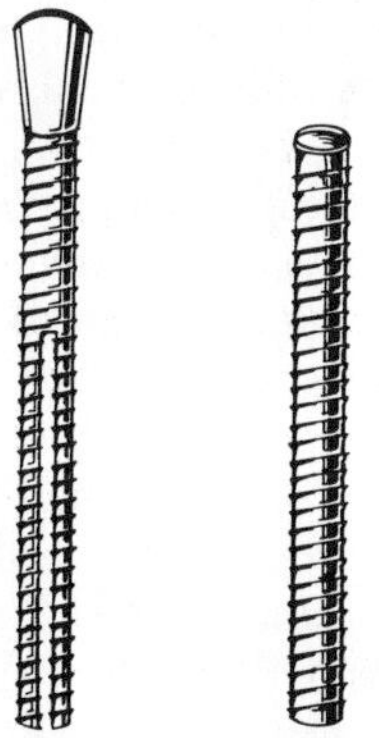

B. Taper type (Fig. 23)

In this type, the sides taper from one end to the other, usually with the same degree of taper of the root canal reamers, files or gutta-percha points.

C. Parallel-tapered type

This is a combination type, with the occlusal one-half to two-thirds being parallel-sided, and the apical portion being tapered.

Each of these three main types can come in one of the following surface textures:

1. Smooth-surface posts (Fig. 24A)

These are used in a cemented technique procedure. In other words, the post channel will be larger in diameter than the post diameter itself.

2. Serrated surface posts (Fig. 24B)

These are also used in cemented technique procedures as (1).

3. Threaded surface posts (Fig. 24C)

This type is used with a screw-in procedure that necessitates the post channel to be slightly narrower in diameter than the post itself. It can be threaded into the root canals clockwise or counter-clockwise.

Within this group, the number, distribution, sharpness, and lateral limits of the threads differ, so the indications of each vary accordingly. Some of the threaded posts have very limited (hardly recognizable) excess diameter than their corresponding post chambers. After these are threaded, they can be unscrewed and then rethreaded with an intervening cementing medium. Any threaded post can be supplied as a solid mass or with a split along its length (Fig. 25A). Also, any of these posts might be supplied as a full-circle diameter, faceted or grooved along one or more sides. Any of the aforementioned types of posts could be centrally hollowed or tube form (Fig. 25B). This is to facilitate post-restorative re-entering into the root canals without the necessity to remove the posts.

Root Canal Post Sizes

Most types of root canal posts are furnished in at least three to six sizes, usually approximating the numbers 60 to 120 reamers or files.

Before insertion, posts usually have to be adjusted, espe-

Fig. 11-25 **A,** Split-threaded. **B,** Hollow-threaded.

cially lengthwise, according to the needs of the restoration, specific root canal and prepared post channel.

That portion of the post which does not engage the root canal might have a variety of configurations (Fig. 25) which serve as a handle during insertion of the post into the canal and, most importantly, as a retentive feature facilitating adaptation to surrounding restorative material. Sometimes, posts in two adjacent canals may be continuous (Fig. 26). This is called a staple post.

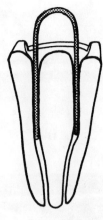

Fig. 11-26

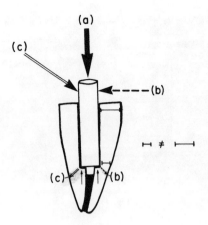

Fig. 11-27

III. Mechanical Aspects of Post-Retained Restorations and Foundations

A. Stressing capabilities of posts

The following features and factors of posts and the involved tooth will govern the stress pattern induced in the surrounding tooth structures due to the use of posts as retentive means:

1. *Type of posts*

Parallel-sided posts will have the tendency to evenly distribute the forces it receives at and around its cavity end onto the root canal walls, if these forces are applied parallel (a) to the post axis (vertical occlusal loading) (Fig. 27). This assumes that a circumferential ledge has been prepared in the root canal to accommodate the post. If the forces applied are at a right angle (b) or oblique (c) to the post axis, the induced stresses in the root canal walls will be unevenly distributed, i.e., (Fig. 27) there is a great possibility of stress concentration due to uneven thickness of the root canal walls around the post (root taper) while the post remains the same diameter. This leads to a thin-sectioned wall at the very apical end of the post.

On the contrary, taper-sided posts and combination type posts (Fig. 28) will concentrate stresses due to apical loading (a) in the root canal walls resulting from its wedge shape. Lateral loading on and around cavity ends of the post, however, will induce evenly distributed stresses in the root canal walls for the taper of the post will correspond with the root and root canal taper, leading to an even thickness of walls occlusoapically.

2. *Method of inserting root canal posts*

During insertion of a post into the root canals, highly threaded posts can induce ten times the amount and extent of stresses as smooth-sided posts. Serrated surface posts will induce about one and a half to two times the stresses that are induced by smooth-surfaced posts. This can be explained by the cemented technique utilized by the serrated and smooth-surfaced posts.

3. *Bulk of dentin in root canal walls*

Naturally, the bulkier that the dentin surrounding a root canal post is, the less will be the induced stresses per unit volume during the post insertion and functional use of the post-retained restoration. It has been estimated that a minimum of 2 mm (Fig. 27) of dentinal root canal wall should surround a post,

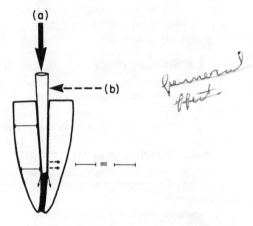

Fig. 11-28

so that the stresses induced there will not lead to dentinal failure in the form of cracks and gross fracture.

4. *Length of clinical root involved with the root canal post* (Fig. 27 and 28)

Although the tooth to receive a root canal post should be non-vital and endodontically treated, the clinical crown portion of the tooth is much more dehydrated than the clinical root portion as the dentin portion of the root still receives some fluids from the adjacent periodontal ligament. The more dehydration that there is, the less will be the modulus of resilience and elasticity of the dentin, and consequently the less will be the dentin's ability to abosrb and resist stresses without failure.

5. *Ferrule or embracing features of the restoration* (Fig. 29)

Post-core and dowel-coping foundations for endodontically treated teeth will always induce stresses in the root canal walls and remaining tooth structures which can only be counteracted by embracing the buccal and lingual cuspal elements of the tooth and/or banding (circumferential embracing) the tooth at its most apical part of the clinical crown (i.e., area of maximum stresses). Such bracing is referred to as the Ferrule effect. The Ferrule feature of the restoration should involve at least 2 mm of crown length to counteract stresses induced by the post. Using less than 2 mm of crown tooth structure, the counter-

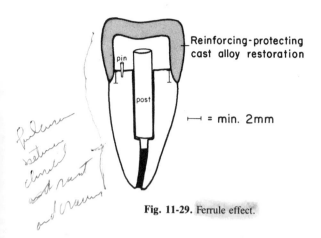

Fig. 11-29. Ferrule effect.

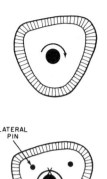

Fig. 11-30

acting Ferrule effect will be reduced. The closer this embracing feature is to the junction between the clinical crown and the root, the more effective it will be. This is the major protecting feature against induced stresses in a restoration for endodontically treated teeth.

6. Lateral locking mechanisms for the post and restoration (Fig. 30)

Because most premade posts are rounded in cross-section there is a great tendency for the post and the restoration retained by the post to rotate under torsional forces. This rotational tendency can induce unnecessary stresses in remaining tooth structures. The presence of a method to lock the post and the restoration against such rotation (e.g., a lateral pin, internal boxes, opposing walls, etc.) will drastically reduce the effect of torsional forces.

7. Presence of a pulp chamber with pronounced walls

Walls of the pulp chamber, especially if they are opposing each other, will increase the frictional retention of the foundation or restoration, minimizing the retention demands on the post and thereby minimizing stresses in the root canal walls.

8. Presence of intact marginal or crossing ridges

These ridges will act as a binder between the buccal and lingual cuspal elements, resulting in better distribution and resistance of induced stresses.

9. Proximity of the post to the root canal filling

Root canal fillings should not be involved in the mechanical problems of the posts. For this reason, there should be a space between the apical end of the post and the occlusal end of the root canal filling. If the post approximates the root canal filling, forces can be transmitted to that filling, which mechanically is made of very weak materials, and lead to profound straining. This can move the post in an undesirable direction, and it may induce unnecessary stresses in the remaining tooth structure. In addition, the direct or indirect loading of the root canal filling may change its relationship to the surrounding walls and apical anatomy, resulting in endodontic failure.

10. Presence of flat planes in the remaining tooth structures, at a right angle to occluding forces

Flat planes, in the form of tables, gingival floors and ledges, etc., which will be able to receive and resist occluding forces before arriving to the post, are the second major feature used to reduce induces stresses in the remaining tooth structure.

Besides partially protecting the post from direct loading, these flat planes will protect a very weak subpulpal floor from being directly loaded.

11. Presence of lateral walls in the remaining tooth structure

Extra- or intracoronal axial walls, that will receive and resist laterally applied forces on the restoration before they arrive at the post, will drastically reduce stresses in the remaining weakened tooth structure, primarily in the root canal walls.

12. The root-post portion relative to the crown post portion

The ideal ratio is to have the root portion of the post twice as long as the crown portion, i.e., a ratio of 2:1 (Fig. 29). Less than that, especially less than a ratio of 1:1, will definitely concentrate intolerable stresses on the lateral walls of the root canal adjacent to the apical end of the post.

13. Hydraulic pressure during post cementation

If there are no lateral vents in the post, or if the post diameter is very close to that of the post-channel diameter, the semi-liquid cement mix, during the cementation of the posts, may exert tremendous amounts of hydraulic pressure that exceed the elastic limit of the surrounding dentin or prevent complete seating of the post.

14. Surface texture and shape of the root end of the post

Greater post surface roughness and/or the presence of a chisel, wedge, or irregular configuration on the root end of the post, increases the possibilities of stress concentration on the root canal walls. The concentration of these stresses will increase with increasing proximity of the post to the involved root canal anatomy.

15. The length of the post relative to the entire length of the root (Figs. 27, 28, 29)

Generally speaking, the more that the root canal length is involved with a post, the more evenly distributed and the better resisted the stresses will be in the root canal walls. On the other hand, the apical one-third of root canals usually have a very limited thickness of dentin walls. By placing the tip of the root post there, with attendant possibilities of substantial stresses being concentrated at that tip, catastrophic failures become inevitable. As a rule from one-half to two-thirds of the root canal should encapsulate the post if the forces transmitted by the post are to be adequately dissipated.

16. Shape of the post in cross-section relative to the shape of the post channel

A post should have a circumference that coincides with the post channel. Differences, e.g., rounded post in an oval post channel, will concentrate stresses at isolated locations in the root canal wall, possibly exceeding the local breaking point of the dentin.

17. Loose post in the post channel

Unconfined movements of a post within a root canal can exaggerate stresses in the root canal walls up to the fracture point of dentin.

18. Post ending apically at the junction of the clinical root with the clinical crown

This specific location is an area of appreciable stress concentration in normal, sound teeth. With root canal therapy, the strength of the area is decreased. If, in restoring a tooth, the apical end of the root canal post is placed at this junction, as when the clinical crown is far longer than the anatomical crown, three problems will be concentrated at these locations: less strength than normal (due to a decrease in bulk resulting from the post's taper), above normal stress concentration resulting from a reduced crown, root ratio and maximum stresses from the apical end of the post, as it is, in effect, the end of a lever. These stresses may approach the failure level of the dentin.

19. Central slitting of posts (Fig. 25 A)

Length-wise slitting of a post involving one-half or more of its length will make the post elastically collapsible in a lateral direction. If such a post is a threaded type, and during threading into the root excessive stresses are induced at the post-dentin interface, instead of these stresses being consumed in detrimental deformation of dentin, they may be consumed, in part, to partially close the central slit. The rigidity of the two parts of the post at this area will keep the post engaged in dentin for retention, and their elasticity will reduce the stress concentration in that dentin.

20. Thread numbers and patterns

Continuous threads from one end of a post to another create more stresses than interrupted threading. The greater that the spacing is between threads, the less will be the attendant stresses. The sharper that the threads are, the less will be the stresses. Circumferentially interrupted threading creates less stresses than continuous threading. The wider and more frequent that the interruptions are, the less will be the stresses. Interruptions (cross-cuts) further serve to facilitate escape of debris during post insertion. The more extended that the threads are laterally, the more the surface interfacial contact with dentin will be and consequently, the higher the stresses.

B. Retention of Posts in Tooth Structures

Because retention is almost the only reason for using posts in a restoration, it is important to recognize those factors which influence post-retention in a prepared tooth.

1. Mode of insertion and surface configuration of posts

Threaded posts are almost six to eight times more retentive in root canals than smooth surfaced posts, and serrated posts are about three to four times as retentive as smooth surface posts. It has been shown that surface configuration is the most important factor in post retention.

2. Depth of root canal involvement

For threaded posts with continuous threading, retention will arrive to a plateau between 5-8 mm inside the root canals. For clinical success, 2-3 mm engagement supplies adequate retaining power. For non-continuous and circumferentially interrupted threaded posts, more than 2-3 mm canal engagement is necessary. For serrated, cemented posts, the maximum retention can be attained by 12-15 mm canal engagement, but 10-12 mm engagement supplies the needed retention for regular use. For smooth cemented posts, retention is directly proportional to root canal engagement.

3. Type of applied forces

Torsional forces are the most disengaging type for a post within a root canal. It has been estimated that from 6 to 8 times more tensile forces than torsional is required to disengage a post from a canal. For this reason, every rounded post should be accompanied by an antirotarional device, e.g., lateral pins, roughened root face, grooves, etc.

4. Type of posts

Generally speaking, parallel sided posts are almost 2-3 times more retentive than tapered ones, while retention of combination posts is 1-2 times greater than that of tapered ones, provided all other variables are constant.

5. Post diameter

The greater that the diameter of the post is, the more will be the retention. It has been observed that there is no increase in retention after 0.075″ post diameter, yet there is a drastic increase in retention between 0.060-0.065″ post diameter.

6. Proximity of the posts to the root canal walls

The greater the proximity that the post is to dentin, the more will be the frictional retention components. Therefore, posts should be as snugly fitting within their post channels as possible to attain their maximum retention.

7. Degree of taper of the posts

The faster the post changes diameter from one end to the other, i.e., the greater the degree of taper, the less will be retention, because it will be easier to dislodge.

8. Type of cementing agents

Copper phosphate cement is the most luting of all cements, followed by zinc phosphate cement, polycarboxylate cement and alumino-silicate polyacrylate cement, all of which can be used but with less expected retention in the mentioned sequence.

9. The ratio between the crown and root portion of the post

The smaller that this ratio is, the greater will be the retention.

10. Discrepancy between the post shape and root canal shape (Fig. 31)

Any discrepancy between the two shapes will lead to an uneven contact between the post surface and the root canal walls, decreasing retention.

11. Nature of circumferential threads

The more continuous the threads are, the more they will be retained in dentin. Retention will increase with an increased number of threads to a certain limit, where retention will then decrease as a result of non-self resistant bulk of inter-thread dentin.

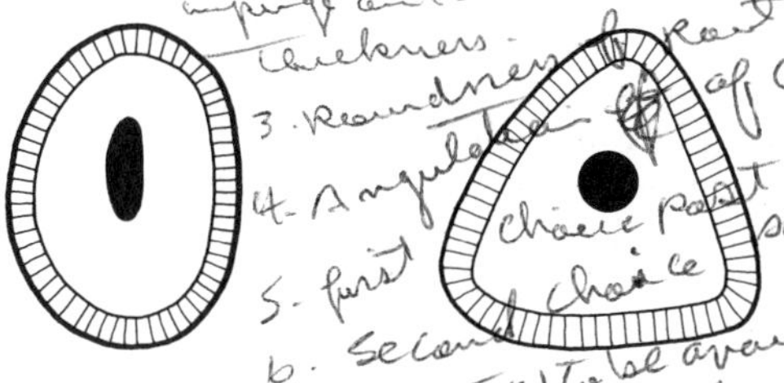

Fig. 11-31

(Handwritten notes surrounding figure:)
1. Root (s) and Root canal(s) anatomy accommodability for premade posts
2. Root (s) fluting that could impinge on the 2mm mesial wall thickness
3. Roundness of Root canal (s)
4. Angulation of crown from Root
5. First Choice post
6. Second choice
7. post (s) to be avoided
8. Alternatives
9. Anti-Rotational devices
10. three dimensional configuration of Root with Root canal

12. Reciprocation

A post cannot solely retain a restoration (foundation), and it must be mated with an opposing retention item (e.g., another post, pin, lateral walls, axial surfaces, etc.) to function effectively. The power of reciprocation is very well exhibited with a staple post in two adjacent canals, as it will increase the retention of the post to the root under torsional forces (Fig. 26).

C. Posts and restorative materials

Posts will affect the restorative material strengths and retention in a manner similar to pins. The only differences are the diameter of the post which, being much larger than that of a pin, increases the retention of the restorative material to the post.

Also, the coronal configuration of the post may be in different patterns. The more complicated and locking this pattern is (assuming it is readily wettable by the restorative material), the more retentive will be the post to surrounding restorative material. Staple posts will retain restorative material more efficiently than straight, separate posts. This assumes that the horizontal part of the staple will not interfere with the proximity of the restorative material to the post during insertion.

There is a slight difference in the effect on strengths when compared to pins.

IV. The Anatomical Aspects of Post-Retained Restorations and Foundations

Naturally, successful endodontic therapy is a prerequisite to using posts as retentive means for a restoration or foundation. Inserting a post in a root canal is supposed to be the last intracanalicular instrumentation from the pulp chamber side, for it is usually impossible to remove these posts without detrimentally affecting the surrounding tooth structures. Posts and post channels should be confined to the root canal space without encroaching or perforating to the root surface. There should be at least 2 mm thickness of dentin circumferentially around the post after insertion to avoid unfavorable sequelae. The following diagnostic items will help in planning and arriving at an acceptable post channel and post placement:

A. Knowledge of anatomy of the root and root canal system

This is a basic condition before attempting any procedure in root canals. Of special importance is knowledge of possible concavities, or surface fluting, or grooving of the involved root which may decrease the dentin bulk encompassing the post.

B. Radiographs

Radiographs, especially post-endodontic ones, indicate the root canal's size, taper, and its relation to the size and taper of the root. Also, they can show root curvatures in the mesio-distal direction, as well as the thickness of the subpulpal floor. A radiograph with the post in the root canal is the best verification for these correlations.

C. Endodontic procedures

Intracanal procedures, when done by the same operator restoring the tooth, will give an insight to any deviation from what appears in the radiograph. A good starting point for the type and size of the post is the size of the last reamer or file used in the root canal debridement.

D. Inclinations

Any inclination in the tooth should be investigated to avoid root canal perforation or gouging of the canal walls. It may be necessary to change the location and angulation of access and instrumentation into the root canals.

E. Anatomical anomalies

These should be thoroughly investigated. They include surface grooves, concavities, dilaceration, curvature, change of root canal shape midway apically, and abrupt taper of the root canals. All of these will influence the root canal instrumentation, the post choice, and post insertion procedures.

V. Mechano-Anatomical Principles of Post Placement

A. Maxillary central incisor (Fig. 122 Chapter 1)

In this tooth there is no demarcation between the pulp chamber and the root canal. At a CEJ cross-section, the root canal will appear triangular with rounded corners in young teeth, but gets more rounded with age, until it becomes circular or crescent shaped. The root canal becomes more rounded in the apical direction, even in young teeth. The root always has a bulky amount of dentin surrounding the root canal. The roots have a very slight tendency for distal curvature and the root canals have some tendency for labial curvature within the root, which cannot be seen in a radiograph. The root has very limited tendency for mesial and distal fluting. The longitudinal axis of the crown, which passes with incisal angles and ridge of the tooth, makes a slight angle with that of the root.

Post-indications and precautions

The root is bulky and tapers very gradually apically so the tooth has an ideal root and root canal to receive a post. As long as the post is engaging the middle or apical one-third of the root canal, a rounded diameter root canal is assured. Tapered sided posts are ideal for use in this tooth, despite the fact that they may leave a space between the post and surrounding walls at the very incisal end of the root canals. If this interferes with the necessary retention, a combination post may be indicated instead. A parallel-sided post can be used in this tooth under limited circumstances, if retention remains a problem. Its apical end, however, should not exceed the middle third of the root canal. Although root surface fluting, which cannot be seen radiographically, is possible, it impinges only very slightly on the 2 mm minimum thickness of root canal walls surrounding the post. Antirotational devices are essential when using posts in this tooth.

B. Maxillary lateral incisor (Fig 123 Chapter 1)

In a cross-section, the root canal of this tooth resembles the central incisor, but on a smaller scale. The roots have much less dentin surrounding the root canals than the central incisor, and in some locations it may be less than the 2 mm limit. The roots are slender and taper evenly for about two-thirds of their length, after which they taper more rapidly forming a pointed tip apically. In most cases this tip will curve somewhat, usually in the distal direction. Still, the root canal, as in the central, has a tendency to curve labially. The roots have limited tendency for proximal surface fluting, especially at the middle and apical thirds. The longitudinal axis of the crown, which passes through the incisal ridge, makes a slight angle with that of the root.

Post-indications and precautions

Each lateral incisor should be studied carefully before deciding to use a post in it, because the minimum limit for root canal wall thickness around the post may not be fulfilled in many situations. Parallel-sided posts are definitely contraindicated here because of the lack of dentin bulk in the root canal walls. Tapered-sided posts are most often indicated. If the apical one-third of the root canal can be avoided, the problems from curvature and possible root perforation are greatly reduced. The side flutes of the root surface are not extensive enough to create the situation of post encroachment or perforation to the root surface, if parallel-sided posts are avoided. In most instances, the taper of the premade tapered post will coincide with the root canal taper, resulting in maximum contact between the root canal walls and the post surface.

C. Maxillary cuspid (Fig. 124 Chapter 1)

The root of this tooth is the longest and the most important in the dentition. The junction of the pulp chamber with the root canal is very well defined and is apical to the CEJ. In cross-section, the root canal in young teeth at its cervical end is triangular with rounded corners. It is wider labio-lingually than mesio-distally. The diameter of the root canal will taper gradually as the root tapers. However, very seldom will it come to a rounded cross-section even at its apical one-third. In older teeth, the root canals become rounded, proceeding apico-incisally. The root tapers very gradually apically to a markedly blunt end, and it may end slightly distally. The root canals have a tendency to lean facially within the root as the apical region is approached. The mesial and distal surfaces of the root always have a very shallow, but broad, developmental indentation or fluting. The bulk of dentin in the surrounding walls of the root canal is considerable. The longitudinal axis of the crown, which passes through the canine tip, makes a definite angle with a long axis of the root.

Post-indications and precautions

Roots and root canals of upper canines are ideal to accommodate posts, including parallel-sided posts. Thickness of surrounding walls, even with the largest size posts, will exceed the 2 mm limit. Proximal fluting will not greatly interfere with the bulk of the dentin encompassing the post.

There are only two problems to be observed. One is in creating a rounded-diameter channel for at least the apical one-half of the post, a situation which may necessitate the removal of internal root structure. The second problem is the possibility of spacing occuring between the perfectly rounded post and the walls of the surrounding canal at the incisal one-half. This will especially occur in tapered posts. These two problems become less severe in older teeth.

The most indicated post in this tooth is the tapered post, followed by the combination type, especially if circumferential spacing incisally will drastically interfere with retention. Parallel-sided posts are the least indicated. Anti-rotational devices are essential in conjunction with any post for this tooth.

D. Maxillary first premolar (Figs. 125 and 126, Chapter 1)

In this tooth there is a distinct constriction where the pulp chamber joins the root canals, of which there are almost always two: one buccal and one lingual. This junction is located at a considerable distance apical to the CEJ, and it leaves a pulp chamber with pronounced occluso-apical length. In most cases, the roots will be in one of three forms:

1. Well separated roots, one buccal and another lingual, starting from the junction of the pulp chamber with the root canal.
2. A single root for half or more of its length, with the apical portion bifurcated. The single rooted portion is always kidney-shaped in cross-section.
3. A single root which is broad bucco-lingually, ending in a bluntly tapered apical end, in which case it is kidney-shaped in any cross-section apico-occlusally. All roots have a slight tendency for distal inclination.

In the kidney-shaped cross-section part of the root, the fluting deepens in the occlusal direction. The longitudinal axis of the crown always coincides with the longitudinal axis of the root or roots. The root canal orifices start deep in the cervical one-third of the root. Although the pulp chamber is a crescent and/or rectangular with rounded corners, the root canals are narrow, small, and rounded in any cross-section. Both canals can be the same size, with a tendency of the lingual canal to be slightly wider than the buccal. The amount of dentin circumferentially around root canal walls is not as bulky as in anterior teeth, but still exceeds the 2 mm limit.

Post-indications and precautions

Upper first premolars are not ideal teeth to receive premade posts if the root canals have to be used for retention. Cemented pins may be a better choice because of the size of the root canals (Fig. 32D). It is not advisable to mechanically widen the root canal or canals to accommodate posts, as this will detrimentally reduce the bulk of dentin in surrounding canal walls. Fortunately, the first bicuspid pulp chamber is deep and has pronounced walls, so it can accommodate enough bulk of restorative material to retain the restoration. An ideal arrangement, if there is not enough retaining pulp chamber dimension, is to use a U-shaped cemented post with each end involved in one root canal (Fig. 32C). If this cannot be accommodated, the smallest post sizes, preferably parallel-sided, should be used.

When using a staple post, antirotational devices are unnecessary. If other type posts are used, antirotational devices are needed.

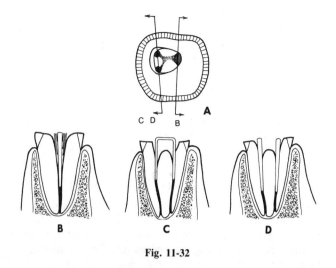

Fig. 11-32

E. Maxillary second premolar (Fig. 127, Chapter 1)

These teeth are almost always single-rooted, with longer roots than those of the first premolars. Axial surfaces of the root are almost parallel to each other for more than half of the root, then they taper to a very blunt apex. There is a tendency for distal curvature of the root at its apex, but it is much less pronounced than in the first premolar. In cross-section, the root is almost oval. Very rarely will there be mesial fluting. The pulp chamber is apically deviated, as in the first premolar. Most of these teeth have one broad canal bucco-lingually for a considerable distance before it bifurcates or narrows to one slender rounded canal. It has a much bulkier root than the first premolar, with more dentin surrounding the pulp chamber and root canals.

Post-indications and precautions

This is not a good tooth to properly accommodate premade root canal posts without possible failure, because of the broad oval-shaped root canal over most of the root length. Only when the canals are sufficiently obliterated by dentin deposition, can they be instrumented to a rounded shape for a premade post. For bifurcated root canals, the staple post could be used. For single root canals, a post could be used provided it would be in contact with a rounded portion of the canal for at least one half its length. Although it is not advisable, rounded-shaped posts can be used in oval-shaped root canals, even though they will contact only the mesial and distal aspects of the root canal walls. Such posts should be accompanied by other retention and resistance forms in the rest of the cavity preparation. Furthermore, the dimension of the pulp chamber can accommodate a retentive bulk of restorative material. Of all posts used in maxillary second premolars, parallel-sided posts are the most indicated, and tapered posts are the least indicated. Antirotational devices are seldom needed because of the pulp chamber pattern in these teeth.

F. Maxillary first molar (Fig. 128, Chapter 1)

This tooth has three roots. The palatal root is the longest and, although tapered, is smoothly and generously formed. The mesio-buccal root is not as long as the palatal root in most cases, but is broader bucco-lingually. It usually has a flat mesial and distal aspect which is often fluted. The disto-buccal root

is the smallest, and is slender and rounded. The pulp chamber is very pronounced, having a high roof and a junction with the root canal that is very apical to the CEJ. Consequently, the surrounding walls have considerable surface area. The palatal root always accommodates a pronounced root canal which corresponds in proportion to the size of the root. It has the most direct access of all three canals. Curvature is seldom encountered, but when it occurs, it is never abrupt. The canal is surrounded by a generous bulk of dentin. According to Wheeler, 50% of the population has a single root canal of some form (rounded to oval) in the wide, fluted mesio-buccal root. The other 50% cannot be standardized with respect to the number of canals, branches or foramina that may be found. The disto-buccal root canal is always rounded and centrically located within its slender root. The pulp chamber always constricts as it joins the buccal root canals. From there the root canals always have a sharp angulation from the chamber until the mid-root is approached. Apical to this point, root canals will adapt themselves to the center of their respective roots or portions of those roots. The sharp angulation of the root canals from the pulp chamber does not correspond to any angulation in the root, and there is no pattern for this angulation. Buccal root apices may curve—usually distally, but apex curvature in the lingual root canal or roots is seldom found.

Post-indications and precautions

Considering their access, size, shape, bulk of circumferential dentin, and absence of lateral surface fluting, the palatal roots and canals are almost as ideal as those of an upper cuspid for accommodating a post. Parallel-sided posts are the most indicated. Tapered and combination posts are the least indicated. The buccal roots and canals, especially the mesio-buccal, are unsuitable for retentive posts, because of the abrupt angulation of the root canals as they leave the pulp chamber. Such angulation could lead to inward, lateral, or outward surface perforation of the root during preparation of a post-channel. Also, these canals should not be used because of their size and location relative to their root, with the possibility of surface thinning or perforation in trying to widen them to accommodate even the smallest of the posts. The buccal root canals could be used to accommodate pins as antirotational devices or as reciprocal retention in conjunction with a post in the palatal root canals (Fig. 32). It is always advisable to avoid the mesio-buccal root canal in any post-retention attempts. The two buccal root canals could accommodate a staple post if the buccal wall of the pulp chamber is lost. This staple could be used as an antirotational device or as a reciprocal retention means. Usually, however, such antirotational devices are not needed in this molar due to the configuration of the pulp chamber. The extensive surface area of the pulp chamber's walls as well as its sizable dimension makes the pulp chamber in the upper first molar an ideal principal retaining mode negating the need of posts.

G. Maxillary second molar (Fig. 129, Chapter 1)

This tooth is very similar to the first molar, but the root canals are more open and accessible because of their age difference. The buccal roots are straighter than those of the first molar and closer together with some tendency for root fusion (but not root canal fusion). The pulp chamber is as generous in size as the first molar, relative to the tooth size. The mesio-buccal root canal is less complicated than that of the first molar. Because of the more acute mesio-buccal axial angle in the second molar, the mesio-buccal root canal opening is in a more extreme mesio-buccal portion than that of the first molar. The disto-buccal and lingual root canal openings are rather evenly centered on the root base. The openings to the three root canals make a distorted Y shape. Other than these differences, second molars closely resemble first molars.

Post-indications and precautions

Indications and precautions for posts are exactly as in first molars, with the palatal root as the ideal location for a post. In the second molars, however, the buccal root canals can be more accommodating to antirotational devices than those of the first molars.

H. Maxillary third molars

These teeth vary greatly in their anatomy, so it is not wise to describe specific root and root canal anatomy for them. Generally, the root canals are shorter and more curved than those of the second molar, and in many cases show a slow tendency toward fusion. Because they are the youngest teeth, third molar's root canals are readily accessible. However, these canals have a tendency to join together and separate from each other with no pattern.

Post-indications and precautions

Every third molar should be studied carefully before deciding whether or not to use a post, primarily because the root canal system anatomy is so unpredictable. In many cases, the lingual root canal can accommodate a post although a rounded cross-section of the post channel, even after substantial instrumentation, is very difficult to attain. The two or more buccal root canals should be avoided completely in any post or pin insertion.

I. Mandibular central incisor (Fig. 130, Chapter 1)

Although it is the smallest tooth in the mouth, the labio-lingual dimension of the root of this tooth is very pronounced compared to its mesio-distal dimension. The mesial and distal sides of the root taper evenly for two-thirds of the root length, whereupon the taper is accelerated, ending in a relatively sharp point. The labial and lingual sides of the root are almost parallel to each other for over one-half of the root length. At about the junction of the middle and apical thirds of the root, the labial and lingual sides taper very rapidly, coming to a blunt point. Many of the teeth will have parallelism of labial and lingual sides of the root surface to the apex. This means that this tooth has more dentinal bulk facially and lingually than mesially and distally. A radiograph will not give a true picture of the labio-lingual anatomy, as occasionally the root canal will divide at mid-root, forming two canals: one labial and another lingual. These can end separately apically, or go around a dentin island there, and then join again before they end in one apical foramina. In cross-section, the root canals are crescent or oval in shape. They become rounded only at the very apical section. They are much wider labio-lingually than mesio-distally in about the incisal two-thirds of the root.

Post-indications and precautions

This tooth is not a good candidate for posts because of the minimal bulk of dentin around the root canal, especially mesially and distally, and because of the non-rounded shape of the root canal section throughout most of its length. Only the smallest size tapered root canal posts can be used here in older teeth and only when the root accommodates one root canal; otherwise, posts will touch only the mesial and distal walls of the root canals, leaving a space of variable dimension labially and lingually. This will be especially true at the incisal part of the root canal and would reduce post retention, necessitating incorporation of other retention means. If an effort is made to create circular canals, detrimental thinning of canal walls mesially and distally will occur. Anti-rotational devices are needed in these teeth.

J. Lower lateral incisor (Fig. 131, Chapter 1)

These teeth are identical to the lower centrals, with slightly greater dimensions in all their anatomical features. The root apices have more tendency for curvature—either mesially or distally, and there is a greater possibility for two root canals (labial and lingual).

Post-indications and precautions

Indications and precautions are the same as for the lower central incisors, with a slight increase in safety in using posts due to the slight increase of bulk.

K. Mandibular canine (Fig. 132, Chapter 1)

These teeth have some similarity to both upper cuspids and lower incisors. They are of smaller dimension in their anatomy than upper cuspids, but greater than that of the lower incisors. The root canals are wider labio-lingually than mesio-distally, but because of the tooth dimension, there will be a sufficient bulk of dentin mesially and distally to exceed the 2 mm minimum requirements for a root canal wall thickness. In the incisal two-thirds of the root, the root canals seem larger labio-lingually than in the upper canines.

For relatively young teeth, rounding of the root canals in cross-sections does not happen, except in very apical portions of the root. The root apices (with the root canals) show a tendency for mesial angulations, as well as for root bifurcation, forming a separate labial and lingual part of the root and canals. Sometimes there will be one blunt root with labial-lingual furcating root canals. There is some tendency for inciso-apical fluting of the mesial and distal surfaces of the root, but this will not drastically affect the 2 mm minimum dentin bulk of root canal walls.

Post-indications and precautions

The lower canine is one of the most suitable teeth to accommodate a post, although not as suitable as the upper cuspids, because in young teeth, trying to round the root canal cross-section will involve a greater bulk of dentin. This is not a problem in older teeth. The operator must usually be satisfied with less than continuous contact between the root canal posts and the walls of the root canals. When using posts in lower cuspids, it is necessary to arrive at the apical one-third of the root canal where roundness is expected. It is advisable to avoid posts in cases of double root canals with or without double roots, unless the root canals can be rounded in cross-sections without impinging on the minimum integrity of the root canal walls, or the post channel can be kept incisal to the furcation. Other than that, it is exactly the same as for the upper cuspid, including the need for anti-rotational devices and the prime indication for tapered-sided posts.

L. Lower first premolar (Fig. 133, Chapter 1)

These teeth will resemble the canine except with less dimension in their root canals and pulp chamber anatomy. In addition, the premolar root will be broader facially than lingually. The facial and lingual sides of the root are almost parallel to each other for two-thirds of the root length, then they taper to a pointed apex. The mesial and distal sides of the root taper evenly and gradually until the apical third, where they taper abruptly to a pointed end. In young teeth the root canals in cross-sections are oval, with some tendency for rounding apically. With increasing age, circular canals replace this pattern. It is not unusual to have a constriction in the root canals of this tooth at about the halfway point on the root length. However, this is usually eliminated by endodontic therapy.

Like the lower cuspids, the first premolars have a tendency for root canals and/or root furcations to end in one or two apical foramina. There is seldom any fluting on the mesial or distal surfaces of these roots. The root apex always curves distally with the root canals.

Post-indications and precautions

If the oval and irregular nature, as well as the midway construction, of the root canals can be overcome, this tooth is much more suitable for posts than the lower cuspid, especially if smaller size posts are used. Parallel sided posts are most indicated in these teeth. Because of the small size of the pulp chamber, lateral pins for antirotation will always be needed.

It should be remembered that the long axis of the crown of this tooth is not coincident with the long axis of the root; rather they make an obtuse angle with each other. Therefore, the post should follow the long axis of the root.

M. Mandibular second premolar (Fig. 134, Chapter 1)

The root of this tooth is broader in all directions and usually longer than that of the first premolar. Also, the pulp chamber is more pronounced, and it has more definite walls. The root has the same pattern as the first premolar, only on larger scale. The transition from the pulp chamber to the root canal is quite abrupt and apical to the CEJ. Although, in young teeth, the root canals are oval in cross-section they become rounder faster and more abruptly than in the case of the first premolar. These minor differences not withstanding, second premolars are very similar to the first premolars and cuspids.

Post-indications and precautions

Indications for posts in the second premolars are stronger than for first premolars. The same scheme for post usage is applied in both premolars, except the pronounced size and wall dimension of the pulp chamber in the second premolar can be a greater help in preventing rotation of the posts.

N. Mandibular first molar (Fig. 135, Chapter 1)

These teeth have two roots: one mesial and another distal. The roots are well formed and separated from each other, flat and broader bucco-lingually than mesio-distally. This is more marked in the mesial root than in the distal one.

The mesial roots show a tendency for curvature, while the distal ones tend to be straighter. Both roots tend to incline distally. The pulp chamber is very sizeable, and has the most pronounced surrounding walls of all teeth in the mouth. The subpulpal floor is very deep and quite apical to the CEJ. In a cross-section at the CEJ, the pulp chamber will be quadrilateral in form, with the buccal wall wider than the lingual wall. The mesial wall is perpendicular to the buccal wall, but the distal wall will incline lingually-mesially from the buccal wall.

There is a marked constriction at the juncture of the pulp chamber with the root canal. This is more obvious in the mesial than in the distal root. Furthermore, the mesial root has a more complicated root canal system than the distal root. In some young teeth the mesial will have a single broad canal which is very thin mesio-distally, but remains quite wide bucco-lingually until it approaches the apical end of the root where it narrows down to a pointed apical foramen. Most of the time, the mesial root will accommodate two separate rounded canals. They may join in one apical foramen or open separately apically. Usually, the distal root accommodates one root canal which, in young teeth, is oval in cross-section at its cervical one-third, and assumes a rounded shape in apical two-thirds. Sometimes, the distal root will accommodate two rounded root canals throughout its length cervico-apically. In cross-section, the mesial root is always kidney-shaped. The distal root is shaped the same way, but with the mesial and distal flutes (concavities) of the kidney less pronounced.

In the distal root, the thinned bulk of dentin coincides with the middle of the root canal in the bucco-lingual direction. The entrance to the distal root canal is always direct, without any curvature or inclination away from the root apex. For the mesial root canals, there is sometimes an angulation in the entrance to the root canal, away from the long axis of the root. This is more pronounced in the mesio-buccal than in the mesio-lingual root canals.

Post-indications and precautions

The distal root canals are a very suitable location for posts, especially when the distal root contains one and not two canals. The huge size of the pulp chamber and the dimensions of the surrounding walls will prevent rotation of the posts. There is always a great danger of lateral perforation of the distal root canals, especially at their mesial wall, due to the presence of flutes. That is why parallel-sided root canal posts (usually indicated for posterior teeth) are to be used here very cautiously or not at all. Instead, tapered-sided or combination type posts are more indicated, to avoid the possibility of perforation. The mesial root canals are usually suitable only for staple posts or pins for regular retention, reciprocation or antirotation. In many situations, posts are not even needed due to the substantial dimensions of the pulp chamber.

O. Mandibular second molar (Fig. 136, Chapter 1)

The mandibualr second molar is very similar to the mandibular first molar, but with much straighter and shorter roots which have a tendency to be closer together. The pulp chamber is less pronounced and less square than in the first molar. Also, the distal root is less kidney-shaped and has less flutes than in the first molars. Other than this, first and second molars are quite similar.

Post-indications and precautions

Indications and precautions are the same for the first molar, except that there is less chance for lateral wall perforation of the distal root canal.

P. Mandibular third molar

A great number of variations can be found in the mandibular third molars. Therefore, every case should be studied carefully before using a post in these teeth. It is usually the distal root canal that can accommodate a post but this is not necessarily the rule. Sometimes there may only be one huge root canal in the tooth that tapers apically.

Post-indications and precautions

It is advisable to avoid posts in the lower third molar because of their unpredictable anatomy. Due to the relative age of the pulp chamber, root canal dimensions are sizable enough to accommodate plastically introduced retaining restorative material without the need of a post.

Techniques for Inserting Pins

I. Pin Channel Preparations

Three basic instruments are needed for pin channel preparations:

A. The twist drill (Fig. 33)

This is an end cutting, revolving instrument with two blades, bibevelled in longitudinal section at precisely the same distance from the tool's center. The sides of the drill are helix-fluted, allowing the escape of debris formed during end cutting. The drill is always made of steel, not carbide, so that there can be some slight plasticity in the drill substance.

There are five rules in using this drill:

1. It should be used at ultralow speed (300-500 RPM) because coolant cannot be used at such depths of dentin engagement. Also, some tactile feeling is needed during cutting. Time is also needed to allow debris to travel out of the channel.

2. It should be used in direct cutting acts, with forces applied parallel to the long axis of the drill. Lateral cutting acts can widen the pin channel and lead to drill fractures.

3. The drill should be revolving while inside the pin channel. Inserting or withdrawing it from the channel while it is not revolving will lead to drill or tooth structure fracture.

4. Do not use pumping strokes (several up and down strokes). This will widen the pin channel more than is required. Plan the cutting, and use one stroke to the full designated depth, then one stroke out of the channel.

5. Never use the drill in enamel. These drills will not cut enamel and will be dulled, even fractured by it.

Generally speaking, each size of drill is furnished in one of three types or a combination of types:

1. Drill with cutting parts 4 mm and more in length (top of Fig. 33), without any self-limiting devices.

2. Drill with cutting parts ending in a button or self-limiting shoulder (bottom of Fig. 33), which can be adjustable or fixed. Usually, when fixed, it is located at 2 mm from the cutting edge of the drill.

3. Drill for parallelometer attachment, which fits loosely in the handpiece and has a sleeve to fit in the parallelometer. It is mainly used for pins in cast restorations to assure parallelism of pin channels (see chapter on cast alloy restorations).

B. No. 1, 2, or 3, round burs, with which a leading hole is established, in the center of which the pin channel drilling is started. This aids in avoiding any skidding of the twist drill.

C. Measuring probes or depth gauge (Fig. 34)

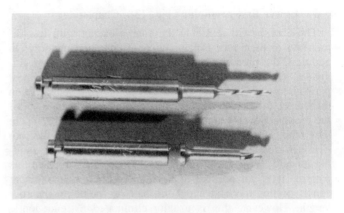

Fig. 11-33

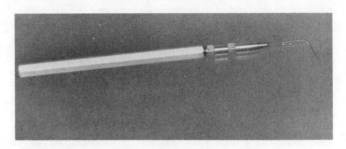

Fig. 11-34

This can be similar to the perio explorer, or it can have a sliding scale in its handle, and is used to verify the depth of the pin channel.

II. Cemented Pin Technique

A. Indications

1. This technique is ideal for all pin-retained restorations, as it creates the least crazing and stresses in the remaining tooth enamel and dentin.

2. It is the only technique to be used for endodontically treated teeth.

3. It is the only technique to be used when the available location for the pin is very close to the DEJ.

4. It is the only technique to be used for U- and L-shaped pins in Class IV restorations and foundations.

5. It is used when the bulk of dentin to accommodate a pin is limited.

6. It is the ideal technique for a sclerosed, tertiary, calcific barrier or any other highly mineralized or dehydrated dentin.

7. It is the only technique for cross-linkage of two parts of the same tooth.

Cemented pins come in the form of wires, which can be cut into the specific required (Fig. 1) lengths.

B. Procedure

The procedure advocated by Markley, with subsequent modifications, is as follows:

Prepare the pin channel as mentioned. If the area of the pin channel is easily and readily accessible, cut a piece of the wire to the designated length, using a wire cutter or, preferably, a dial-a-pin cutter (Fig. 35). Hold it with a lock-in or magnetized tweezer or a hemostat, and try it in the pin channel for proper fitting and protrusion in the restoration. If access is difficult, and there is a possibility of losing or mislocating the pin while trying it in, do not cut the wire completely to the desired pin length. Establish a groove (shear line) at the desired length and use the rest of the wire as a handle to try and seat the pin. The rest of the wire can be separated from the pin after cementation by simply bending it.

If there is any roughness or irregularities in the pin ends, they should be smoothed using a carborundum disc. If several pins are to be used, they should be prepared separately and put aside in a way to define their location at the cementation step. Be sure to mark each pin channel end as well as the cavity end of every pin.

Slow setting zinc phosphate cement, polycarboxylate cement or, in the case of endodontically treated teeth, copper phosphate cement is mixed and then introduced swiftly into the pin channel using a root canal or perio explorer tip or a lentulo-spiral at slow speed. All walls and floors of the pin channel must be properly coated with the cement. Using a hemostat, or a magnetized tweezer, the right pin for the specific pin channel is held firmly from its cavity end, dipping the pin-channel end into the cement and seating it firmly into the pin channel. A plugging act on the pin head, using a large amalgam plugger, may be needed to verify complete seating. After the cement has completely set, flake excess off with an excavator and/or explorer.

If a pin with the same diameter as the pin channel is used, as advocated by Courtade, the same procedure can be followed, except that a lateral facet is placed on the side of the pin, using a carborundum disc to create an escape way for the cement during cementation and to reduce friction during seating into the channel. As claimed by Courtade, this procedure will increase the retention of the cemented pins within the pin channel.

In the case of Class IV restorations-foundations, where it may be necessary to bend pins to conform with the incisal angles, bending should be done prior to cementation. Bending a pin while it is in the tooth will loosen the cement joint and it may stress the surrounding dentin beyond recovery.

III. Threaded Pin Technique

A. Indications

This is the most applicable and feasible of all the techniques for the following indications:

1. It is used for vital teeth.

2. Dentin to engage the pin is primary or secondary dentin properly hydrated.

3. Available pin location is at least 1.5 mm from DEJ.

4. A minimal number of pins is needed for the restoration.

5. Maximum retention of pin to dentin and restoration is needed for one reason or another.

Each pin will have a wrench attachment portion where the driving wrench device can firmly hold it while driving the pin into the pin channel (Fig. 36B).

Each pin is furnished in one of four designs:

1. The standard design, 7 mm in length (Fig. 36A Bottom), should be shortened after seating.

2. The selfshearing design automatically shears off at 4 mm

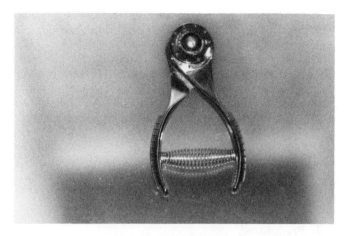

Fig. 11-35

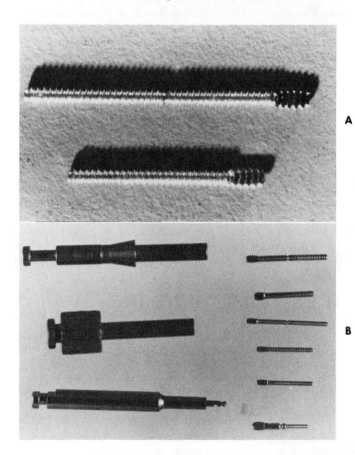

Fig. 11-36

(Fig. 36B) from the dentinal end, when this end comes in contact with the pin channel floor.

3. The twin stage (two in one) design (Fig. 36, A Top), in which two pins are joined together, end to end, but separated by a shear line. The wrench attachment part is on one end only. After threading in the peripheral stage (peripheral pin) it will separate from the wrench attachment stage (pin) as soon as it contacts the pin channel floor. Another pin complete with its wrench attachment will remain, to be used in another pin channel. This design may even possess a shear line (groove)

[handwritten at top: we use pins in anterior teeth when we don't have enough Dentine to produce retention or we need teeth as foundation of cast]

4 mm from its tip, but this shear line should be more resistant (less-grooved) than the shear line between the two pins, in order to avoid losing one pin.

The above three designs can fit in a reusable hand-wrench, (Fig. 36 B middle) a hand-piece wrench to be used in a decelerated (geared down) handpiece, (Fig 36 B top) or a disposable wrench (Fig. 37), which comes attached to the pin so as to shear off automatically or be cut off after complete seating.

4. Pins with a disposable latch-head (Fig. 37) usually have a plastic head to fit a geared-down slow speed contrangle handpiece. At the point where there is resistance for further threading, i.e., touching the pin channel bottom, the disposable latch-head will separate from the pin.

B. Procedure

The procedure for using these pins can be expected from describing their designs. The pin channel is prepared as usual. The pin is then engaged with its driving device (if it does not already have one), and the pin is threaded continuously until it offers the resistance initiated by touching the pin channel floor. This resistance may lead to self-shearing or disengagement of the driving device. If further threading can be stopped without shearing the pin, back up for a quarter to a half turn. One can cut the pin by nicking it at the desired length, using a very small bur in a high speed handpiece. The cutting should be applied clockwise (threading direction), with very light intermittent touches. Give the pin one additional turn (energy will not be used for threading, it will be consumed in shearing the excesses) and bend it to separation. Finally, smooth the cavity end of the pin using some light touches with the same bur that was used to nick it.

No bending should be performed. Simple or slight alignment of the pin into the cavity preparation could be done to prevent it from the impinging on the restoration surfaces, but it is not advisable.

IV. Friction Grip Pin Technique

A. Indications

This is the least used of all pin techniques because of the following strict requirements:

1. Use in vital teeth only.
2. Very bulky dentin should be available to encompass the pin (at least 4 mm in three dimensions).
3. Pin should be located at least 2.5 mm from the DEJ.
4. Use only in accessible areas of the mouth, so the seating force will be parallel to the pin axis.

This deisgn of pins come in 4-5 mm precut lengths, but they may come in wire forms. If in the wire form, they can be cut and shaped the same way as the cemented pins.

B. Procedure

The procedure can be predicted from the previous discussion (Fig. 1B). The pin channel is prepared to the designated depth as described, and a countersink is prepared at the pin orifice to the depth of 0.5 mm using a 168 bur. The correct length of the pin is then cut from the supplied wire or precut pins using cutting pliers or carborundum discs. Both ends of the pin are squared up and smoothed. The pin is held by a hemostat or a

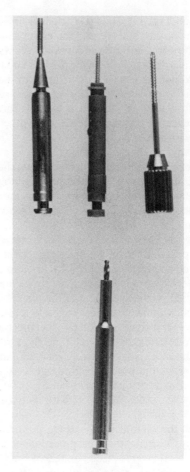

Fig. 11-37

magnetized or lock-up tweezer, just shy of its cavity end, being sure that this end will be well exposed and accessible. Put a mark on the pin with a colored marker to show the exact depth of the pin channel as prepared. The measuring probe can help in obtaining this figure. The pin is then seated at the pin channel orifice (the countersink will help hold and attach it). While the pin is being held there, a specially made seater with a concave head is firmly applied on the pin head, being sure that its axis is parallel to that of the pin in three dimensions. With a hammer, apply light strokes to the seater, parallel to its longitudinal axis, until the established mark on the pin comes to the cavity floor.

Finally, remove all holding devices and check the cavity floor, walls and surrounding tooth surfaces for any cracks, chipped pieces, or gross fractures.

Cavity Preparations, Designs and Indications for Pin-Retained Restorations

I. Class II

A. Indications

In addition to the general indications, previously mentioned, pins are indicated for Class II cavity preparations in shallow and wide cavities where the contemplated axial wall of the preparation will be short or absent completely, in posterior teeth with missing cusps where retention is not adequate in the rest of the cavity preparation, and in a cavity preparation for a foundation, where many of the possible retention forms will be lost during the tooth preparation for a future cast restorations.

B. Design features (Figs. 38 and 39)

It must be emphasized that pins are auxillary means of retention, i.e., the cavity preparation should have principal means of retention before adding pins to augment this retention. All possible surrounding walls, especially opposing ones, boxes, and dove-tails should be prepared in the remaining parts of the tooth before placement of any pins is planned.

The following are some design features in a Class II cavity preparation which have a pin as one of the retention means.

1. As much as possible, pins should be put in the apically deepest and most peripheral parts of the cavity preparation, without violating any of the previously mentioned principles.

2. Although most of the facio- and linguo-proximal corners of the tooth are choice locations for pins, they should be placed slightly mesial or distal and/or slightly facial or lingual to the actual axial angle there in order to avoid additional stresses in these critical locations.

3. The worst location for a pin is on a table replacing or capping a cusp, exactly under the tip of the cusp, for it will not be possible to achieve the minimum 2 mm restorative coverage for the pin without the possibility of impinging or involving the pulp horns. Also, this location would ensure that the pin will encounter maximum loading.

4. An ideal arrangement is to have as many flat planes in the cavity preparation as possible, either surrounding the pin or close to it. The more the surface area of these flat planes, the less the chance for stress concentration in the dentin around the pins.

5. Reciprocation for the pin retention by another retentive form, i.e., another pin, groove, box, etc., at the other side and opposite to the pin is essential in any design for this kind of restoration.

6. As much as possible, avoid putting pins in the gingival floor proximally, as it could be an isthmus area. If the gingival floor is deep apically, although the pin may not encounter the isthmus area, it may encounter the root canal or root concavities at its tooth end.

7. It is a good idea to establish external boxes (proximally, facially and/or lingually) adjacent to a pin, as this will immobilize the restoration, at least laterally, minimizing the stresses on the pin. It does not matter how short the walls of these boxes are, even half a mm will create some immobilization.

8. In locating pins for foundations, consider the future reduction for the cast restoration and estimate the minimum amalgam or composite resin coverage of the pin. Pins will be placed more axially in teeth receiving future cast preparations, than when the pins will be retaining a final restoration.

9. Try to use the minimum number of pins possible, but strategically locate them. Remember, it is not the number of pins that will enhance the retention, it is their location.

10. Analyze and estimate the direction of displacing forces on the contemplated restoration, and try to locate pins at the

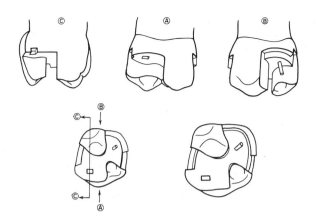

Fig. 11-38. Upper molar for cemented pin.

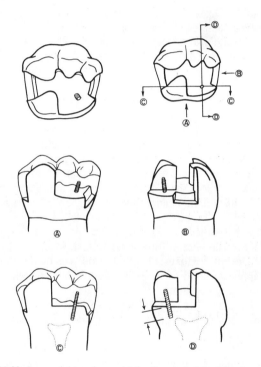

Fig. 11-39. Lower right molar model for threaded pin and amalgam.

starting and the terminating points of these possible movements, rather than in between.

11. Use the minimum size (diameter) of pin possible, relative to the size of the restoration and remaining tooth structures. Remember, it is not only the increase in size that will effectively enhance retention, but also, most importantly, the location of the pins.

12. In case one side of the pin is close to a wall, usually the axial wall, enough space between the pin and this wall should be left (prepared) to accommodate a bulky amount of the restorative material for it to be self-resistant as well as to grip the pin. Remember, there should be at least 1.5-2 mm of restorative material lateral and occlusal to a pin.

13. All other features of the cavity preparation may be exactly similar to the different designs of Class II cavity preparations previously described.

II. Class III and IV Cavity Preparations

A. Indications

Since the introduction of enamel acid etching, pins in Class III and IV tooth-colored restorations are rarely used. However, rare situations are encountered when the cavity preparation is for a foundation that is to be subsequently covered with a permanent restoration or is to be used as a provisional restoration for an extended period of time. In these cases, conditioned enamel retention is contraindicated, as the retaining enamel will be eliminated during the tooth preparation for the final restoration. In addition, pins are indicated when the defect is much greater than the anticipated reduction for that permanent restoration.

Pins are also indicated if the Class III or IV cavity preparation involves two-thirds or more of the inciso-gingival length of the clinical crown, or if the labial, incisal and lingual walls are either completely lost or have no dentin.

Pins would also be indicated if the remaining tooth structure cannot accommodate retentive grooves or boxes compatible in bulk to the size of the foundation, without encroaching on vital pulp or root canals. It is to be emphasized here that direct tooth-colored materials are not ideal foundations for cast or cast-based restorations. Therefore, if esthetics is not of major concern, it is preferable to build the foundation in amalgam.

Sometimes pins are used for final restorations in Class III and IV lesions in situations where there is little or no remaining enamel on the tooth (e.g., due to structural disorders in its formation, or loss thereafter), or the restoration is going to be directly loaded in centric and excursive mandibular movements, or the available enamel to be etched cannot be strategically distributed around the defect to warrant adequate resistance and retention for the future restoration.

B. Design features (Figs. 40 and 41) include the same principles applied in Class II situations, but in addition, there will be the following:

1. For Class III (Fig. 40) and IV (Fig. 41) cavity preparations, establish as pronounced a gingival floor in its two dimensions as possible.

2. Create labial and lingual walls even as little as 1 mm long. Sometimes it is necessary to extend the gingival floor apically, or the axial wall must be deepened to accommodate these walls. Each wall may not be continuous inciso-gingivally, so there may be incisal and gingival portions separated with an area of no wall labially and lingually. These walls are very important in immobilizing the future restoration.

3. If cavity margins approach the incisal angle, try to support it as much as possible by avoiding retention forms there (Fig. 40).

4. Placement of only one pin per gingival floor is sufficient.

5. For unilateral Class IV's, the L-shaped cemented pin is the most efficient (Fig. 41A). It is to be emphasized that the short arm of the L will fit incisally, not in a pin channel, but within a "step" which should not exceed 1 mm in depth. These L-shaped pins are used only when there is sufficient dentin bulk between the labial and lingual enamel plates to accommodate them (2 mm and more). If the bulk is not sufficient, use a gingival pin only, as in Class III designs.

6. For bilateral Class IV the U-shaped cemented pin (staple) is ideal. The two ends of the U-pin will be located gingivally. (Fig. 41B)

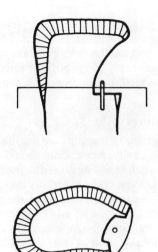

Fig. 11-40. Class III. Cavity preparation for a pin-retained restoration.

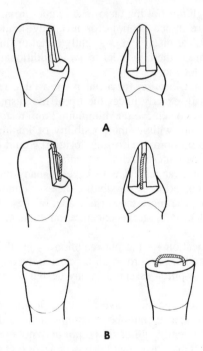

Fig. 11-41. Class IV cavity preparation for pin-retained foundations. **A,** Unilateral. **B,** Bilatera.

7. In the L-shaped and the U-shaped cemented pin techniques, sufficient space should be left between the vertical or horizontal arms of the pins and the internal parts of the cavity preparation to accommodate a bulky amount of the restorative material.

8. The bending of the pins in the L- or U-shaped cemented pin technique should be gradual and very rounded to avoid fracture and stress accumulation, and to improve adaptability of the restorative material at these corners.

9. For esthetic purposes, pins should be located as internally as possible, away from direct observation, and covered with an opacifier if this is possible.

10. Other design principles mentioned for any Class III or

IV cavity preparation may be followed, including conditioning of available enamel.

III. Class V

A. Indications

Seldom are pins used in Class V restorations, but they may be indicated in the following situations:

1. Both the mesial and distal walls of a Class V cavity preparation are lost.

2. Class V cavity preparations involve half or more of the facial or lingual surface of the tooth.

3. Remaining tooth structure cannot accommodate occlusal and gingival retention grooves large enough to be compatible with the size of the future restoration without compromising the integrity of the pulp, root canals, or furcation areas.

4. The gingival floor is lost due to fracture or furca involvement.

B. Design features (Fig. 42)

The same general principles to any class V are applicable. In addition, observe the following:

1. Pins are placed axially, paralleling the adjacent proximal surface. In the mesio-distal direction, pins should be located between the axial angle and the pulp or root canal periphery. In the inciso- (occluso-) gingival direction, pins should be midway in the preparation, but as close to the gingival wall as possible.

2. Pin protrusion within the cavity should be minimal (maximally 1 mm) to allow for restorative material bulk between the pin and restoration surface.

3. Place as many bulky and deep retentive grooves occlusally and/or gingivally as possible.

4. It is essential to have as pronounced occlusal and gingival walls as possible in order to immobilize the future restoration.

The Biologic Form

It is necessary to ask the same three questions as mentioned for each restorative technique:

A. Are pins and pin-retained restorations irritant to the P-D organ? The answer is "yes".

B. What are the irritating ingredients and characteristics? They are:

1. Cracks

If cracks connect the cavity preparation wall surfaces or tooth surfaces with the pulp chamber or root canal system, they will be direct avenues for irritants from the leakage space and the oral environment to the pulp tissues. Even if cracks do not directly connect any surface to the pulp chamber or root canal system, their presence in multiple patterns will increase the permeability of the underlying dentin, bringing the irritants more proximal to the pulp tissues.

2. Vibrations

Movements from the slow speed rotary instrument used to establish the pin channel will have the effects on the P-D organ as discussed earlier.

3. Cement

Zinc phosphate and copper phosphate cement are particularly irritating, and will have an effect on the P-D organ as described in the chapter on intermediary basing. However, the quantity

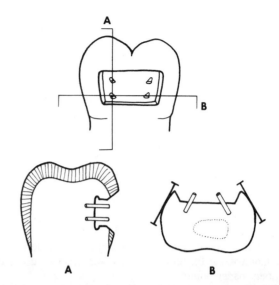

Fig. 11-42 Class V Cavity Preparation For Pin-Retained Restoration. Pins drawn here show possible locations for pins. By no means are they the indicated number of pins to be used.

of cement needed to lute a pin in place is very small compared to that needed for a base or for a casting cementation.

4. Stress concentration

Stresses can occur during function or insertion and pin manipulation within the tooth. Stresses propagating toward the pulp may be a stimulant for further dentin formation within the pulp or they may reversibly or irreversibly irritate the pulp tissues, leading to an unhealthy reparative reaction or destruction. This depends on their intensity and location relative to the pulp horns. (There is no available data to correlate these items.)

5. Conductivity

Thermal and galvanic irritation can be transmitted through the pin to the underlying pulp, as the pin in the restoration may be the closest to the pulp tissues. The greater that the pin diameter is, the higher is its thermal conductivity.

6. Irritants from the restorative material

Composition, methods of insertion, and post-insertion irritants may all irritate the pulp. (Refer back to materials' irritating qualities in the chapters on amalgam and direct tooth-colored materials.)

C. What are the effects on the P-D organ?

A healthy reparative reaction is expected to occur if there are no cracks, the induced stresses do not exceed the modulus of resilience of the dentin, and no cement was used with the pin. However, if the pin creates microcracks which directly connect the cavity preparation anatomy with the pulp chamber, or if the induced stresses and cracks increase the permeability of the underlying dentin, there can be a reparative reaction (mostly healthy) if the original pulp-dentin organ is sound and healthy, no cement was used (zinc phosphate or copper phosphate), and no microorganisms penetrated the dentin from the leakage space to the pulp tissues.

A destructive reaction may be expected if the pin induced cracks between the clinical crown surface and the pulp chamber or root canal system, the dentin permeability has increased accompanied by a degenerating P-D organ, or the dentin permeability has increased accompanied by cement with the pin.

Destruction may also be expected if microorganisms are allowed to travel through cracks directly connected to the pulp chamber or root canal system, or if the tooth end of the pin penetrated to the pulp chamber or root canal through its roof or lateral walls.

If the pin penetrates to the pulp or root canal system, there is a chance for an unhealthy reparative reaction if the P-D organ is sound, the penetration is confined to the peripheral superficial layer of the pulp tissues, the penetration is at the roof of the pulp chamber, and not the lateral walls of the root canals, no cement is involved with the pin insertion, and the procedure is carried out under fairly sterile conditions.

In the event that the pulp chamber is penetrated with the twist drill or the pin, in order to enhance the possibilities of healing, the following procedures are encouraged:

1. Create a sterile field, pin, and pin armamentarium.

2. Control the bleeding from the pin channel using blunt absorbent paper points.

3. Take a bead of calcium hydroxide paste on the tip of absorbent paper points and apply as deep as possible in the pin channel, placing several applications.

4. Soak the tip of the pin in calcium hydroxide paste and insert the pin very gradually into the pin channel, stopping short of pulpal penetration.

5. Do not use the cemented pin technique.

6. Be sure the pulpal end of the pin is smooth.

Many times, non-cemented pins impinge on the pulp tissues, and the P-D organ heals unnoticeably. This is probably due to the fact that the pulpal end of the pin becomes encapsulated by a blood clot, which organizes to granulation tissue. This tissue fibroses, then calcifies, and is finally paved with odontoblasts. This process can be greatly accelerated by the presence of calcium hydroxide, provided the P-D organ is healthy originally.

Techniques for Inserting Posts

Successful root canal therapy is a prerequisite for a post-retained restoration. For each type of post, there are a number of available varieties, and each variety has its own armamentarium. Generally speaking, however, any of these armamentariums fall under one of the following headings (Figs. 43, 44, 45):

A. Instruments which remove the root canal filling, mostly gutta-percha (Figs. 43 and 46)

B. Instruments which grossly shape the root canals to the specific dimensions and shape of the posts (Fig. 43)

C. Instruments which refine the established post channel (Fig. 44)

D. Measuring devices (Fig. 34)

E. Threading devices for the threaded post technique (Fig. 45)

F. Instruments to adjust the post shape and dimensions

G. Cement carrying or applying instruments

H. Instruments to remove excess cement

A. Preparing the Post Channel

Removal of part of the root canal filling to accommodate a post is to be accomplished first.

Gutta-percha is easily removed by a hot spreader in small

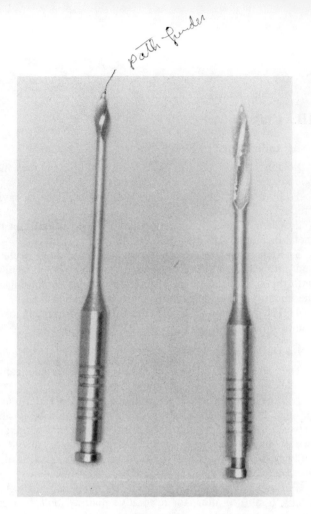

Fig. 11-43

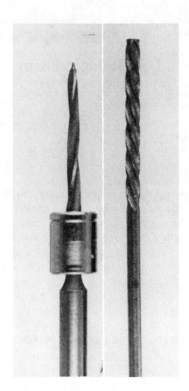

Fig. 11-44

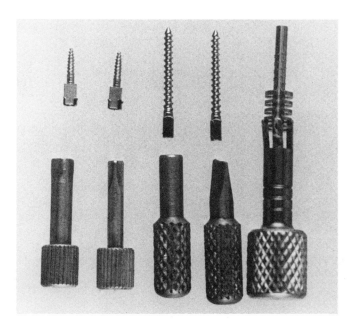

Fig. 11-45

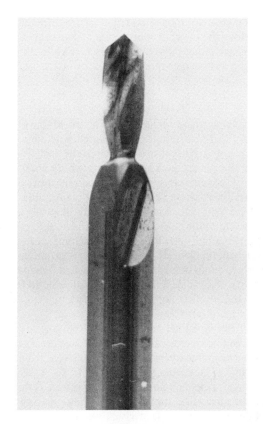

Fig. 11-46

increments, frequently wiping the spreader with a 2″ × 2″ gauze soaked in alcohol or chloroform, until the proper depth of the future post channel has been reached. The depth gauge, or a root canal file with a rubber stop, will help in recording the attained depth. If the root canal is filled with a silver point, it is ideal to remove the cone completely and fill the root canal with gutta-percha. If this is not possible, drill the post channel past the silver point to the desired depth, then nick the silver point at that level and remove the separated occlusal part by a simple twisting motion.

It is always advisable, if the restoring dentist performs the root canal therapy, to fill only the canal's apical one-third to one-half, if it is going to accommodate a post or to remove the root canal filling from the portion of the canal that is to receive a post immediately after the therapy. This will eliminate any unpleasant surprises if done in the post-insertion visit, where conditions for endo therapy are not quite adequate.

Sometimes, a revolving, bibevelled blade bur with tapered sides (Fig. 46) can be used to remove the gutta-percha. The bur can be frequently soaked in chloroform or warmed to facilitate the gutta-percha removal. At least the apical 5 mms of the root canal should be left obliterated.

B. Gross preparation for the post channel

The pesso reamers or the gates-glidden reamers are ideal engine reamers (Fig. 43) for shaping post channels. First of all, note the file or reamer size to which the root canal has been debrided, then choose the corresponding size of either pesso or gates-glidden reamer. Both reamers are used at slow speed with apical pressure at the beginning, then light lateral touches for all surrounding walls, then forceful occlusal dragging, wiping the reamer frequently with a 2″ × 2″ gauze and irrigating the root canal with distilled water. Repeat these steps with larger and larger reamers until arriving to the desired diameter, depth, and taper of the root canal.

C. Final shaping and refinement of the post channel

Usually the pesso and gates-glidden reamers are quite adequate for final shaping, but when using parallel sided posts, a special cylindrical fissure bur or parallel sided engine reamer (Fig. 44 Right), coinciding with the post diameter should be used in the canals to create comparably parallel sides in the post channel (Fig. 22). Final refinement and smoothing can be done with the same instruments mentioned in (B) and (C), using very light touches.

D. Fitting the post

The post with the same number or color code as the last reamer or bur that operated in the post channel is held with the hemostat and fitted into the post channel. The post may need some adjustment, such as shortening a very pointed tip, lateral grinding, etc., until the maximum proximity of the post to the post channel walls is obtained.

For staple (U-shaped) posts, especially those that are pre-made, adjustment will involve increasing or decreasing the horizontal part of the "U" so the two ends of the post can be seated in the canals. Sometimes these "U"-shaped post can be made from orthodontic wire (.050″). In both situations contouring pliers are needed. A radiograph is taken with the post inside the root canal to verify its location and engagement, relative to the root anatomy and the root canal filling. If everything is adequate as previously described, each post should be shortened from its coronal portion, so that no more than 3-4 mm of it is protruding into the pulp chamber, and the crown cavity preparation. It should be smoothed at both ends and put aside for cementation or threading into the channel.

Shortening the protrusion of the ''U''-shaped post is accomplished by trimming the root canal ends. Ideally, there should be 2-3 mm between the horizontal arm of the post and the cavity floor.

E. Cementing the post

Copper phosphate cement is mixed on a cold slab to a creamy consistency and carried to the post channel with a lentulo-spiral or a root canal explorer. The root side of the post is adequately soaked in the cement and inserted with steady apical pressure until it is fully seated. In snugly fitting posts, especially parallel sided posts, it is advisable to cut a longitudinal side groove in the post prior to cementation. This will allow the cement to escape during seating, thus minimizing hydraulic pressure on the dentin. For hollow (tube) posts the central space should be temporarily obliterated with paper points, appropriate root canal file or wire until cementation is completed, when the post's internal space is vacated. The cement is allowed to set and the excess is flaked off using sharp excavators or explorers.

F. Threading a post into post channel

The threading device can be different shapes of engine and hand wrenches, and screw drivers. Simply seat the post at the post channel orifice, then wrench it or screw it into the root canal. (Usually the wrench or the screw will act as the carrying device.) Be sure, after threading a post into the root canal, to inspect the root side and face visually and with radiographs to ascertain whether any cracks or fractures have been incurred.

Design Features for Tooth Preparations Accommodating Posts and Post-Retained Restorations and Foundations (Fig. 47)

The following are some usual features in cavity or tooth preparations to receive a post:

A. Close to the post, there should be an antirotational device in the form of a pin, box, groove, pronounced pulp chamber, etc.

B. Gingival floors should be prepared as pronounced and bulky as possible even with a step occlusally which arrives to the gingival margin.

C. The post should be surrounded by as many flat planes at right angles to the occluding forces as can possibly be created, so as to reduce stresses on the post and its encompassing dentin. The flat planes can and should be in the form of:

1. Tables (especially occlusal ones)
2. Gingival floors
3. Ledges in the pulp-chamber walls or peripheral to them
4. Pulpal floor if it is still present

D. Avoid any loading on the subpulpal floor. For this reason, ledges (shelves) should be placed at any bulky part of the pulp chamber walls if undermining tooth structures there can be avoided.

E. As many of the pulp chamber walls as possible should be left intact to help the post in its retention. Also, the pulp

chamber should be evacuated from any root canal cements or filling to accommodate the maximum bulk of amalgam or other non-cast restorative materials.

F. The crown portion of the root canal post should be surrounded with at least a 2 mm space in both lateral and occlusal directions to accommodate a restorative material properly engaged with the post.

G. The gingival margin of the amalgam foundation should be located at a level such that there is a minimum of 2 mm of tooth surface apical to them for the reinforcing cast restoration to grip on the tooth (Ferrule).

H. The post channel should be drilled to the minimum depth necessary to satisfy retentive features.

I. If substantial space is observed surrounding the fitted post at the junction of the root canal with the pulp chamber, it is advisable to evacuate that space from luting cement, and to prepare it as a ''countersink'' to accommodate bulk of restorative material.

J. The usual features as described for the other designs of cavity preparation previously described may also be applied.

Factors in the Choice Between Tapered, Parallel Sided, Combination Type Threaded or Cemented Posts

Although personal preference, skill and experience will be important factors in the choice of one type of post over the other, the following criteria can help in deciding which post is to use for which case:

A. If the foundation or restoration to be retained by a post

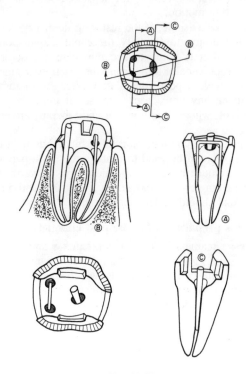

Fig. 11-47

is extremely deficient in retention at other parts of the tooth except the root canal(s) and, the root canal(s) space available for a post is very short, a cemented parallel sided, or (in extreme situations) a threaded post can be indicated, provided either one will not compromise the integrity of the surrounding walls of the root canals.

B. If the occluding forces are almost always applied vertically, paralleling the post (posterior teeth), a parallel-sided post is indicated. Here again, this is provided that such a post will not drastically weaken or affect the surrounding root canal walls.

C. If the bulk of the dentin surrounding the available root canal space for a post is limited, the smallest size of tapered-sided, cemented post is indicated.

D. If the pulp chamber is pronounced in volume and has intact walls, some of which are opposing each other, a post is not indicated at all. In other words, if enough retention forms can be created in the remaining tooth structures, avoiding using the root canals as one of the locations, a post is not needed, provided both that these retention forms will not be involved or minimized during the tooth preparation for the reinforcing cast restoration and that they will not compromise the integrity of tooth structures accommodating them.

E. Purely solid threaded posts should be confined to root canals surrounded by bulky resilient dentin walls, and, insofar as possible, inserted into the trunk of the root (junction between pulp chamber and root) where the bulkiest dentin is located.

F. Paralleled-sided posts should be avoided in roots where there is any possibility of fluting or root surface concavities.

G. Root canal posts should not exceed the middle third of the apical portion of the root.

H. Solid threaded posts should not be threaded to their maximal limit. 2-3 mm into the root trunk is adequate.

I. Inserting posts (especially parallel-sided and threaded) to their end location in the root canal should be done very slowly to allow for stress relief and close observation of any cracks or fractures that may occur.

J. Tapered-sided and combination-type cemented posts should be used as much as possible in anterior teeth. Similarly, cemented parallel-sided posts should be used for posterior teeth. Threaded posts (tapered, parallel-sided, and combination type) should be reserved for cases with special indications as mentioned earlier.

K. A centrally slitted threaded post may be the one of choice when there is any doubt about the resilience of the dentinal walls of the root canal, yet threaded posts are deemed necessary.

L. Staple posts are usually indicated where two adjacent canals are available with minimal intra-canalicular dimensions. Such a post is enhanced by the reciprocating retention provided by such a situation.

M. Tube type posts should be used when there is any possibility that the involved root canal could be re-entered for one reason or another.

N. In teeth indicated for posts that have very shallow and wide defects, with limited occlusal space for the post to protrude enough to retain the foundation material, it is advisable to use a combination of vertical and staple posts or a staple post and pin superimposed on each other.

BIBLIOGRAPHY

Antonoff, S.J., Gulker, I.A., and Kaufman, E.G.: A survey of post and core designs for endodontically treated teeth. Quintessence Int. 1978 Apr; 9(4):79-83.

Baraban, D.J.: The restoration of pulpless teeth. Dent. Clin. North Am. 67: 633-653.

Barkmeier, W.W., and Cooley, R.L.: Self-shearing retentive pins: a laboratory evaluation of pin channel penetration before shearing. J. Am. Dent. Ass. 1979, Sep; 99(3):476-479.

Barkmeier, W.W., and Cooley, R.L.: Temperature change caused by reducing pins in dentin. J. Prosthet. Dent. 1979 Jun; 41(6):630-633.

Baum, L.: Helpful hints in restorative dentistry. Pin build-ups in composite resin. J. Conn. State. Dent. Assoc. 1978 Winter; 52(1):30.

Baum, L.: Helpful hints in restorative dentistry. Retentive pins. I. J. Conn. State. Dent. Assoc. 1978 Summer; 52(3):124-125.

Boyde. A., and Lester, K.S.: Scanning electron microscopy of self-threading pins in dentin. Oper. Dent. 1979 Spring; 4(2):56-62.

Caputo, A.A., and Standlee, J.P., Collard, E.W.: The mechanics of load transfer bu retentive pins. J. Prosthet. Dent. Apr 73; 29(4):442-449.

Caputo, A.A., and Standlee, J.P.: Pins and posts—why, when and how. Dent. Clin. North Am. Apr 76; 20(2):protec.

Chan, K.C., and Svare, C.W.: Comparison of the dentinal crazing ability of retention pins and machinist's taps. J. Dent. Res. Jan-Feb 73; 52(1):178.

Chan, K.C., Svare, C.W., Williams, R.H., and Khowassah, M.A.: Comparison of the retentive property and dentinal crazing ability of retention pins and machinist's taps. J. Dent. Res. Nov-Dec 74; 53(6):1425-1427.

Christian, G.W., Button, G.L., Moon, P.C., England, M.C., and Douglas, H.B.: Post core restoration in endodontically treated posterior teeth. J. Endod. 1981 Apr; 7(4):182-185.

Colman, H.L.: Restoration of endodontically treated teeth. Dent. Clin. North Am. 1979 Oct; 23(4):647-662.

Cooley, R.L., and Barkmeier, W.W.: Temperature rise in the pulp chamber caused by twist drills. J. Prosthet. Dent. 1980 Oct; 44(4):426-429.

Courtade, G.L.: Pin pointers, 3. Self-threading pins. J. Prosthet. Dent. Oct 1968; 20(4):335-338.

Currens, W.E., Korostoff, E., and von Faunhofer, J.A.: Penetration of shearing and nonshearing pins into dentin. J. Prosthet. Dent. 1980 Oct; 44(4): 430-433.

Davy, D.T., Dilley, G.L., and Krejci, R.F.: Determination of stress patterns in root-filled teeth incorporating various dowel designs. J. Dent. Res. 1981 Jul; 60(7):1301-1310.

D'erand, T.: The principal stress distribution in a root with a loaded post in model experiments. J. Dent. Res. 1977 Dec; 56(12):1463-1467. Dhuru, V.B., McLachlan, K., and Kasloff, Z.: Axial stiffness of retention pins in human dentin. J. Dent. Res. 1979 Mar; 58(3):1055-1059.

Dhuru, V.B., McLachlan, K., and Kasloff, Z.: A photoelastic study of stress concentrations produced by retention pins in amalgam restorations. J. Dent. Res. 1979 Mar; 58(3):1060-1064.

Dilts, W.E., and Coury, T.L.: Conservative approach to the placement of retentive pins. Dent. Clin. North Am. Apr 76; 20(2):397-402.

Dilts, W.E., Duncanson, M.G. Jr., Collard, E.W., and Parmley, L.E.: Retention of self-threading pins. J. Can. Dent. Assoc. 1981 Feb; 47(2):119-120.

Dilts, W.E., and Mullaney, T.P.: Relationship of pinhole location and tooth morphology in pin-retained silver amalgam restorations. J. Am. Dent. Assoc. May 68; 76(5):1011-1015.

Dilts, W.E., Welk, D.A., and Stovall, J.: Retentive properties of pin materials in pin retained silver amalgam restorations. JADA Nov 68; 77(5):1085-1089.

Duperon, D.F., and Kasloff, Z.: The effects of three types of pins on the tensile strength of dental amalgam. J. Can. Dent. Assoc. Feg 73; 39(2): 111-119.

Durney, E.C., and Rosen, H.: Root fracture as a complication of post design and insertion: a laboratory study. Oper. Dent. 1977 Summer; 2(3):90-96.

Fusilier, C.N.: Cross-pinning for added retention. J. Prosthet. Dent. Apr 74; 31(4):397-402.

Galindo, Y.: Stress-induced effects of retentive pins. A review of the literature. J. Prosthet. Dent. 1980 Aug; 44(2):183-186.

Glantz, P.O., Jendresen, M.D., and Wittbjer, J.E.: Retention of zinc phosphate cement as influenced by post material. CDA J. 1981 Feb; 9(2):36-41.

Goldstein, P.M.: Retention pins are friction locked without use of cement. J. Am. Dent. Assoc. Nov 66; 73(5):1103-1106.

Gutmann, J.L.: Preparation of endodontically treated teeth to receive a post-core restoration. J. Prosthet. Dent. 1977 Oct; 38(4):413-419.

Guzy, G.E., and Nicholls, J.I.: In vitro comparison of intact endodontically treated teeth with and without endo-post reinforcement. J. Prosthet. Dent. 1979 Jul; **42**(1):39-44.

Hanson, E.C., Caputo, A.A., and Travert, K.C.: The relationship of dental cements, pins, and retention. J. Prosthet. Dent. Oct 74; **32**(4):428-434.

Henry, P.J.: Photoelastic analysis of post core restorations. Aust. Dent. J. 1977 Jun; **22**(3):157-159.

Johnson, J.K., and Sakumura, J.S.: Dowel form and tensile force. J. Prosthet. Dent. 1978 Dec; **40**(6):645-649.

Khera, S.C., Chan, K.C., and Rittman, B.R.: Dentinal crazing and interpin distance. J. Prosthet. Dent. 1978 Nov; **40**(5):538-543.

Krupp, J.D., Caputo, A.A., Trabert, K.C., and Standlee, J.P.: Dowel retention with glass-ionomer cement. J. Prosthet. Dent. 1979 Feb; **41**(2):163-166.

Kwan, E.H., and Harrington, G.W.: The effect of immediate post preparation on apical seal. J. Endod. 1981 Jul; **8**(7):325-329.

Larson, T.D., and Jensen, J.R.: Microleakage of composite resin and amalgam core material under complete cast crowns. J. Prosthet. Dent. 1980; **44**(1): 40-44.

Lau, V.M.: The reinforcement of endodontically treated teeth. Dent. Clin. North Am. April 76; **20**(2):313-328.

Leggett, L.J.: Restoration of non-vital posterior teeth. J. Br. Endod. Soc. 1979 Jul; **12**(2):73-82.

Lovdahl, P.E., and Nicholls, J.I.: Pin-retained amalgam cores vs cast-gold dowel cores. J. Prosthet. Dent. 1977 Nov; **38**(5):507-514.

Markley, M.R.: Pin-retained and pin-reinforced amalgam. J. Am. Dent. Assoc. Dec 66; **73**(6):1295-1300.

Markley, M.R.: Pin-retained and reinforced restoration and foundations. Dent. Clin. North Am. Mar 67; 229-244.

Messing, J.J., and Wills, D.J.: Investigation of resistance to stress of screw-threaded crown posts. J. Prosthet. Dent. Sep 73; **30**(3):278-282.

Moffa, J.P., Going, R.E., and Gettleman, L.: Silver pins: their influence on the strength and adaptation of amalgam. J. Prosthet. Dent. Nov. 72; **28**(5): 591-599.

Moffa, J.P., Razzano, M.R., and Doyle, M.G.: Pins—a comparison of their retentive properties, JADA Mar 69; **78**(3):529-535.

Moffa, J.P., Razzano, M.R., and Folio, J.: Influence of cavity varnish on microleakage and retention of various pin-retaining devices. J. Prosthet. Dent. Dec 68; **20**(6):541-551.

Mondelli, J., and Vierira, D.F.: The strength of Class II amalgam restorations with and without pins. J. Prosthet. Dent. Aug 72; **28**(2):179-188.

Motta, A., and Motta, R.: Provisional coronal preparation to root canal therapy. J. Endod. 1980 Sep; **6**(9):749-751.

Nayyar, A., Walton, R.E., and Leonard, L.A.: An amalgam coronal-radicular dowel and core technique for endodontically treated posterior teeth. J. Prosth. Dent. 1980 May; **43**(5):511-515.

Outhwaite, W.C., Garman, T.A., and Pashley, D.H.: Pin vs. slot retention in extensive amalgam restorations. J. Prosthet. Dent. 1979 Apr; **41**(4):396-400.

Perel, M.L., and Muroff, F.I.: Clinical criteria for posts and cores. J. Prosthet. Dent. Oct 72; **28**(4):405-411.

Podshadley, A.G.: Post and core buildup for endodontically treated posterior teeth. J. Ky. Dent. Assoc. 1981 Jan; **33**(1):26-28.

Ruemping, D.R., Lund, M.R., and Schnell, R.J.: Retention of dowels subjected to tensile and torsional forces. J. Prosthet. Dent. 1979 Feb; **41**(2):159-162.

Schlissel, E.S., Hmelo, A.B., Bilello, J.C., and Gwinnett, A.J.: The failure of self-threading retentive pins under tensile load. J. Dent. Res. 1979 Nov; **58**(11):2105-2108.

Schuchard, A., and Reed, O.M.: Pulpal response to pin placement. J. Prosthet. Dent. Mar 73; **29**(3):292-300.

Simonsen, T.L., Nilsen, G.N., and Hals, E.: A follow-up study of post- or pin-retained amalgam fillings with special reference to possible corrosion. Scand. J. Dent. Res. 1973; **81**(6):415-424.

Standlee, J.P., Caputo, A.A., Holcomb, J., and Travert, K.C.: The retentive and stress-distributing properties of a threaded endodontic dowel. J. Prosthet. Dent. 1980 Oct; **44**(4):398-404.

Standlee, J.P., Collard, E.W., and Caputo, A.A.: Dentinal defects caused by some twist drills and retentive pins. J. Prosthet. Dent. Aug 70; **24**(2):185-192.

Stern, N., and Hirshfeld, Z.: Principles of preparing endodontically treated teeth for dowel and core restorations. J. Prosthet. Dent. Aug 73; **30**(2): 162-165.

Takahashi, N., Kitagami, T., and Komori, T.: Effects of pin hole position on stress distributions and interpulpal temperatures in horizontal nonparallel pin restorations. J. Dent. Res. 1979 Nov; **58**(11):2085-2090.

Tilk, M.A., Lommel, T.J., and Gerstein, H.: A study of mandibular and maxillary root widths to determine dowel size. J. Endod. 1979 Mar; **5**(3):79-82.

Trabert, K.C., Caputo, A.A., Collard, E.W., and Standlee, J.P.: Stress transfer to the dental pulp by retentive pins. J. Prosthet. Dent. Nov 73; **30**(5):808-815.

Wheeler, R.: Pulp, cavities of the permanent teeth. Philadelphia, Saunders Co., 1976.

Winstanley, R.B.: Pin-retained amalgam foundations for anterior crowns. Quintessence Int. Sep 76; **7**(9):13-22.

Winstanley, R.B.: Pin—a review. Quintessence Int. May 76; **7**(5):15-18.

Zmener, O.: Adaptation of threaded dowels to dentin. J. Prosthet. Dent. 1980 May; **43**(5):530-535.

Zmener, O.: Effect of dowel preparation on the apical seal of endodontically treated teeth. J. Endod. 1980 Aug; **6**(8):687-690.

CHAPTER 12

Contacts and contours

From the cariogenic aspect there may be only twenty occlusal surfaces but there are sixty contacting proximal and sixty-four facial and lingual surfaces that are susceptible to decay in the full complement of teeth. Occlusal surfaces are predisposed to decay by faulty fissures and grooves. Decay on the proximal, however, occurs mainly due to the faulty interrelationship between the contact areas, the marginal ridges, the embrasures, and the gingiva.

Decay is predisposed facially and lingually, especially in the gingival one-third of the teeth, primarily by faulty interrelationship between tooth contour and items as the dimensions and interrelations of the periodontal components, including the free, attached, and unattached gingiva as well as the vestibule; and the surrounding musculature and its capability for impeding or enhancing plaque adhesion and growth.

From the periodontal aspect, periodontitis also will be enhanced and accelerated both interproximally and in the facial and lingual periodontium by these faulty interrelationships.

The key to these "proper" relationships interproximally is the contact area in relation to its location, extent, and size, while the proper relationships facially and lingually are the occluso-gingival and mesio-distal configurations.

The failure to comprehend these relationships will cause not only premature failure of restorations but also periodontal problems, as well as the carious involvement of adjacent tooth surfaces.

Although the contacts and contours of each tooth will vary from one individual to another, or from one tooth to another, the following provides a brief description of the general physio-anatomical features of the normal contact, contour, and related structures. These can be used as guidelines in reproducing contacts and contours in restorations, but, by no means, should they be imitated indiscriminately.

I. Proximal Contour, Contact Areas and Related Structures

According to their general shape, teeth can be divided into three types, with each having its own physical characteristics in the contact area and related structures.

A. Tapering teeth (Fig. 1)

In an inciso-apical direction contacts of tapered maxillary central and lateral incisors start incisally near the incisal edges. In a labio-lingual direction they start slightly labial to the incisal edges.

Tapered cuspids are very angular, with the mesial contact area close to the incisal edges and the distal contact area near the center of the distal surface.

The tapering type of bicuspid is also angular, possessing crowns, constricted cervically and with long cusps. The latter may form from one-third to one-half the entire height of the crown. As those crowns taper lingually, the contact areas occur bucally starting almost at the buccal axial angle of the tooth. Since nearly all these contact areas begin approximately 1 mm gingivally from the crest of the marginal ridges, the bicuspid contacts of this type of tooth will be found just gingival from the junction of the occlusal and middle third of the crown.

Mesial contacts of tapered molars approach the mesio-buccal axial angle of the tooth, in a bucco-lingual direction, and from one-third to one-half the distance from the occlusal surface to the cemento-enamel junction of the tooth occluso-gingivally. The distal contacts of molars shift lingually to the middle third bucco-lingually, and are midway on the length of the crown occluso-gingivally. Lingual shifting of the contacts is more noticeable in mandibular than in maxillary molars.

No definite position can be set for the mesial contacts of tapered mandibular second molars and the distal contacts of

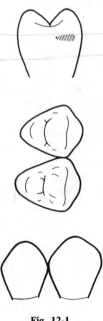

Fig. 12-1

the approximating first molar, owing to the fact that the third buccal cusp of the first molar presents many variables in contour and position.

The proximal contour of the tapering type of teeth has one common feature: starting at the cemento-enamel junction, the surface presents a concavity almost to the contact areas, and they are decidedly convex from there to the crest of the marginal ridges. The concavities are more pronounced on the mesial than on the distal surfaces, the latter being a diverging plane bucco-lingually. Concavities occur most frequently on the mesial surfaces of teeth having buccal and lingual roots, the most pronounced being the mesial of the first upper premolar.

The tapering type of tooth presents embrasures with greater variations in shape than any of the other types do. Incisal and labial embrasures are almost negligible. The gingival embrasures between anterior teeth are very extended incisally and wide at the gingival crest, while the lingual embrasures are almost the full depth of the labio-lingual dimensions of the crown and almost as wide as the distance from the center of one tooth to the center of the approximating one. The gingival and lingual embrasures are the largest to be found anywhere in the mouth.

The buccal embrasures are very small. The occlusal embrasures are comparatively wider and deeper. The gingival embrasures between posterior teeth are broad and have their bases more apically located than those associated with other types of teeth. The lingual embrasures in posterior teeth are very wide bucco-lingually, but diverge somewhat more than those found between teeth of a square type.

B. Square type (Fig. 2)

This type of tooth is bulky and angular, with little rounded contour. Since there is little cervical constriction, their proximal surfaces are almost devoid of curves.

The incisor contacts are in a line with the incisal edges, labio-lingually and extend almost to the incisal angle incisally. These teeth are frequently in contact with their neighbor in a plane instead of point, which varies from 0.5 to 3 mm. Cuspid contacts are relatively close to the incisal edges and in line with them labio-lingually. The posterior contacts are broad areas on the square type of teeth. Since the teeth have relatively short cusps, the occlusal limit of the posterior contacts will be found in the occlusal ⅓ of the crown. The configuration of the bicuspids and molars places the buccal extent of the contact well into the buccal ⅓.

The lingual extent of the contact of maxillary molars usually stops in the middle ⅓, while the gingival extent is seldom more than 1 mm from the CEJ.

Mesial contacts are nearer the buccal axial angle than the distal. Mesial contacts of the mandibular molars may measure from 1 to 4 mm bucco-lingually and be from a mere line contact to including half the height of the crown occluso-gingivally. Contacts originate in the bucco-occlusal section of the crown. The distal contacts originate more lingually. If they are small areas, they will be found at the midline of the crown, bucco-lingually, and in the occlusal third, occluso-gingivally. If they are large areas, they will occupy from one-third to two-thirds of the bucco-lingual dimension and extending from the lower

border of the marginal ridge to the CEJ occluso-gingivally.

Incisal, labial, occlusal, and buccal embrasures are almost nil. The gingival embrasures may be barely noticeable or they may extend about one-third of the height of the crown. When the buccal embrasures are present, they are very narrow and flat. The lingual embrasures may be narrow or wide in their bucco-lingual extension but they are always narrow mesio-distally.

The proximal contours of square type teeth have a tendency to become a plane instead of a curved surface. Bucco-lingual concavities are found occasionally on the mesial surfaces of maxillary first bicuspids, first and second molars, and the mesial surface of the mandibular first molar. The distal surfaces are generally either flat or slightly convex from the buccal to the lingual surface. The convexity which creates the marginal ridges disappears at the contact and the remainder of the surface in the gingival direction is usually flat.

C. Ovoid type (Fig. 3)

The ovoid type of tooth is a transitional type between the tapering and square types. Its surfaces are primarily convex, but infrequently they may be concave.

In an inciso-gingival direction, the mesial contacts of the incisors start at about one-fourth the height of the crown from the incisal edges. In a labio-lingual direction they start slightly lingual to their mesial edges. The distal contacts of the incisors have the same labio-lingual position, but may be found from one-third to one-half the height of the crown from the incisal edge in an inciso-gingival direction.

While ovoid posterior teeth have comparatively short cusps, it will be found that the convexity of the marginal ridges carries the contacts almost to the middle of the crown height. In mo-

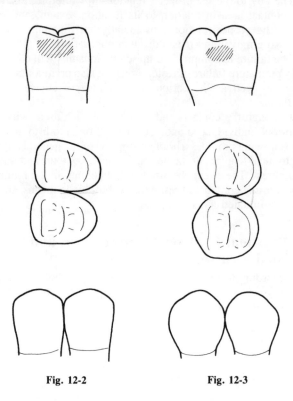

Fig. 12-2   Fig. 12-3

lars, the prominence of the mesio-buccal cusp, coupled with the bucco-lingual convexity, places the buccal extent of the mesial contacts at the junction of the buccal and middle thirds of the crowns. Bucco-lingually the buccal extent of the distal contacts is found in line with the central grooves on the occlusal surface of the crown.

The labial, incisal and buccal embrasures of ovoid teeth are larger and more extensive than those found in other types. Gingival embrasures are relatively short occluso-gingivally and broad mesio-distally at their bases. Lingual embrasures are comparatively short labio-lingually and broad mesio-distally.

Proximal contours of ovoid anterior teeth are decidedly con-vex from the incisal angle to the cervix. Bicuspids of the ovoid type are frequently bell-shaped with the convex surface running from the crests of the marginal ridges almost to the cervix, where they merge via a slightly concave surface to a union with the root surfaces. The bicuspids are likewise convex from the buccal to the lingual axial angles. The mesial surfaces of ovoid molars present convex areas which are less extensive than those found on the distal surfaces. The latter are usually convex in all directions. Generally, there is a tendency in all three types of teeth for the distal contacts to move in a lingual direction, progressing further back in the arch.

To summarize the anatomical features of contact areas and associated surface anatomies, refer to the following table:

Contact	Tapering (wide crowns and narrow cervices)	Square (boxed)	Ovoid (transitional)
1. Between incisors	Contact starts at the incisal ridge incisally and a little towards the labial, labio-lingually	Start at incisal ridge incisally and in line with it labio-lingually	1. Slightly lingual to the incisal ridge, labio-lingually 2. Mesial contacts start at ¼ of the crown inciso-gingivally 3. Distal contacts start ⅓ to ½ of the crown inciso-gingivally
2. Canine	1. Mesial contact at the incisal ridge 2. Distal contact near the middle 3. Very angular	1. Close to incisal ridges incisally 2. In line with them labio-lingually	1. The same as square type
3. Bicuspids	1. Buccal periphery almost at buccal axial angle (buccal third) of the tooth 2. Occlusal periphery at the junction of occlusal and middle third of the tooth 3. Contact is deviated buccally 4. Cusps form ¼-⅓ of the crown	1. Buccal periphery more towards buccal axial angle (buccal third) 2. Occlusal periphery is at occlusal third 3. Short cusps	1. Convexity of MR carries occlusal periphery towards middle third 2. Buccal periphery at junction of buccal and middle third
4. Molars mesial contact	1. Buccal periphery almost at the buccal axial angle of the tooth 2. O-periphery, at junction of occlusal and middle third of the crown 3. Large cusps	1. The same as premolar 2. Extension lingually stops in the middle third (1-4 mm)	Same as bicuspids
5. Molar distal contact	1. Buccal periphery at the middle third 2. Occlusal periphery at the middle third 3. Distal contact of first molar is variable due to position of distal cusps	More lingually deviated than the mesial but not to the extent of the tapering teeth	Buccal periphery in line with the central groove in the occlusal surface

Continued.

Contact	Tapering (wide crowns and narrow cervices)	Square (boxed)	Ovoid (transitional)
6. Embrasures	1. Wide variations 2. Incisal and labial are negligible 3. Gingival and lingual embrasures between anterior teeth are the widest and longest in the mouth 4. Buccal embrasures are small 5. Lingual embrasures are long, with medium width 6. Gingival embrasures between posterior teeth are broad and long	1. Incisal, lingual, occlusal and buccal embrasures are nil 2. Gingival embrasures are almost not noticeable; if found, they are very narrow and flat 3. Lingual embrasures are very narrow (may be slit) and long	1. Incisal, buccal, labial and occlusal embrasures are wider and deeper than the others 2. Gingival and lingual are short and broad

Contact areas and embrasures are associated with an interdental col following the apical outline of the contact area. The relationship between adjacent teeth at their contact areas is not absolutely static, as there is an allowance by the periodontal ligament and bone elasticity for slight tooth movement in three dimensions. However, for practical purposes, this relationship can be considered fixed. The contact area should create a positive tight relationship between adjacent teeth, unyielding to physiologically functional forces in order to preserve intact the mesio-distal dimension of the dental arch and to protect the investing periodontium. These features should also be assimilated in such a way as to discourage the accumulation of plaque and cariogenic material at and around the involved surfaces. With age, the surface dimensions of the contact areas are increased as a result of proximal abrasion and attrition. This leads to a decrease in proximal convexities, i.e., creating contact areas similar to the box-shaped teeth. This enlargement of the contact area will subsequently decrease the dimensions of the adjoining embrasures.

II. Marginal Ridges

It is imperative to have a marginal ridge of proper dimensions, i.e., compatible to the dimension of the occlusal cuspal anatomy, creating a pronounced adjacent triangular fossa and producing an adjacent occlusal embrasure. A marginal ridge should always be formed in two planes bucco-lingually, meeting at a very obtuse angle. This feature is essential when an opposing functional cusp occludes with the marginal ridge.

A marginal ridge with these specifications is essential for the balance of the teeth in the arch, the prevention of food impaction proximally, the protection of the peridontium, the prevention of recurrent and contact decay, and for helping in efficient mastication. Some marginal ridges function as working occluding cuspal elements.

The following diagram (Fig. 4) illustrates how a proper marginal ridge will perform these functions.

Forces 1 and 2, acting on two adjacent marginal ridges, will have their horizontal components, 1H and 2H drive the two teeth towards each other, thus preventing any impaction proximally, maintaining the mesio-distal dimension of the dental arch and anchoring the teeth against each other. But, as men-

tioned, with age, the dimensions of the marginal ridges and occlusal embrasures are reduced, due to vertical occlusal attrition and proximal flattening of the contact areas.

III. Facial and Lingual Contours and Related Structures

In a vertical direction, all tooth crowns will exhibit some convex curvatures occlusal to the cervical line. This curvature is sometimes called the cervical ridge. Although the extent of the curvature will vary in different individuals, it is not normal for a curvature on a completely erupted permanent tooth to extend more than 1 mm beyond the cervical line. Usually the extent is much less.

The curvatures on the labial, buccal and lingual surfaces of all maxillary teeth and on the buccal surfaces of mandibular posterior teeth will be rather uniform. In any mouth, the average curvature is about 0.5 mm or less.

Mandibular posterior teeth will have a lingual curvature of approximately 1 mm, with the crest of the curvature at the middle third of the crown instead of at the cervical third, which is caused mainly by the lingual inclination of these teeth. It is not uncommon for maxillary posterior teeth to have similar curvatures on the lingual aspects, especially when the buccal inclinations of these teeth are less than normal.

Mandibular anterior teeth will have less curvature on the crown above the cervical line than any other teeth. Usually it is less than 0.5 mm, and occasionally it is so slight that it is

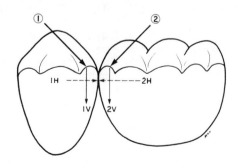

Fig. 12-4

hardly distinguishable. The canines may show a little more curvature than the central and lateral incisors.

Although inciso-apical curvature of the facial and lingual surfaces of all teeth is convex, the incisal one-half to two-thirds of the lingual surfaces of anterior teeth displays some concavities, a feature more pronounced with upper central and lateral incisors. These concavities are less pronounced in lower central and lateral incisors, and least pronounced in cuspids (both upper and lower). For upper anterior teeth the concavities are an essential anterior determinant for mandibular movement. For upper and lower anterior teeth, concavities serve to reduce the tooth bulk from its gingival third (maximum dimension) to its incisal third (minimal dimension). These concavities may exist as one concavity per tooth or as two separate concavities per tooth, according to the tooth's role in guiding mandibular movements. In the mesio-distal dimension tooth crowns also exhibit certain curvatures. At some locations they are convex and at others they are concave.

In posterior teeth there will be a mesio-distal convexity, corresponding to each cusp in the anatomical crown portion of the tooth. In molars where there is more than one cusp bucally and lingually, the facial or lingual convexities are interrupted by concavities at the occlusal one-half to two-thirds of the crown. However, the convexities are uninterrupted apical to these concavities creating a continuous convex surface mesio-distally. This convexity on the facial and lingual areas decreases in magnitude as we approach the CEJ. At the CEJ, or slightly occlusal to it, the facial or lingual surface will flatten or become concave, especially if the crown surface joins a bifurcation.

In anterior teeth, the entire labial surface always has a pronounced convexity mesio-distally. The magnitude of this convexity increases gradually from the incisal ridge apically, reaching its maximum just incisal to the CEJ (gingival line), then decreases to an almost flat surface at the CEJ.

The lingual surface of an anterior tooth exhibits a mesio-distal convexity only at its apical one-third to one-half. From that point incisally it is concave, completing a dish-shaped surface started by the incisal guidance concavities. Each tooth accommodates one or two concavities at this location, completing the incisal guidance configuration.

The proper mesio-distal contour at different levels and locations of the facial and lingual surfaces is vital for the health of the investing periodontium. A comparison between the contour of the teeth and periodontium contour mesio-distally will reveal that both contours should be the same to ensure physiologic movement of the structures and materials.

IV. Hazards of Faulty Reproduction of Physio-Anatomical Features of Teeth in Restorations

A. Contact size

Creating a contact that is too broad, bucco-lingually or occluso-gingivally (Fig. 5), in addition to changing the tooth anatomy, will change the anatomy of the interdental col. The normal "saddle-shaped" area will become broadened. The epithelium of the col, like that lining the gingival sulcus, is non-keratinized, and, as a result, the area for the development of incipient periodontal disease, is markedly increased. Furthermore, the broadened contact produces an interdental area

that the patient is less able to clean, i.e., increases the areas susceptible to future decay. The microbial plaque develops more readily and as a result, the papillary area becomes inflamed and edematous.

Broadening the contact area will of necessity, be at the expense of the dimensions and shapes of the buccal and lingual embrasures. This usually leads to improper movement or flow of masticated material. In turn, this leads to adhesion of debris and possible intraproximal impaction of that debris.

Finally, broadening the contact area could also be at the expense of the gingival embrasures, so that the restoration could encroach physico-mechanically on the interdental periodontium, predisposing to its destruction.

Creating a contact that is too narrow bucco-lingually or occluso-gingivally (Fig. 6), besides changing the anatomy of the tooth, will allow food to be impacted vertically and/or horizontally on the delicate non-keratinized epithelial col area. Of course, this will lead to greater susceptibility for microbic plaque accumulation, which, in turn, predisposes to the same periodontal and caries problems.

A contact area placed *too occlusally* will result in a flattened marginal ridge at the expense of the occlusal embrasures (Fig. 7). A contact area placed *too bucally or lingually* will result in a flattened restoration at the expense of the buccal or lingual embrasures (Fig. 8, A and B). A contact area placed *too gingivally* will increase the depth of the occlusal embrasures at the expense of the contact area's own size or at the expense of broadening or impinging upon the interdental col (interdental papillae) (Fig. 8C).

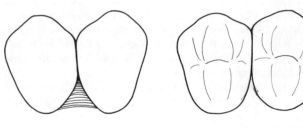

Fig. 12-5

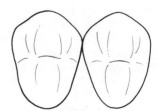

Fig. 12-6

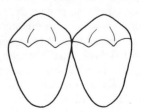

Fig. 12-7

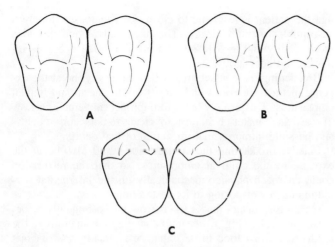

Fig. 12-8

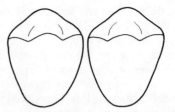

Fig. 12-9

A loose (open) contact creates continuity of the embrasures with each other and with the interdental col (Fig. 9). All of these defects in the contact area will allow for the impaction of food and the accumulation of bacterial plaques, with the accompanying periodontal and caries problems (Figs 10 A and B). Therefore, the proper reproduction of the size and location of the contact areas to imitate the natural dentition is essential for the success of the treatment and restoration of the proximal surface.

B. Contact configuration

Creating a contact area that is flat (deficient convexity) can make it too broad buccally, lingually, occlusally, and/or gingivally. On the other hand, a contact area with excessive convexity will diminish the extent of the contact area. Both will predispose to the aforementioned problems of decay and periodontal destruction (Fig. 11).

A concave contact area in a restoration usually occurs in restoring adjacent teeth simultaneously. It is accompanied by an adjacent restoration with a convex proximal surface. Besides broadening and mislocating the contact area, the interlocking between the concavity and the adjacent convexity can immobilize the contacting teeth, depriving them of normal, stimulating physiologic movements, resulting in peridontitis and/or mechanical breakdown. Also, in the restoration with a concave contact area, it is impossible to create the proper size of marginal ridge or adjacent occlusal anatomy (Fig. 12).

C. Contour

1. Facial and lingual convexities

It was previously theorized that the vertical convex curvatures on the facial and lingual surfaces of teeth hold the gingiva under definite tension and also protect the gingival margin by deflecting food material away from this margin during mastication. It was also suggested that the proper degree of curvature is that which could deflect food over the gingival margin, thereby preventing undue frictional irritation, while allowing stimulation of the soft tissues enabling them to keep their tone. Recent experimental and clinical data do not fully support this theory. It has been revealed that there is always more inherent danger in overconvex rather than underconvex facial and lin-

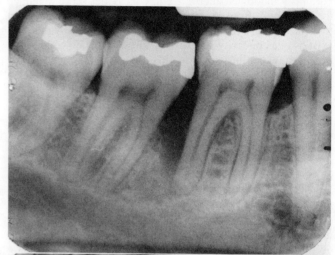

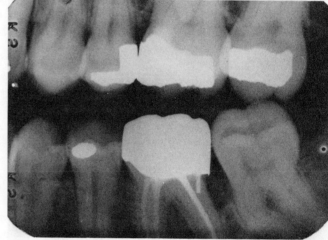

Fig. 12-10. A, Flattened, opened contact area with incompatible MR in the MO amalgam of tooth #31 led to infraboney pocket between teeth #30 and #31. **B,** Treated infraboney pocket between teeth #19 and 18. Recurrence is possible if crown proximal contour, contact, (flat distal contact area of tooth #19) and MR are not corrected.

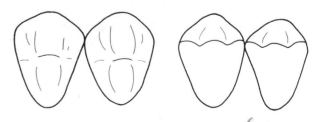

Fig. 12-11

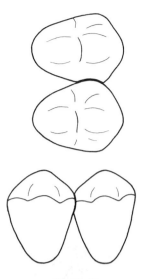

Fig. 12-12

gual surfaces of teeth. The overconvex curvatures can create an undisturbed environment for the accumulation and growth of cariogenic and plaque ingredients at the gingival margin, apical to the height of contour. Additionally, this deprives the free and attached gingiva facially and/or lingually from the massaging-stimulating-keratinizing effect of the apical components of the food stream. Also from these data it is known that there are no apparent hazards from underconvex curvatures of the facial and lingual surfaces.

2. Facial and lingual concavities

Those concavities occlusal to the height of contour, whether they occur on anterior or posterior teeth, are involved in the occlusal static and dynamic relations, as they determine the pathways for mandibular teeth into and out of centric.

Deficient or mislocated concavities will lead to premature contacts during mandibular movements, which could inhibit the physiologic capabilities of these movements. On the other hand, excessive concavities can invite extrusion, rotation, or tilting of occluding cuspal elements into non-physiologic relations with opposing teeth.

Concavities apical to the height of contour, therapeutically or pathologically exposed, are essential for the proper maintenance of the accompanying new components of the adjacent periodontium and must be imitated in a restoration. Deficient concavities at these locations can create restoration overhangs, and excessive concavities decrease the chance for successful plaque control in these extremely plaque-retaining areas. In other words, the mesio-distal curvatures of a restoration should recreate the original tooth contour, insofar as these curvatures are a necessary compliment to the occluso-gingival curvatures.

3. Areas of proximal contour adjacent to the contact area

In addition to creating a contact area of proper size, location, and configuration, it is also essential to restore to a proper contour that portion of the proximal surface not involved in the contact. This would include the areas occlusal, buccal, lingual, and gingival to the contact area. Fabricating a restoratoin that does not reproduce the concavities and convexities which occur here naturally will lead to restoration overhangs

and underhangs, vertical and horizontal impaction of debris, and impingement upon the adjacent periodontal structures.

D. Marginal ridges

The following examples will illustrate the consequences incurred by the creation of a faulty marginal ridge:

a. Absence of a marginal ridge in the restoration (Fig. 13)

By the absence of a marginal ridge, force 1 will be directed toward the proximal surface of the adjacent tooth. 1H and 2H, the horizontal components of forces 1 and 2, will tend to drive the two teeth away from each other. Meanwhile, the vertical components, 1V and 2V, can impact food and other intraoral materials interproximally.

b. A marginal ridge with an exaggerated occlusal embrasure (Fig. 14)

Exaggerating the occlusal embrasure will direct forces 1 and 2 toward the adjacent proximal surfaces, with the horizontal components, 1H and 2H, separating the teeth and the vertical components, 1V and 2V, driving debris interproximally.

c. Adjacent marginal ridges not compatible in height (Fig. 15, A, B, C)

Constructing a restoration with a marginal ridge higher than the adjacent one (Fig. 15A), will allow force A to work on the proximal surface of the restoration. The horizontal component, AH, will drive the restored tooth away from the contacting tooth, and the vertical component will drive debris interproximally. Even in the presence of force B, with its horizontal component acting on the adjacent marginal ridge, there will be some separation of teeth as the surface hold for force B is too small to counteract that of force A. By constructing a restoration with a marginal ridge lower than the adjacent one (Fig. 15B), the same thing will occur, but the major movement will be in the non-restored tooth.

d. A marginal ridge with no adjacent triangular fossa (Fig. 16)

In this situation there are no occlusal planes in the marginal ridges for the occlusal forces to act upon, so there are no horizontal components to drive the teeth toward each other, closing the contact. Furthermore, the vertical force will tend to impact food interproximally.

e. A marginal ridge with no occlusal embrasure (Fig. 17)

In this case, the two adjacent marginal ridges will act like a pair of tweezers grasping food substance passing over it. Although debris may not be forced interproximally, it will be very difficult to remove once it is thus trapped.

f. A one-planed marginal ridge in the bucco-lingual direction (interrupted line, Fig. 18)

Usually, the facial and lingual inclines of a marginal ridge are part of the occluding components of the tooth. Therefore, making them one-planed can create premature contacts during both functional and static occlusion. A one-planed marginal ridge increases the depth of the adjacent triangular fossa magnifying stresses in this area. Moreover, the one-planed marginal ridge could increase the height of the marginal ridge in the center, making it amenable to the adverse effects of horizontal components of force. Likewise, a one-planed marginal ridge will deflect the food stream away from normal, proximal embrasure movements (spill away).

g. A thin marginal ridge in its mesio-distal bulk (Fig. 19)

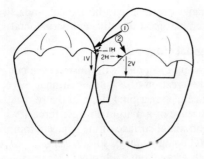

Fig. 12-13

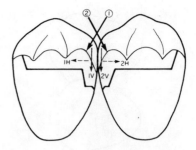

Fig. 12-14

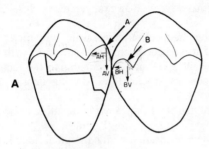

A

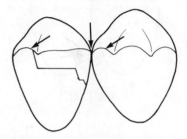

Fig. 12-16

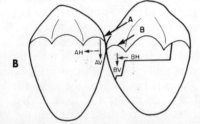

B

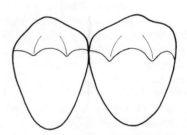

Fig. 12-17

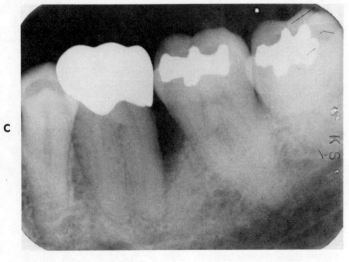

C

Fig. 12-15. C, Boney defect between tooth #18 and tooth #19 due to incompatibility of marginal ridge heights.

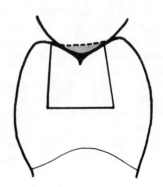

Fig. 12-18

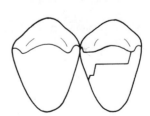

Fig. 12-19

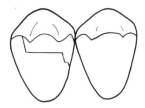

Fig. 12-20

will be susceptible to fracture or deformation leading to the problems of the previously mentioned faulty marginal ridge. Also, this thinness may leave either shallow or deep adjacent fossa or bulky occlusal anatomy with their aforementioned inherent problems.

h. Marginal ridges not compatible in dimension or location with the rest of the occluding surface components predisposes to similar problems (Fig. 20). As the marginal ridge is frequently a part of occluding anatomy, it should have the same occlusal pattern that dictates the shapes, locations, and inter-relationships of the rest of the occluding components. (This is discussed in detail in the chapter on single tooth restorations and the stomatognathic system).

Procedures for the Formulation of Proper Contacts and Contours

Intraoral Procedures for the Creation of Contacts and Contours

For the proper reproduction, with a restorative material, of the previously described physio-anatomical features of teeth, two operative acts must precede or accompany the restorative procedure: tooth (teeth) movement and matricing.

I. Tooth Movement:

It is the act of either separating the involved teeth from each other, bringing them closer to each other, and/or changing their spatial position in one or more dimensions. This is done in order to facilitate the creation of a physiologically functional contact, contour and occluding anatomy in the restored tooth.

The objectives of tooth movement are:

1. To bring drifted, tilted or rotated teeth to their indicated physiologic positions as a prerequisite for proper reproduction of the proximal surfaces in restorative materials. This should be done to avoid flat or concave proximal surfaces and contact areas in the restoration, to regain the mesio-distal dimension of the dental arch, and to assure physiologic loading of the restored tooth.

2. To close space between teeth not amenable to closure by the contemplated restoration.

3. To move teeth to another location, so that when restored, they will be in a position most physiologically acceptable by the periodontium.

4. To move teeth occlusally (extrusion) or apically (intrusion) in order to make them restorable.

5. To move teeth from a non-functional or traumatically functional location to a physiologically functional one.

6. To move teeth to a position, so that when restored, they will be in the most esthetically pleasing situation.

7. To move teeth in a direction and to a location to increase the dimensions of available tooth structure for the resistance and retention forms of the contemplated restoration.

8. To create a space sufficient for the thickness of the matrix band interproximally. This space should be *in addition* to the mesio-distal dimension of the restoration, *not* at its expense. This is necessary to create a positive, (plus) tight contact.

Besides, the use of tooth separation preparatory to and during the formulation of the proximal contacting surfaces, it can also be used as convenience means for facilitating access to proximal cavity preparations, especially Class III preparations. In addition, it can be used to detect proximal decay, to facilitate adequate polishing of the restoration's proximal surfaces, and to remove foreign bodies impacted proximally that are not dislodgeable by floss or brushes.

There are two principal methods of tooth movement: rapid or immediate tooth movement and slow or delayed tooth movement.

A. Rapid or immediate tooth movement

This is a mechanical type of separation that creates either proximal separation at the point of the separator's introduction and/or improved closeness of the proximal surface opposite the point of the separator's introduction (Fig. 21).

Indications

Besides the general indications, it can be used preparatory to slow tooth movement, or to maintain a space gained by slow tooth movement. This type of tooth movement should not exceed the thickness of the involved tooth's periodontal ligament, as more separation can tear these ligaments at one site and crush them at the other. In other words, it should not exceed 0.2-0.5 mm. Rapid tooth movement can be done by one of the following methods.

1. Wedge method

Separation is accomplished by the insertion of a pointed wedge-shaped device between the teeth, in order to create separation at that point or closure on the opposite proximal side of the involved teeth. The more the wedge moves facially or lingually, the greater will be the separation. The following are examples of these types of separators:

a. Elliot separator (Fig. 22) is indicated for short-duration separation that does not necessitate stabilization. It is useful in examining proximal surfaces or in final polishing of restored contacts.

Procedure

Adjust the two opposing wedges of the separator interproximally so that they are positioned gingival to the contact area, not impinging on the interdental papillae or the interceptal rubber dam. Move the knob clockwise so that the wedges move towards one another establishing the desired separation.

b. Wood or plastic wedges (Fig. 23)

These are triangular shaped wedges, usually made of medicated wood or synthetic resin. In cross-section the base of the triangle will be in contact with the interdental papillae, gingival to the gingival margin of the proximal cavity. The two sides of the triangle should coincide with the corresponding two sides (mesial and distal) of the gingival embrasure. The apex of the triangle should coincide with the gingival start of the contact area.

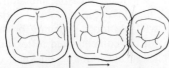

Prior to Separation

Note Open Distal Contact Caused by Mesial Drifting
of First Molar Due to Mesial Carious Lesion

After Separation

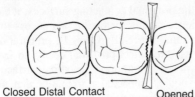

Closed Distal Contact

Opened Mesial Contact to
Facilitate Instrumentation
and Restoration

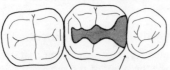

Normal Physiological Contacts Restored

Fig. 12-21

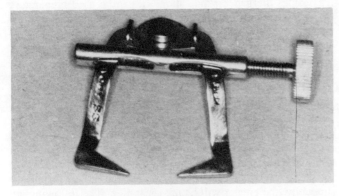

Fig. 12-22

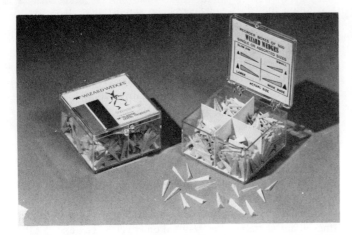

Fig. 12-23

The wedge is used in conjunction with matrices for inserting plastic restorative materials. Wedges perform the following functions:

i. They assure the close adaptability of the matrix band to the tooth, gingival to the gingival margin of the preparation, thus preventing plastic restorative materials from accumulating between the band and the tooth below the gingival extremity of the cavity preparation.

ii. They occupy the space designated to be the gingival embrasure, preventing the restorative material from impinging on it, thus assuring proper health for the gingival interdental col (papillae).

iii. They define the gingival extent of the contact area as well as the facial and lingual embrasures, thereby assuring the health of the proximal periodontal tissues.

iv. They create some separation to compensate for the thickness of the matrix band and minor drifting of the teeth.

v. They establish atraumatic retraction of the rubber dam and the gingiva from the gingival margin of the cavity preparation, thereby producing a temporary hemostasis and minimizing moisture in an area which will receive moisture-sensitive dental materials.

vi. They assure the immobilization of the matrix band against movement both facial-lingually and cervico-occlusally during insertion of the restorative material.

vii. They protect the interproximal gingival from unexpected trauma.

Although wedges are supplied in different sizes to suit different locations, they should not be used as supplied. Because of infinite variations in the configuration of the gingival embrasures they are to occupy, the wedges should be trimmed to exactly fit each gingival embrasure.

The main advantages of wood wedges are that they are easily cut and trimmed and they absorb water intraorally. This causes them to swell, improving their interproximal retention. The man advantage of resin wedges is that they can be plastically molded and bent to correspond with the configuration of the interdental col.

c. For instantaneous separation of teeth during operative procedures in anterior teeth, e.g., planing the axial walls, accentuating the line angles, or polishing in Class III restoration, wedging the nail of the thumb or the first finger between the teeth will make rapid separation which is usually sufficient for these purposes.

2. Traction method (Fig. 24, 25)

This is always done with mechanical devices which engage the proximal surfaces of the teeth to be separated by means of holding arms. These are mechanically moved apart, creating separation between the clamped teeth.

Examples of the traction method include:

a. Non-interfering true separator (Fig. 24)

This device is indicated when continuous stabilized separation is required during the dental operation. Its advantages are that the separation can be increased or decreased after stabilization, and the device is non-interfering.

Procedure

Insure that the jaws of the separator are closed together. Apply the jaws closest to the bow against the tooth to be operated upon. The jaws further from the bow will move later in the adjustment. Apply a piece of softened compound to the teeth under the separator, locking it there by introducing it in their buccal and lingual embrasures. Also cover the incisal or occlusal surface under the separator with the compound. Another piece of softened compound is applied occlusal to the separator so that it is enclosed within the compound, attached to the underlying tooth, i.e., stabilized. No compound should be permitted to interfere with the movements of the jaws or the screws.

A wrench is now used to move the far (movable) jaws over the approximating tooth there, exerting the pressure of separation. The nut on the facial side should be moved first until the jaw touches the surface needed, then that of the lingual side, then repeat the adjustment until the desired amount of separations (closure) is obtained. A beaver-tail burnisher may be used during the process to move any septal part of the rubber dam, so it does not become engaged in the jaws of the instrument.

b. Ferrier double-bow separator (Fig. 25, A and B)

With this device, the separation is stabilized throughout the operation. Its advantage is that the separation is shared by the contacting teeth, and not at the expense of one tooth, as with the previous type of instrument.

Procedure

The four arms are adjusted so that each will hold a corner of the proximal surface of the contacting teeth. The arms will be gingival to the contact area, yet will not impinge upon the rubber dam or gingiva.

A wrench applied to the labial and lingual is used to make the desired separation.

Compound is applied gingival and occlusal to the mesial and distal bows, as described for the previous separator, thereby stabilizing it by attaching it to the underlying teeth.

B. Slow or delayed tooth movement

1. Indications

When teeth have drifted and/or tilted considerably, rapid movement of teeth to the proper position will endanger the periodontal ligaments. Therefore, slow tooth movement, over a period of weeks, will allow the proper repositioning of teeth in a physiologic manner.

2. Methods

a. Separating wires

Thin pieces of wire are introduced gingival to the contact, then wrapped around the contact area. The two ends are twisted together to create separation not to exceed 0.5 mm. The twisted ends are then bent into the buccal or lingual embrasure to prevent impingement upon soft tissue or interference with food flow. The wires are then tightened periodically to increase the separation. This is a very effective method of slow tooth movement, although the maximum amount of separation will be equivalent to the thickness of the wire.

b. Oversized temporaries

Resin temporaries that are oversized mesio-distally may achieve slow separation. Resin is added to the contact areas periodically to increase the amount of separation, which will not exceed 0.5 mm per visit.

c. Orthodontic appliances

For tooth movement of any magnitude, fixed orthodontic appliances are the most effective and predictable method available. Comparable end results may be achieved by removable

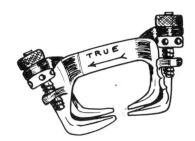

Fig. 12-24

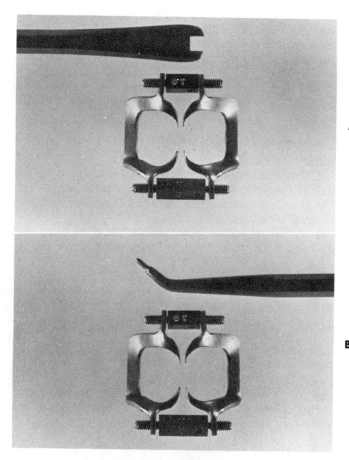

A

B

Fig. 12-25

orthodontic appliances, but they require longer treatment (see chapter 28).

After repositioning of the tooth (teeth) by any of the aforementioned delayed tooth movement techniques, it is necessary to use one or more of the immediate tooth movement techniques, just before or during the restoration fabrications, to create space and to compensate for the thickness of the band material, if a proximal matrix is involved.

II. Matricing

Matricing is the procedure whereby a temporary wall is created opposite to axial walls, surrounding areas of tooth structure that were lost during preparation. It is used with restorative materials that are introduced in a plastic state. The matrix wall should possess the exact three-dimensional contour (including the contact area) of the future restoration. More importantly, the matrix should be capable of imparting this configuration to the inserted restorative material during its plastically deformable state. Not only should it be immobile during the setting of the restorative material, but also it should not react with or adhere to the restorative material. On the other hand, it should be easily removed after hardening of the restorative material, without compromising the created contact and contour or the restorative material's characteristics.

The matrix is always formed of two parts; the band, which is a piece of metal or polymeric material used to support and give form to the restorative material during its introduction and hardening, and the retainer, which is a device by which the band can be retained in its designated position and shape. The retainer could be a mechanical device, a wire, dental floss and/or compound.

The matrix is essential for the proper reproduction of the proximal, facial and lingual anatomy in any restoration of plastic nature.

A. Objectives

The matrix should:

1. Displace the gingiva and rubber dam away from the cavity margins during introduction of the restorative material. This will assure maximum wetting and adaptation of the restorative material to the preparation details.

2. Assure dryness and non-contamination of the details and the space to be covered with and occupied by the setting restorative material.

3. Provide shape for the restoration during the setting of the restorative material, i.e., the band materials should be unyielding to the energies of insertion.

4. Maintain its shape during hardening of the material.

5. Confine the restorative material within the cavity preparation and predetermined surface configuration. Therefore, the matrix should provide a temporary wall of resistance during introduction of the restorative material. It should also resist and compensate for the dimensional change in the material during its setting by applying a positive pressure against it at this stage.

B. Types of matrices

1. Matrices for Class I cavity preparations to receive a restorative material inserted in a plastic state (Double-banded Tofflemire for Class I, Designs 4, 5, 6, 7, and 8 cavity preparations (Fig. 26).

Procedure

Acquire a working understanding of the Tofflemire retainer (see next section).

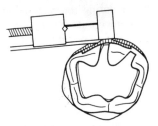

Fig. 12-26. Occlusal view: lower molar, double-banded tofflemire matrix.

Turn the large vice-moving knob until the slotted vice is about ¼ inch from the inner end of the retainer (Fig. 26). Loosen the vice screw until its pointed end is clear of the slotted vice (Fig. 27). Make a loop out of the universal band creating an edge with a narrow circumference and an edge with a wide circumference. The narrow circumference edge is placed gingivally and the wide circumference edge is placed occlusally. Insert the occlusal edge of the universal matrix into the slotted vice first. The free ends of the band are inserted into the vice while the looped end of the band extends away from the retainer. (The band is inserted until it is in contact with the arched top of the vice slot.) Always be sure that the slotted end of the vice is facing gingivally. This will facilitate easy occlusal removal of the retainer.

Tighten the vice-screw to lock the band in the vice. Guide the looped end of the band gently over the tooth. The size of the loop may be increased or decreased by turning the vice-moving knob. With the band in position around the tooth, tighten the vice moving knob. Ideally, the retainer should be parallel and adjacent to the facial surfaces of the quadrant of teeth being operated on.

An additional small piece of matrix band material is then contoured to the facial or lingual axial configuration of the contemplated restoration and inserted between the tooth and the previously positioned and retained matrix in the area of the facial or lingual extension of the cavity preparation. This piece of material should lap over the margins of the extension by about 1.5-2 mm circumferentially.

With a beaver-tail burnisher, create a separation between the two bands. Select a wedge that will create and maintain the proper separation between the two bands and thereby enable the formation of the proper contour facially and/or lingually. Cover the wedge(s) with softened compound and insert it between the two bands and cool to harden.

Check the stability of each component of the matrix and be sure of its unyielding resistance to the insertion energy necessary for the restorative material.

2. Matrices for Class II cavity preparations to receive a restorative material inserted in a plastic state.

a. single-banded Tofflemire for Class II Designs 1, 2, 3, 6, 7, 8 cavity preparations (Fig. 27).

This is the most practical matrix for Class II cavity preparations, making a very stable device against which restorative materials can be condensed. Its use is made universal by the easy application and removal of the band to and from its holder without disturbing the condensed material.

Procedure

Repeat the basic steps from the previously described double-banded arrangement. Usually (especially in Designs, 1, 2, and 3 cavity preparations) the band will go to its destination clear of the cavity margins and adjacent soft tissues. However, in some cases of Designs 1, 2, 3, and in most cases of Designs 6, 7, and 8, the following modifications should be performed.

If the cavity preparation involves one proximal surface only and there is a substantial difference between the heights of the interproximal gingiva on the mesial and distal sides of the tooth, the matrix band should be trimmed so that it is narrower (occluso-apically) on the side where the interproximal gingiva is more occlusally located. It may also be possible to use matrix bands with only one gingival projection, which should coincide

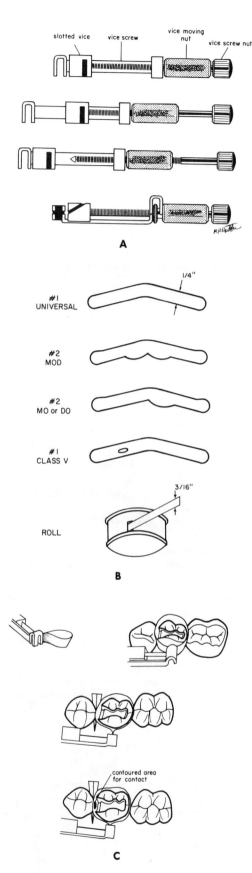

with the proximal side where the interproximal gingiva is more apically located (Fig. 27B, # 2 MO and DO).

If the gingival extension of the proximal portion of the cavity preparation is more apically located than gingival lines facially and lingually, there is danger of cutting the gingival tissues facially and lingually in using a band with a straight gingival edge. In this situation, it is necessary to either reduce the occluso-apical width of the band facially and lingually or to use a band with apical projections which coincide and cover the gingival extension of the proximal portion of the cavity preparation. The latter bands are supplied precut, but they always need further trimming facially, lingually or even proximally in order for them to fit, exactly, the outline of the proximal preparation without injuring gingival tissues (Fig. 27B, # 2 MOD).

In preparations with subgingival margins, especially at the axial angles or any surface protrusion of the tooth, the edges of the band occasionally encounter the gingival margin and become bent inward, preventing further seating of the band. For this reason there should be unprepared, exposed tooth surface apical to the gingival margin of the preparation to support the band in its apical path and to prevent its inward collapse or bending. This may necessitate gingival retraction or cutting. Also, in these situations, the band edges should be guided in their apical path by placing a flat-bladed, blunt instrument between the band and the adjacent unprepared tooth surface apical to the gingival margin. This will enable the band to pass by the gingival margin without encountering it or the gingival floor.

Although it is preferable to put the retainer in the buccal vestibule, parallel to the adjacent teeth, sometimes, due to shallow sulcus or sizable buccal involvement of the tooth in a cavity preparation, the retainer is placed on the lingual. This usually necessitates a contrangled retainer. However, the retainer should never be located at a right angle to the facial or lingual surfaces of the teeth operated upon as this will drastically change the occluso-apical contour of the band.

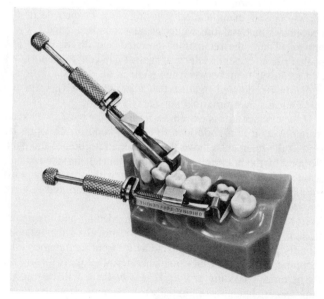

Fig. 12-27. A, Tofflemire retainer: bottom view (note various exits from vice). **B,** Bands for tofflemire matrix. **C,** Single-banded tofflemire matrix for a Class II cavity preparation.

[handwritten at top: For adding eye should burnish it to bring mercury to surface and if it is not shiny the adding can't produce.]

The junction between the retainer and the band should always be located next to unprepared intact tooth surface to insure its stability and prevent unnecessary accumulation of excess restorative material at that location.

As soon as the band is in place and all cavity margins can be seen inside the matrix, a wedge, comparable to the dimensions of the future gingival embrasure, is chosen and tried (always from the opposite side of the retainer attachment). The wedges should be trimmed using sharp knives. Plastic wedges could be trimmed with sand-paper discs and molded, after softening in warm water. Sometimes the wood wedge is dipped in warmed compound and tried until it exactly fits the contemplated space for the future gingival embrasure.

Usually one wedge from the opposite side of the retainer is sufficient. However, more than one wedge could be necessary if the configuration of the gingival embrasure cannot be created by one wedge only. More than one wedge could also be necessary in the following situations: the gingival margins are located very apically, proximal preparations adjacent to a very exaggerated interdental col, the gingival margin is located in a proximal surface concavity or defect, more separation is needed than can be supplied by one wedge, or in extraordinarily large gingival embrasures resulting from extensive taper of the tooth or from gingival recession.

More than one wedge can be used, but usually two will suffice—one from the buccal and one from the lingual. Sometimes, more may be needed, and they should be inserted and located where they best fulfill their objectives. Each should be handled in the same manner as a single wedge. If more than one wedge is to be used, it is advisable to dip each in softened compound before the final insertion in order to assure their immobility.

Using a ball burnisher from within the cavity preparation, shape the matrix band material to create the outline of the contact and contour of the future restoration. If the cavity has buccal or lingual extensions, repeat the modifying steps in the double-banded Tofflemire application. Check the stability and the details of the matrix before the insertion of the restorative material.

For all Tofflemire applications after the insertion and initial hardening and manipulation (carving—see chapter 4) of the restorative material the wedges and secondary band are removed. Then, the retainer is loosened and disengaged. The primary band is bent (reflected) against adjacent tooth surfaces and removed from between the teeth in an occlusal direction while being pressed against the adjacent tooth (not on the restoration's own proximal surface).

If the contact area is extremely tight and the band is resistant to removal, it is a good idea to cut the band on the opposite side of the retainer, remove the roughened portion of the band (formed by the holding screws of the retainer); and then to pull it bucco-lingually (or linguo-buccally) with pressure against the adjacent tooth. This creates some separation and reduces friction with the restoration.

In MOD restorations, after initial hardening and manipulation of the restorative material and removal of the retainer, slightly pull one side of the band away from the retainer side, stopping just short of the roughened terminal parts formed by the retainer's holding screw. This way there will be enough band material facially or lingually to separately move the mesial or distal part of the band occlusally without moving the opposite proximal part of the band. As soon as you release one side of the band from the interproximal area, proceed with the other side as in a proximo-occlusal arrangement. If the contact is very tight, cut the band and drag each piece of the band faciolingually, (or vice versa) with positive pressure against the adjacent contacting teeth.

b. Ivory matrix No 1 (Fig. 28)

The band encircles a posterior proximal surface so it is indicated in unilateral Class II cavities. The band is attached to the retainer via a wedge-shaped projection which engages with the tooth at the embrasures of the unprepared surface.

c. Ivory matrix No 8 (Fig. 29)

The band encircles the entire crown of the tooth, so it is indicated for bilateral Class II cavities. Both ivory matrices are remnants of old techniques, so their operating instructions are not presented here. They are indicated for Class II, Designs 1, 2, and 3.

d. Black's matrices

Of all the different designs for matrices presented by Black to the profession, only two will be described. Both are indicated for Class II, Designs 1, 2, and 3 only.

i. Black's matrix for simple cases (Fig. 30) is recommended for the majority of small and medium size cavities.

Procedure

Cut a metallic band so that it will extend only slightly over the buccal and lingual surfaces of the tooth, beyond the buccal and lingual extremities of the cavity preparation. To prevent a

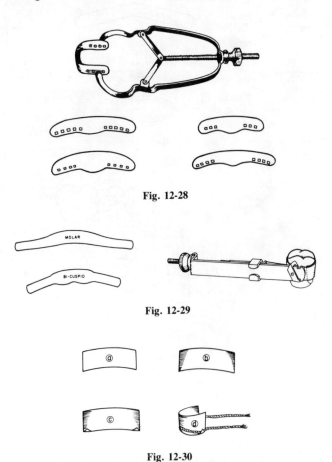

Fig. 12-28

Fig. 12-29

Fig. 12-30

wrap around holding ligature (a wire or dental floss) from slipping off the band and the band sliding gingivally, the corners of the gingival ends are turned up (occlusal) to hold the ligature.

ii. Black's matrix with a gingival extension (Fig. 31) to cover the gingival margin of a subgingival cavity

In this form, an extension is created in the occluso-gingival width of the band to cover the gingival margin of a subgingival cavity. The retaining procedures are the same as for the previous type of Black's matrix. All matrix bands should be trimmed, smoothed, and have corners rounded to prevent cutting of the ligatures and wounding of soft tissues. The ligature should be securely tied with a surgical knot on the side, after wrapping it around the tooth. A wedge should be carefully adjusted to produce and maintain the proper separation and to hold the band tightly over the gingival margin of the restoration.

e. Soldered band or seamless copper band matrix (Fig. 32)

These are indicated for badly broken down teeth, especially those receiving pin-retained amalgam restorations, with large buccal and lingual extensions, i.e., in Class II, Designs 6, 7 and 8 cavity preparations.

Procedure

A stainless steel band is cut according to the measured diameter of the crown of the tooth. Then the two ends are soldered together. Or, a seamless copper band is selected so that it barely clears the diameter of the tooth in the cervical area. Either band could be heated in a flame until it glows light red. It is then quenched in alcohol, thus softening the band for easier

handling. With curved scissors, festoon the band so its gingival periphery corresponds to the gingival curvature and the CEJ. The band is then smoothed to remove rough edges cervically and occlusally. With contouring pliers, contour the band to reproduce the proper shape in the contact area, as well as the buccal and lingual contours to be restored. Areas of the band in the contact area are reduced to a paper thinness using a coarse sand paper disc. They are then recontoured. Next, the band is seated on the tooth and tightened at the cervical end by pinching up a "tuck", using a flat-bladed plier at the gingival edge in an area accessible to the plier.

To stabilize the band and prevent cervical flashes of amalgam, wedges are placed gingival to the cervical margin of the preparation. Use the same procedures in choosing and adapting the wedges as described with the Tofflemire matrix. The external portions of the matrix and the wedges are covered with compound to further stabilize the matrix in the same way as applied to the double-bow separator (embrasures and surrounding occlusal surfaces). A wire "staple" is inserted facio-lingually in the compound to further stabilize it.

Apply a heated ball burnisher from the inside of the cavity to the band, softening the external compound and insuring the proper contour, contacts, and embrasures. After condensation and initial carving, the compound is removed and the matrix is cut at the area of the tuck. The matrix band is opened and then slipped far enough occlusally to cut its edges with a crown scissors over each contact area. With a plier or hemostat, grip the band at either side of the scissor's, cut and tear through each thinned contact portion to remove the band without damaging the proximal region of the amalgam.

f. The anatomical matrix (Fig. 33)

This is the most efficient means of reproducing contact and contour. It is entirely hand-made and contoured specifically for each individual case. It is especially useful in mutilated teeth or teeth requiring unique anatomy to be reproduced in the restoration. It is indicated for Class II, Designs 1, 2, 3, 6, 7, 8 cavity preparations.

Procedure

A piece of 0.001-0.002" stainless steel matrix band ⅛" in width is drawn between the handle of a pair of festooning

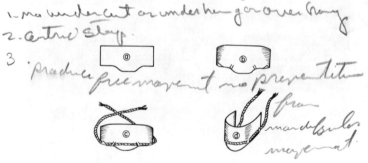

Fig. 12-31

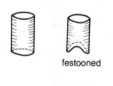

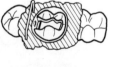
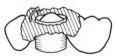

thinned area for contact

festooned   edge crimped in

Seamless copper band matrix
welded band matrix

Fig. 12-32

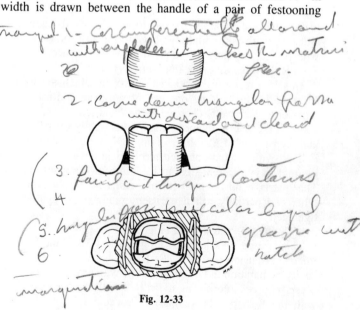

Fig. 12-33

scissors. This procedure facilitates the adaptation of the free ends of the matrix to the proximal surface of the tooth by curling the band.

The matrix is then cut to proper length. It must extend well beyond the cavity margins. To obtain the proper length, the centers of the proximo-buccal and proximo-lingual cusps are used as a guide. The matrix band is contoured with contouring pliers. Light pressure should be used and the process repeated until a suitable vertical, as well as horizontal, convexity is obtained. The band is then trimmed so that the matrix will extend well below the gingival margin of the cavity and at least 2 mm beyond the buccal and lingual margins of the cavity.

A wedge is selected and shaped to conform to the gingival embrasures, and it is then placed in warm water to soften it slightly. This procedure facilitates adaptation of the wedge to any irregularities of the proximal surface of the tooth. The wedge is forced into position, to insure adequate gingival adaptation, as well as to provide adequate separation.

Two small cones of compound are warmed in hot water. The tips are heated in a flame to further soften them and make them adhesive. These compound cones are foced one at a time, using thumb and finger pressure, into the buccal and lingual embrasures. The pressure is maintained until the compound has flowed evenly over the entire buccal and lingual surface of the adjacent teeth.

A wire staple is constructed from a metal paper clip, such that the length of the staple is slightly shorter than the crown of the tooth. The staple is heated in a flame and forced into the compound in the buccal and lingual embrasures. This adds to the stability of the matrix by locking together the two pieces of the blocking compound.

A warm ball burnisher is used to soften any compound that has been forced between the matrix and the adjacent tooth. The matrix is burnished lightly against the contacting tooth. The matrix is now ready for condensation of the restorative material.

After initial hardening of the inserted restorative material the compound is cracked at its occlusal junctions using a sharp chisel or knife. Then the separated pieces are removed using the attached staple, if it is still present. The wedges are removed using a hemostat and the band is curled backwards against the adjacent tooth and withdrawn bucco-lingually (or vice versa) with pressure against the adjacent proximal surface.

g. Roll-in band matrix (auto-matrix) (Fig. 34)

This is a recently introduced matrix in which the band is self-retained by holding one end of the band and rolling the other end over itself, decreasing the band length and, consequently, the matrix diameter until it fits tightly over the tooth and preparation. This rolling of one end of the band over itself is done with a hand-operated mechanical device. The matrix is supplied in different sizes to accommodate varieties of teeth. The matrix band comes with one end held in place and the other end partially rolled on itself, ready to be applied and tightened.

h. S-shaped matrix band (Fig. 35)

This is used for Class II, Designs 4 and 5 and the facial or lingual extension part of Class II, Design 7. The rest of the cavity preparation in Design 7 is done with any of the previous seven matrices after filling the very apically located extension with the S-shaped band matrix. Procedural instructions are exactly as described in Class III cavity preparations.

i. T-shaped matrix band (Fig. 36)

These are premade T-shaped brass or stainless steel matrix bands. The long arm of the T is bent or curled to encompass the tooth circumferentially and to overlap the short horizontal arm of T. This section is then bent over the long arm, loosely holding it in place. Wedges and stabilizing compound can be applied as in the anatomic matrix to add further stability.

3. Matrices for a cavity preparation for amalgam restorations on the distal of the cuspid

a. The S-shaped matrix (Fig. 35)

This is the ideal matrix for Class III cavity preparation on the distal of the cuspid, with either a labial or lingual access. The procedure for its construction is similar to that of the anatomic matrix.

Procedure

One half to one inch of regular strip matrix 0.001-0.002'' in thickness is used. A mirror handle is used to produce the S-shape in the strip. The band is contoured over the labial surface of the cuspid and the lingual surface of the adjacent bicuspid.

With contouring pliers, the strip is contoured in its middle part to create desired form for the restoration. It is then placed interproximally and wedged firmly apical to the gingival margin and covered with compound at its facial and lingual ends. The compound should lock into adjacent embrasures for stability.

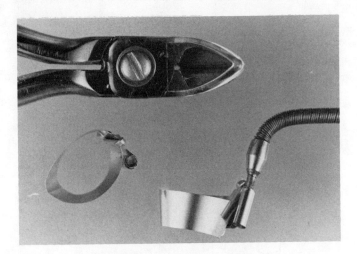

Fig. 12-34

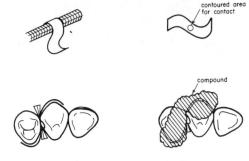

Fig. 12-35. S-shaped matrix.

If the lingual opening of the cavity preparation is blocked by this process, the compound can be removed with a warm instrument. (The previous arrangement is for lingual approach preparation. For a preparation with a labial approach, the exact reverse should be performed.) To insure proper contour of the band, a burnisher is heated, placed within the matrix and pushed towards the mesial surface of the bicuspid.

The remaining instructions are identical to those of the anatomic matrix. If this band is to be used for Class II, Designs 4, 5, or 7, it should wrap around the operated tooth on its non-access side. At the access side the band should be away from the cavity and adapted on the adjacent tooth to the nearest embrasure.

b. For a cavity preparation with incisal access on the distal of the cuspid the regular Tofflemire could be used efficiently.

4. Matrices for Class III direct tooth-colored restorations

These are usually transparent plastic matrix strips. For silicate cements they are usually celluloid strips and for resins they are cellophane strips. Mylar strips may be used for either material.

a. Matrix for Class III preparations with teeth in normal alignment (Fig. 37)

Procedure

The suitable plastic strip is burnished over the end of a steel instrument, e.g., handle of a tweezer, to produce a "belly" in the strip. This will allow for a curvature which, if properly contoured and designed, will reproduce the natural proximal contour of the tooth.

The strip is cut to allow the belly to be placed where the contact is desired. In placing a plastic strip between the teeth, it should be cut as wide as the tooth is long. Bear in mind that the tooth is cone-shaped, which will cause the apical corners of the strip to bend on the rubber dam, the gingival tissues or the palate. The corners of the strips should be trimmed therefore, to allow for better adaptation to the tooth and to prevent any excess material from forming on and beyond the facial or lingual margins. The length of the strip should be just sufficient to cover the labial and lingual surfaces of the tooth. If the strip extends onto an adjacent tooth, it will buckle and allow unnecessary excesses of restorative material to escape.

A wedge is trimmed and applied to hold the strip in place. This prevents the strip from slipping when it is brought over the inserted restorative material. The wedge also closes the avenue of escape for the material toward the gingiva and helps create the separation necessary to produce approximate contact. Wedges are introduced from the side opposite to that of access. Any portion of the wedge protruding toward the access side should be trimmed, so that it will not interfere with the convenient insertion of the restorative material.

For a labial approach preparation, use the fingers of the left hand for holding the strip firmly against the lingual surface of the tooth while the material is being placed in the cavity. The reverse is true for a lingual approach preparation.

After insertion of the material, reflect the free end of the strip and hold the whole strip firmly against the setting restorative material using the thumb and first finger of the left hand (for a right-handed operator). Mechanical holding devices can also be used.

b. Matrix for Class III preparations in teeth with irregular alignment

Procedure

A suitable plastic strip is contoured and adapted as described previously, and then removed. For a labial approach preparation a compound impression is taken of the lingual surface. The compound is allowed to overlap the adjoining teeth. It is

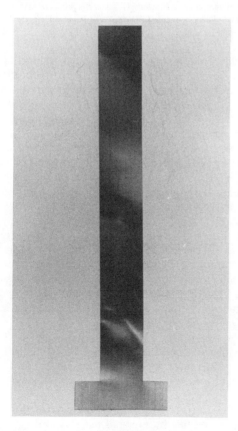

Fig. 12-36

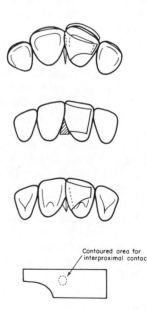

Fig. 12-37. Band strip matrix for a class III cavity preparation.

cooled, then removed. The compound impression should show an imprint of the cavity preparation. This excess of the compound impression from within the cavity is trimmed off to produce a flat surface.

The compound impression is then warmed. The surface is softened without distorting the form of the entire impression. This is done by holding the impression close to a flame only for a moment.

The strip is then placed into position again, followed by the compound impression against the strip, assuring a perfect adaptation of the matrix to the cavity on the lingual surface. The material is then introduced from the labial. The reverse can be done for a lingual approach cavity preparation.

c. Matrix for two small proximal preparations in contact with each other (Fig. 38)

An appropriate plastic strip is folded with one end slightly longer than the other to facilitate their separation after the insertion of the strip between the teeth. A loop ½'' in diameter is formed in the matrix strip. This loop is flattened and creased with a finger, making a ''T-shape'', and trimmed. The trimmed matrix is then placed between the teeth. For labial approach preparations the strip is held over the lingual surfaces with the fingers while the cavities are filled. After the insertion of the material each wing of the strip is folded over the setting restorative material and held with the thumb of the left hand. These instructions are for Class III cavities with a labial approach. For those with a lingual approach, reverse the position of the strip.

5. Matrices for Class IV preparations for direct tooth-colored materials

a. The plastic strip for inciso-proximal cavities (Fig. 39)
Procedure

A suitable plastic strip is folded at an angle into an L-shape, then sealed with a plastic cement or any adhesive that does not react with the tooth-colored material. One side of the strip is cut so that it is as wide as the length of the tooth. The other side is cut so that it is as wide as the width of the tooth. The strip, with a wedge in place, is adapted to the tooth. It is important that the angle formed by the fold of the strip approximates the normal corner of the tooth and supports the matrix on the lingual surface, which is held by the forefinger of the left hand. The cavity is then filled to a slight excess, and one end of the strip is brought across the proximal surface of the filled tooth. When this is completed, the other end of the strip is folded over the incisal edge. The matrix is held with the thumb of the left hand.

b. Aluminum foil incisal corner matrix (Fig. 40)

These are ''stock'' metallic matrices shaped according to the proximo-incisal corner and surfaces of anterior teeth. They can be adapted to each specific case. These types of matrix cannot be used for light cured resin material.

Procedure

A corner matrix closest in size and shape of the lost area of tooth is selected. It is trimmed gingivally, so that it coincides with the gingival architecture and covers the gingival margin of the preparation. As it is readily deformable, shape it with the thumb and first finger until it fits the mesio-distal and labio-lingual dimensions of the tooth, with a sufficient overlap of unprepared surface areas. Loosely place the wedge, allowing space for the matrix band thickness. Partially fill the preparation

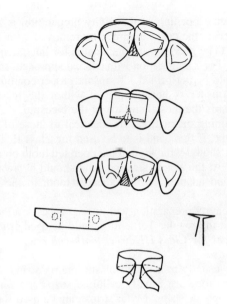

Fig. 12-38. T-shaped band strip matrix for two adjacent small Class III cavity preparations

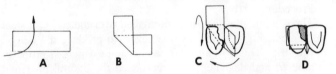

Fig. 12-39. A, The matrix is folded at 90° forming. **B,** The L-shaped matrix. The matrix is measured and sized. **C,** Insuring proper shape of the incisal angle. **D,** The matrix is adapted, wedged and held under pressure while the restorative material sets.

and then the corner matrix, preferably after venting the corner. Apply the partially filled matrix over the partially filled tooth preparation at its predetermined location between the loosened wedge and the tooth. Tighten the wedge and wipe off excess material.

c. Transparent crown form matrices (Fig. 41)

These are ''stock'' plastic crowns which can be adapted to tooth anatomy. In bilateral Class IV preparations use the entire crown form, but in a unilateral Class IV cut the plastic crown inciso-gingivally into two halves and use only the side corresponding to the location of the preparation.

Procedure

Choose the crown form with the size and shape closest to the tooth to be restored. For a unilateral Class IV, after cutting the crown form inciso-gingivally, so that the correct incisal angle of the crown form matches the lost tooth incisal angle, allow the lateral peripheries of the crown form to overlap the lateral extension of the preparation. If for bilateral Class IV's, keep the crown as it is.

Trim the crown form (or its half) gingivally, so that it coincides with the gingival architecture and completely covers the gingival margin of the preparation. Then choose and trim a wedge and loosely fit it interproximally without the matrix in place.

Check the matrix to insure that it will recreate proper contact and contour, and that it covers all margins of the preparation. Then remove the matrix and thin it at its contact area with a

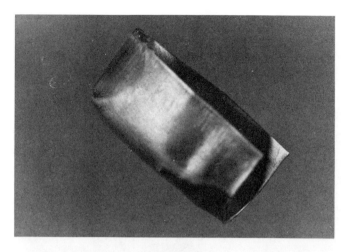

Fig. 12-40

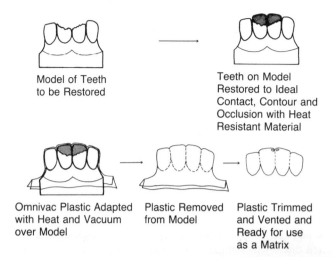

Fig. 12-42

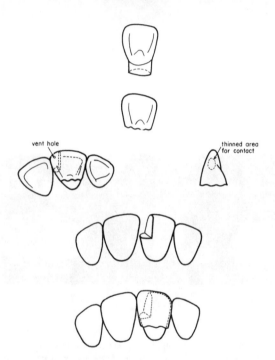

Fig. 12-41. Crown form matrix for a Class IV cavity preparation.

sand paper disc. It should also be perforated at the incisal angle. Completely fill the matrix with the restorative material and partially fill the preparation with the restorative material. Place the filled crown form on the tooth in the desired location. The wedge is then tightened, excess material is wiped off the matrix peripheries and the material is allowed to set while it is under finger pressure.

d. Anatomic matrix (Fig. 42)

Prior to preparing the teeth (tooth), study model for the affected tooth (teeth) together with at least one intact adjacent tooth on each side is made. It is preferable, especially in multiple involvement where the restoration(s) is (are) part of the disclusion mechanism, to make full arch study models and mount them in CO.

The defective area(s) is (are) restored on the study model in

a fairly heat resistant material (plaster, acrylic resin, blocking compound, plasticine, etc.) to the appropriate configuration. A plastic template is made for the restored tooth (teeth) on the model using a combination of heat (to thermoplastically soften the template material) and suction (vacuum) consequently to draw the moldable material onto the study model. The template is trimmed gingivally to fit the tooth (teeth) and adjacent periodontal architecture. It should seat on at least one unprepared tooth on each side. This is the matrix, which should be vented by perforating the corners of its part corresponding to the future restoration. The restorative material is inserted into the preparation, then the matrix is filled with the material and inserted over the prepared and partially filled tooth, ready for curing.

e. Modified S-shaped band

Procedure

A strip of dead metal (a metal with no elastic deformation, malleable, with no memory, usually copper, tin, or aluminum foil) is cut ⅛'' in length and made S-shaped with a mirror handle. Apply the band so that one arm will go over the labial surface of the contacting tooth and the other will go over the lingual surface of the tooth operated upon. Contour and thin the part coinciding with the proximal surface of the restoration. Apply a tailored wedge from the lingual to fulfill all the objectives of wedging.

Flow softened compound on the lingual surface of the matrix and the adjacent tooth surfaces. While hardening, contour the band more from inside the cavity. By now we have a complete matrix with a labial opening but no incisal wall from which we can introduce our material. Overfill toward the labial and incisal so we can contour the restoration after hardening.

6. Matrices for Class V amalgam restorations

These are usually not indicated except for very wide cavities occluso-gingivally and/or mesio-distally.

a. Window matrix

This matrix if formed using either a Tofflemire matrix or copper band matrix (Fig. 43)

Procedure for using the Tofflemire matrix

The contrangle retainer is applied at the side of the tooth that does not have the preparation. A window is cut in the band slightly smaller than the outline of the cavity (preformed

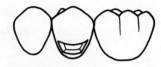

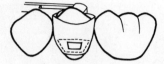

Fig. 12-43. Window matrix.

windowed bands are available). Wedges are placed mesially and distally to stabilize the band.

Procedure for using the copper band

A seamless copper band is selected that is just larger than the prepared tooth. Festoon and adjust the band to the tooth. A window is cut coinciding with the cavity, but smaller in diameter. The edges are smoothed. The band is positioned on the tooth, and wedges are placed.

b. The S-shaped matrix

This is usually indicated for a proximal extension of a buccal or lingual Class V preparation. It is done in the same manner as described for the Class III amalgam preparation with the exception that the buccal and lingual opening of the matrix is not excessively widened.

c. Other options in lieu of matrices in extremely wide Class V cavities

The cavity is prepared in two stages—a mesial half is prepared and filled with amalgam. After the amalgam hardens, the distal half is prepared and restored. If there are sufficient mesial and distal walls in the Class V cavity preparation, condense the mesial one-third of the amalgam mesio-axially and the distal one-third disto-axially, allow to partially harden, then condense the middle third axially with a flat-bladed instrument.

7. Matrices for Class V preparations for direct tooth-colored restorations

a. Anatomic matrix (Fig. 44) for *non-light* cured, direct tooth colored materials

Procedure

The Class V cavity may be preliminarily filled with inlay wax or gutta-percha and trimmed to the proper contour. The wax (gutta-percha) and the tooth are then coated with cocoa butter or mylar strip and compound impression is taken of the tooth surface to be restored. Adjacent surfaces are to be included in the impression. After the compound has cooled, it is removed and the wax is removed from the cavity.

A mix of the restorative material is made and placed into the cavity, and the compound matrix is placed into position and held securely in place under pressure until the material sets. In using resins, the impression surface of the compound must be lined with a tin-foil substitute, or mylar strip.

b. Aluminum or copper collars (Fig. 45) for non-light cured direct tooth colored restorations

Aluminum or copper bands are preshaped according to the gingival third of the buccal and lingual surfaces. They can be adjusted to each specific case so that the band will cover 1-2 mm of the tooth surface circumferential to the cavity margins.

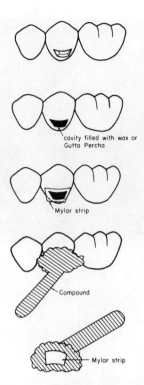

Fig. 12-44. Anatomic matrix for Class V tooth-colored restorations.

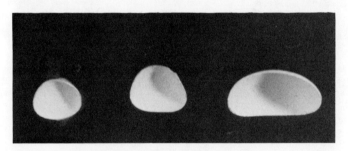

Fig. 12-45

They are then mounted on the tip of a softened stick of compound, which is used as a handle. Fill the cavity with restorative material and apply the adjusted collar onto the tooth.

c. Anatomic matrix for light and *non-light* cured, direct tooth-colored materials

The same as anatomic matrix for Class IV, study models for the defected tooth (teeth) with at least one intact tooth on each side is made. After restoring the defects on the model, a plastic template is made, as described before. The template is cut mesio-distally, keeping its occlusal (incisal) portion and the facial and lingual parts where the defects are. It is then trimmed gingivally and used as a matrix for applying pressure and keeping the restorative material while being cured.

Evaluation of Different Matrix Techniques

Although there have been very few investigations conducted on this subject, the following observations can be summarized from information that is presently available. It is clear that no matrix technique is capable of the exact replication of normal anatomic contours of restored teeth. However, deviations from normal are slight in any matricing procedure if proper contouring and wedging are utilized. Overall, the anatomic matrix procedure most closely reproduces normal tooth contours.

Wedging is universally imperative in order to eliminate cervical flash of restorative material (Fig. 46). This is true with all three types of tooth shape. Although matrix contouring, in the absence of wedging, produces a more rounded contour (especially on square-type teeth), it does not reduce cervical overhangs. With tapering type teeth, however, an accurate reproduction of the proximal surface can be achieved without contouring; i.e., using wedging alone. Ovoid-type teeth are the most difficult to reproduce, so that, like square teeth, contouring, in addition to wedging, is required.

Too many human variables come into play in trying to trim overhangs and to change proximal contours after the removal of a matrix. In fact, since proper contouring and complete flash removal at this stage of the restorative process is impossible to predict, it would behoove the operator to utilize a matrix technique which will minimize these cervical overhangs and improper contours. Even with the properly chosen technique, using floss after condensation of amalgam definitely improves proximal contour as well as reduces overhangs.

Of some clinical significance is the fact that circumferential matrix bands retained by tightening devices (e.g., Tofflemire) have been shown to elastically deform tooth structures. Immediately after removal of the matrix bands, tooth structures then regain their original dimension, resulting in gaps between the tooth and the hardened restorative material. These gaps may range from 11.4 to 25 microns. The width of this gap is directly proportional to the width of the preparation, the pressure applied with the matrix, and the post-operative contraction of the particular restorative material used.

Passively inserted matrix bands, like anatomic matrix and T-shaped bands, etc., have no deformative effect on the remaining tooth structures.

For matrices and formulation of contact and contour in direct gold restorations, refer to the chapter on direct gold restorations.

Extraoral Formulation of Contacts and Contours (for Cast Restorations)

The procedure is facilitated and made convenient through wax pattern and cast adjustments.

A. Wax pattern

This is usually built in a slightly overcontoured condition, especially at the contact area to allow for the finishing and polishing surface losses. Removable dies make the procedure very feasible as they will allow additions or removal of small increments of waxes at or from indicated areas. (Refer to the chapter on cast restorations.)

B. Cast adjustments

These are usually done with rubbery stones incrementally removing cast material surfacewise to obtain the exact dimensions, configuration and interrelationship of the contact and contour. It is partly done on the working models, that are

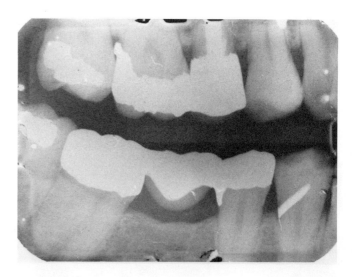

Fig. 12-46

mounted on articulators, and partly, and finally, intraorally. Use dental floss around the contact area with its ends pulled buccally parallel to each other, to estimate the occluso-apical shape and dimensions of the contact area, it is then pulled occlusally, also parallel to each other, to estimate the buccolingual dimensions and shape of the contact area (refer to the chapter on cast restorations).

BIBLIOGRAPHY

Bell, J.G.: An elementary study of deformation of molar teeth during amalgam restorative procedures. Australian Dental Journal, 22, 177-181, 1977.

Black, G.V.: Textbook of operative dentistry. Chicago, Medico-Dental Pub., 1917.

Bossert, W.A.: Relation between shape of occlusal surfaces of molars and prevalence of decay. II. J. D. Res. **16**:63, February 1937.

Fee, A.H.: Anatomy of contacts. JADA **27**:1038, 1940.

Gilmore: Textbook of operative dentistry. St. Louis, The C.V. Mosby Co., 1977.

Hollenback, G.: The most important dimension. J. of Southern Calif. State D.A. Vol. 29, p. 2, 1961.

Ingraham, R., and Koser, J.: The anatomic matrix. JADA vol 51, p. 590, Nov. 1955.

McGhee, True, and Inskipp.: Textbook of operative dentistry. McGraw-Hill, 1956.

Parel, M.L.: Axial crown contour, J. Prosthet. Dent. **25**:642, 1971.

Parel, M.L.: Periodontal considerations of crown contours. J. Prosthet. Dent. **25**:627, 1971.

Phillips and Castaldi.: Further studies on the contour of Class II restorations with various matrix techniques. JADA **36**:462, 1957.

Phillips, R.W., and Castaldi, C.: A study of the proximal contour of Class II amalgam restorations using various matrix band techniques. JADA **53**:391, 1956.

Powell, G., Nicholls, J., and Molvar, M.: Influence of matrix bands dehydration and amalgam condensation on deformation of teeth. Operative dentistry, 5, p. 95, 1980.

Powell, G., Nicholls, J., and Shurtz, D.: Deformation of human teeth under the action of an amalgam matrix band. Operative Dentistry, 2, 64-69, 1977.

Stein, M.R.: Decline of human dentition. JADA **22**:1372, Aug. 1935.

Stuart, C.W., Knudson, W.N., and Arnold, Lloyd: Self-protecting mechanism of mouth against endogenic bacterial flora, and movements of extrinsic organisms within oral cavity. J.D. Res. **15**:41, Feb. 1935.

Wheeler, R.C.: Complete crown form and the periodontium. J. Prosthet. Dent. **11**:722, 1961.

Yuodelis, R.A., Weaver, J.D., and Sapkos, S.: Facial and lingual contours of artifical complete crown restorations and their effects on the periodontium. J. Prosthet. Dent. **29**:61, 1972.

CHAPTER 13

Intermediary bases and basing

Most tooth preparations involve dentin. The majority of this dentinal portion has been irritated not only by the disease process itself, but also by the mechanical process of cavity preparation. Restorative materials, themselves, even have irritating effects on the P-D organ. Therefore, after removing the diseased tissues and completing the cavity preparation it is essential to try to prevent further irritation of the P-D organ as well as to improve the defensive capabilities of that organ. This is accomplished by intermediary basing. Before describing any specific details regarding the procedures for intermediary basing it is vitally important to comprehend:

A. The physio-anatomical relationships of the P-D organ mentioned in chapter 1, namely, the correlation between the pulp tissues and dentin components; the types and nature of the P-D organ defensive mechanisms as a function of the intensity and duration of the irritants; and the conditions in the P-D organ that may modify the effects of these irritants. Also, one should recall the clinical signs of a directly involved pulp chamber or root canal system and the significance of those signs relative to the reparative capacity of the P-D organ.

B. The three possible reactions of a vital P-D organ to irritation, as mentioned in Chapter 1.

C. The irritating capabilities of the diseases affecting the tooth, the possible irritation from operative procedures, including tooth preparation, restoration and the materials involved. In addition, one should have a general idea regarding the physiologic status of the P-D organ prior to proceeding with intermediary basing and subsequent restoration placement. For information concerning these subjects refer to Chapter 1 and also to the sections regarding biologic form in each chapter describing a restorative technique.

D. The chemical irritation to the P-D organ resulting from the diffusion of irritating agents through the dentin. Proper understanding of the nature of the diffusability and the factors affecting it is essential. Dentin permeability differs from one person to another, from one tooth to another, and from one area of a tooth to another area of the same tooth. There are twelve factors governing dentin permeability:

1. The type of dentin

It is well documented that calcific barrier dentin is the most impermeable type of dentin, and that dead tract dentin is the most permeable. The different types of dentin, in order from lowest to highest permeability, are: calcific barrier dentin, sclerosed dentin, primary dentin, secondary dentin, tertiary (reparative) dentin, globular dentin, granular dentin, and dead tract dentin.

Recognizing calcific barrier dentin and sclerotic dentin is easily done by radiographic observation. The calcific barrier dentin layer will appear quite radiopaque, more closely resembling enamel in its radiopacity, than normal primary dentin. Sclerosed dentin is more radiopaque than adjacent dentin, but its radiopacity is closer to that of normal, primary dentin than to enamel. Explorer palpation will reveal a consistency as hard as enamel for calcific barrier dentin, while sclerotic dentin is softer than enamel even though it is more resistant to penetration than primary dentin.

Primary and secondary dentin are readily recognizable by their normal texture, radiopacity, and regular pattern. They are the control for any differential comparison. Tertiary (reparative) dentin can be recognized by its location pulpal to a surface defect or caries cone, the irregularities of its pulp peripheries compared to the surrounding pulp chamber or root canal walls and its localized occupation of the pulp chamber. Its radiopacity differs greatly from one lesion to another.

Globular and granular dentin are very difficult to recognize by radiographs or explorer palpation. They can be anticipated only in certain locations, globular dentin occuring in the coronal portion of the tooth, close to the DEJ. Granular dentin occurs in the root, adjacent to the cementum.

Dead tract dentin can be recognized radiographically by a slightly radiolucent appearance, compared to the adjacent primary or secondary dentin, especially if the dead tract is of long standing duration. It can also be recognized by the presence of tertiary dentin pulpal to it if the P-D organ is vital. Clinically, the dead tract dentin appears more grayish and is less resistant to indentation than normal dentin. If the tooth is not anesthetized the area of the dead tract will be less sensitive than surrounding normal primary or secondary dentin. It should be mentioned here that burnt dentin, usually resulting from rotary instrumentation, allows diffusants to penetrate even more easily than dead tract dentin. This dentin can be recognized by the burnt protein odor during its cutting and the surface carbonization of the burnt area.

2. The types and nature of penetrants (diffusants)

A variety of materials can diffuse through dentin, depending upon their compatibility and reactivity with the dentinal constituents, their valencies, degree of ionization, molecular size, molecular mobility, wetting ability, and the driving forces.

Generally, plaque acids and other highly dissociable acids can penetrate dentin quickly and extensively. Salivary ions can penetrate dentin to a degree dependent upon their molecular size and reaction potential with dentinal ingredients that may either enhance or prevent further progress. Calcium and fluoride ions can penetrate dentin, but the reaction product will decrease dentin permeability. Conversely, acid penetrants result in reaction products that increase dentin permeability drastically. Corrosion products from metallic restorations can readily penetrate dentin. The degree of penetration is dependent upon the factors governing salivary ion diffusion.

3. The degree of mineralization of the dentin

Dentinal perfusion occurs primarily through the dentinal tubules, although some penetration does occur through the organic matrix. The greater mineralization of the organic matrix and the attendent partial or complete mineral obliteration of the dentinal tubules is, the less will be the dentin permeability. This is most readily observed in sclerotic and calcific barrier dentin.

4. Dentin exposed during tooth preparation

The greater the surface area of the dentin exposed to preoperative, operative, and post-operative irritants, the greater the potential intensity of the irritant.

5. Effective depth (dentinal bridge)

The less the effective depth of dentin is, the faster the penetrants will arrive to the pulp tissues. Additionally, they will have had little of their toxicity diminished, resulting in a greater destructive reaction in the P-D organ.

6. Induced stresses

Mechanically, thermally, or electrically induced stresses can enhance and accelerate the diffusion of penetrants into the P-D organ. Examples of mechanical stresses are premature occlusal contacts, the energy of inserting restorative materials, and the pressure and vibration of preparation instrumentation. Examples of thermal stresses are temperature cycling in the oral environment, thermal conductivity of metallic restorations, and frictional heat during tooth preparation. An example of electrical stress is a galvanic current in the oral cavity, especially one involving a restored tooth.

7. Hydraulic pressure

Hydraulic pressure is capable of forcing liquids or semiliquids into the P-D organ, greatly increasing the dentin permeability. One example would be the hydraulic pressure of the cementing media during the seating of cast restorations, especially those for teeth with extensive intracoronal preparaion. Another example would be the percolation of the restoation (expansion and shrinkage) due to the difference in thermal expansion between the restorative material and tooth structure.

8. Deficient resistance and retention form

Deficient resistance and retention form in a preparation will allow micro- and macromovements of the restoration facilitating the pumping of fluids from the oral cavity through the microleakage space into the dentin.

9. Microleakage

The greater that the dimensions and extent of the leakage space between the restorative material and tooth structure are, the greater will be the availability and potential penetration of irritants into the dentin.

10. Cracks and microcracks in the dentin and enamel

The presence of cracks and microcracks, arranged in a connecting and penetrating fashion will readily allow maximum penetration of the P-D organ.

11. Type of intermediary base or restorative material

Both intermediary bases and restorative materials are capable of affecting dentin permeability. Some decrease permeability while others will increase permeability. Their effects will be described as each material is discussed.

12. Desiccation of dentin

Heat or air desiccation of vital dentin, by eliminating fluids from dentinal tubules, will greatly enhance the potential for dentin permeability.

E. The functions of intermediary bases. After removing the diseased and unwanted tooth structure, prior to insertion of the restoration, we apply protective and healing agents to the cut dentin to prevent further irritation to the P-D organ and to allow healing to occur within the P-D organ. These agents are the intermediary bases and they should meet certain criteria. *The basing procedure should:*

1. Be able to cover a pulp chamber, pulp horn, or root canal system exposure, first mechanically, and subsequently by dentinal bridge formation.

2. Create an environment in the P-D organ conducive to repair and healing.

3. Impart a sedative action on an irritated P-D organ. This effect is produced either directly, by a pharmacological action, or indirectly, by physically intercepting the pain transmission path within dentin.

4. Possess the ability of sealing the dentinal tubules to some degree. Sealability is precipitated either mechanically, by obliterating the dentinal tubules, or biologically, by stimulating the underlying odontoblasts to participate in a mechanism to seal the preparation ends of the tubules with mineral deposits.

5. Diminish the extent of microleakage for a sufficient length of time to allow the P-D organ or the restoration to minimize the effects of microleakage.

6. Provide thermal insulation for the P-D organ, reducing the potential for pain and pathological deterioration in the pulpal tissues. The ability to provide thermal protection will differ from one material to another, but will always be directly proportional to the thickness of the material.

7. Provide electrical (galvanic) insulation, especially under metallic restorations. This insulating quality is directly proportional to the thickness of the base and inversely proportional to the fluid content and porosity of the base materials.

8. Provide chemical insulation, i.e., prevent or minimize the penetration of chemicals into dentin. This is accomplished by either creating a physical barrier or by chemically reacting with the irritant producing non-penetrating products.

9. Seal off the dentin's own moisture, preventing it from contaminating restorative materials during setting, thereby insuring proper behavior and adhesion of the set materials.

10. For esthetic reasons, either mask discolored areas of a tooth preparation and/or prevent discoloring agents from the oral environment or restoration from penetrating into the underlying dentin.

Classification of Intermediary Bases

A. Varnishes

A material of this class is applied in a thin film, the thickness of which will not exceed the leakage space at the restorative material-tooth substance interface. Its film thickness is usually 5-10 micrometers. Varnishes are applied to all prepared dentin surfaces and frequently on prepared enamel.

B. Liners

Although much thicker than varnishes, liners still will not exceed the leakage space around the restoration. These materials are usually made of film forming materials like varnish, but they carry therapeutic agents which create their greater film thickness (up to 25 micrometers). They are usually applied to dentin only.

C. Subbases

These are therapeutic materials placed in deep portions of the cavity preparation. They possess specific pharmacological actions. They should be covered with or carried in a supporting base.

D. Bases

Bases are insulating materials that can be used directly on certain areas of the dentinal parts of the preparation. They may also be used indirectly as supporting, retaining modes for subbases.

Ideal Requirements for Intermediary Base Materials

To create any of the previously mentioned healing-protecting effects in a P-D organ, the following ideal requirements for these materials should be met. Although no available material possesses all of these properties, some of them have most of the properties and can be used effectively. However, by combining materials, all ideal requirements can be achieved:

A. The material should be capable of creating an impervious layer on cut vital dentin in a thickness which neither impinges on the bulk of the restorative material nor compromises the mechanical properties of the restoration. It should be impervious to toxins, salivary ions, tarnish and corrosion products of metallic restorations, acids, and chemicals from the restorative materials.

B. The material should be biologically compatible with the P-D organ.

C. The material should be chemically compatible with both the P-D organ and the restorative material.

D. The material should discolor neither the tooth nor the restorative material.

E. The material should harden (set) quickly to allow for the subsequent insertion of the restorative material.

F. The set material should withstand, without changing shape or location, the condensation forces involved in placing permanent restorative material.

G. The material should stabilize or diminish dentin permeability.

H. The material should be able to be easily manipulated in its preparation and insertion.

Materials Used for Intermediary Bases and Basing

Intermediary bases are usually mechanically weak materials, but they are used for their non-mechanical properties. As mentioned, we frequently utilize different combinations of these materials to satisfy the ideal objectives of intermediary basing.

Presently, there are six materials that can be used in a variety of ways as intermediary bases:

A. *Zinc oxide and eugenol (ZOE)*
B. *Calcium hydroxide*
C. *Zinc phosphate cement (ZPC)*
D. *Polycarboxylate cement (PCC)*
E. *Varnishes and film-forming resinous materials*
F. *Glass ionomer cement or aluminosilicate-polyacrylate cement (ASPA)* (This cement is discussed at length in the chapter on direct tooth colored restorative materials.)

We shall briefly discuss the composition of each of the materials, their setting reactions, their properties and behavior both during and after setting, their compatibility with the P-D organ and restorative materials, their therapeutic effect on the P-D organ, and the principles and procedures for creating intermediary bases with them.

I. Composition and Setting Reaction

A. ZOE

ZOE is supplied in the form of a powder and liquid. In its unmodified form the powder is primarily zinc oxide which is partially hydrolyzed; or, if prepared from hydrated compounds, the water will not be completely eliminated, insofar as water is essential to start the setting reaction.

The unmodified liquid is primarily eugenol or oil of cloves (85% eugenol). Mixing powder with the liquid creates a paste that will set to a hard mass. The setting reaction is mainly a physical reaction of wetting the zinc oxide particles with eugenol. A limited chelation reaction occurs wherein the eugenol chelates zinc and gives water as a by-product, which stimulates further setting.

The unmodified ZOE is used only as a therapeutic agent. To improve the physical and mechanical properties of ZOE, thereby making it suitable for use as a base, the material is mixed with modifiers. Some of these are physically imbedded in the final structure, while others are chemically bonded. Examples of modifiers are:

1. Rosin, which is used to improve the strength, homogencity, and smoothness of the mix while decreasing flow, brittleness and solubility. Hydrogenated rosin is bonded better and imparts more predictable properties within the structure than natural rosin. Rosin in a ZOE mass may physically bond to the other components or react chemically with the eugenol.

2. Ethoxy benzoic acid increases the strength of the material, but also increases the solubility. It participates in a saponification reaction with the zinc oxide.

3. Fillers, which are physically imbedded within the mass, substantially improve the mechanical properties of the material by reducing slip and increasing friction within the mass. Multiple fillers can be used. Examples of fillers are polystyrene, silica, alumina, diatomaceous earth, cotton fibers, etc.

4. Chemical setting accelerators shorten the setting time of the material. A variety of chemicals can be used, e.g., zinc acetate, proprionate or succinate, calcium chloride, or low molecular weight primary alcohols.

5. Medicaments, including coagulants and bactericidal and bacteriostatic agents, may be incorporated.

The microstructure of the set material is composed primarily of the original particles of zinc oxide and modifiers joined with a continuous matrix of eugenol, zinc eugenolate, and zinc benzoate (if ethoxy benzoic acid takes part in the reaction). Compared to the other intermediary bases, this material displays the lowest porosity and a very high packing factor.

B. Calcium hydroxide

Calcium hydroxide is in a powder form and can be carried to the tooth in a variety of ways. The powder can be mixed with distilled water or a sterile saline solution to form a thick paste and applied as such. The powder can also be suspended in plasma, distilled water, or chloroform and applied on the tooth surface with a syringe. Or, calcium hydroxide may be applied in the pure powder form, without any carrier whatsoever.

It can be carried in methylcellulose (or any biologically compatible and degradable polymeric material). This is supplied in the form of a two-paste system. One paste contains the monomer of the methylcellulose, a chemical initiator, and calcium hydroxide particles. The other paste contains the catalyst and calcium hydroxide particles. By mixing equal portions of each paste, methylcellulose monomers will polymerize creating a porous meshwork matrix. In this carrier system there is chemical coherence of the ingredients, i.e., the bonding that occurs between the polymer macromolecules. The calcium hydroxide does not enter into the chemical reaction. The polymer meshwork carries the calcium hydroxide to the P-D organ, where it is available to engage in its therapeutic action.

The non-polymer carried calcium hydroxide mass is very porous and lacks any reasonable packing. Those carried in a polymeric matrix also have high porosity and low packing ability. For these reasons they are used almost exclusively for their therapeutic action in the form of a subbase.

However, the most common way of introducing calcium hydroxide into a cavity preparation is through calcium hydroxide cements, where calcium hydroxide enters a chemical reaction with other ingredients. They are supplied in a two-paste system. An acidic paste, which is mainly composed of alkyl salicylate (iso-butyl salicylate, or 1-methyl triethylene disalicylate) and inert fillers such as titanium oxide (12-14%) and/or barium sulfate (32-35%) for radiopacity, or calcium tungstate or sulfate (14-15%); and a basic paste, which is basically composed of calcium hydroxide (50-60%). It also contains a plasticizer which could be a sulfonamide or paraffin oil. Mixing equal parts of the two pastes together will start an acid-base reaction resulting in a weakly bonded (mostly secondary forces) composite structure. Chelates of calcium alkyl salicylate and water (the reaction by-product) will form the continuous phase and the unreacted ingredients will form the interrupted phase. The mass is hydrolytically unstable and contains a large percentage of unreacted calcium hydroxide. Calcium ions, hydroxyl ions and salicylate ions are released continuously from the mass. The release is mostly controlled by the percentage of the continuous phase and the type of plasticizer (sulfonamides allow more erosion and ion release than paraffin oil). Anyway, the packing factor is very low, and the mass is porous. Porosity increases with time, due to the continuous erosion of the mass. With time, the entire cement mass may disappear under restorations. However, their packing factor is higher and the porosity is lower than other types of calcium hydroxide. That is why calcium hydroxide cement could be used as a base under certain restorative materials, otherwise they should be used as subbases only.

C. Zinc phosphate cement

ZPC is supplied in the form of a powder and a liquid. The powder is almost 90% zinc oxide, with magnesium oxide and traces of tribismuth oxide and silicone dioxide. The last three ingredients are essential for creating a workable mix and reasonable setting time. The reactivity of the powder is controlled by the calcination temperature and time, and by the particle size and shape. The liquid is a buffered 45-55% aqueous solution of orthophosphoric acid. Almost one-third of the phosphate groups in the liquid are combined in the form of aluminum, zinc, and bismuth phosphates to reduce the reactivity of the liquid and give a reasonable working time.

The setting reaction, which is mainly between the zinc oxide and phosphoric acid, is an ordinary acid-base reaction. This results in a composite structure of reacted (chemically bonded) and unreacted (physically bonded) powder particles bound to a continuous amorphour matrix of hydrated zinc phosphate. The mass has very poor packing characteristics and is extremely porous. The material is used only as a base or as a luting agent.

D. Polycarboxylate (polyacrylate) cements

PCC is supplied in the form of a powder and liquid. The powder is primarily zinc oxide, with small amounts (10%) of magnesium oxide and traces of alumina. Like zinc phosphate cement, the powder is calcined-sintered and pulverized to decrease its reactivity and establish reasonable working properties.

The liquid is an aqueous (40-50%) solution of polyacrylic acid. The setting reaction is a type of chelation reaction between the outer portion of the powder particles and polyacrylic acids that results in a structurally composite two-phase mass (an interrupted phase and a continuous phase). The interrupted phase is comprised of the unreacted portion of the powder particles. The continuous phase is a matrix gel comprised of hydrated cross-linked polyacrylate macromolecules, which is the product of chelated cations (mainly zinc) lengthening and cross-linking the liquid polymer molecules. The two phases are bonded together by the cation-depleted portion of the original powder particles. Water is a by-product of the recation and is a part of the hydrated matrix. Sodium fluorides are added to some cements. They do not enter the setting reaction, but they can be released to surrounding tooth structure. As we can predict, the matrix structure is amorphous and porous to some extent, but it has better packing characteristics than ZPC. The material is used only as a base or as a luting agent.

E. Film-forming resinous materials

Film-forming resinous materials can be either natural gums or resins, e.g., copal or rosin, or synthetic resins, e.g., nitrated cellulose or polystyrene. The gum or resin is dissolved in an organic solvent which is readily volatalizable in the oral environment, e.g., chloroform, acetone, alcohol, etc. The solution is painted on cut tooth surfaces and the organic solvent is allowed to vaporize. The gum or resin will remain forming a thin film. This is called a varnish. The varnish film will not be continuous with only one application, so several applications should be done to insure minimal porosity.

The gum or resin may have suspensions of zinc oxide, calcium hydroxide, sodium monofluorophosphate or other therapeutic agents which will be incorporated in the residual film. These therapeutic agents create specific actions within the tooth substance or P-D organ. They constitute a cavity liner, which will have a greater film thickness than varnish.

There is no chemical reaction in creating these films, and the bonding between their precipitated components is principally physical. They display porosity on atomic, microscopic, and macroscopic levels.

II. Setting Time and Factors Affecting It

ZOE

The normal reactivity between zinc oxide and eugenol is very limited and must be accelerated in order for the material to have a practical clinical application. Acceleration of the set may be achieved by:
1. Incorporating chemical accelerators in the mix (the most efficient and predictable way of controlling the setting time).
2. Reducing the powder particle size, providing for accelerated reactivity.
3. Increasing the powder:liquid ratio (of limited effect in reducing the setting time).
4. Increasing the percentage of rosin and fillers.
5. Increasing the temperature and/or humidity.
6. Adding water to the original mix or after mixing is complete and seated into the preparation.
7. Introducing greater energy in the mixing procedure (pressure-movement and time).

A delay in setting is rarely needed. This is accomplished by adding vegetable oils or glycerin which keep the mass plasticized for a long period of time.

B. Calcium hydroxide

The setting time for polymer-carried calcium hydroxide can be increased by increasing the ration of catalyst to base paste. The setting of Ca(OH)$_2$ alkyl salicylate cement can be accelerated by moisture and heat. Conversely, the setting time will be retarded by dryness and cold.

C. ZPC

The normal reactivity between the cement powder and liquid is violent and fast. The reaction must be retarded to allow for a reasonable working time and for maximum incorporation of the powder in the liquid. The manufacturers control this by altering the powder particle size and shape and by calcination of the powder to reduce the surface energy of the particles. They also buffer and alter the water contents of the liquid to control the amount of phosphate groups available for the reaction. The dentist can control the setting time by one or more of the following:
1. Use of a glass slab at temperature between the atmospheric dew point and 20° C. Such a low temperature will retard the reaction and neutralize the exothermic heat of the reaction.
2. Add the cement powder to the liquid in small increments, mixing on a large surface area of the cool slab. This allows the reaction to proceed only partially, with limited exothermic heat.
3. Accelerate the reaction by increasing the powder:liquid ratio, adding water to the liquid, decreasing the particle size of the powder and/or increasing the temperature of the mixing environment.

D. PCC

The setting reaction between the powder and liquid, like ZPC, is very violent and fast. It must be retarded to allow for a reasonable working time. This is controlled by the manufacturer in the same way the powder of ZPC is controlled. The dentist can control the setting time by:
1. Use a cool glass slab, thereby retarding the chemical reaction
2. Most or ALL of the powder should be incorporated into the liquid in one large increment because the reaction is *not* delayed by incremental mixing.
3. Adding water and increasing the temperature of the mixing environment are the most efficient means of accelerating the setting time. These may, however, deleteriously affect other properties of the cement.

E. Film-forming resinous materials

For film forming resinous materials, an indirectly applied stream of air, a vacuum, or an increase in temperature will conveniently accelerate the evaporation of the organic solvent.

III. Dimensional Stability and Factors Affecting It

A. Setting shrinkage

ZOE exhibits the least amount of shrinkage of all intermediary base materials (0.1% by volume). The maximum setting shrinkage is that of polymer carried calcium hydroxide (5% by volume). However, in the dimensions and locations that these materials are used such shrinkage is of no clinical significance.

B. Fluid and water absorption

The more porous the material is, the greater will be the chance of absorbing fluids with subsequent dimensional increase. This is observed more with non-carried calcium hydroxide and zinc phosphate cement than with the other materials.

C. Coefficient of thermal expansion

The material with the coefficient of thermal expansion closest to that of tooth structure is ZOE (11 PPM/1° C). Although the other materials have higher coefficients of thermal expansion, in the thickness and the locations in which they are used, this is of no clinical significance.

D. Solubility and disintegration

There is quite a discrepancy between laboratory and clinical test results in evaluating these properties. Clinical tests reveal that calcium hydroxide in any form is the most soluble material followed by PPC, ZOE containing ethoxy benzoic acid, unmodified ZOE, then ZPC. It should be emphasized that in most cases it is not the material per se that will be responsible for its degree of solubility, but rather that the solubility will be the result of the following factors:
1. For all materials, the greater that the percentage of original (or dispersed) particles bound to the matrix (dispersion phase) is, the less will be the solubility, i.e., increasing the powder:liquid ratio (the dispersed relative to the dispersion phase) to the full bonding capacity of the liquid (dispersion

phase) will definitely decrease the solubility and disintegration.

2. For all materials, the solubility is directly proportional to time.

3. For all materials, the solubility is directly proportional to the acidity of the environment.

4. With the exception of ZOE, the earlier during the setting reaction that the materials are exposed to moisture, the greater will be the solubility.

5. For ZOE, the incorporation of ethoxy benzoic acid drastically increases the solubility, but this can be compensated for by the addition of rosin and fillers.

6. For ZPC and PCC, increasing the water content of the liquid increases the solubility of the cement.

7. For calcium hydroxide alkyl salicylate cement, paraffin oil plasticizer reduces solubility as compared to sulfonamide one.

8. Chelating acids increase the solubility of PCC, ZOE, and calcium hydroxide cements.

E. Flow (viscosity)

Although high flows are needed during the insertion of the intermediary base materials into the cavity, low flows are necessary for the mechanical well-being of these materials.

With the exception of uncarried calcium hydroxide, unmodified ZOE has the highest flow of all these materials. ZOE flow is decreased by increasing the powder:liquid ratio and by the addition of the fillers, rosin, and ethoxy benzoic acid. Polymer-carried and cement type calcium hydroxide, consequently, has the next highest flow, and it is decreased by increasing the degree of polymerization of the carrying polymer or the percentage of calcium alkyl salicylate in the mix. PCC ranks next, although there is quite a difference between its flow and that of the two previously mentioned materials. The three aforementioned polymeric-physically bonded materials will have their flow increased by shearing energy induced during the manipulation. Set ZPC has the lowest flow of all intermediary base materials. This is understandable, due to the ionic bonding in the mass. Flows in each of PCC and ZPC can be decreased by increasing the powder:liquid ratio and by reduction of pores. Because of the thermoplastic nature of ZOE, PCC, and calcium hydroxide cement, the flow increases with temperature increase.

IV. Strength

ZPC has the highest ultimate compressive strength of all the materials (12-17,000 PSI), followed by PCC (7-9,000 PSI). PCC has the highest ultimate tensile strength, almost 10% higher than ZPC, but both tensile strengths are drastically lower than the compressive strengths.

Strength properties in both cements could be increased by increasing the powder:liquid ratio to the maximum accommodation of the liquid. Strength properties will be decreased by increasing the water content of the liquid, by early exposure to moisture, or by voids or early exposure to mechanical stress.

Because of the differences in composition there are a variety of strength figures for ZOE. Unmodified ZOE can have compressive strength figures of 800-5,000 PSI, while modified ZOE can have a compressive strength as high as 12,000 PSI. Strength properties are inversely proportional to the particle size of the powder, but directly proportional to the powder:liquid ratio, the percentage of rosin and ethoxy benzoic acid, and the percentage of fillers in the mass.

Carried calcium hydroxide and those with the continuous phase in the form of calcium alkyl salicylate chelate can have compressive strength up to 800 PSI, while non-carried calcium hydroxide has virtually no strength. PCC, ZOE, and calcium hydroxide cements are visco-elastic. That is why they react more favorably in resisting deformative failures with high rates of stressing rather than lower ones. Due to their thin film thicknesses, it is not possible to ascertain strength figures for film forming materials.

V. Adaptability

Adaptability and adhesion of these materials to underlying dentin are governed by the following factors:

A. Film thickness

The lower that the film thickness of the material is, the better its wetting ability for the minute, irregular areas of the tooth preparation, and the better its adaptability will be.

Excluding film-forming resinous materials (which can create film thicknesses in the range of 5-10 micrometers), zinc phosphate cement can produce the lowest film thickness of all intermediary and cementing materials. Although the lowest thickness according to the ADA test is 25 microns, ZPC can produce a film as low as 8-10 microns in practice. Calcium hydroxide has the highest possible film thickness, ranging from 70-90 microns, followed by ZOE in the range of 35-40 microns. Polycarboxylate cement is next to ZPC in low film thickness. According to the ADA tests its film thickness is 30 microns, but it can be made in films with thicknesses as low as 20 microns. From this we can realize why of all the intermediary basing materials, ZPC is the most mechanically adhering material to tooth structure.

B. Viscosity

The lower that the viscosity of the material is, the better its wetting ability and the greater its adaptability will be. That is why, for cementation, a mix with the lowest viscosity which can be biologically and mechanically acceptable should be used. For basing purposes, thick consistencies (viscosities) have to be made for biologic reasons.

The apparent viscosity of polycarboxylate cement is the highest of all intermediary base materials, but it decreases under shearing forces (mixing and insertion seating forces). Excluding film forming resinous materials, zinc phosphate cement can have the lowest viscosity of all intermediary base materials.

Besides the types of materials, the viscosity is a product of powder:liquid ratio, temperature, particle size, and energy used in mixing and inserting. It is directly proportional to the first three and inversely proportional to the last factor.

C. Physico-chemical bonding to tooth structure

Only polycarboxylate and alumino-silicate-polyacrylate cements have the ability to chelate calcium from tooth structure, creating an adhesive bridge between the hydroxy-apatite crystals and the set cement bases. For such a reaction to occur, however, there are strict requirements, namely: cleanliness of tooth structure, exposing hydroxy-apatite crystals in the proper plane, dry field, and the availability of COOH groups from the cements. Obviously, such bonding is not continuous over all the surface area of contact between the cement and tooth structure, but the fact that it *can* happen increases the chance of adhesion between the base (cementing material) and the tooth.

D. Self-etching

Self-etching is achieved by using zinc phosphate cement, creating irregularities in the tooth surface (as mentioned with direct tooth-colored materials) and increasing the adaptability and retentive adhesiveness of the base (cement) to tooth structure, especially enamel.

E. Coefficient of thermal expansion

Similar coefficients of thermal expansion between the base material and tooth structure can enhance adhesion, especially when the structure is subjected to thermal cycling during function. The phenomenon is well demonstrated by zinc oxide and eugenol, since it has the closest coefficient of thermal expansion (K_t) to that of tooth structure of all intermediary base materials. It has the best physical adaptability of these materials to dentin. That is why it is the best sealer of all restorative materials, if it is not subjected to dissolution and mechanical stressing.

F. Strength properties

The higher the strength of a basing material, the more permanent will be its adaptation. For example, ZPC will have the highest adaptability to tooth structure over a long period of time.

Considering all these factors, we conclude that every intermediary base material has some characteristics that enhance its adaptability and the possibility of adhesion to tooth structure. For example, zinc phosphate cement has low film thickness, high strength, is self-etching, and has low viscosity.

ZOE has a favorable coefficient of thermal expansion and initial low viscosity. Polycarboxylate cements possess physico-chemical adhesion and strength.

Film-forming resinous materials have the lowest viscosity and film thickness of all materials. The only material that has none of the adaptability enhancing properties is calcium hydroxide, and thus it demonstrates the lowest adaptability to tooth substance.

VI. Biological compatibility with the P-D Organ

To biologically evaluate the intermediary base materials, the following four questions should be asked:

1. Is the material itself an irritant to the P-D organ? And, if so, what are the irritating ingredients and characteristics, and what is the material's effect at different effective depths?

2. Can the material create an impervious layer on cut vital dentin? And, if not, how porous is the formed layer?

3. What is the effect of the material on the permeability of the underlying dentin?

4. Is the material thermally and electrically (galvanically) insulating, and, if it is, what should be the minimal thickness that it should have to be clinically effective?

A. Zinc oxide and eugenol

1. Biological irritation

ZOE is the least irritating to the P-D organ of all intermediary base materials. If mild irritation is generated, it is due to the eugenol or to impurities (modifiers) within it.

2. The biological effect at different effective depths

Whenever there is any effective depth between the unmodified ZOE and the pulp tissues, the pulpal reaction will be a healthy reparative reaction provided the pulp is healthy. The underlying pulp-dentin organ will have odontoblastic activity stimulated, increasing the dimensions of the peritubular dentin peripherally (sclerosed dentin) and depositing secondary dentin.

When the unmodified ZOE comes in direct contact with the pulp tissues, there are four possible reactions from which several subreactions can occur within the P-D organ.

a. If the pulp is healthy and sound, the exposure site is controlled microbiologically, and the size of exposure is reparable considering the vital capacity of the P-D organ, the pulp tissues in contact with the ZOE will undergo limited chronic inflammation. The chronic inflammation will persist and eventually evolve into one of the following:

i. If the inflammation remains limited, the area will be walled off by fibrous tissues followed by matrix formation, mineralization, and bridging of the exposure. This process may take more than a year.

ii. Chronic inflammation may propagate to involve all the pulp and root canal tissues with slow, symptomless necrosis.

iii. The chronic inflammation may lead to complete fibrosis of the pulp and root canal tissues, without any bridging of the exposure, leaving the P-D organ very susceptible to any irritation, and with little or no defense.

iv. The chronic inflammation may change to acute inflammation through changes in the microbial condition (as from anachoresis or externally induced infections at the exposure site), leading to necrosis of the pulp and root canal tissues.

b. If the pulp is undergoing acute inflammation and the microbial condition of the exposure site controlled, the acute condition is suppressed (due to different pharmacological actions of ZOE to be discussed later). Chronic inflammation will supplant the acute status. The fate of the pulp can be any one of those mentioned in (a), but dentinal bridging is unlikely to occur.

c. If the P-D organ condition is as described in (a), and in addition to unmodified ZOE, we implant sound dentin chips at the exposure site, fibrotic walling off and bridging of the exposure with a deposited mineralizable matrix will occur, utilizing the dentin chip as a nucleus for formation. Deposition of reparative dentin will be reasonably fast (8 weeks on the average).

d. Any mechanical impingement of the unmodified ZOE on the pulp tissues, either by forceful insertion, inadequate reinforcement, or placement of a thin ZOE mix in contact with pulp tissues, will definitely interfere with the healing-bridging reaction. Among the reasons for these are the increased surface area to be bridged, the mechanical irritation to additional pulp tissues, and increased possibility of infection at the repair site.

Any modifications in ZOE, especially incorporating mobile and penetrating modifiers, can have irritating actions on the P-D organ up to an effective depth of 1 mm.

In answer to the second question—ZOE material can create a completely impervious layer to elements normally present in the oral environment, if it is applied in 0.5 mm thickness, provided it is not disturbed either mechanically or by dissolution.

In answer to the third question—although ZOE decreases the hardness of a very minimal thickness of underlying dentin (possibly due to chelation), it does not increase the penetrability of the underlying dentin. On the contrary, with its multiple pharmacological actions it can enhance the sclerosing of underlying dentin.

Regarding the fourth question—ZOE is an excellent thermal insulator with a coefficient of thermal conductivity and thermal diffusivity, slightly less than that of the tooth structure. 0.25 mm thickness layer is sufficient to impart this property. ZOE can conduct minimal electric energy, probably due to its moisture contents. Although its electric insulating ability is the best of all intermediary base materials, it is not an electric insulator in any thickness.

B. Calcium hydroxide

1. The answer to the first biologic inquiry for calcium hydroxide is "Yes, it can be an irritant to the P-D organ, if it comes in contact with it." The irritating ingredients and characteristics could be the forces with which the material is introduced into the pulp tissues and the high alkalinity of the material.

2. Effect at different effective depths

Provided the pulp and root canal tissues are healthy and devoid of any degeneration, the following pulpal reaction to calcium hydroxide can occur:

a. Whenever there is an effective depth of 100 micrometers and more, a healthy reparative reaction can be expected.

b. With less than 100 microns effective depth, expect an unhealthy reparative reaction (Fig. 1).

c. When calcium hydroxide comes in contact with the pulp or root canal tissues, the layer of tissues that it contacts directly will undergo chemical necrosis (coagulation). The subsequent response of the entire P-D organ will depend upon several factors. To anticipate a favorable pulpal reaction, the following criteria must be met:

i. The pulpal tissue must exhibit no signs of degeneration, and have sufficient cellularity and vascularity, indicating an adequate reparative capacity.

ii. The calcium hydroxide must not be pushed inside the pulp chamber and root canal space, thereby increasing the area to be bridged by reparative dentin as well as decreasing the vital capacity of the P-D organ (Fig. 2E).

iii. The calcium hydroxide must not be located opposite to areas in the pulp chamber or root canals where deposition of tertiary dentin will interfere with proper vascular circulation and fluid recovery, i.e., the calcium hydroxide will not precipitate strangulation of the pulp tissues. Examples of these areas (Fig. 2, A, B, C, and D) are: constricted areas of the pulp chamber (e.g., junction between pulp chamber and root canals (Fig. 2, A and C), almost all root canals, especially narrow ones, lateral walls of pulp horns (Fig. 2B), and aged pulp chamber walls or floors (Fig. 2D).

iv. The microbial status at the exposure site must be controlled.

v. The exposure diameter should be comparable in size to

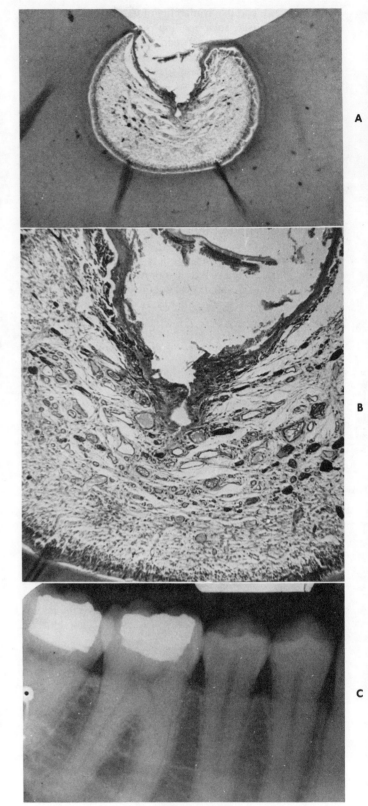

Fig. 13-1. A, Effects of calcium hydroxide on a vital, healthy sterile P-D organ. Original pulp exposure was 2000 microns diameter. **B,** Higher magnification of (A). Notice bridging calcified dentin that occured 6 weeks after application of the calcium hydroxide. **C,** Calcium hydroxide on a degenerating P-D organ of tooth #30 and 31 led to uncontrolled intrapulpal calcification.

A—Calcium hydroxide
B—Tertiary dentin

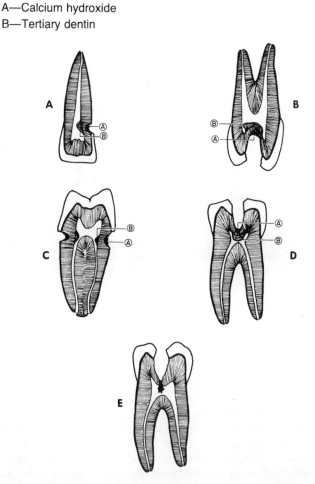

Fig. 13-2. Examples of strangulating calcification. **A,** Strangulation of pulp chamber in maxillary incisor (Class III or V). **B,** Strangulation of pulp horns in maxillary premolar (Class I). **C,** Strangulation of pulp chamber in mandibular molar (Class II or V). **D,** Strangulation of pulp horns and chamber in maxillary molar in aged previously retracting pulp. **E,** Calcium hydroxide has been forced through an exposure site increasing the surface area to be bridged and strangulation of pulp chamber and pulp horn.

the dimensions and reparative capacity of the pulp and root canal tissues.

If all these five criteria are fulfilled, the pulp-root canal tissues next to the coagulated surface area in contact with calcium hydroxide will deposit an organic matrix which will mineralize within 4-6 weeks (Fig. 1B). This will bridge the exposure without interfering with the normal, physiologic-formative function of the pulp-dentin organ. The high calcium ion concentration, alkalinity and antibacterial potential of calcium hydroxide will induce and create the environment for this type of healing by precipitating calcium ions from contacting tissue fluids and by counteracting any activities inducing or producing possible inflammation (microorganism and acidity of inflammation).

d. If calcium hydroxide comes in contact with degenerating pulp tissues, the degeneration will be converted to a calcific type of degeneration that will proceed in an uncontrolled and unpredictable fashion. This situation will lead to multiple local isolations of the pulp and root canal tissues which will be devitalized. The calcification may isolate large segments or the entirety of the pulp tissues from their nutrient sources, leading to their devitalization. Root canal therapy will be indicated, and will be complicated by these calcified masses, insofar as it is sometimes impossible to negotiate root canals through them.

e. A strangulating type of calcification may occur, if calcium hydroxide is placed next to narrow areas of the pulp chamber and root canal system (Fig. 2, A, B, C, D, and E). (The situations mentioned in (d) and (e) can occur even with an effective depth of 100 microns or less.)

In answer to the second question—calcium hydroxide is porous at any thickness on dentin, but its penetrability is reduced to some extent by its neutralizing effect on acids from restorative materials which could penetrate the dentin.

In answer to the third question—calcium hydroxide, in contact with vital dentin, will encourage the formation of a calcific barrier in that dentin by means of its alkalinity and high calcium ion concentration, thus decreasing the permeability of that dentin.

In answer to the fourth question—calcium hydroxide can be a thermal insulator, especially if carried in a methyl cellulose polymer or used in alky salicylate cement form. The clinically effective thickness for proper insulation is 0.5 mm. Calcium hydroxide in any form is not an electrical insulator at any thickness.

C. Zinc phosphate cement

In answer to the first biologic question—zinc phosphate cement is the most irritating of all the intermediary base materials.

1. The irritating ingredients and characteristics are:
a. Acidity during setting.

This will be in the range of a pH of 3-4 in the first hour after mixing. The pH will increase to neutrality in 48 hours. Acidity during the first 48 hours can be very detrimental to the P-D organ as the penetrability of the phosphoric acid is substantial. Some mixes have residual phosphoric acid for more than a week.

Acidity can be reduced by increasing the powder:liquid ratio of the mix, increasing the surface area of contact with the dentin to take full advantage of the buffering capacity of the dentin, and accelerating the setting of the cement.

b. Microleakage.

While microleakage is maximum at the margins of a restoration and minimal internally, both areas can allow passage of oral environment irritants.

c. Exothermic reaction heat.

This is the least irritating characteristic of ZPC. However, if the cement base is bulky enough, the accumulated calories of the setting reaction can be detrimental to the P-D organ.

2. Effect at different effective depth
a. At an effective depth of 2.5 mm and more, zinc phosphate cement will usually create a healthy reparative reaction but occasionally will precipitate an unhealthy reparative reaction.

b. At effective depth of 1.5-2.5 mm, we can anticipate an unhealthy reparative reaction in most cases, but sometimes destruction will occur.

c. At effective depth less than 1.5 mm, there will always be destruction in the pulpal tissues.

In answer to the second question, ZPC can create a partially impervious layer on cut dentin in thicknesses of more than 1 mm. Thinner applications will be completely pervious.

In answer to the third question, zinc phosphate cement depletes underlying dentin from part of its calcium content, thereby increasing dentinal permeability to incoming elements, especially the cement's own phosphoric acid.

In answer to the fourth question, ZPC is an excellent thermal insulator, but in thicknesses of 1 mm or more. It is not an electric insulator, mainly because of its porosity which accommodates moisture, thus encouraging electron transport.

D. Polycarboxylate cements

The answer to the first biologic inquiry about polycarboxylate cement is "Yes, it is minimally irritating to the P-D organ, similar to ZOE."

1. The irritating ingredients, if present, may be the exothermic heat of the polymerization reaction (especially if used in a bulky dimension), porosity, and, to some extent, the polyacrylic acid in deep cavities. Although the pH of the setting cement is in the range of 1.5 for the first day or so, it is minimally irritating to the P-D organ compared to ZPC. This is because of the giant dimensions of polyacrylic acid macromolecules and their attachment to the main bulk of the cement mass. The acid has low diffusion mobility into the underlying dentin due to its immediate complexing with dentinal fluoride, calcium, and some proteinaceous components. The complexed product will prevent further penetration of the acid. This will result in minimal effects on the P-D organ, unless it comes in actual contact with the pulp tissues.

2. The effect at different effective depths

a. Whenever the P-D organ has a 1 mm effective depth or greater, a healthy reparative reaction can be expected.

b. Whenever the effective depth is less than 1 mm, we can expect either an unhealthy reparative reaction, or more frequently, destruction.

c. Whenever the material comes in contact with the pulp or root canal tissues (0 effective depth), a destructive reaction will definitely be initiated.

In answer to the second question—PCC can create a partially impervious layer on cut vital dentin at 1-1.5 mm thickness.

Regarding the third question—PCC does not increase the permeability of the underlying dentin. This may be due to the decreased microleakage at the interface with underlying dentin.

Regarding the fourth question—PCC is a good thermal insulator in thickness of 1.5 mm, but much less so than zinc phosphate cement and ZOE. At less than 1.5 mm it is not an effective thermal insulator. The material is electronically conductive at any thickness.

E. Film-forming resinous materials

The answer to the first question is "Yes, film-forming resinous materials are irritant to the P-D organ at certain effective depths."

1. Irritating ingredients are always the organic solvents and their cooling effect when they evaporate.

2. Effect at different effective depths

a. Applied to a P-D organ with an effective depth of 0.5-1 mm or more, there will be no reaction or a healthy reparative reaction.

b. With less than 0.5 mm effective depth, one should expect either an unhealthy reparative reaction or, infrequently, destructions, which will be sure at zero effective depth.

In answer to the second question—these resinous-based materials do not make an impervious film layer on cut dentin, neither in vitro nor in vivo, although they can make an impervious layer on a glass slab. This indicates that specific problems are related to the cut dentinal surface preventing the continuity of these films. These interfering agents could be crushed microscopic layers of hydroxy apatite crystals, coagulated and desiccated collagen and cytoplasm, and/or water. A varnish layer applied over these contaminants will have porosities.

Nevertheless, a varnish (liner) layer can hinder the penetration of 70% of the acids and irritating elements from the restorative materials and oral environment. The use of hand instruments to scrape away these contaminant layers and use of cavity cleaners as EDTA, or low concentration of citric acid (see Chapter 1) will enhance the continuity of the varnish (liner) film. The major advantage of varnish is that it can decrease microleakage if used under amalgam and zinc phosphate cement. There are several explanations for this phenomenon. The created film may act as a semi-permeable membrane, selectively passing elements and ions; or the film may reduce the irregularities of the cavity details, thereby improving the adaptability of the amalgam and zinc phosphate cements, thus decreasing leakage; or the film may occupy part or all of the microleakage space, thus minimizing or eliminating the microleakage space dimensions.

In answer to the third question—varnishes do not directly affect the permeability of the underlying dentin, but through their microleakage reduction and their 70% effective imperviousness, they can reduce the dentin permeability. Liners, on the other hand, can decrease the permeability of the underlying dentin if they contain calcium hydroxide or fluorides, or phosphates (sodium monofluorophosphate), as these materials can stimulate mineralization in the underlying dentin.

In answer to the fourth question—varnishes (liners) are not thermal or electrical insulators at any thickness used clinically.

Principles of Intermediary Basing

By now, it should be obvious that intermediary base materials are applied on dentin only to change certain properties of tooth structure and to impart certain protective or therapeutic characteristics. They should not be concerned with the resistance and retention form of the restoration, i.e., intermediary bases should be mechanically passive in any restorative combination. The following are the principles used to achieve these objectives.

If the layer of the intermediary base material is less than the dimensions of the microleakage space around the contemplated restoration (20 microns or less), and the permanent restorative material will not possess chemical and/or physical adhesion capabilities to tooth structure (e.g., ASPA or resin materials using enamel etching), nor have any therapeutic effect on tooth structures (fluoride exchange), the intermediary base could be applied all over the preparation details without interfering with the restorative therapy or with the resistance and retention forms. However, if the layer to be applied will exceed the dimensions of the microleakage space or if the permanent restorative material will depend mainly on physico-chemical adhesion for retention, the following rules must be followed:

A. Do not apply the intermediary base material on margins

or surrounding walls, rather, confine it to pulpal and axial walls only. If placed on surrounding walls and on margins, bases will occupy a space intended for the permanent restorative materials, which are less susceptible to failure mechanically and physically.

B. Confine the intermediary base material to the deepest part of the pulpal and/or the axial walls (the deepest part of the excavated dentinal caries cone) so that the peripheries of these walls and/or floors are in dentin or, at the very least, the restoration will be seated on two opposite points (areas) in dentin (Figs. 3 and 4). In other words, the entire pulpal or axial wall is not to be covered with the intermediary base, because if this is done, the weak intermediary base materials will yield to stresses induced from occlusal loading on the restorations, leading to micromovement of the restoration with all its sequelae (recurrent decay, tooth fracture, increased microleakage, tooth hypersensitivity and cracks, etc.).

C. Apply the minimal thickness of base material to fulfill the objectives (Figs. 4 and 5), as spaces unoccupied by intermediary bases can be occupied by the permanent restorative material, thereby adding to its bulk and improving its mechanical and physical properties.

D. Therapeutic intermediary bases are always very weak, even in their mechanically passive role. They should be either carried in an inert, biocompatible, reinforcing carrier (Fig. 4), forming a suitable base; or used as a subbase, to be covered with a stronger, more durable and compatible base (Figs. 3 and 6).

E. Operators should strive in designing and executing the dimensions, location, extent, and relationship of the intermediary base so as not to involve the base in the mechanical problems of the restoration.

F. If the subsequent restorative procedure involves substantial mechanical energy that may distort the dimension, location, extent, and relationship of the intermediary base, every effort should be made to locate the intermediary base material in areas that will receive the least energy, and/or to reinforce or cover it with a base that can withstand these types of energy with minimal disturbance (Figs. 3 and 6).

G. If the intermediary base material is to be directly loaded during subsequent restorative procedures, it should be securely retained in dentin to avoid subsequent displacement. Retention should be mechanical, physical, or chemical. Mechanical retention (Fig. 6) should be confined to bases only, as attempts to create mechanical locks for subbases will irritate or involve the pulp or root canal systems. Subbases can be immobilized in location by a retained base. The mechanical locks for the base should be at the very external peripheries of the defect and in the bulkiest area of the circumferential dentin (Fig. 6).

Determination of the Effective Depth

One of the basic factors in determining the choice of the intermediary basing materials and techniques is the thickness of the dentin bridge at the deepest portion of the preparation. The following procedures can be an aid in obtaining this information, although there is no absolutely reliable method.

A. From a radiograph of the tooth we can measure the dentin bridge at its deepest portion and the thickness of any clinically measurable anatomical part of the tooth, e.g., enamel thickness at the periphery of the preparation. On the tooth we can measure

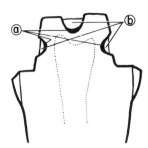

Fig. 13-3. a. Subbase of UNM, ZOE or calcium hydroxide. **b,** Base of modified ZOE, ZPC, or PCC.

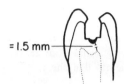

Fig. 13-4. Modified ZOE base.

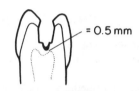

Fig. 13-5. Alkyl-salicylate calcium hydroxide cement base.

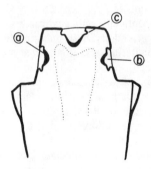

Fig. 13-6. Bases for cast and direct gold restorations. **a,** Subbase of UNM, ZOE or calcium hydroxide. **b,** Base of ZPC or PCC, **c,** Retentive grooves.

the same anatomical landmark. Then, using the following equation:

$$\frac{\text{Effective depth in the radiograph}}{\text{Enamel thickness in the radiograph}} = \frac{\text{Actual effective depth}}{\text{Actual enamel thickness}}$$

$$\text{Actual effective depth} = \frac{\text{Effective depth in radiograph} \times \text{actual enamel thickness}}{\text{Enamel thickness in the radiograph}}$$

This is a very reliable procedure. The only disadvantages are that we have to take a radiograph after excavating all irreparable dentin, and that it is a two-dimensional measure, rather than three-dimensional.

B. Correlate the actual depth of the lesion (as measured from the dentino-enamel junction) at its deepest location with the available dentin encasing the pulp chamber and root canal system. This procedure depends on complete comprehension of the tooth anatomy in three dimensions and extensive clinical experience.

C. Although sonic probes are still only available for research use only, they are the most reliable tools. They send ultrasonic waves through the dentin bridge at its thinnest location and then recover them. From this information the actual dentin thickness can be determined.

D. By correlating dentinal items with items recognizable in the preoperative radiograph, e.g., sclerotic dentin, dead tract, etc., we can estimate the thickness of the dentinal bridge. Also, from this observation we may encounter the shadow of the underlying pulp tissues. In the latter case we are assured that we are at least as close as 0.5 mm from the pulp chamber (the maximum thickness of dentin that can be transparent).

Compatibility of Intermediary Base Materials with Restorative Materials and Techniques

To evaluate the compatibility of intermediary base materials with restorative materials the following questions should be asked:

1. Does the intermediary base material interfere with the setting (hardening) reaction and the properties of the permanent restorative material? And if it does, what are the precautionary measures to prevent this interference if the intermediary base is the only therapeutically indicated material?

2. Can the intermediary base material discolor the permanent restorative material, and if so, what are the measures to prevent this effect?

3. Knowing the physical and mechanical properties of the intermediary base material, can its adaptation to underlying dentin, its dimension and its location be disturbed by the subsequent restorative procedures; and if they can, what are the measures to prevent this disturbance?

4. If combinations of intermediary base materials are used in the same preparation in contact with each other, can any one of them affect the setting (hardening) reaction of the other or any of its properties? If it does, what are the measures to prevent that?

A. ZOE

The eugenol of ZOE interferes with the setting reaction of any polymer and, to some extent, can even depolymerize already set polymeric materials. That is why it should not be brought into contact with resinous direct tooth-colored materials. Also, it can discolor other non-polymeric direct tooth-colored materials as a result of its diffusion through such porous materials. If ZOE is the only intermediary base material to be used (due to the condition of the P-D organ), it should be covered with zinc phosphate cement to minimize the amount of eugenol seeped to the resinous restorative material.

Under the manipulative energies anticipated in amalgam, direct gold, and cast alloy restorations, unmodified ZOE is not sufficiently rigid, tough, or durable. So, if used as a subbase,

it should be covered with a modified ZOE or zinc phosphate cement base. Modified ZOE bases, especially those containing EBA or reinforcements, perform adequately under such stresses.

Zinc oxide and eugenol can interfere with the setting of polycarboxylate cements, ASPA cements, and methyl cellulose carried calcium hydroxide, if they polymerize in contact with it. That is why ZOE subbases or bases should not come in contact with any of these materials.

B. Calcium hydroxide

Calcium hydroxide has no effect on the setting reaction or properties of any permanent restorative material. It does not discolor permanent restorative material. However, in translucent tooth-colored materials, especially with thin cross-sections, calcium hydroxide will show through as a chalky patch.

Calcium hydroxide carried in any carrier (other than methyl cellulose or one of its equivalents) cannot stand restorative manipulative energies without interfacial or bodily failure. Calcium hydroxide carried in methyl cellulose or in the form of alkyl salicylate chelate cement base can be used as a base under amalgam restorations and direct tooth-colored materials, but for direct gold and cast restorations any form of calcium hydroxide should be covered with a retaining-protecting-reinforcing base of zinc phosphate cement or polycarboxylate cement.

Calcium hydroxide in any other form than in methyl cellulose carried does not react or interfere with other intermediary base materials coming in contact with it. As mentioned, calcium hydroxide carried in methyl cellulose can be affected by ZOE. The organic solvent of varnishes (liners) and some of the monomers of resinous direct tooth-colored restorations could dissolve part of calcium hydroxide cements and carrier. The dissolution is incomplete because of the fast evaporation of the solvent and consumption of the monomer. Consequently, the effect is of little clinical significance except if applied in copious amounts.

C. Zinc phosphate cement

ZPC does not interfere with the setting or physical properties of any permanent restorative material. It does not discolor restorative materials per se, but if it is used in any other color than yellowish, its color will show through translucent or thin sections of direct tooth-colored materials. ZPC is the most rigid, tough and durable intermediary base material and will efficiently withstand all manipulative energies. It is completely compatible with other intermediary base materials. That is why it is more frequently used as a base over subbases than all the intermediary base materials.

D. Polycarboxylate cements

PCC does not interfere with the setting reaction of any permanent restorative material. It does not discolor restorative materials per se, but its color will show through translucent or thin sections of direct tooth-colored materials. PCC is durable enough to withstand manipulative forces during restorative procedures. Physico-chemically it is compatible with all intermediary base materials with the exception of ZOE and film-forming resinous materials.

E. Film-forming resinous intermediary base material

These resins do not interfere with the setting reaction of permanent restorative materials. They can be dissolved by the monomer of polymeric restorative materials, creating a dark line around the restoration, thereby making them esthetically unacceptable. As was mentioned, organic solvent carriers of this film-forming material could, to a very limited extent, dissolve calcium hydroxide carriers and cement. Film-forming resinous materials are not affected by the manipulative forces of restorative procedures.

In a practical sense, physically and chemically film-forming resinous materials are compatible with all intermediary base materials, except ASPA and polycarboxylate cement, as they may be dissolved by either. On the other hand, varnishes can interfere with the physico-chemical adhesion expected between each of these two materials and the tooth structures.

Indications and Uses of Intermediary Base Materials

Other chapters describe the indicated intermediary basing materials and designs with each permanent restorative technique. Here, a general view of the indications, rationale and use of different intermediary base materials will be provided.

A. ZOE

In its unmodified form, this is the oldest and most effective intermediary base material. It is one of the best insulators and sealers of the P-D organ. It has multiple pharmacological actions. It has an antiseptic effect upon microorganisms remaining in the dentin and it has sedative and anti-inflammatory action upon the P-D organ. Its hygroscopic action removes excessive moisture that may add to the irritation of the P-D organ. Its sealing ability minimizes microleakage and the ingress of irritants. And it insulates against thermal and galvanic shocks. All these effects and actions will give the P-D organ the best possible chance to undergo a healthy reparative reaction if ZOE is used as an intermediary base component.

Unmodified ZOE is the only base which can guarantee a favorable reaction in the P-D organ when the effective depth is less than 1 mm, even if the P-D organ has a history of degeneration or is undergoing a mild one. In its unmodified form, it is the only subbase used where Ca(OH)$_2$ is contraindicated for a P-D organ with a history of degeneration (Fig. 3). In its modified form, it can be ideal for bases under amalgam and cast restorations (Fig. 4). It is contraindicated as a base for polymeric restorative materials.

B. Calcium hydroxide

Calcium hydroxide can stimulate the fastest healing response in the P-D organ in certain situations, but it can also be the most destructive intermediary base material if used in contraindicated situations. Pharmacologically it is an extremely potent alkaline calcifying agent. It has a substantial antibacterial effect on carious dentin flora. It has some insulating properties as well as the ability to neutralize acids diffusing from an overlying material. As mentioned before, a healthy, sound P-D organ is a basic requirement for using calcium hydroxide as an intermediary basing component. In alkyl salicylate cement or methyl cellulose carried form it can be used

as a base under amalgam (Fig. 5) or direct tooth-colored materials, and as a subbase to be covered with zinc phosphate cement or polycarboxylate cement under direct gold and cast restorations. In any other form it should be used as a subbase followed by an appropriate base.

C. Zinc phosphate cement

ZPC is used as a base with or without an underlying subbase. Varnish films should always precede it on cut dentin. It is indicated when significant forces are anticipated during the subsequent stages of the restorative sequence, e.g., direct gold and cast restorations. Also, being compatible with all subbase materials, it can be used when other base materials are not compatible with subbase materials. It should not be used on effective depths of less than 2 mm without an intervening subbase. There is no therapeutic benefit from zinc phosphate cement bases; they are only a mechanical diffusion barrier and thermal insulator for the underlying parts of the P-D organ.

D. Polycarboxylate cement

PCC can also be used as a base either with or without underlying subbases. It could be used as a base for preparations with effective depths as low as 0.5 mm. There should not be any intervening varnish between it and underlying dentin. The only therapeutic subbase to be used under polycarboxylate cement is calcium hydroxide. There is usually no need for prepared mechanical modes in surrounding dentin to retain a base made of this material, as it has the ability of chemico-physical adhesion to tooth structure. Also, there is no therapeutic value of polycarboxylate cement bases. It, too, provides only a mechanical diffusion barrier and thermal insulation for underlying portions of the P-D organ.

Film-forming resinous material

Varnish films on cut dentin can hinder the passage of acids and most of the diffusing ions from overlying restorations or intermediary base materials. Also, on cut enamel and dentin it substantially decreases the microleakage space around amalgam restorations and, to some extent, around direct gold and cast alloy restorations. Varnishes should always be applied on cut tooth structure under amalgam restorations, under zinc phosphate cement, and on dentinal walls only under silicate cement and direct gold restorations. Varnishes have no therapeutic effect on the P-D organ. They only provide a diffusion barrier and antileakage effect. Cavity liners have the same effect and use as varnishes. In addition, however, they do have therapeutic effects, e.g., dentin mineralizing and acid neutralizing effects if they contain calcium hydroxide or zinc oxide, and anticariogenic effects if they contain fluoride components.

Preparation and Application of Intermediary Base Materials

A. Application of varnishes and liners

Dry the cavity properly with short blasts of warm air and dry cotton pellets. Hold a small cotton pellet in a tweezer, soak it in the varnish or liner. Carry it to the cavity. Starting at one corner, squeeze the varnish (liner) out of the pellet without moving it. Soak the pellet again and squeeze in another corner, and so on, until there is a continuous film over the cavity walls, floors, and margins. Usually three applications are sufficient. Let it dry for 2-3 minutes before inserting amalgam. To remove film from enamel walls, use a sharp chisel or resin solvents in light, gentle rubbing acts. It is always preferable to avoid film formation at contraindicated locations during the application of the materials.

B. Application of calcium hydroxide base or subbase

Dry the cavity. If it is calcium alkyl salicylate cement or methyl cellulose (or other equivalent polymer) carried calcium hydroxide, follow the following steps:

1. Squeeze equal parts from the base (basic) tube and catalyst (acidic) tube on a paper pad. Incorporate the two parts in each other with a stiff spatula, until there is homogeneous mix. Take a bead from the mix using a calcium hydroxide applicator and carry it to the cavity, flowing it on the surface of the concavity created by decay. Allow to dry for 1-3 minutes. Another bead to cover the concavity may be added, but before taking another bead, clean the applicator.

2. If the calcium hydroxide is in powder form, carry a small amount between the beaks of a tweezer and deliver it to the indicated area by releasing the tweezer beaks. Repeat the procedure several times, until the material occupies the desired dimensions.

3. If carried as a suspension in a liquid carrier, it is usually supplied in an injecting applicator. Shake the suspension, then inject a bead at the indicated area. The carrying fluid can be blotted with a cotton pellet or allowed to evaporate or left to coagulate in place, according to its composition and the manufacturer's instructions.

4. If $Ca(OH)_2$ is to be mixed with distilled water or other liquid to create a paste, mix on a paper pad to a thick consistency and carry it to the area in beads using a plastic instrument or calcium hydroxide applicator.

C. Application of ZOE base or subbase

Dry the cavity. Dispense a drop of eugenol and two measures of zinc oxide on a glass slab or a paper pad. Incorporate half of the powder in the liquid until there is a homogeneous mix. Add small increments of the powder and continue mixing after each addition, acquiring the proper consistency for the specific indication. Carry a small piece of the mix with a plastic instrument (flat-bladed side) to the desired location in the cavity. Compact a cotton pellet and carry it with a tweezer and load it with zinc oxide powder. Adapt the ZOE to the cavity walls with this cotton pellet. Another piece may be added, if desired, in the same fashion. Allow it to dry for five minutes. Remove excess with a spoon excavator and explorer soaked in alcohol or water. To accelerate setting, apply water to the surface of the base and leave it there.

D. Application of zinc phosphate cement base

Dry the cavity. Dispense one large and one small measure of the powder, then dispense one drop of the cement liquid on a cool glass slab. Divide the powder into 6-8 parts. Incorporate the first part in the liquid, mix it heavily on a large area of the slab until it is completely dissolved in the liquid. Repeat the

same with the second part, and so on, until there is a consistency thick enough to handle with your fingers. Soak first finger and thumb in alcohol or cement powder and take a piece from the cement mix and form a small ball out of it. Carry the cement ball to the cavity preparation with a plastic instrument, wet the plastic instrument in alcohol, and adapt cement to the desired areas. Allow it to set for 5 minutes, then flake away the excess with a sharp excavator.

E. Application of polycarboxylate cement

Dry the cavity. Dispense one drop of the liquid and one measure of the powder on a pad. Incorporate half of the powder in the liquid in patting and folding motions, using a small area of the pad surface. Add small increments of the powder to the mix, using the same mixing motions until acquiring the proper consistency. With a plastic instrument dusted with powder, pick up a piece of the mix large enough to fill the caries concavity. Apply it to the desired area in the cavity preparation adapt, and shape it with the plastic instrument. Remove excess using a sharp excavator and explorer.

BIBLIOGRAPHY

Barry, T., Clinton, D., and Wilson, A.: The structure of a glass-ionomer and its relationship to the setting process. J. Dent. Res. **58**(3):1072-1079, 1979.

Batchelor, R.F., and Wilson, A.D.: Zinc oxide-eugenol cements: I. The effect of atmospheric conditions on rheological properties. J. Dent. Res. **48**:883-887, 1969.

Berk, H.: Preservation of the dental pulp in deep seated cavities. JADA **54**:266, 1957.

Bernier, J.L., and Knopp, M.J.: New pulpal response to high speed dental instruments. Oral Surg., Oral Med. and Oral Path. **11**:187, 1958.

Bertenshaw, B.W., and Combe, E.C.: Studies on polycarboxylate and related cements. I. Analysis of cement liquids. J. Dent. **1**:13, 1972.

Bertenshaw, B.W., and Combe, E.C.: Studies on polycarboxylate and related cements. II. Analysis of cement powders. J. Dent. **1**:65, 1972.

Bertenshaw, B.W., Combe, E.C., and Grant, A.A.: Studies on polycarboxylates and related cements. 4. Properties of cements. J. Dent. **7**(2):117-125, 1979.

Braden, M.: Heat conduction in teeth and the effect of lining materials. J. Dent. Res. 315, 1964.

Bränström, M., and Nyborg, H.: Pulpal protection by a cavity liner applied as a thin film beneath silicate restorations. J. Dent. Res. **50**:90, 1971.

Brauer, G.M., Simon, L., and Sangermano, L.: Improved zinc oxide-eugenol type cements. J. Dent. Res. **41**:1096-1102, 1962.

Brauer, G.M., White, E.E., and Moskonas, M.G.: The reaction of metal oxides with o-ethoxybenzoic acid and other chelating agents. J. Dent. Res. **37**:547-560, 1958.

Carbini, R.C., Maisto, O.A., and Frodi, E.E.: Internal resorption of dentin histopathological control of 8 cases after pulp amputation and capping with calcium hydroxide. Oral Surg., Oral Med. and Oral Path. **10**:90, 1957.

Causton, B.E., and Johnson, N.W.: The role of diffusible ionic species in the bonding of polycarboxylate cements to dentin: an in vitro study. J. Dent. Res. **58**(4):1383-1393, 1979.

Charbeneau, G.T., and Bozell, R.R.: Clinical evaluation of a glass ionomer cement for restoration of cervical erosion. J. Am. Dent. Assoc. **98**(6):936-939, 1979.

Civjan, S., and Brauer, G.M.: Clinical behavior of o-ethoxybenzoic acid-eugenol-oxice cements. J. Dent. Res. **44**:80, 1965.

Copeland, H.I., Brauer, G.M., Sweeney, W.T., and Forziati, A.F.: Setting reactions of zinc oxide and eugenol. J. Res. N.B.S. **55**:134-138, 1955.

Craig, R.G., and Peyton, F.A.: Thermal conductivity of tooth structure, dental cements, and amalgam. J. Dent. Res. **40**:411, 1961.

Crisp, S., Abel, G., and Wilson, A.D.: The quantitative measurement of the opacity of aesthetic dental filling materials. J. Dent. Res. **58**(6):1585-1596, 1979.

Crisp, S., Lewis, B.G., and Wilson, A.D.: Characterization of glass-ionomer cements. 6. A study of erosion and water absorption in both neutral and acidic media. J. Dent. **8**(1):68-74, 1980.

Dennison, J.B., and Powers, J.M.: A review of dental cements used for permanent retention of restoration. I. Composition and manipulation, Mich. Dent. Assoc. J. **56**:116, 1974.

Eames, W.B., and others: Proportioning and mixing of cements: a comparison of working times. Op. Dent. **2**(3):97-104, 1977.

Eames, W.B., Hendrix, K., and Cleveland, D.: Pulpal protection of liners against zinc phosphate and 50% phosphoric acid: a primate study. Ga J. Autumn, 1978.

Eames, W.B., Hendrix, K., and Mohler, H.: Pulpal response in rhesus monkeys to cementation agents and cleaners. J. Am. Dent. Assoc. **98**(1):40-45, 1979.

Edwall, L.: Methods of measuring dentinal, pulpal, and periapical reactions to dental materials. Int. Dent. J. **24**(2):251-257, 1974.

El-Kafrawy, A.H.: Secondary dentin and pulp reactions to silicate cement in the teeth of monkeys. Thesis, Indiana University School of Dentistry, 1962.

El-Tahawi, H., and Craig, R.: Thermal analysis of zinc oxide-eugenol cements during setting. J. Dent. Res. Vol 50, #2, 1970.

Fairbourn, D.R., Charbeneau, G.T., and Loesche, W.J.: Effect of improved Dycal and IRM on bacteria on deep carious lesions. JADA **100**:547-552, 1980.

Fédération Dentaire Internationale, Specification for Dental Zinc Phosphate cement. Int. Dent. J. **13**:138-145, 1963.

Friend, L.A.: Handling properties of a zinc polycarboxylate cement. Br. Dent. J. **127**:359, 1969.

Gilson, T.D., and Myers, G.E.: Clinical studies of dental cements, II. Further investigation of two zinc oxide-eugenol cements for temporary restorations. J. Dent. Res. **48**:366, 1969.

Going, R.: Status report on cement bases, cavity liners, varnishes, primers, and cleaners. JADA **65**:694, 1972.

Gordon, S.M.: Gum copal solution for cavity lining and varnish. J. Am. Dent. Assoc. **23**:2374, 1936.

Hess, W.: The treatment of teeth with exposed vital pulp. Inter. D. J. **1**:10, 1950.

Hotz, P.R.: Experimental secondary caries around amalgam, composite and glass ionomer cement fillings in human teeth. SSO, **89**(9):965-986, 1979.

James, V.E., and Defenbach, O.B.: Prevention of histopathologic changes in young dog's teeth by the use of zinc oxide and eugenol. JADA **29**:583, 1942.

Jorgensen, K.D.: Factors affecting the film thickness of zinc phosphate cement. Acta Odont. Scand. **18**:479-490, 1960.

Jorgensen, K.D., and Petersen, G.F.: The grain size of zinc phosphate cements. Acta Odont. Scand. **21**:255-270, 1963.

Kawahara, H., Imanishi, Y., and Oshima, H.: Biological evaluation on glass ionomer cement. J. Dent. Res. **58**(3):1080-1086, 1979.

Kent, B.E., Lewis, B.G., and Wilson, A.D.: Glass ionomer cement formulations: I. The preparation of novel fluoroaluminosilicate glasses high in fluorine. J. Dent. Res. **58**(6):1607-1619, 1979.

Kozan, G., and Burnett, O.W.: Blood circulation in the dental pulp. JADA **59**:458, 1959.

Langeland, K.: Biologic considerations in operative dentistry. Dent. Cl. North Am., 125, March 1967.

Langeland, K.: Management of the inflamed pulp associated with deep carious lesion. Journal of Endodontics, Vol. 7, #4, April 1981.

Langeland, K.: Tissue changes in the dental pulp. An experimental histologic study. Oslo, Oslo University Press, 47, 1957.

Larson, G.H., Moyer, G.N., McCoy, R.B. and Pelleu, G.B.: Effects on microleakage of intermixing intermediary bases and cavity varnish. Operative Dentistry **4**:51-55, 1979.

Maldi, J., Wynn, W., and Culpepper, W.D.: Dental pulp fluid - I- relation between dental pulp fluid and blood plasma in protein glucose and inorganic element content. Arch. Oral Biol. **3**:201, 1961.

Manley, E.B.: Experimental investigation into the early effect of various filling materials on the human pulp. Roy. Soc. Med. Sect. Odont. Proc., **34**:693, 1941.

Manley, E.B.: Investigation into the early effect of various filling materials on the human pulps. Den. Res. **62**:1, 1942.

Manley, E.B.: Preliminary investigation into the reaction of pulp to various filling materials. Brit. D. J. **60**:321, 1936.

Marzouk, M.A.: Effect of deep cavity preparation on the tooth pulp using the operating microscope as well as serial histologic sections. Thesis submitted to Indiana University graduate school of Dentistry in partial fulfillment for the Master in Science in Dentistry degree, 1963.

McCabe, J.F., Jones, P.A., and Wilson, H.J.: Some properties of a glass ionomer cement. Br. Dent. J. **146**(9):279-281, 1979.

McLean, J.W.: Status report on the glass ionomer cements. Council on dental materials and devices. J. Am. Dent. Assoc. **99**(2):221-226, 1979.

Messing, J.J.: A polystyrene-fortified zinc oxide-eugenol cement. Brit. Dent. J. **110**:95-100, 1961.

Mitchell, D.F. and Jensen, J.R.: Preliminary report on the reaction of the dental pulp to cavity preparation using ultrasonic device. JADA **55**:57, 1957.

Mitchem, J.C., and Gronas, D.G.: Clinical evaluation of cement solubility. J. Prosthet. Dent. **40**:453, 1978.

Molnar, E.J., and Skinner, E.W.: A study of zinc oxide-rosin cements: I. Some variables which affect the hardening time. JADA **29**:744-751, 1942.

Negm, M.M., Combe, E.C., and Grant, A.A.: Factors affecting the adhesion of polycarboxylate cement to enamel and dentin. J. Prosthet. Dent. **45**(4):405-410, 1981.

Nordenvall, K.J., Brannstrom, M., and Torstensson, B.: Pulp reactions and microorganisms under ASPA and concise composite fillings. ASDC J. Dent. Child. **46**(6):449-453, 1979.

Norman, R., Phillips, R., and Swartz, M.: The effect of particle size on the physical properties of zinc oxide-eugenol mixture. J. Dent. Res., May-June, 1970.

Norman, R.D., Swartz, M.L., and Phillips, R.W.: Studies on film thickness, solubility and marginal leakage of dental cements. J. Dent. Res. **42**:950-958, 1963.

Norman, R.D., Swartz, M.L., Phillips, R.W., and Sears, C.R.: Properties of cements mixed from liquids with altered water content. J. Prosth. Dent. **24**:410-418, 1970.

Norman, R.D., Swartz, M.L., Phillips, R.W., and Virmani, R.: A comparison of the intraoral disintegration of three dental cements. JADA **78**:777-782, 1969.

Oilo, G., and Espevik, S.: Stress/strain behavior of some dental luting cements. Acta Odontol. Scand. **36**:45, 1978.

Oldham, D.F., Swartz, M.L., and Phillips, R.W.: Retentive properties of dental cements. J. Prosth. Dent. **14**:760-768, 1964.

Patterson, S.S., and Van Huysen, G.: The treatment of pulp exposure. Oral Surg., Oral Med. and Oral Path. **7**:194, 1954.

Phillips, L.J., Schnell, R.J., and Phillips, R.W.: Measurement of electric conductivity of dental cement. III. Effect of increased contact area and thickness; values for resin, calcium hydroxide, zinc oxide-eugenol, J. Dent. Res. **34**:597, 1955.

Phillips, R.W., and Love, D.R.: The effect of certain additive agents on the physical properties of zinc oxide-eugenol mixtures. J. Dent. Res. **40**:294-303, 1961.

Phillips, R.W., Swartz, M.L., and Rhodes, B.F.: An evaluation of a carboxylate adhesive cement. J. Amer. Dent. Assn. **81**:1353-1359, 1970.

Powers, J.M., Johnson, Z.G., and Craig, R.G.: Physical and mechanical properties of zinc polyacrylate dental cements. J. Am. Dent. Assoc. **88**:380, 1974.

Reader, A., and Foreman, D.: An ultrastructural qualitative investigation of human interdental innervation. Journal of Endodontics, Vol. 7, #4, 1981.

Seltzer, S., and Bender, I.B.: Early human pulp reaction to full crown preparation. JADA **59**:915, 1959.

Servais, G.E., and Cartz, L.: Structure of zinc phosphate dental cement. J. Dent. Res. **50**:613-620, 1971.

Shroff, F.R.: Effect of filling materials on the dental pulp. A critical review. J.D. Education **16**:216, 1952.

Silvey, R.G., and Myers, G.E.: Clinical studies of dental cements. V. Recall evaluation of restorations cemented with a zinc oxide-eugenol cement and a zinc phosphate cement. J. Dent. Res. **55**:289, 1976.

Smith, D.C.: Dental cements. Dent. Clin. North Am. **15**(1):3-31, 1971.

Smith, D.C.: A review of the zinc polycarboxylate cements. J. Canad. Dent. Assn. **37**:22-29, 1971.

Soremark, R., Hedin, M., and Rojmyr, R.: Studies on incorporation of fluoride in a cavity liner (varnish). Odontol. Rev. **20**:189, 1969.

Swartz, M.L., Niblack, B.F., Alter, E.A., Norman, R.D., and Phillips, R.W.: In vivo studies on the penetration of dentin by constituents of silicate cement. J. Amer. Dent. Assn. **76**:573-578, 1968.

Swartz, M.L., and Phillips, R.W.: In vitro studies on the marginal leakage of restorative materials. Journal of the American Dental Association, 62, 141-151, 1961.

Swartz, M.L., Phillips, R.W., Norman, R.D., and Niblack, B.F.: Role of cavity varnishes and bases in the penetration of cement constituents through tooth structure. J. Prosthet. Dent. **16**:963, 1966.

Swartz, M.L., Phillips, R.W., Norman, R.D., and Oldham, D.F.: Strength, hardness and abrasion characteristics of dental cement. J. Amer. Dent. Assn. **58**:367-374, 1963.

Swartz, M.L., Sears, C., and Phillips, R.W.: Solubility of cement as related to time of exposure in water. J. Prosth. Dent. **26:**501-505, 1971.

Swerdlow, H., and Stanley, H.R.: Response of the human dental pulp to amalgam restorations. Oral Surg. **15**(4):499-508, 1962.

Truelove, E.L., Mitchell, D.G., and Phillips, R.W.: Biologic evaluation of a carboxylate cement. J. Dent. Res. **50:**166, 1971.

Van Hassel, H.J.: Physiology of the human dental pulp. Oral Surg. **32**(1):126-134, 1971.

Van Huysen, G., and Boyd, D.A.: Operative procedures and the tooth. J. Pros. Den. **3:**818, 1953.

Virmani, R., Phillips, R.W., and Swartz, M.L.: Displacement of cement bases by condensation of direct gold. J. Amer. Acad. Gold Foil Oper. **8:**39-43, 1970.

Voth, E.D., Phillips, R.W., and Swartz, M.L.: Thermal diffusion through amalgam and various liners. J. Dent. Res. **45:**1184-1190, 1966.

Wilson, A.D., Kent, B.E., and Lewis, B.G.: Zinc phosphate cements: Chemical study of in vitro durability. J. Dent. Res. **49:**1049-1054, 1970.

Wilson, N.A., and Batchelor, R.: Zinc oxide-eugenol cement. II. Study of erosion and disintegration. J. Dent. Res. Vol. 50, 1970.

Yates, J., Murray, A., and Hembree, G.: Cavity varnishes applied over insulating bases: Effect on microleakage. Operative Dentistry, Vol. 51, 1980.

Zach, I., and Brown, G.N.: Pulpal effect of ultrasonic cavity preparation preliminary report. New York D.J. **22:**9, 1956.

Zander, H.A.: The effect of self-curing filling resin on the dental pulp. J.D. Education **16:**241, 1952.

Zander, H.A.: Reaction of the pulp to calcium hydroxide. J.D. Res. **18:**373, 1939.

Zander, H.A.: The treatment of dentin before insertion of restorations. Int. D.J. **4:**693, 1954.

CHAPTER 14

The management of deep carious lesions

One of the basic steps in a restorative operative procedure is the removal of carious dentin. Unfortunately, this procedure is still empirical, resulting in a great deal of inconsistency. It is a well documented fact that recurrence of decay under and around restorations is primarily caused by the mishandling of carious tooth structure at the time of tooth restoration, i.e., iatrogenically created problems. In this chapter we will try to give the reader some insight into these problems and establish possible solutions.

I. Types and Layers of Dentinal Carious Lesions

There are two types of carious processes, *acute* and *chronic*. They differ in the dynamics of their creation, the reaction of tissues to them, and the resultant end-products of their activity.

Any dentinal carious lesion in a vital P-D organ will exhibit five layers, or zones, when undecalcified tooth sections (ground sections) are examined under an optical microscope (Figure 1A and 1B). The zones are not neatly arranged with definite demarcations. There is some overlap and some zones may be missing in certain sections. They differ in their dimensions, contents, nature, and activities in the two types of carious processes. The five zones are:

A. Decayed zone
B. Septic zone
C. Demineralized zone
D. Transparent zone
E. Opaque zone

We shall examine each zone separately, starting with the most superficial, and distinguish differences between acute and chronic decay exhibited in each zone.

A. Decayed zone (Figs. 1 and 2A)

The dentin in this zone is almost completely devoid of minerals, more so in acute than in chronic lesions. The organic matrix is completely decomposed to an unrecognizable state. Collagen fibers, if found, have completely lost their cross-striations and links. There is a high concentration of microorganisms in the destructured dentin mass with substantial amounts of residual plaque deposits. The only activity in this layer is microbial. Its thickness will vary depending upon whether it is an opened, partly opened, or closed lesion. The maximum thickness is found in closed lesions (Fig. 1). The decayed zone is clinically similar in acute and chronic lesions,

with the exception that chronic lesions may be more odiferous, due to extensive lysis, and darker in color, due to the longer duration of the decay process, which allows for greater activity of chromogenic bacteria.

Zones of decay in acute decay.

Zones of decay in chronic decay.

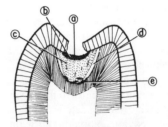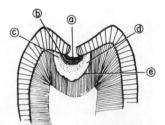

Fig. 14-1. a, Decayed zone. **b,** Septic zone. **c,** Demineralized zone. **d,** Transparent zone. **e,** Opaque zone.

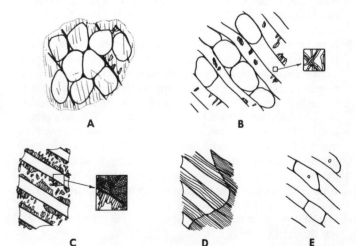

Fig. 14-2. Zones of decay in dentin. **A,** Decayed zone. Accumulation of microorganism, plaque, complete loss of structure. **B,** Septic zone. Invasion by microorganisms, irregular crystal formation, deformed tubules, loss of collagen banding structure and intermolecular connection. **C,** Demineralized zone. **D,** Transparent zone. **E,** Opaque zone.

B. Septic zone (Figs 1 and 2B)

The highest concentration of microorganisms is found here. Although the dentin is very well decalcified (more so in acute than in chronic decay), its framework structure can still be recognized, but the collagen fibers have fewer cross-band striations than normal, and intermolecular links are lost. The remaining mineral crystals are deformed, irregularly scattered, and show no relation to the collagen fibers. The dentinal tubules are extremely widened and cavitated. This layer may have slightly greater dimensions in chronic than in acute decay and, again, only microbial activity is found in this layer. The color resembles that of the first zone (ranging from a light yellow to a dark reddish brown, depending upon the presence and duration of chromogenic bacterial activity).

The previous two zones have the softest consistency of all the zones, and the consistency is softer in an acute lesion than in a chronic lesion.

C. Demineralized zone (Figs. 1 and 2C)

Clinically this is the most significant zone, both diagnostically and therapeutically. Here the dentin is only demineralized, with the dentinal matrix still intact. Collagen fibers still have their normal cross-band structure striations and intermolecular cross-links, and the remaining mineral crystals are still attached to collagen fibers. The dentinal tubules still have their normal dimensions. In this zone, although there are destructive activities in the form of decalcification, there are also repair activities in different forms of remineralization, precipitating a variety of phosphate crystals in different shapes and compositions, e.g., tricalcium phosphate (white lockite), large rhombohedric crystals, regular apatite crystals, caries crystals, and others. Acute and chronic decay differ greatly in this zone.

The dimension of this zone is greater in an acute lesion than in a chronic lesion. According to Fusiyama, a maximum width for this layer is 1750 micrometers in acute decay, with a minimum of 50 micrometers width in chronic decay. Remineralization activities are much less pronounced in acute decay, with a lower percentage of deposition of new phosphate crystals. Microorganisms will be confined to the superficial $1/3$-$1/2$ of this zone in acute decay, but will be found throughout this zone in chronic decay. The color of this zone in acute decay is straw yellow, the color of decalcified dentin that does not exhibit microbial or environmental staining. For chronic decay, however, the color is always yellow-brown or dark brown, depending upon the amount of time it has been subjected to microbial and environmental staining activity. The consistency and hardness of the dentin in acute decay in this zone will be much less (possibly more than 15 times less) than in chronic decay. Repair activities will be more noticeable at the sides of the dentinal caries cone, decreasing gradually to the tip of that cone. This contrast is more pronounced in acute than in chronic decay, for in chronic decay it is occasionally observed that crystal deposition activities will be evenly distributed throughout the caries cone.

D. Transparent zone (Figs. 1 and 2D)

This zone appears transparent in ground sections, but will definitely appear radiopaque in a radiograph. It is the area of undisturbed mineralization repair. It is the zone of dentinal sclerosis and the calcific barrier, the two most impermeable and impenetrable types of dentin. This zone is more pro-

nounced in chronic decay. Although present in acute decay, it will be of smaller dimensions and will occasionally be interrupted. The discontinuity of this zone in acute decay is almost always at the tip of the dentinal caries cone, which defines the maximum advancement of the lesion and the extent of bacterial toxins and destructive agents. This zone may contain a few microorganisms in a chronic lesion. Clinically, this zone may be slightly discolored compared to the surrounding unattacked dentin due to the remineralization of decalcified stained dentin. The dentin in this zone is extremely hard when compared with normal dentin (19 times greater on the average) and is found to be harder in chronic lesions.

E. Opaque zone (Figs. 1 and 2E)

This zone is usually found pulpal to the transparent zone. It is characterized by intratubular fatty degeneration with lipid deposits being precipitated from fatty degeneration of the peripheral odontoblastic processes. This type of degeneration predisposes to the sclerosis of the dentinal tubules. This zone is more pronounced in acute lesions and will appear radiolucent in a radiograph.

The process of decay advances until each of these zones, starting with the opaque zone, arrives at the pulp. The maximum resistance to pulpal penetration occurs with the arrival of the transparent and demineralized zone. However, if the septic zone penetrates the pulp chamber, the P-D organ will be unable to offer any resistance, and will suffer complete collapse.

One should bear in mind that the chronic or acute status of a lesion can be changed if there is a change in the environment encouraging one condition over the other. For example, by diminishing or eliminating the presence of bacterial substrates, an acute lesion may become chronic in nature. Conversely, by increasing the presence of bacterial substrates, a chronic lesion may become acute in nature.

II. Effects of Caries on the P-D Organ

The carious process creates three distinct forms of irritants: biological irritants (microorganisms and their metabolites), chemical irritants (acids), and physico-mechanical irritants (the gradual diminution of the effective depth of the P-D organ due to the advancing carious process). Each of these irritants will precipitate a reaction in the P-D organ at one stage of its progress. It has been demonstrated by some investigators that the P-D organ will react to caries as early as the stage of enamel caries. Conversely, other investigators proved that no actual reaction will start until the caries is 2 mm or less from the pulp chamber. These diverse results merely confirm that many factors are involved in the type, extent, and destructive-protective nature of the P-D organ reaction toward the caries irritation. Therefore, for proper therapy, it is essential to correctly diagnose the type, extent and nature of the pulp-dentin reactions to the decay process. The following factors are guidelines for this essential information.

A. Type of decay

Understandably, the more acute the decay process is, the less effective the defensive reparative mechanisms will be, with a greater tendency towards a destructive reaction in the P-D organ. Chronic decay is usually accompanied by substantial repair provided it has not involved the pulp or root canal system. However, should the microorganisms involved in chronic decay, which are present even in the transparent zone, directly contact the pulpal tissues, the potential for a destructive pulpal reaction will be initiated. Some of these microorganisms are anaerobic and can maintain activity even when isolated from the oral environment.

B. Duration of the decay process

The longer the duration in acute decay, the more massive the destruction of tooth structure. The longer the duration in chronic decay, the greater the chances for repair, provided the pulp chamber and root canal system are not directly involved. Again, however, chronic decay possesses the potential to be irritating, considering the microbial population and virulence in these lesions. Whenever the carious lesion is isolated from the underlying pulpal tissues by sound dentin (original or reparative), the carious process in chronic decay can stimulate repair. In acute lesions, however, due to the high diffusion of microbial irritants, the carious process can be very destructive.

C. Depth of involvement

It is simple mechanics and physics that the deeper the caries cavity is, the nearer the sources of irritation are to the pulp. This creates greater intensity of irritation with a greater possibility of pulpal destruction. For peripheral involvements (Fig. 3A), we would anticipate either no pulpal reaction at all, or a reparative reaction in both acute and chronic lesions. For moderate depth involvement (Fig. 3B), we can expect the same reaction from chronic decay as was observed in peripheral involvement. For acute lesions of moderate depth we would observe some resolved pulpal destruction. For profound depth involvement (Fig. 3C), we can expect some repair and perhaps resolved pulpal destruction in chronic decay, but definite pulpal destruction (resolved or unresolved) in acute decay. For perforating lesions (Fig. 3D), we can expect pulpal destruction in both types of decay. Whether it is resolved or unresolved will be dependent upon the other factors mentioned in this section.

D. Number and pathogenecity of microorganisms

The greater that the virulence and population of microorganisms are, the greater is the likelihood of the pulpal reaction ultimately being destruction.

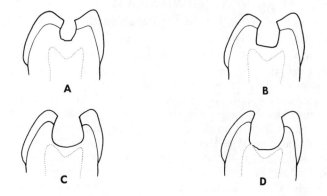

Fig. 14-3. Depth of involvement. **A,** Peripheral involvement–outer one third, or less of dentin. **B,** Moderate involvement–outer two thirds, or less, of dentin. **C,** Profound involvement–more than two thirds of dentin short of perforation. **D,** Perforating involvement.

E. Tooth resistance

This involves an infinite number of factors, ranging from the thickness of dentin through which the decay must pass to initiate a recognizable effect, to the permeability of the involved dentin, the solubility of the involved dentin, the fluoride and calcium content of the involved dentin, the susceptibility of the tooth, and so forth.

F. Individual reaction of the P-D organ

Myriad factors, both known and unknown, which can influence the individual reaction of the P-D organ, include tooth age, patient's age, cellularity and vascularity of the pulpal and root canal system tissues, population group differences, etc.

One should recognize, then, that factors (E) and (F) constitute the basis for the differences observed in the reactions of pulp-dentin organs to seemingly the same type and extent of a carious process. Some generalizations must be made, however, and following are average figures from well documented investigations. They are to be used as diagnostic and therapeutic guidelines—bearing in mind that individual cases may vary according to the modifying effects of the previously described factors (A) through (F).

We should now define "effective depth". The effective depth is the area of minimum thickness of sound dentin separating the pulpal tissues from the carious lesion. This is usually found in the deepest portion of the caries activity.

1. When we have an effective depth in the P-D organ of 2 mm or more, we can expect a healthy reparative reaction.

2. When the effective depth is from 0.8 to 2 mm, we can expect an unhealthy reparative reaction.

3. When the effective depth is less than a 0.3-0.8 mm range, we can expect pulpal destruction.

III. Effect and Fate of Microorganisms Sealed in a Cavity with an Inert Sealer

Several experiments were done (Besic) where the superficial and peripheral carious dentin was removed from a caries cavity, leaving carious dentin only in the deepest portions of the cavity (Both pulpally and axially). Population types and distribution were established for the microorganisms remaining in the carious dentin. The cavities were then sealed with a sealer that was totally inert, both in terms of pulpal and microbial response. After varying intervals of time, the cavities were reopened and the types, numbers, and condition of the microorganisms still present were evaluated and compared to the original microbial population. The results of these experiments revealed that:

A. There was a sharp decrease in the number of microorganisms.

B. There were no traces of lactobacilli or spirochetes.

C. The residual microorganisms (mainly staphylococci and streptococci) had undergone morphological changes.

D. No carious activity in the form of demineralization was observed. On the contrary, in certain cases there were some signs of remineralization.

It must be emphasized here that the cases were well chosen, with an established history of the P-D organ in each case. There were periodic check-ups to insure the potency of the seal of the cavity obliterants. Due to the nature of the experiments, the respective populations and activities of anerobes were not established.

IV. Incidents of Macroscopic Direct Pulp Exposures

It has been well documented that whenever a carious lesion extends 3-4 mm pulpally or axially to the DEJ, visible perforation to the pulp chamber can be expected in 75% of the cases. This figure will increase the younger the chronologic or physiologic age of the tooth. Also, perforation incidents are more inevitable the further apically the lesion occurs on the axial wall; or if the carious lesion is the first irritant to which the tooth is subjected, i.e., there is no history of previous restorations, periodontal disease, occlusal disease, etc.

V. Incidents of Microscopic Direct Pulp Exposures

As previously mentioned, the peripheral pulpal tissues (the odontoblastic layer, subodontoblastic layer, and layer of Weil) are partially or completely avascular. Blood vessels, if present, have very narrow, tortuous lumen, which severely impede the passage of both red and white blood cells. Therefore, if these layers are involved in excavating carious dentin from a deep carious lesion (which would constitute a direct pulp exposure), there will be no hemorrhage observed from the perforation. The only evidence of a perforation of the pulp chamber will be the oozing of the colorless dental pulp fluid, which, regrettably, can only be observed microscopically. The unaided eye will not detect the perforation. One can surmise, then, that pulp exposures occur with far greater frequency than we are able to detect, for preparations which we assume end in sound dentin may, in fact, be microscopic pulp exposures, and our subsequent intermediary basing and restorative efforts will be entirely misdirected.

VI. The Lack of Reliable Clinical Devices Either to Differentiate Between Remineralizable and Non-Remineralizable Affected Dentin or to Assure Complete Removal of Irreparable Carious Dentin

We frequently depend upon our tactile sense, using explorers, excavators, or round burs, to verify the soundness of the dentinal walls and floors in tooth preparation, i.e., to insure that we have removed all the undesirable non-remineralizable dentin. These techniques are mainly uncontrollable, unmeasurable tests of the hardness and abrasive resistance of the remaining dentin. They are diagnostic tools with inherent human errors, with inconsistent and usually unreliable results. Fusiama and his coworkers demonstrated by hardness testing that the Knoop Hardness Number (KHN) of the remaining dentin following clinical removal of carious dentin using a spoon excavator was 22.8 ± 9.95 KHN; using a round bur for excavation, the remaining dentin was to have a KHN of 28.4 ± 16.36. When compared to the KHN of sound dentin, which is 69, it becomes abundantly apparent that this present type of testing procedure is, indeed, completely unreliable. Additionally, it should be emphasized that there is no correlation between dentin abrasive resistance or hardness and its ability to remineralize. Obviously, there is a great need for the development of more consistent diagnostic tools in the treatment and removal of carious dentin.

VII. The Relationship Between Discolored Attacked Dentin and its Soundness or Reparability

As was discussed in the previous section, relying on the hardness of dentin as an indication of its capacity to remineralize can be misleading and totally unreliable. The same observation can be made in attempting to correlate the color of dentin with its capacity to remineralize. We find, for example, areas in chronic decay which have been demineralized, stained by chromogenic bacterial activity, but have subsequently remineralized to a far greater extent than sound dentin. The calcific barrier and sclerotic dentin, in fact, are usually darker in color than sound, unattacked dentin. Conversely, in acute decay, there may be areas of dentin demineralized to the point of irreparability which are the same color of sound unattacked dentin. Sound unattacked dentin may have different colors in the same tooth, perhaps even in the same wall of the preparation, depending upon the concentration and arrangements of the contents in each area. So the traditional philosophy of establishing dentinal walls and floors of uniform color should be abandoned. It should not be the color, but rather the soundness and reparability of the dentin that determines the removal or inclusion of that dentin in the cavity preparation.

VIII. The Disinfection of Dentin

Another remnant of traditional technique is to sterilize the preparation walls and floors to prevent new carious activity. As mentioned before, the sterilizing effect will not be permanent insofar as the leakage space around and under the restoration will allow any size of oral microbia to ingress to any portion of a cavity preparation. Also, effective disinfectants can interfere with the physiologic function of the P-D organ, which is badly needed for both the repair of attacked dentin and the maintenance of the defensive mechanisms which are responding to the offending microbia. Finally, impregnation of microbia into sound or repaired dentin occurs only in chronic decay, where the microorganisms have been walled off from the pulpal tissues by a well established transparent zone of dentin. In acute decay, the reparable areas of dentin are almost totally devoid of microorganisms. So in either chronic or acute decay, there is really no need for disinfectants to ensure or aid the reparative capacity of the P-D organ.

IX. The Correlation Between the Symptomatology and Histopathology of the P-D Organ

A basic requisite for correct therapy is to know both the type and nature of the disease as well as the reparative capacity of the host organ. In our case the host organ is the P-D organ. Its reparative capacity depends on its physio-pathologic condition. Many attempts have been made to correlate the actual histopathology or histology of the P-D organ and recognizable symptoms, but none have been completely successful. We will be confronted with patients who show no symptoms of pain or discomfort, yet whose pulpal tissues are undergoing acute degenerative changes. Conversely, other patients may have simple pulpal hyperemia (engorgement of blood vessels) but will complain of a severe toothache. It is safe to say there is no absolutely reliable correlation between the symptoms and histopathology of the P-D organ. Any symptoms should be verified by other diagnostic means, insofar as symptoms are frequently not indicative of either the condition or the reparative capacity of the P-D organ.

X. Frequency of Location of Direct Pulp Exposures

Documented research has revealed that in excavating carious dentin that is directly continuous with either the pulp chamber or root canal system (i.e., a direct carious exposure), operating on teeth with little or no previous symptomatology, the exposure will occur in the demineralized zone in 90% of the cases. Further, the cases have demonstrated that the dentin peripheral to the perforation will exhibit both the transparent and opaque zones pulpal to the demineralized zone. This indicates that the P-D organ still may retain reparative capacity even if there is direct continuity between the caries cone and the pulpal and/or root canal system tissues.

XI. Diagnosis and Prognosis of Deep Carious Lesions

From the previous discussion it is obvious that an adequate and detailed diagnosis of the following items is essential for proper therapy in the management of deep carious lesions:

A. Reparative capacity of the P-D organ

B. Soundness of the dentin in the preparation floors and walls

C. Reparative capacity of unsound attacked dentin

D. Type and extent of any degeneration in the P-D organ

E. Sealability of the restorative materials to be used

F. Potential further irritation to the P-D organ resulting from preparation instrumentation, restorative materials and restorative procedures. If possible, the nature and extent of their irritation should be estimated.

Unfortunately, our available diagnostic tools are not sufficiently reliable to get an exact picture of the involved tissues and tooth. However, by combining the results of the following clinical tests and observations, we can gain a good diagnostic perspective.

1. Pain

The absence of a toothache cannot be used as a deciding criterion for the status of the P-D organ insofar as pain thresholds differ from one individual to another. Also, teeth with non-vital P-D organs are frequently painless.

The presence of pain may serve as a guiding criterion for the status of the P-D organ, although this is not very reliable. For example, pain at night or spontaneous pain not initiated by thermal or chemical stimulation of the P-D organ could indicate possible destructive degenerative changes in the P-D organ. However, pain initiated by thermal or chemical stimulation of the P-D organ that disappears immediately after the removal of the stimulation is a possible indication of a much lesser degree of degenerative changes. There are, of course, degrees of pain that lie between the aforementioned examples. Any symptoms of pain should be recorded, in the patient's own words, to be used in conjunction with other diagnostic tools.

2. Radiographs

Although they give a two-dimensional image of three-dimensional structures, radiographs, especially periapical radiographs, can be a very practical supporting tool. A radiograph can indicate:

a. The proximity of the carious lesion to the pulp chamber and root canal system. From this, the thickness of the dentinal bridge (effective depth) can be estimated. It should be emphasized that the extent of the carious lesion as shown in the radiograph will always be less than the actual size of the lesion.

b. Any pulpal changes in the form of intrapulpal and peripulpal calcification, which will denote the consumption of and reduction of the reparative capacity of the pulp. If these calcified tissues are deposited in areas which will restrict or prevent the flow of fluids into or out of the pulp and/or root canal system, we can be assured of either lessened or lost reparative capabilities of the P-D organ. If the calcified tissues are evenly distributed, but to an extent that we observe an exaggerated physiological age of the tooth, we are assured of maximum consumption of the reparative capabilities and maximum decrease in the space (pulp chamber and root canal system) for the reparative tissues to function. Further irritation to such a pulp-dentin organ may easily lead to the destruction of any remaining reparative tissues.

c. The thickening of the periodontal ligament space with an intact lamina-dura, especially periapically, will indicate increased vascularity and consequently increased activities of the P-D organ. Discontinuity in the lamina-dura may indicate more advanced activities of the P-D organ, possibly destructive in nature.

d. The vital capacity of the P-D organ as a function of the size of the pulp chamber compared to the size of the tooth. The higher the pulp size/tooth size ratio is, the better will be the reparative capabilities of the P-D organ. However, it must be mentioned that an unusually high ratio in comparison to the adjacent, opposing, and contra-lateral teeth may indicate complete cessation of the reparative capabilities of the pulpal tissues of the involved tooth.

e. The location of the caries cone tip relative to the anatomy of the pulp chamber and root canal system. Caries cones proximate to constrictions in the pulpal or root canal tissues will profoundly affect the design of the cavity preparation and the choice of an intermediary base.

f. The relative size of the apical foramen to that of the pulp and root canal system tissues. The higher the ratio is, the better will be the reparative potential of the P-D organ.

g. The size (diameter) of a pulp exposure relative to the dimensions of the pulp chamber and root canal system. This is a major factor in determining the repairability, via dentinal bridging, of the exposure.

h. The gross evaluation of mineralization, and consequently the permeability, of the involved dentin. We can radiologically identify sclerotic dentin, which will appear radiopaque; the calcific barrier which, again, will appear radiopaque; and tertiary dentin, which will appear as a localized thickening of the dentinal bridge, pulpal to the lesion, creating irregularities in the pulp chamber or root canal walls and/or roof. This data is very important in determining the reparative capability of the P-D organ and the type of intermediary base to be used.

3. Pulp testing

a. Thermal pulp testing

This can be accomplished by simple application of heat or

cold on the tooth. Examples of cold stimuli would be cotton pellets soaked in ethyl chloride or liquid nitrogen, or simply chips or sticks of ice. Heat stimuli would include heated compound or gutta percha sticks, or, in the case of teeth with full coverage crowns, the use of a rubber cup or wheel under pressure generating frictional heat. A positive response from any of these stimuli merely denotes that there is some pulpal vitality. Make note, however, that a negative response does not indicate a non-vital pulp. The thermal conductivity of enamel and dentin is extremely low, and if these structures are bulky in thickness, they will prevent the transmission of hot and cold stimuli.

b. Electric pulp testing

This is performed with instruments employing battery or alternating current powered electrodes to transmit electric stimuli through the P-D organ. When a positive response is obtained, comparisons should be made with the adjacent, opposing, and contra-lateral teeth. Notation should be made for the minimum energy required to elicit a response in these control teeth. If the required energy is higher in the control teeth, this is an indication of possible acute changes in the P-D organ of the affected tooth. If the required energy is lower in the control teeth, this may indicate possible progressive chronic changes, advance repair, or walling off of the P-D organ from the offending lesion.

A positive response, however, does not always indicate vitality in the P-D organ. The inflammatory exudative fluids and pus that may fill the pulp chamber and root canal system of recently devitalized teeth are good electric conductors and may generate a false response. Conversely, negative responses may also be misleading, insofar as dehydrated or hypermineralized dentin may be poor electric conductors. Therefore, electric pulp testing should not be the sole diagnostic tool in recording or verifying the vitality or the degenerative status of the P-D organ.

4. Direct pulp exposure

The direct exposure of the pulp or root canal system is usually accompanied by symptoms which are the most indicative of the actual condition of the P-D organ. The following is the data that can be collected from observation of a direct pulp exposure and its clinical significance:

a. A pin-point exposure having sound dentin at the periphery of the exposure, with no hemorrhage, in a vital P-D organ, is an indication of either no pulpal inflammation or a mild degree of pulpal inflammation restricted to the exposure site. This can be successfully repaired, if properly treated.

b. A pin-point exposure having sound dentin at its periphery, but accompanied by a drop of blood that coagulates immediately on the cavity floor in the form of a button is also an indication of a healthy, reparable P-D organ. Mild pulpal inflammation will be restricted to the exposure site.

c. An exposure having decayed or infected carious dentin at its periphery would indicate considerable inflammation in the pulpal or root canal tissues far beyond the exposure site. The reparability of this type of exposure is doubtful.

d. An exposure accompanied by profuse hemorrhage could be an indication of great involvement (usually mechanical) of the pulpal and root canal tissues. This type of exposure is usually beyond repair.

e. An exposure accompanied by inflammatory fluids or pus is evidence of extensive inflammation and destruction of the pulpal and root canal tissues. This indicates the P-D organ is definitely beyond repair.

f. The lower that the ratio of the exposure diameter relative to the dimensions of the pulpal and root canal tissues is, the greater will be the possibility of repair and healing of the P-D organ.

g. The closer the exposure is to anatomical constrictions in the pulpal chamber or root canals the less will be the reparability locally, because of the diminished availability of nutrients. Also, repair in these areas may occlude the adjacent pulpal vasculature causing total destruction of the pulpal and root canal tissues.

5. Percussion sensitivity

Tenderness to percussion is of little value in determining the degree of inflammation in the pulpal and root canal tissues. Although teeth with extensive inflammation often exhibit tenderness to percussion (especially when directed laterally), teeth in which the inflammation is restricted only to the coronal portion of the pulp, or even to the exposure site, frequently exhibit pain to percussion. The psychological reaction of a patient in pain makes this response quite unreliable in evaluating the pathology of the P-D organ. Tenderness to percussion, therefore, merely demonstrates the likelihood of some type of pathology in the P-D organ.

6. Type of dentin

Visual examination and tactile evaluation by use of an explorer can give us an idea of the type of dentin present in the preparation walls and floors. The presence of a calcific barrier or sclerotic dentin close to the pulp chamber indicates reparative activity. Generalized discoloration of the dentin, not arising from a previous amalgam restoration, and which ranges from grayish to grayish-pink or grayish-brown, may indicate a devitalized or dying P-D organ that has lost all reparative capacity.

7. Removal of tooth structure without anesthesia

The removal of tooth structure without anesthesia, whether it is the removal of soft dentin using a spoon excator, or hard dentin using rotary instrumentation, is a very reliable, albeit potentially painful, test to verify the vitality of the P-D organ.

8. Selective infiltration or ligamental anesthesia

If pulpal symptoms described by the patient involve a total side or a quadrant, local or periodontal infiltration anesthesia for the most suspected tooth should stop the pain if the anesthetized tooth is the offending one.

9. Use of dyes to differentiate between reparable and irreparable dentin.

Suggested method to guide an operator as to where to stop in excavating dentin from cavity walls and floors is to apply a solution of 0.5% basic fuchsin in propylene glycol to the dentin for 10 seconds, then thoroughly wash the preparation with water. The irreparable areas of dentin will distinctly stain red. Fusiama and his coworkers have shown that the banding between the reparable and irreparable areas will be very clear to the unaided eye. They claim that the nature of the collagen fibers constitutes the difference in the stainability in the two layers of dentin. The reparable attacked dentin will have intact collagen fibers oriented for remineralization and will not stain with the fuchsin solution. However, the irreparably attacked dentin will have its collagen fibers denatured to the extent of being non-receptive to remineralization and can be stained red by the fuchsin solution. Another dye which creates the same effect is a 1% acid red solution in propylene glycol.

10. To differentiate between pain coming from upper teeth or from maxillary sinus, a swab soaked in topical anesthetic ointment or gel is introduced through the nostrils into the middle conchae upwards, medially and backwards for about ¾ of an inch, applying the topical anesthesia to the mucous membrane of the walls of the conchae. If the pain is of a sinus origin, it will disappear momentarily. If it is from dental cause, it will not.

XII. Treatment of Acute Decay

Deep lesions (deeper than 2 mm from the DEJ) confirmed as acute decay using the aforementioned criteria, can be treated in the following sequence.

A. All possible information regarding the status of the P-D organ should be collected using the previously mentioned diagnostic tools.

B. All undermined or unwanted enamel in the preparation should be removed.

C. If it is safe to remove all softened dentin without creating an exposure, this should be done using a spoon excavator. The reparability of the remaining dentin should be verified using the basic fuchsin or red dye solutions. Any non-reparable dentin should be removed.

D. If there is imminent danger of creating a pulp exposure by removing all softened dentin, the deepest layer should be left, provided:

1. The P-D organ has been established as being healthy.

2. The remaining dentin has been established as being reparable. (This dentin would constitute the deepest portion of the demineralized zone.)

3. The softened dentin that is to remain should be located in the deepest part of the pulpal and/or axial wall. The surrounding walls and at least a portion of the pulpal and axial walls should be in hard sound dentin.

E. If there is any doubt about (1) or (2) in (D), treat the lesion and the P-D organ as you would in chronic decay.

XIII. Treatment of Chronic Decay

Deep carious lesions proven to be chronic in nature, or any lesion whose acute nature is suspected should be treated in the following sequence:

A. The physiologic status of the P-D organ should be evaluated using as many of the aforementioned diagnostic tools as possible.

B. All undermined or unwanted enamel in the preparation should be removed.

C. All softened dentin should be removed, using either spoon excavators or large round stainless steel burs in a slow-speed handpiece. The soundness of the remaining dentinal matrix should be evaluated using the appropriate dyes, and any non-reparable dentin should be removed.

D. If removal of softened dentin leads to an exposure of the pulpal or root canal tissues, proceed either with the appropriate pulp capping procedure or with endodontic therapy.

In both acute and chronic decay, after removing undesirable dentin from the cavity preparation, proceed with the proper selection and application of intermediary bases (see chapter on intermediary bases and basing).

XIV. Indirect Pulp Capping (Gross Caries Removal, or Caries Control) (Fig. 4A, B, C, D)

When we are confronted with multiple carious lesions in which the removal of all carious dentin will invariably lead to several pulp exposures, it is a prudent idea to first attempt indirect pulp capping.

Dynamics of Indirect Pulp Capping

The caries formula consists of three items, each of which is essential for the caries process to be active and progressive. They are: tooth structure, microorganisms, and substrates. If any of these items is missing, the caries process will stop. By indirect pulp capping, we are removing two items, namely, microorganisms and substrates.

In acute decay, the excavation of softened dentin will remove all microorganisms. In chronic decay, minimal numbers of microorganisms will remain, but they will be rendered inert by effectively sealing them off from their source of substrates via an appropriate therapeutic temporary restoration. Therefore, the only element remaining in the caries formula will be tooth structure. A favorable environment will have been created for the repair of damaged tooth structure, which will proceed in two dimensions.

First, remineralization of part or all of the remaining decalcified dentin in the cavity floor will occur; and, secondly, deposition of secondary and/or tertiary dentin pulpal to the carious lesion will be initiated as dictated by the medicaments used and the physiological condition of the P-D organ. Indirect pulp capping should be limited to those teeth that have been evaluated to be free from any form of pulpal degeneration insofar as the success of the operation is dependent upon the reparative capacity of the P-D organ. The technique is as follows:

A. Data regarding the condition of the P-D organ should be collected and recorded using as many diagnostic tools as possible.

B. The decayed and infected zones and the external part of the decalcified zone in the carious lesions are excavated using a spoon excavator. It is not necessary to remove all undermined enamel, especially if losing the enamel will diminish the retention of the temporary restoration. All surrounding walls should be cleared of softened tooth structure to improve the sealability of the temporary restoration (Fig. 4B).

C. Suitable capping material (according to the condition of the P-D organ and the location of the lesion) is flowed over the remaining softened dentin on the pulpal and/or axial walls (Fig. 4C).

D. Modified ZOE, ZPC, PCC, or amalgam temporaries are placed so as to be in occlusal function, insofar as functional use of the tooth will accelerate the repair process in the P-D organ (Fig. 4C).

E. A radiograph is taken, the patient is made familiar with the signs and symptoms of degeneration in the P-D organ, and asked to report if any are experienced. The patient is recalled in 4-6 weeks if the capping material is calcium hydroxide, or 6-8 weeks if the capping material is unmodified ZOE.

F. After the designated period, a radiograph is taken and the same diagnostic data is collected and compred to the pretreatment data. If signs and symptoms indicate no degeneration

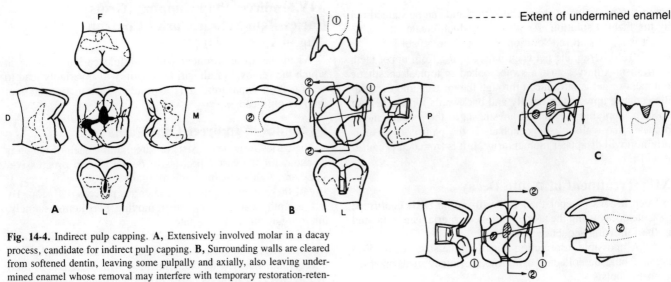

- - - - - Extent of undermined enamel

Fig. 14-4. Indirect pulp capping. **A,** Extensively involved molar in a dacay process, candidate for indirect pulp capping. **B,** Surrounding walls are cleared from softened dentin, leaving some pulpally and axially, also leaving undermined enamel whose removal may interfere with temporary restoration-retention. **C,** Indicated indirect capping material placed. Tooth is ready for temporaray restoration. **D,** After the designated recuperation period for the P-D organ the tooth is prepared for permanent restoration, using part of the indirect capping material as an intermediary base (acute decay), or total cavity re-entry procedure is persuaded (chronic decay).

in the P-D organ, the indirect pulp capping procedure can be considered a clinical success and we can proceed with (G).

G. All undesirable and/or undermined enamel is removed and the tooth is prepared for permanent restoration. The capping material and part of the temporary may be left as an intermediary base in the case of acute decay (Fig. 4D). However, in the case of chronic decay, all the temporary and capping materials should be removed. The underlying softened dentin should be excavated and the appropriate intermediary base is placed prior to creation of the permanent restoration.

H. If repair is not apparent and there are signs of a degenerated or degenerating P-D organ, endodontic therapy should be instituted immediately.

I. If the removal of the softened remaining dentin under the capping material leads to a pulp exposure, proceed with direct pulp capping or endodontic therapy.

XV. Direct Pulp Capping (Fig. 5, A, B, C and D)

If a perforation of the pulp chamber or root canal system occurs during the removal of the decay, the tooth can be considered a candidate for direct pulp capping provided:

A. There are no signs or symptoms of degeneration in the P-D organ and there is sufficient evidence of reasonable reparative capacity.

B. The exposure has the following characteristics:
1. The exposure is pin-point in size or has a small diameter relative to the pulp size
2. There is either no observable hemorrhage from the exposure site, or, if there is hemorrhage, the blood immediately coagulates in the form of a small button at the exposure site
3. The dentin at the periphery is reparable as verified by different visual and tactile tests.

4. The exposure site is not at a constricted or potentially constricting area in the pulp chamber or root canal system (Fig. 6).

C. The field of operation is completely aseptic.

The basic idea of direct pulp capping is to generate a dentin bridge composed of secondary or reparative dentin. The mechanism is precipitated by either a dentin chip and unmodified ZOE or calcium hydroxide being placed directly over the exposure site. The procedure is as follows:

1. All previously described data regarding the physiologic status of the P-D organ should be collected and recorded.

2. All undesirable and/or undermined enamel and unsound dentin should be removed (Fig. 5B).

3. The cavity floor and exposure site should be gently washed and irrigated with sterile water. Drying should be done with sterile cotton pellets, not an air spray.

4. Either calcium hydroxide or unmodified ZOE can be used as a capping material, depending on the health of the P-D organ and the location of the exposure site (Fig. 5C).

5. When using ZOE, sound dentin shavings are cut from surrounding walls and deposited at the exposure site, and then covered with a creamy mix of unmodified ZOE.

6. When using calcium hydroxide, a creamy mix is prepared and placed directly on the exposure site.

7. The unmodified ZOE and calcium hydroxide are handled the same way as intermediary bases in regard to location, dimensions, etc.

8. The permanent restoration should then be placed. However, in the case of cast restorations, the casting should be temporarily cemented until the status of the P-D organ is well established (Fig. 5D).

9. The patient should be informed of the signs and symptoms of pulpal degeneration and advised to report if any are experienced.

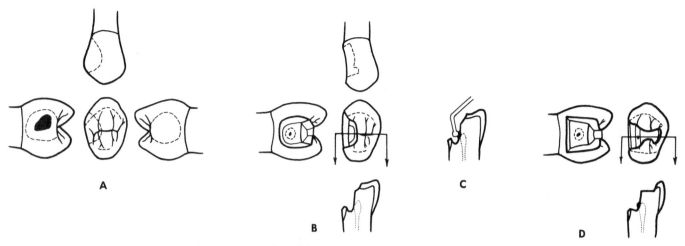

Fig. 4-5. A, Interproximal lesion on distal of right maxillary second premolar. **B,** Lesion is excavated, resulting in pulp exposure. **C,** Appropriate direct capping material is applied to exposure site. **D,** Tooth is prepared for permanent restoration.

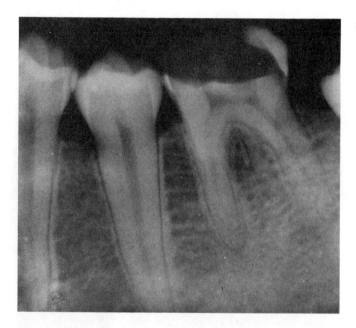

Fig. 14-6. Tooth #19 with a perforating lesion. Poor candidate for direct pulp capping, as perforation is opposite to a constriction and the exposure diameter:pulp chamber dimension, ratio is very high.

10. The patient is recalled after 6-8 weeks if calcium hydroxide is the capping agent, or 8-9 weeks if the capping agent is unmodified ZOE and dentin shavings. Data will be obtained to evaluate the status of the P-D organ and compared with the data that was gathered prior to treatment, and a prognosis for the P-D organ will be established. If the pulp is degenerated or degenerating, endodontic therapy should be instituted immediately.

It should be emphasized here that after the indicated treatment of deep carious lesions the optimum healing environment should be created for the P-D organ. This implies that the P-D organ should be protected from further unnecessary tooth preparation, irritating cementing agents, biologically toxic restorative materials, and so forth. For further discussion concerning the effect of the intermediary base material on cut dentin or exposed pulpal or root canal tissues, refer to the chapter on intermediary bases and basing.

BIBLIOGRAPHY

Anderson, D.M., and others: Criteria for the assessment of dental pulp beneath deep caries. Proceedings, International Association for Dental Research, J. Dent. Res. **59**(Spec. Issue A):467, Abstract No 799, 1980.

Anderson, A.W., Sharav, Y., Massler, M.: Reparative dentin formation and pulp morphology. Oral Surg. Med. Path. **26**:837-847, 1968.

Berggren, H., and Cederberg, I.: The translucent zone of reaction in the dentin. A radioautographic study, Ark. Pys. **4**:565, 1952.

Bernick, S., Warren, O., and Baker, R.F.: Electron microscopy of carious dentin. J. D. Res. **33**:20-26, 1954.

Besic, F.C.: Fate of microorganisms in deep carious lesions. J. Dent. Res. **22**:349, 1943.

Black, G.V.: Operative Dentistry, Vol. I. The pathology of the hard tissues of the teeth, Glossary and Index, Vol. II. Technical procedures in filling teeth. Chicago: Medico-Dental Publishing Co. 1908.

Bradford, E.W.: The dentin, a barrier to caries, Brit. Dent. J. **109**:387-398, 1960.

Brannstrom, M., and Lind, P.: Pulpal response to early dental caries, J. Dent. Res. **44**:1045-1050, 1065.

Burkman, N.W., Schmidt, H.S., and Crowley, M.C.: A preliminary report of an investigation to study the effectiveness of certain drugs for sterilization of carious dentin, Oral Surg. **7**:647, 1954.

Burnett, G.W., Scherp, H.W.: Bacteriologic studies of the advancing dentinal lesion. J. D. Res. **30**:766-777, 1951.

Dirksen, T.R.: Lipid components of sound and carious dentin. J. D. Res. **42**:123-132, 1963.

Dowden, W.E., and Langeland, K.: A correlation of pulpal histopathology with clinical symptoms, J. Dent. Res. Proceedings **48**:183, Abstract No. 569, 1969.

Dowden, W.E., and Lange and, K.: A correlation of dental caries, bacterial penetration, and pulpal histopathology, J. Dent. Res. Proceedings **49**:179, Abstract No. 523, 1970.

Fusayama, T.: Two layers of carious dentin diagnosis and treatment, Operative Dentistry **4**:63-70, 1979.

Fusayama, T., Okuse, K., and Hosoda, H.: Relationship between hardness, discoloration and microbial invasion in carious dentin, J. Dent. Res. **45**:1033-1046, 1966.

Fusayama, T., and Terashima, S.: Differentiation of two layers of carious dentin by staining, Bulletin of Tokyo Medical and Dental University **19**:83-92, 1972.

Johansen, E., and Parks, H.F.: Electron-microscopic observations on soft carious human dentin, J. Dent. Res. **40**:235-248, 1961.

Kato, S., and Fusyama, T.: Recalcification of artificially decalcified dentin in vivo. J. Dent. Res. **49**:1060-1067, 1970.

Kuboki, Y., Ohgushi, K., and Fusayama, T.: Collagen biochemistry of the two layers of carious dentin. J. Dent. Res. **56**:1233-1237, 1977.

Langeland, K.: Biologic considerations in operative dentistry. Dental Clinics of N.A., Phil. & London, W.B. Saunders Co., p. 125, 1967.

Langeland, K.: Biologic considerations in operative dentistry, Dent. J. North Am. 125, March 1967.

Langeland, K. (Editor): International conference on deep carious lesions, A.D.A. F.D.I., New York, 1969.

Langeland, K.: Management of the inflamed pulp associated with deep carious lesion, Journal of Endodontics. Vol 7, No. 4, April 1981.

Langeland, K.: Tissue changes in the dental pulp. An experimental histologic study, Oslo, Oslo University Press, p. 47, 1957.

Langeland, K., and Langeland, L.K.: Indirect capping and the treatment of deep carious lesions, Int. D. J. **18**:326, 1968.

Lichtenberg, Crone, Fr.: Deep dentinal caries from a microbiologic point of view, Int. D. J. **18**:481, 1968.

Lundy, T., and Stanley, H.R.: Correlation of pulpal histopathology and clinical symptoms in human teeth subjected to experimental irritation, Oral Surg., Oral Med., and Oral Path. **27**:187, 1969.

MacGregor, A.B., Marsland, E.A., Batty, L.: Experimental studies of dental caries. I. The relation of bacterial invasion to softening of the dentin, Brit. D. J. **101**:230, 1956.

Marzouk, M.A.: Effect of deep cavity preparation on the tooth pulp using the operating microscope as well as serial histologic sections, Thesis submitted to Indiana University Graduate School of Dentistry in partial fulfillment for the Master in Science in Dentistry degree, 1963.

Massler, M.: Pulpal reactions to dental caries, Int. Dent. J. **17**:441, 1967.

Mechanic, G.L.: The intermolecular cross-link precursors in collagens as related to function. Israel Journal of Medical Sciences, **7**:458-462, 1971.

Nyborg, H.: Healing processes in the pulp on capping, Acta Odont. Scand. 13, Luppl 16, 1955.

Ohgushi, K., and Fusayama, T.: Electron microscopic structure of the two layers of carious dentin, J. Dent. Res. **54**:1019-1026, 1975.

Reeves, R., and Stanley, H.R.: The relationship of bacterial penetration and pulpal pathoses in carious teeth, Oral Surg. **22**:59, 1966.

Sato, Y., and Fusayama, T.: Removal of dentin by fuchsin staining, J. Dent. Res. **55**:678-683, 1976.

Schroeder, A.: Indirect capping and the treatment of deep carious lesions, Int. D. J. **18**:381, 1968.

Shimizu, C., Itoh, K., Yamada, T., Hachiya, Y., Iwaku, M., and Ohba, J.: Pulp reactions to the fuchsin solution for caries diagnosis, Japanese Journal of Conservative Dentistry **20**:140-143, 1977.

Shovelton, D.S.: Studies of dentin and pulp in deep caries, Int. Dent. J. **18**:392, 1968.

Takuma, S., Kurahashi, Y.: Electron microscopy of various zones in a carious lesion in human dentin. Arch Oral Biol. **7**:439-453, 1962.

Terashima, S., Watanabe, M., Kurosaki, N., and Kono, A.: Hardness of dentin after clinical excavation of soft dentin, Japanese Journal of Conservative Dentistry **11**:115-120, 1969.

Walkoff,: Dentisterie Opératoire, 3rd Ed., J.B. Ballierére et Fils, Paris. 1891. (Quoted from Marmasse, A. 1963).

Wei, S.H., Kaqueler, J.C., and Massler, M.: Remineralization of carious dentin, J. Dent. Res. **47**:381-391, 1968.

Yoshida, S., and Massler, M.: Pulpal reactions to dental caries, N.Y. State D. J. **34**:215-222, 1964.

CHAPTER 15

Single tooth restorations and the periodontium

To be biologically acceptable, a restoration must be compatible not only with the pulp-dentin organ but also with the periodontium. It is a paradox that despite the fact that destroyed root canal tissues are replaceable with inert materials, and destroyed periodontal tissues are virtually irreplaceable, vast amounts of research deals with the effect of operative procedures on the pulp, while little is written or researched on the effects of operative procedures on the periodontium.

The purpose of this chapter will be to elucidate the cause-effect relationship that exists between procedures for single-tooth restorations and their influence on adjacent periodontal tissues. For this discussion, the following physio-anatomical facts concerning the peridontium are re-emphasized.

A. Physiologically, the periodontium should be considered as one organ, composed of the gingiva, dento-gingival attachment, periodontal ligament, and alveolar bone. Therefore, any irritation to one element, e.g., the gingiva, will be followed by a reaction in underlying and surrounding components of the entire organ.

B. The normal free gingival margin has a knife-edge relationship to the facial and lingual surfaces of the teeth. This discourages the accumulation of plaque and food substrates in these areas. In contrast, edematous inflammation of these structures would predispose to accelerated plaque accumulation.

C. The normal gingival crevice, which is lined with a non-keratinized epithelium, should be envisioned as a "potential" space. If an instrument or other foreign body is forced into a healthy crevice, the space thereby created will regain its non-dimensional status once the intervening object is removed. If, however, the crevice space is violated by the foreign object for a long period of time, it will remain accommodable to other available environmental materials.

D. Healthy crevicular epithelium is relatively immobile in relation to the adjacent tooth. Therefore, any physical or mechanical manipulation of this epithelium as during tooth preparation, can lead to destructive reactions in underlying components of the periodontium. Such destruction begins as denudation of the non-keratinized epithelium lining the crevice.

E. Interproximal contact of teeth is defined by the "contact area". Depending upon physiological, chronological, and pathological processes, the gingiva will, for a period of time, extend up and around the contact area. The maximum extent will be at the buccal and lingual papillae. This creates a col-shaped area of gingiva, like a saddle, between adjacent teeth. Even this col has a knife-edged relationship with adjacent tooth surfaces. When adjacent teeth erupt, the col is covered with a layer of tissue 1-2 cells in thickness known as "reduced enamel epithelium". This tissue possesses a formative, not a protective, function, and as it lacks the capacity of repair or keratinization, it is normally replaced by stratified squamous epithelium derived from the oral mucosa. However, under abnormal circumstances, such as the failure of the reduced enamel epithelium to unite successfully in the col, or damage to the reduced enamel epithelium by operative procedures, any subsequent inflammatory reaction will fail to resolve, and chronic inflammation will ensue. Under the best conditions, this could lead to interdental crater formation; in the worst conditions, pocket formation and periodontitis could result.

F. Passive eruption of teeth is an age-related, physiologic process that reaches a plateau between the ages of 25 to 30 years. The process changes the spatial relationship between the cemento-enamel junction, the attachment epithelium, the apical extent of the crevice, and the alveolar bone crest. Ultimately, the last three of these end-up apical to the cemento-enamel junction. Identifying the topographical relationship between these four components is essential in designing restorations.

G. With advancing age, the facial and lingual papillae can undergo atrophy. When this is combined with gingival recession, the proximal gingiva acquires a convex surface with a varying distance between it and the contact area. This geriatric apical migration of the periodontium exposes unusual anatomical variations in surface topography (e.g., concavities, flat facets, etc.). That become a part of the clinical crown which must be considered when designing restorations.

H. In the healthy periodontium, the crevicular fluid is alkaline in nature (see Chapter 1).

I. The normal facial and lingual contours of teeth are designed to distribute food during mastication to the facial and lingual gingiva in a physiologic manner. This means that the mechanical energy of mastication is distributed to the tissues in such a manner that it will massage them, stimulating circulation and keratinization. Restorative procedures must reproduce physiologic contours in order to facilitate these same beneficial effects.

J. The normal occluding anatomy of teeth should not only serve for proper incision and grinding of food and its deflection away from the occlusal surfaces and contact areas, but also should be able to direct functional forces parallel to the long axes of the teeth. In this way, such forces will be most favorably received by the periodontium, with a stimulating and maintaining effect on that organ. Any restoration should be designed to deliver such loading forces in the proper direction, as improper (e.g., lateral) loading on the periodontal ligament can hasten its demise.

K. Properly restored contact areas, with their accompanying marginal ridges and embrasures, preserve the integrity of the periodontium by

1. Preventing food impaction proximally.
2. Allowing physiologic, tissue stimulating, food streams during mastication.
3. Maintaining the mesio-distal dimensions of the arch and preventing teeth from tilting.

L. The normal mandibular movements allow protection of the periodontium in lateral excursions via a disclusion mechanism. Laterally applied forces are minimized and the teeth with high periodontium:tooth dimension ratios receive the majority of these lateral forces. This is accomplished through canine protection, group function, or mutually protected occlusion.

M. Even though, clinically, the gingival margin and wall of a restoration appears to coincide perfectly with the gingival margin and wall of a cavity preparation, microscopically there will be discrepancies (overhangs or underhangs) of from 20-200 micron. In addition, there will be microscopic microleakage spaces, which vary in size with every restorative material and procedure. Both of these marginal discrepancies will harbor bacterial plaques, especially if they are found subgingivally, removed from natural and artifical cleansing mechanisms.

N. It is essential to have a suitable zone of attached gingiva and a comparable depth of adjacent vestibule to maintain the integrity of the facial and lingual periodontium. This is accomplished by discouraging the accumulation of plaque and food substrates at the free gingiva and thereby resisting their entry to the underlying periodontal components.

I. Irritating Factors for the Periodontium

Unfortunately, the periodontium is irritated not only *prior* to the operative procedure by the disease process itself, and *during* the operative procedure by even the most meticulous instrumentation, but also *long after* the operative procedure by the mere presence of the restoration in close proximity to soft tissues. The following summarizes all the irritating factors involved:

A. Caries

The gingivae will react to caries in a stage as early as superficial enamel decalcification, primarily due to the roughening of the enamel or dentin predisposing to enhance plaque accumulation. Of course, the soft tissue inflammation will increase with more advanced cavitation of tooth structure. The reaction of the periodontium can range from marginal gingivitis to periodontitis, depending upon the nature of tooth destruction, population of microorganisms in the plaque, and host resistance. Periodontal reaction will be more severe with cariogenic loss of physiologic contact and contour of the tooth. The closer the carious lesion to the periodontium and the more plaque retaining the lesion is, the more destructive will be the reaction of the periodontal tissues.

So, whenever we treat a lesion approximating adjacent gingiva, we must realize that the periodontal tissues are in a state of inflammation and that our operative procedures and materials must not enhance that condition. It is best, therefore, to try to solve any periodontal problems *before* undertaking any operative procedure.

B. Teeth separation

Although it is sometimes required by the restorative procedure, separation of teeth for access should not exceed the width of the periodontal ligament space (0.2-0.5 mm). If separation does exceed this, the periodontal ligament will be compressed on one side of the tooth and possibly torn on the other side. Failure to immobilize a separator can cause further trauma to the ligaments. Prolonged separation can cause irreversible ischemia, so proper massaging of the area is important to restore circulation to the periodontium. Even under favorable circumstances, separation beyond that achieved with wooden or plastic wedges should be discouraged.

C. Rubber dam

The rubber dam affords protection from instrumentation and chemicals for the gingiva and underlying periodontal tissues *when it is properly applied*. However, it could just as easily be hazardous to these tissues if:

1. There is insufficient interseptal rubber, causing compression ischemia of the interdental gingiva and facial and lingual papillae, or separation of the interdental gingiva from the adjacent tooth.
2. The clamps are incorrectly chosen and/or applied, traumatizing already inflamed gingiva.
3. The dental floss or tape used to seat interseptal rubber is pushed with detrimental force against periodontal tissues; or if the floss serves to force intracrevicular rubber during inversion of the dam causing separation of tissues from tooth surface; or if floss is used as a ligature, strangulating or lacerating entrapped gingiva.

D. Preparation instrumentation

During tooth preparation itself, the following items should be considered in an effort to avoid detrimental effects to the periodontal tissues:

1. Of all the insulting factors resulting from tooth preparation, vibration is the most irritating to the periodontum. Vibration can lead to laceration of periodontal ligament fibers; it can create dilaceration or cessation of root formation in a developing tooth; or it can cause compression and ischemia of ligament fibers and their blood vessels.
2. Preparation of gingival cavosurface margins is most effectively and atraumatically accomplished with properly utilized hand instruments. Unfortunately, using rotary instruments in this area will almost invariably result in laceration and bruising of tissue, with healing by secondary intention.
3. Injury to adjacent gingival tissues can usually be avoided if an effort is made to preserve the proximal plate of enamel during gross cavity preparation.
4. Before preparing the proximal portion of any tooth, placement of wedges from the facial and/or lingual, apical to the contact area, will assure protection of the

underlying periodontium from the mechanical and physical trauma of instrumentation. In addition, the wedges can not only create some separation for access, but they can also aid in controlling gingival fluids.

5. Handling of the periodontium in subgingivally extended lesions is covered in the chapter on principles of the restoration of badly broken down teeth.

6. If there is very limited attached gingiva and/or vestibule adjacent to a cervical lesion facially or lingually, avoiding recurrence of decay can only be accomplished by free gingival grafting or laterally repositioned flap to establish an indicated thickness of attached gingiva; or by surgically deepening the sulcus if adjacent anatomy allows.

E. Matricing

Matrices for amalgam, direct gold, and direct tooth-colored materials should not only be firm and unyielding, but they must also be biologically acceptable. To fulfill these requirements, the matrix must be:

1. Properly contoured mesio-distally and bucco-lingually to reproduce normal tooth form.

2. Properly contoured occluso-gingivally, so that its gingival end does not exceed the apical extent of the gingival crevice. It does not involve the gingiva or any component of the periodontium between it and the tooth, and it reproduces the tooth shape occluso-gingivally.

3. Properly stabilized by the appropriate retainer, wedges, and/or compound to avoid slippage apically and laterally, which might cause laceration and contusion of the gingiva and underlying periodontal tissues.

F. Gingival retraction

Some destruction can happen as a result of procedures designed to control the peripheral components of the periodontium prior to any restorative procedure requiring a completely dry gingival sulcus. Physical retraction methods (see chapter on cast restorations) are not usually responsible for tissue destruction unless retracting items are forced past the apical extent of the gingival crevice, or if they involve strangulating gingival tissue against the tooth surface. In both cases, gingival laceration and contusion can occur, which may be followed by gingival and/or alveolar bone resorption.

The three chemical methods of retraction (see chapter on cast restorations) differ in their effects on the periodontium. Physiologically constricting chemicals have no local tissue after-effects. Fluid coagulant chemicals may leave the gingiva in an inflamed condition, but healing by primary intention could occur within a week, with only slight residual recession. Surface layer tissue coagulants may leave the gingiva in a state of severe inflammation, with surface ulceration or even partial loss of sulcular epithelium. Healing by secondary intention occurs within two weeks, with considerable residual recession.

Electrosurgical procedures to retract the gingiva will leave the tissues covered with a coagulum, possibly accompanied by minute ulcerations. The gingiva recovers from the mild to moderate inflammation by both primary and secondary intention, with only slight residual recession. The degree of inflammation and the fate of the periodontium after any of these procedures is not only dependent on the nature of the retraction procedure, but also on the post-retraction environment. Sub-

sequent impression procedures, plaque control, temporary restorations, and permanent restorations can either promote healing or aggravate the initial inflammatory process.

G. Impression procedures

In fabricating cast restorations, the periodontium could be affected by impression procedures and materials. Examples include:

1. Heat from hydrocolloid sols and exothermic polymerizable impression materials

2. Catalysts and chemical by-products of rubber base elastomeric impression materials causing allergic reactions

3. Mechanical trauma caused by repeated insertion and removal of impression compounds

H. Temporary restorations and their fabrication

The trauma from this procedure to the periodontium could result from:

1. Excessive or residual monomer of a resinous temporary material.

2. Exothermic heat of polymerization.

3. Irritating qualities of the cementing medium.

4. Physico-mechanical irritation from temporary restoration try-in, intraoral adjustment, cementation and removal of excess cement.

J. Restorations

In any of the previous steps, even the most meticulous operator cannot avoid some irritation to the periodontium. However, such irritation is reparable and reversible provided:

a. The gingival tissues were previously healthy.

b. The restoration itself will create an environment suitable for healing.

The effect of the restoration on the periodontium may be considered in relation to eleven factors:

1. The first is the shape of the restoration with respect to its contour, occlusal form, and contact areas. The facial and lingual surfaces of a restored tooth can predispose to food stagnation and heavy plaque accumulation if those surfaces are overcontoured, thereby deflecting the food stream away from the gingiva. By contrast, occluso-apical undercontouring of those surfaces, especially if the resulting shape is box-shaped or tapered, can lead to atrophy and abrasion of the gingiva. The mesio-distal contour of the facial and lingual surfaces is actually more influential in regulating plaque accumulation on these surfaces. A restored tooth should have the indicated convexities and concavities to coincide with the configuration of the adjacent periodontium.

The restoration is required to have an occlusal form which will:

a. Direct the functional forces parallel to the long axis of the tooth.

b. Allow maximum freedom in all functional jaw movements.

c. Provide maximum masticatory efficiency.

d. Deflect the food stream away from contact areas by proper size, shape, and position of marginal ridges.

e. Protect the periodontium from lateral loading by proper discluding mechanisms.

f. Re-establish the proper mesio-distal and occluso-apical

dimensions of the tooth in order to prevent tilting or supere-ruption of not only the restored tooth, but also of adjacent or opposing teeth.

The shape of the restoration also exerts its influence on the periodontium by the size, extent, shape and location of restored contact areas. A contact that is too broad bucco-lingually or occluso-gingivally changes the anatomy of the interdental col, increasing the surface area of irritation-prone, non-keratinized epithelium. In addition, such an area becomes more difficult to clean, markedly increasing the chances for inflammation. A contact that is too narrow will allow adverse vertical stresses on tissues unaccustomed to such energy. Narrow contacts also invite food impaction. A contact that is placed too occlusally results in a flattened marginal ridge at the expense of the occlusal embrasures. A contact that is placed too lingually or facially compromises facial or lingual embrasures. A contact placed too gingivally diminishes the gingival embrasure and exaggerates the occlusal embrasures. All of these contact area deficiencies will predispose to food impaction and concomitant periodontal harm.

2. The surface finish of the restoration is directly related to its capacity to retain plaque. At this time, there is no restorative material available which can duplicate the surface glaze of tooth enamel. Bear in mind, however, that gingival irritation in proximity to rough surfaces is a function of bacterial, rather than mechanical irritation. Soft tissues may adjust themselves equally well to a rough, unpolished surface as to a highly polished one, as long as plaque accumulation is scrupulously controlled.

3. Marginal discrepancies, e.g., overhangs and underhangs, are minor factors in gingival irritation, especially when they are microscopic. Nevertheless, their irritation stems, again, from their enhancement of plaque accumulation in proximity to soft tissues.

4. Poor marginal adaptation of restorations allows the formation of a crevice between the gingival wall of the prepared tooth and the restoration. Such a crevice harbors bacterial plaque predisposing to a full spectrum of periodontal inflammation. A classic example of such a fault occurs when a cast restoration is seated without proper cavity debridement, frequently trapping granulation or gingival tissue between the restoration and the gingival floor. Such tissues will degenerate and become necrotic, serving as a good culture for bacteria. The poor marginal adaptation, therefore, becomes a continuous source for bacterial toxins that are injurious to periodontal tissues.

5. Electrical potentials and galvanism between restorations of dissimilar metals can create atrophic degeneration in the adjacent gingiva or sometimes encourage gingival recession.

6. The chemical effects of restorative materials on the periodontium include: corrosion products, phosphoric acid of silicate cement and zinc phosphate cement, and monomers of tooth-colored resins. All of these cause varying inflammatory responses in the gingiva contacting them. Generally, inflammation resulting from chemical irritation to the gingiva is reversible, and seldom are the chemicals in a sufficient concentration to create irreparable damage.

7. Some restorative materials, or certain of their ingredients, can precipitate a local or systemic allergic reaction. Typical lesions (vesicles, rashes, erythemas, ulcers) can occur in adjacent gingiva or in specialized mucous membranes of the mouth. Rarely are gold alloys and amalgams etiologic factors in such reactions. They are most frequently caused by resinous materials or casting alloys containing nickel.

8. Porosity is an inherent property of agglomerated materials, such as amalgam and direct tooth-colored resins. Although it is not a direct irritant to the periodontium, porosity indirectly contributes to inflammation by retaining plaque and its metabolic by-products.

9. Physical and mechanical trauma from the insertion of the restoration does directly affect the periodontium. Such trauma can result from subgingival removal of excess restorative material, finishing and polishing, exothermic heat of impression and temporary materials, and heat from uncontrolled electrosurgery.

10. Solubility, disintegration and corrosion of restorative materials, besides releasing irritants to the adjacent periodontium, will leave the restoration deficient in shape, compromising the integrity of the surrounding periodontium. Also, they will result in a rougher surface and increased marginal leakage space, both of which invite more plaque accumulation.

11. Restorations undergoing micromovements can impinge on the periodontium causing traumatic irritation. Also, these movements can enhance marginal discrepancies and invite greater plaque accumulation.

II. Periodontal Evaluation of Restorative Materials

To reiterate, no restoration or restorative material can imitate the compatibility of intact tooth structure to the periodontium. The inherent irritating qualities of restorative materials, coupled with iatrogenically introduced defects in final restorations can predispose to, and/or actively participate in periodontal breakdown. The following will specify the shortcomings of currently available materials adjacent with respect to periodontal tissues:

A. Amalgam

1. Surface roughness, especially subgingivally, where a biocompatible polish is impossible
2. Marginal discrepancies, usually clinically undetectable, become more pronounced through tarnish, corrosion, creep and flow
3. Marginal adaptation, although usually improving with time, can be adversely affected by corrosion, micromovements, fatigue failure, creep, etc.
4. Galvanism, especially in the presence of restorations in the immediate proximity containing dissimilar metals
5. Chemical irritation, specifically from mercury which is leached out with corrosion products

B. Direct tooth-colored materials

With regard to the different insulting factors to the periodontium, all of these materials are unfavorable except in one aspect: their electrical potential, which is almost nil.

1. None of these materials permanently retains its shape under occluding and abrading forces.
2. All of these materials demonstrate surface roughness, even after meticulous polishing, and composite resins have the highest surface roughness of all.
3. Marginal discrepancies are increased with time in all of these materials.

4. The chemical insult from these materials is greatest after initial placement and never diminishes completely.

5. Acid-etching technique for use with these materials is detrimental not only from the standpoint of the direct effect of the acid on the periodontium but also indirectly, as etched non-restored enamel serves to more readily retain bacterial plaques.

C. Zinc oxide and eugenol

Despite the favorable antiseptic and sedative effects of this material, its high solubility in the oral acids causes surface roughness and marginal inadequacies which enhance plaque accumulation. In addition, when this material is used as a temporary, it tends to flow, with the passage of time, causing an eventual impingement on the adjacent periodontal tissues. Nevertheless, its non-existent electrical potential is a major advantage of this material towards the periodontium.

D. Zinc phosphate cement

This material, too, has an inert electrical potential, but this is its only biological advantage for the periodontium. The surface roughness and marginal inadequacies of this material are primary detrimental factors, and these are enhanced by continued erosion of the cement by acidic crevicular fluids. Chemical insult to the periodontium occurs from the phosphoric acid content of the cement. Mechanical trauma from this cement can occur from forcing the material gingivally during the cementation process, and from removal of excess marginal cement after setting. The ultimate trauma to the periodontium would occur by inadvertently leaving attached or unattached set cement within the gingival crevice.

E. Polycarboxylate cement

Being very similar to zinc phosphate cement in its biological effects on the periodontium the solubility of this material is even greater in the oral fluids. Chemical irritation is due to polyacrylic acid.

It should be emphasized that even when ZOE, ZPC, and PCC are used as cementing agents, their surface area at cementation margins (e.g., 2-4 mm^2 in a molar full crown casting) is significant enough to retain sufficient plaque to induce a localized gingival irritation.

F. Cast alloy restorations

The major irritating factors to the periodontium include the previously mentioned cementation margins, inadequacies in the margins of the restorations themselves, the electrical potential of the metals, the mechanical insults that occur from impression taking and casting try-in and adjustment, the previously mentioned pre- and post-cementation trauma, and allergic reactions to certain metals, especially alloys containing nickel. All things considered, the cast alloy restoration can be tolerated very well by the adjacent periodontium, if the aforementioned irritants are properly controlled.

G. Direct gold restorations

In mouths having no other metal and exhibiting good oral hygiene, the gingiva around a properly condensed and polished direct gold restoration will appear very sound. However, in subgingival restorations containing porosity or scratches, the tissue will react in much the same way as to amalgam. The primary insults of the direct gold restoration to the periodontium are the lacerations and contusions which can occur during condensation.

Such trauma can be avoided by:
1. Splinting the operated tooth to at least one adjacent tooth to dissipate the energy of condensation.
2. Immobilizing the operated tooth to prevent vibratory trauma to the periodontium.
3. Avoiding condensation forces at right angles to the longitudinal axis of the tooth.
4. Adjusting condensing instruments for the safest amplitude and frequency commensurate with the pre-existing periodontal and bone conditions.

H. Fused porcelain (ceramic) restorations

Glazed high-fused and low fused porcelain (ceramic) exhibit surfaces with the least amount of scratches and irregularities of all available restorative materials. Therefore, aside from the trauma of preparation and impression taking and post-operative cement lines common to cast restorations, these types of restorative materials are the most biologically acceptable to the periodontium.

III. How to Preserve the Integrity of the Periodontium for a Restored Tooth

One of the major objectives of operative dentistry is to prevent destruction of tooth-supporting structures. It should be obvious from the information presented thus far in this chapter that the most influential factor in determining the reaction of periodontal tissues to single tooth restorations is the proximity of the margins of these restorations to the gingiva.

Historically, it has been a basic rule to place the gingival margins of restorations 1-2 mm apical to the free healthy gingival marginal limit. Such a rule, however, cannot be blindly applied. Rather, the following factors must be considered in order to determine the optimum location for the restoration gingivally.

A. Patient age and relative age of the tooth

As previously mentioned, the gingiva tends to recede apically as a patient matures, with the process decelerating after 25 years of age. So, in younger ages (patient and tooth age), the gingival margins of restorations could be located in greater proximity to the gingiva. With passing time, the interface between the restoration and the gingiva will passively separate.

B. Caries rate

It is a well documented fact that the tooth surface forming the wall of the gingival crevice is an area relatively immune from decay. It would follow, therefore, that placing a restoration margin there could impart some protection from recurrance of decay. Such subgingival placement would be especially indicated in cases of high caries rate or caries susceptibility. Otherwise, locating these margins away from the gingiva would be preferred.

C. Patient plaque control

The more efficiently the patient controls plaque formation, the safer it becomes to locate restoration margins supragingivally. On the other hand, in patients with a high plaque index, we should not risk placing cariogenically susceptible margins occlusal to the free gingival margin.

D. Periodontal index

The more susceptible or involved the tooth's periodontium to disease, the further away from the gingiva should be the location of the margins of the restoration.

E. Type of restorative material

In restorations of all direct tooth-colored materials, gingival margins should be located supragingivally, for none of these materials is biologically compatible with the peridontium.

In amalgam restorations, gingival margins should be located supragingivally or even with the crest of the free gingiva. Subgingival placement of amalgam margins is only indicated in cases of high caries rate or caries susceptibility. For cast restorations, there are fewer hazards in placing their margins subgingivally, provided they are within the gingival sulcus. However, this is not the preferred location for reasons that have been previously discussed. Porcelain restorations, too, are safely placed with margins subgingival or even with the crest of the free gingiva. If the gingiva can be retracted for biologic margination and surfacing of the restoration, direct gold can safely have subgingival margins. Again, however, it is preferable to marginate even with the free gingival crest or supragingivally.

F. Apical extent of the decay

Naturally, this should be the primary determining factor, with all other factors considered secondary.

G. Esthetics

The masking effect of subgingival restorative margins, especially facial margins anteriorly and in the premolar area, is desirable. However, it is essential to also consider other, more important determining factors which might contraindicate esthetic considerations.

H. Gingival extension for retention and resistance form

In certain situations, subgingival location of margins is justified in order to improve the overall retention and resistance of the restoration, e.g., a short coronal tooth preparation with deficient internal retention.

It should be emphasized that the above factors and rules are only guidelines for planning the most appropriate location of gingival margins of restorations. Ultimately, clinical judgment plays a major role in the final decision. In addition to the location of these margins, the other previously discussed criteria for periodontally compatible restorations should be observed and fulfilled. Finally, the placement, finishing, and polishing of a restoration should not be the end of the restorative procedure. The patient should be educated not only in the precarious relationship that exists between the restoration and surrounding soft tissues, but also in the meticulous plaque control measures that are necessary throughout the dentition. Routine follow-up and maintenance are required to intercept any failure and to execute appropriate corrective measures.

Only in this way can we rest assured that a real service has been performed to maintain a healthy relationship between the single tooth restoration and the surrounding periodontium.

BIBLIOGRAPHY

Alexander, A.G.: Periodontal aspects of conservative dentistry, Brit. Dent. J. **125**:111-114, 1968.

App, G.R.: Effect of silicate, amalgam, and cast gold on the gingiva, J. Prosthet. Dent. **11**:522-532, 1961.

Attstrom, R.: Presence of leukocytes in crevices of healthy and chronically inflamed gingivae. J. Periodontal Res. **5**:42-47, 1970.

Bjorn, A-L, Bjorn, H., and Grkovic, B.: Marginal fit of restorations and its relation to periodontal bone level. Part I: metal fillings, Odontologisk Rev. **20**:311-321, 1969.

Black, G.V.: Operative Dentistry. Vo. 2. Pp 142-143. Chicago: Medico Dental Publ. Co., 1908.

Egelberg, J.: Gingival exudate measurements for evaluation of inflammatory changes of gingivae, Odontologisk Revy **15**:381-398, 1964.

Gargiulo, A.W., Wentz, F.M., and Orban, B.: Dimensions and relations of dentogingival junction in humans, J. Periodontology **32**:261-267, 1961.

Karlsen, K.: Gingival reactions to dental restorations, Acta Odont. Scand., **28**:895, 1970.

Larato, D.C.: Effect of cervical margins on gingiva, J. of the Calif. Dent. Assn. **45**:19-22, 1969.

Larato, D.C.: Influence of a composite resin restoration on the gingiva, J. Prosthet. Dent. **28**:402-404, 1972.

Loe, H.: Reactions of marginal periodontal tissues to restorative procedures, Int. Dent. J. **18**:759, 1968.

Marcum, J.S.: The effect of crown marginal depth upon gingival tissue, J. Prosth. Dent. **17**:479-487, 1967.

Renggli, H.H., and Regolati, B.: Gingival inflammation and plaque accumulation by well-adapted supragingival and subgingival proximal restorations. Helvetica Odontologica Acta **16**:99-101, 1972.

Richter, W.A., and Ueno, H.: Relationship of crown margin placement to gingival inflammation, J. Prosthetic Dent. **30**:156-161, 1973.

Silness, J.: Fixed prosthodontics and the periodontal health, Dental Clinics of North Am. vol 24, No 2, April 1980.

Silness, J., and Hegdahl, T.: Area of the exposed zinc phosphate cement surfaces in fixed restorations, Scand. J. of Dental Res. **78**:163-177, 1970.

Sotres, L.S., Van Huysen, G., and Gilmore, H.W.: A hostologic study of gingival tissue response to amalgam, silicate and resin restorations, J. of Periodontology **40**:543-546, 1969.

Trivedi, S.C., and Talim, S.T.: The response of human gingiva to restorative materials, J. of Prosthet. Dent. **29**:73-80, 1973.

Trott, J.R., and Sherkat, A.: Effect of Class II amalgam restorations on health of the gingiva: a clinical study, J. Dent. Assoc. **30**:766-770, 1964.

Valderhaug, J.: Gingival reaction to fixed prostheses, J. Dent. Res., 50 Abstract No 74, p. 728, 1971.

Waerhaug, J.: Effect of rough surfaces upon gingival tissues, J. Dent. Res. **35**:323-325, 1956.

Waerhaug, J.: Effect of zinc phosphate cement fillings on gingival tissues, J. Periodontol. **27**:284, 1956.

Waerhaug, J.: The furcation problem: Etiology, pathogenesis, diagnosis, therapy and prognosis, J. Clin. Periodontol., in press.

Waerhaug, J.: Histologic consideration governing locations of margins of restorations in relation to gingiva, Dental Clinics of North America, March, 161-176.

Waerhaug, J.: The ingrabony pocket and its relationship to trauma from occlusion and subgingival plaque, J. Periodontol. **50**:355, 1979.

Waerhaug, J.: Presence of absence of plaque on subgingival restorations, Scand. J. Dent. Res. **83**:193, 1975.

Waerhaug, J.: Temporary restorations: Advantages and disadvantages, Dental Clinics of North America. Vol. 24. No 2. April, 1980.

Waerhaug, J.: Tissue reactions around artificial crowns, J. of Period. **24**:172-185, 1953.

Wright, W.H.: Local factors in periodontal disease, Periodontics **1**:163, 1963.

Zander, H.A.: Tissue reaction to dental calculus and to filling materials, J. Dent. Medicine **13**:101-104.

CHAPTER 16

Single tooth restorations and the stomato-gnathic system

It is not our intention in this chapter to present detailed information concerning stomato-gnathology or occlusion. The reader is referred to the several publications enumerated in the references for such details. It is our desire here to emphasize the link between and the interdependency of stomato-gnathology and operative dentistry restorative procedures.

Simply stated, a dental restoration, after being attached to a tooth, becomes one of the essential components of the stomato-gnathic system. Previously in this text, two biological bases for tooth restoration were fully explained, i.e., the pulp-dentin organ and the periodontium. However, the tripod for a biologically functional restoration is never complete without the third base for that tripod, namely, "occlusion" (Fig. 1).

An apparently satisfactory restoration, mechanically, pulpo-dentally and periodontally, that nonetheless interferes with the normal physiologic activities of the stomato-gnathic system, can initiate or predispose to a myriad of pathologic processes. These processes could be in remote areas within the stomato-gnathic system and/or in the very pulp-dentin organ and periodontium of the restored tooth. Symptoms for these pathological changes can range from a toothache to earache, headache, sore throat, neck pain, backache, etc.

Every practicing dentist should have complete awareness and comprehension of the components of the stomato-gnathic system as well as their functions, their dynamics, their controls and the interrelationship between these components. The practitioner should be familiar with modes of recording and/or reproducing static and dynamic relationships within this system, as well as have the knowledge to utilize these recordings to create a restoration that will be integral, functional component of the system.

The stomato-gnathic system is a conglomerate of organs which are functionally related to each other. These organs include the mandible, the maxilla, the tempro-mandibular joint, the teeth and their supporting structures, muscles of mastication, muscles of the face, muscles of the neck, muscles of the head, and, to some extent, muscles of the back. Although most of these parts are not involved directly in the oral and intraoral activities of the system, they nevertheless participate in these activities in a reciprocating, supporting and bracing manner.

There will be no attempt here to describe all of these organs. Rather, the following will enumerate the parts of the four major components responsible for the main activity in the system, i.e., "the movements of the mandible."

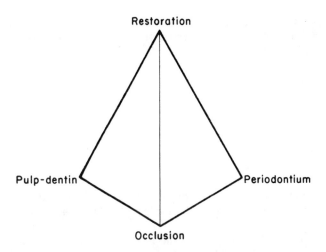

Fig. 16-1. The biological bases for a dental restoration.

I. Muscles of Mastication and their Primary Functions

A. Temporalis—retracts and elevates the mandible. It also helps in rotating the mandible and supplies power on closure.

B. Masseter is the primary power muscle for mandibular closure. It also retracts and protracts the mandible.

C. External pterygoid—has two parts (heads) which may act as antagonists. The superior head attaches to the *articular disc* and the inferior head attaches to the neck of the condyle. The superior head moves the articular disc of the TMJ forward. The right and left ones move either in unison or independently. Both the superior and inferior head together or separately move the mandible forward. The inferior head also depresses and helps rotate the mandible.

D. Internal pterygoid—elevates and rotates the mandible. It also protracts the mandible and helps in the application of power on closure.

E. Suprahyoid muscles—help stabilize the hyoid bone. When this bone is immobilized, the suprahyoids can depress the mandible.

The digastric muscles—have two bellies, both are powerful retractors of the mandible.

F. Infrahyoid muscles—help immobilize the hyoid bone, enabling the suprahyoid muscles to depress the mandible.

291

G. Posterior muscles of the neck—stabilize the craniun for the retractor, protractor, and elevator muscles to act. Also, individually (sterno-cleido-mastoid) they can participate in rotating the mandible laterally.

II. Tempro-Mandibular Joint

This is, indeed, a complex apparatus as it consists of four parts:

A. The glenoid fossa is basically a concavity, with its anterior border defined by the eminentia (a bony elevated convexity facing downwards).

B. The articular disc is an hour-glass shaped, proteinaceous ''gasket-like'' separator, having its posterior part much thicker than its anterior part. The middle section of the disc is the thinnest and least vascular and is almost non-innervated. The disc is attached at its anterior end to the superior head of the external pterygoid muscle, which we now know to contract independently from the inferior head. At its posterior end, the articular disc is attached to a very elastic portion of the capsular ligament (bilaminar zone). The disc thus divides the space between the roof of the fossa and the condyle into two completely separate compartments. The disc can be actively moved forward by the underlying condyle or by the upper head of the external pterygoid muscles. However, it can be passively moved backwards by the elasticity of its attachment to the capsular ligament.

C. The condyle, which is the oblong, doubly convex, superior terminal of the mandible. The condyle almost completely occupies the lower compartment of the fossa. The inferior head of the external pterygoid muscle is attached to its neck, so with contraction, the lateral pterygoid moves the mandible forward.

D. The capsular ligament is the tough fibrous ligament encasing the above three structures, partially immobilizing and restricting (controlling) their movements.

III. Cranio-Mandibular Ligaments

These ligaments are as important as the muscles in guiding, limiting, and controlling the movements of the mandible. They extend from different parts of the base of the skull to the mandible. Examples of these ligaments are: the tempro-mandibular, the stylo-mandibular, tempro-condylar, and spheno-mandibular ligaments.

IV. The Teeth

Besides their morphology, contact and contour, and gross- and micro-anatomy, for the purpose of this discussion, it is also essential to recognize several other positional factors about teeth:

A. The spatial locations of teeth within their bony investments

The lower anterior teeth are eccentrically located within their supporting bones, with more bone labially than lingually. Eccentricity is less noticeable proceeding from the incisors to the cuspid, which may often be centrally located within its bone. The lower premolars are usually centrically placed within their investing bone; however, the lower molars are eccentrically located in the alveolar bone, with more bone buccally than lingually. Eccentricity increases proceeding further distally. Furthermore, in the lower arch, there is some bony thickening

labial to the cuspid and sometimes buccal to the first molar.

The upper anterior teeth are eccentrically located within their investing bone, with the teeth deviated labially. This deviation is less noticeable with the cuspids than the incisors. As in the lower arch, the maxillary cuspids are almost always centrically located within bone.

The maxillary premolars are also deviated buccally, but to a lesser extent than the anterior teeth. Also, the upper molars are eccentrically located with more alveolar bone lingually than buccally. However, this is to a lesser extent than the premolars. In the upper arch, there is substantial thickening of bone facial to the cuspid and first molar.

Recognizing the alveolar bone distribution around teeth is important in order to comprehend the magnitude and direction of stresses on these teeth during function.

B. The three-dimensional spatial inclinations of teeth

Following a tooth from the occlusal (incisal) termination of its crown to the apex of its root, each will show the following spatial angulation pattern.

1. Upper incisors have disto-lingual inclinations.
2. Upper cuspids have a distal and sometimes a disto-lingual inclination.
3. Upper premolars may either be vertically located or have some distal inclination.
4. Upper molars may have lingual inclinations with some mesial tendency. This inclination is increased proceeding distally.
5. Lower incisors and canines have the same inclination as the upper, but it is more exaggerated.
6. Lower premolars are almost vertically located in the mandible with only a slight tendency for a disto-facial inclination.
7. Lower molars are inclined disto-facially. This inclination increases proceeding distally.

These spatial patterns create two types of curves within the occlusal plane:

a. The curve of Spee, which is an anterior-posterior curve, with its convexity on the upper dentition and its concavity on the lower teeth.

b. The curve of Wilson, which is a medio-lateral curve. It is also convex for the upper dentition and concave for the lower one.

C. The relative position of teeth to the power-application musculature (masseter, internal pterygoid and temporalis)

The closer a tooth is to the area of insertion for the musculature, the more stresses it will incur. Therefore, the first molars and second premolars are the teeth that are subjected most to the effect of this power application.

D. The relative position of a tooth to the corner of the arch

The corner of the arch is an area where there exists a general tendency for lateral loading, due to lateral movements of the mandible, and to the concentration there of the anterior components of force. It is no surprise, then, that a tooth with such sturdy structure and durable support as the canine is located there. The closer another tooth is to that corner, the greater will be the possibility that it will encounter this lateral loading, and perhaps resist it less successfully.

E. Tooth positions relative to their resistance to loading

Tooth shapes and their orientation with supporting structures tolerate substantial axial loading (parallel to their longitudinal axis).

Laterally applied loads are detrimental to the teeth and their supporting structures. While axial loads are delivered to the tips of the cusps, crests of ridges, or depths of fossa and grooves parallel to the long axis of the tooth, lateral loads, on the other hand, are those delivered to inclined planes. Tooth orientation is not designed to resist such loading over an extended period of time.

F. Cuspal inclines

In posterior teeth every cusp has four inclines, i.e., two facial and two lingual. Gnathologically, these are classified as working and balancing types. The working inclines are those facing a working (functional) cusp side, e.g., buccal cusps of the lower and lingual cusps of the upper. The balancing inclines are those facing a balancing (non-functional) cusp side, e.g., lingual cusps of the lower and buccal cusps of the upper.

In anterior teeth the working inclines are the lingual inclined planes for the uppers (inclines toward the lingual concavity or the tooth end of the ridges). They are also the labial inclines on the labial surface of the lower anterior teeth including parts of the incisal ridges.

G. Lingual concavity of maxillary anteriors

In upper anterior teeth there is always a lingual concavity starting from the cingulum and reaching the incisal ridge. This anatomic feature is essential for non-interfering gliding protrusive and lateral protrusive movements of the mandible.

H. Proprioceptive terminals

The investing tissues for each tooth are enriched with proprioceptive sensory terminals. Their sensory nerve capsules are pressure sensitive, especially to laterally applied pressure. The number of nerve capsules is inversely proportional to the tooth's tolerance for loading (especially non-axial loads), e.g., the upper cuspids have the least number of proprioceptive sensory terminals, and the upper second molars have the maximum number of these terminals.

I. The relative position of a tooth to the fulcrum of movements

Every mandibular movement has a specific fulcrum. The closer any tooth is to that fulcrum during mandibular movements, the more the stresses will be on that tooth. Also, the more this tooth will affect the nature of the movements.

J. Holding cuspal elements

For teeth to remain stable within their investing tissues there must be certain barriers against their displacement. Examples of these barriers in the facial-lingual direction are the vertical overlaps of the teeth and the musculature. Stabilizing barriers are supplied mesio-distally by the contact areas, and occluso-apically by the opposing teeth. To assure this three-dimensional stability, every tooth must have a holding cuspal element (usually a cusp in posterior teeth) to match a reciprocating fossa (concavity) in the opposing tooth. In a centric occlusion relationship between the mandibular and maxillary teeth, when there will be maximal intercuspation between the opposing teeth, these holding elements (e.g., cusps and fossae) should interdigitate, preventing any movements in any of the three possible directions. For the upper posterior teeth in normal occlusion, these holding cusps are usually the lingual cusps occluding in opposing fossae. For lower posterior teeth, in normal occlusion, they are usually the buccal cusps, frequently with opposing fossae. Of course, some other anatomical items could be the holding elements, provided they are not detrimental to the normal function at that location.

Functional Dynamics

Although the stomato-gnathic system is composed of and participates in multiple functional activities, e.g., respiration, speech, deglutition, expression esthetics, its main activity is in moving the mandible, which is included in most of the other, above-mentioned functions. Therefore, the dynamics of this activity will be discussed in detail here.

Mandibular Movements

The mandible and the TMJ are one of the very few structures and joints in the human body that are capable of three-dimensional (directional) movements. Also, the TMJs and their components are the only joints in the human body which are capable of both translation and rotation concurrently and even bilaterally. Having this capability, the mandible could be moving in more than one or two directions at the same moment. For the purpose of this discussion, it is important to identify and describe each direction of movement.

1. Movements along the saggital plane (parallel to the saggital suture)

This is the most obvious mandibular movement. It may represent rotation around a horizontal axis between the centre of each condyle or it may represent translatory motion—downwards, upwards, forwards, backwards, or a combination of these.

2. Movements along the horizontal plane

These can be rotations around a vertical axis passing superio-inferiorly through the center of each condyle, or they can be translatory, i.e., lateral, medial, forward or backwards, or combinations of these.

3. Movements along the coronal (parallel to the coronal sutures) plane

Such motions can be rotatory, around a saggital axis through the center of each condyle parallel to the saggital plane, or they can be translatory, i.e., lateral, medial, upwards and downwards, or combinations of these.

The following will be a description of the path of the mandible (and its occlusal elements) during its movements in each of the possible three directions. The path will be described to points beyond which the mandible is not capable of further movement. These points are defined as the border limitation of mandibular movements, and moving the mandible to these points is therefore called "border movements of the mandible''. It is to be understood that persons do not arrive to these points during functional use of the mandible, i.e., functional paths of the mandible are always internal to these points (intraborder movements).

I. Pure Protrusive Mandibular Movements-Paths and Termination Along the Saggital Plane

The best description for these paths and their terminations is the Posselt envelope of mandibular movements (Fig. 2). This ''envelope of motion'' describes tracing a point on a lower incisor during opening of the mouth. CR (centric relation) represents a border tracing point where the condyles are at their most upward, sometimes medialward, and anterior locations within their fossae. (Recent research indicates that physiologic centric relation dictates that the condyle heads be in their most superior position, which frequently places them on the anterior wall of the fossa or the inclines of the eminentia, and *not* on the posterior surface of the fossa, as had been traditionally thought). CR is the most reproducible location of the mandible. It is a position of the mandible where the muscles are thought to be in an equilibrium status. The location itself is governed by the musculature and the relative position of the condyle to the disc, and the disc-condyle complex to the superior wall of the fossa and eminentia. It should not be a strained position. Usually, it is not a fixed point anterio-posteriorly, i.e., it has a range of a few mm in that direction. However, it should be a fixed point (area) superio-inferiorly and medio-laterally. CO (centric occlusion), on the other hand, is an intraborder position in the tracing that represents the maximum interdigitation of the cuspal elements participating in holding the stability of the teeth. This position is mainly determined by the teeth. EE (edge-to-edge) is an intraborder position of anterior teeth during the forward translation of the mandible. PC (protrusive contact) represents contact of anterior teeth after the upward translation and rotation of the mandible. This is another terminal point.

The arc defined by TH represents the rotary acts of the

mandibular movement along its saggital plane where the axis is a horizontal hinge axis. During this arcing the condyle is always in centric relation. This is a very important and reproducible arc, as it occurs on a repeatable axis. Midway along the arc is the rest position of the mandible, where the mandible is at its most suspended location. The space between the teeth at this rest position is called the intermaxillary space. Its dimension, as with the hinge axis arc, is under muscle control, and differs from one person to another. This arc ends the maximum vertical departure of the mandible from the maxilla along the saggital plane.

In the saggital plane, translatory disclusions are obvious when the condyles move downward and forward. The nature and extent of these translatory arcs govern and are governed by the following:

A. The degree and extent of the slope of the eminentia

B. The degree and extent of the cusp angle inclination of posterior teeth

C. Cusp height of posterior teeth

D. The degree and extent of vertical overlap of anterior teeth

E. The degree and extent of horizontal overlap of anterior teeth

F. The degree and extent of the lingual concavity of upper anterior teeth

G. Protrusive inclines of posterior teeth (distal of upper and mesial of lower teeth cusps) and their extent, location, and degree of angulation

H. Intercuspal grooves in posterior teeth

I. The degree of curvature, extent, and directions of the compensating curves

J. The distance between the condyle and all above-mentioned items

The interrupted line in the middle of the envelope represents the customary intraborder functional movement of the mandible. The anterior border arc represents border movements of the mandible when it closes at its most forward location.

II. Lateral Movement Paths and Termination

Moving the mandible laterally will involve two sets of motions. Therefore, during such movements it is necessary to identify the working (rotating or functional) side and the non-working (orbiting or non-functional) side. Understandably, these sides are interchangeable according to their respective sets of motions. These two sets of motion can be recognized both at the posterior as well as the anterior segments of the arch.

A. Lateral movements represented in a posterior segment

The best description for this type of movement can be derived from a horizontal and coronal pantographic tracing. Figures 3 and 4 represent the possible condylar movements as recorded by such a tracing. Figure 3 represents lateral movements visualized on a horizontal plane, while Figure 4 represents these movements visualized on a coronal plane. Combining both figures can produce a good idea about the lateral movements of the condyle (and the mandible) in three dimensions.

The tracing from A to C (C′ or C″) represents the condylar movement when it is a working condyle. The tracing from A to D represents the condylar movement when it is a non-

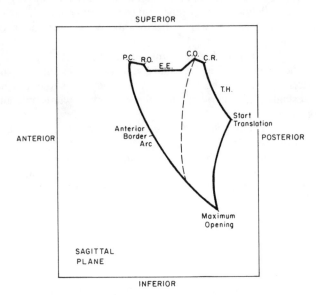

Fig. 16-2. Posselt's envelope of mandibular movements.

working condyle. Let us discuss the graphic representation of these movements first from a horizontal view, and then from a coronal view.

1. Condylar motion path and termination along the horizontal plane (Fig. 3)

"A" represents the location of the working condyle in centric relation. Line A to C (C' or C") represents the side shift of the working condyle (Bennet movement). As shown, there is initially an almost pure common path (from A to I), then the condyle could go backward (latero-retrusive), straight laterally, or forward (latero-protrusive). Each one of these directions can affect and is affected by the following:

a. Intercuspal grooves (location, directions, and dimensions, especially widths)

b. Maxillary anterior lingual concavities (location, direction, and dimensions)

c. Horizontal overlap of maxillary anterior teeth (dimensions, extent, and location)

d. Vertical overlap of maxillary anterior teeth (inclinations, extent, and locations)

e. Occlusal plane versus the angle of the eminentia (relative parallelism)

f. Compensating curves (types, relative curvature, and position to the condyle)

g. Cusp heights

h. Cusp inclinations

i. Lateral walls of the joints (inclinations, extent and directions)

j. Distance between the condyle and the other governing items

The Bennet movement is increased with age and with bite collapse. If excessive, it can be an indication of lateral elasticity (slack) in the capsular ligament.

Again, starting at "A", which is centric relation, the non-working condyle moves almost in a straight line for a short distance to "B", a fraction to a few mm. This is called the "immediate side shift". Straightness of the tracing here differs from one person to another depending upon the elasticity of

the capsular ligaments. The condyle then descends medio-anteriorly as represented by line BD. The incline of the path BD governs and is governed by most of the factors governing the protrusive path of the mandible, besides some of the factors affecting the direction of the lateral shift of the working condyle. Other factors involved in this movement are:

a. Inclination and extent of the balancing cuspal incline

b. Curvature of the curve of Wilson

c. The angle between the pure protrusive path and the orbiting condylar path (Fisher's angle—best observed on a sagittal tracing)

2. Condylar motion path and termination along the coronal plane (Fig. 4)

"A" represents the working condyle in centric relation. The working condyle can travel along A-C (C' or C"), which represents the lateral side shift. It might be an upward (latero-surtrusion) path as in AC, or it can be straight laterally as in AC', or it may be downwards (latero-detrusion as in AC"). The exact nature of the lateral side shift is decided by the same factors that affect the nature of the lateral side shift in the horizontal direction. Especially important, however, are:

a. Cusp height, specifically the working cusps

b. Inclines of the cusps, specifically working inclines

c. Concavity of the upper anterior teeth lingual surfaces

Also, "A" represents centric relation for the non-working condyle. From A to B is almost a straight line, i.e., the immediate side shift. Then the tracing will follow a downward and medial inclination governed by the same factors affecting the motion of the non-working condyle along the horizontal plane.

B. Lateral movements represented in an anterior segment of the arch

Mandibular motion in the anterior is best illustrated by a gothic arch tracing (Fig. 5). Assuming that "A" represents

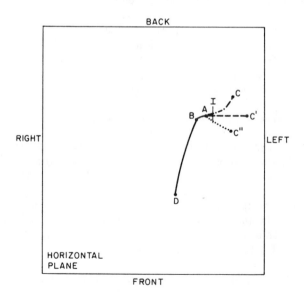

Fig. 16-3. Left horizontal pantographic tracing.

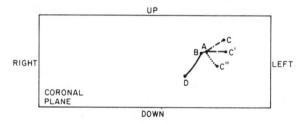

Fig. 16-4. Left coronal pantographic tracing.

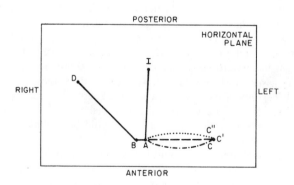

Fig. 16-5. Right anterior gothic arch tracing.

centric relation, A to I represents pure protrusive movement. Movement of the working condyle side is represented on the tracing by line AC (C' or C"). Tracing AC', which is a straight line, represents the tracing anteriorly when the side shift is purely lateral. Tracing AC represents the motion when the side shift is lateroretrusive, while tracing AC" represents the motion when the side shift is latero-protrusive.

Movement of the non-working condyle is designated on the tracing by line ABD. AB is the immediate side shift, and B to D is called the "progressive side shift."

The characteristics of this part of the mandibular movement dictate and is dictated by:

1. The intercondylar distance
2. The amount of immediate side shift
3. The amount of progressive side shift
4. Direction of the lateral shifting of the mandible in 3 dimensions
5. The lingual concavity of anterior maxillary teeth (extent, location and angulation)
6. The timing of the immediate relative to the progressive side shift
7. The inclination of the non-working condylar path
8. All the cuspal factors that influence the path of motion in coronal, horizontal and saggital planes

It should be reemphasized that although the mandibular motion patterns are described here as separate ones, in actual function they are not; i.e., the mandible is capable of instantaneous multiple motions.

III. Disclusion

This is one of the most important features in the functional dynamics of mandibular movement. Because most functional movements of the mandible are intraborder type—i.e., lateral and latero-protrusive movements, mandibular teeth must be disengaged from maxillary teeth to even allow these movements. If, in fact, such movements were to occur with teeth still in contact, substantial lateral loading, with all of its detrimental sequelae, would result. Disclusion is more important for posterior than for anterior teeth primarily because posterior teeth are relatively more incapable of withstanding lateral loading. The proximity of the posterior teeth to the load applicators and to the fulcrums of motion further necessitates disclusion as a vital part of functional dynamics.

The most effective disengaging tooth is a healthy, well-supported canine (for reasons previously mentioned). Therefore, if possible, a sound self-resistant cuspid should be an integral part of any disclusion mechanism during protrusive, lateral, or latero-protrusive motion. Sometimes, the canines may be assisted by premolars, especially the upper premolars during lateral disclusions. Also, one or two anterior teeth might assist in forward disclusion and both premolars and anteriors may assist disclusion in latero-protrusive directions.

When any of these teeth are involved in the disclusion mechanism, the following should be observed:

A. Only their working inclines should be included in the act of disclusion.

B. Minimum load should be applied to teeth further away from the canine. Loads should gradually increase nearer the cuspids, where the maximum load should be applied.

C. The canine should be the last to disengage, and the tooth furthest from the canine should be the first to disengage.

D. Supporting (auxillary) teeth or cuspal elements involved in this group function disclusion should not exceed the mesio-buccal cusps of upper first molars posteriorly and the central on the same side of the canine anteriorly.

E. In pure lateral excursions only posterior teeth (besides the cuspid) should be involved as discluding cuspal elements.

F. More importantly, in pure anterior excursions, only anterior teeth should be involved as auxillary discluding cuspal elements. At no time should there by any contact between posterior teeth during protrusive excursions.

G. In no instance should there be any cross-arch or cross-midline auxillary cuspal elements involved in the disclusion mechanism.

H. In some instances, involving lower incisor teeth gliding along the lingual concavities of upper incisor teeth may be the only functional anterior discluding mechanism, without the canine being involved. However, for lateral disclusion, there can be no substitute for the canine.

I. For auxillary posterior cuspal elements assisting a cuspid in disclusion, the mesial cuspal inclines for the upper teeth and the distal cuspal inclines for lower teeth are the most effective in facilitating disclusion with the least amount of loading and its detrimental effects.

J. If the canine's self-resistance to lateral loading is doubtful, group function should be established, loading the most supported tooth maximally. This choice should be the last resort, however, as failure might be reasonably expected.

K. Regarding the canine itself, the ideal location for the main path of disclusion should be on the mesial aspect of the lingual surface of the upper cuspid, paralleling the marginal ridge. At this location quicker translation of the mandible will be achieved. Also, the discluding forces will be distributed in the most advantageous configuration for the canine to resist them. A diagonal crossing path across the lingual surface of the upper cuspid should be avoided, for this will distress the TMJ capsular ligament and the lateral resistance of the cuspid.

The dimensions of tooth contact as well as the time involved in contact, and concomittantly the amount of lateral loading is determined by the following 12 factors:

1. The amount of vertical overlap
2. The amount of horizontal overlap
3. The inclination of cuspal inclined planes
4. The nature of mandibular side shifts and the factors influencing them
5. The inclination of the eminentia
6. Cusp height
7. The lingual concavity of upper anterior teeth
8. The presence of escaping grooves for opposing cuspal elements, their location, direction, and dimensions
9. The location of the saggital and vertical fulcrum for the rotation of the mandible relative to the discluding tooth (teeth)
10. The intercondylar distance
11. The plane of occlusion, relative to the angle of the eminentia
12. The nature of compensating curves

Control of Mandibular Movements

Mandibular movements are basically muscle controlled motions with two hard tissue mechanical restrictors, i.e., the walls of the glenoid fossae and the teeth. In addition, there may be some minor mechanical limiting factors, e.g., ligaments (especially the capsular ones), facial tissues, etc.

Muscular control is shaped by the same factors that dictate any muscular activity, i.e., reflex mechanisms through stimuli arriving to the central nervous system, followed by signals activating, deactivating, synchronizing, bracing, etc. different muscles of mastication and the rest of the muscles of the stomato-gnathic system. These complex muscular activities are programmed to avoid destructive loading (e.g., lateral loading or loading forces with fulcra on teeth). This can occur to the extent that the muscles themselves are in some state of contraction for a varying period of time in an effort to prevent the undesirable loading. However, this continuous contraction of the muscles can establish certain pathological disorders. The bony control of mandibular movement is always a given situation around which all other controls should operate. On the other hand, the tooth control for mandibular movements is the most acquired and changeable factor. Any modification in the tooth control of movement can elicit a chain reaction of changes in the nature, extent, and effect of mandibular movements. This will consequently affect the physiology of the stomato-gnathic system.

From the previous discussion, the controlling effect of the teeth on mandibular movements should be very clear. It should be emphasized that the effect of the bony controls of the TMJ (condylar guidance) decreases proceeding away from them. Therefore, the controlling effect of bone is very pronounced for mandibular motion at the posterior segments of the arch (posterior teeth), but the more one proceeds anteriorly, the tooth control of motion will play a major role in controlling the mandibular movements. This control is referred to as "incisal guidance," and it is the cumulative effect of:

A. Anterior vertical overlap

B. Anterior horizontal overlap

C. Reverse overlap

D. Disclusion capabilities of anterior teeth

E. Role of the cuspid in these controlling capabilities

F. Lingual concavities in upper anterior teeth

G. Occluding cuspal elements in centric occlusion

H. Angulation of the eminentia relative to the vertical overlap

I. Anterior teeth inclination relative to the curve of Spee

J. Compensating curve angulation relative to the incisal plane angulation

K. Location of the lower anterior teeth cuspal elements in the lingual concavity of the upper anterior teeth (collective cusp fossa relationship)

L. Relationship of the upper and lower anterior teeth in the alert-feed position of the mandible

M. The controlling effect of the ligaments and the facial tissues, always restricting and repositioning in nature

Static and Dynamic Contact Relationship Between Mandibular and Maxillary Teeth

When teeth come in contact with one another, it is in a predetermined, orderly pattern with specific tooth surfaces occluding with each other. If unspecified areas on the tooth come in contact with opposing occluding elements, it may be detrimental not only to that tooth, but also to other parts of the stomato-gnathic system. This contact relationship between the opposing teeth can be stationary, which only occurs in centric occlusion or sometimes in the very lateral and protrusive (or combinations) border locations of the mandible. Or, it can be dynamic, which occurs during the motion of the mandible from centric relation to centric occlusion and from centric locations to lateral and protrusive (or combination) border locations. It can also occur during movements of the mandible from an intraborder location to a border one. The following discussion will summarize these contact relationships. The description will be for situations confirmed to be normal functional occlusions. Understandably, every individual could have some deviation from this mean situation.

I. Static Contact Relationships

A. Centric occlusion contacts

The holding cusp fossa arrangement, previously described should be the prevailing pattern, with the upper lingual cusps firmly seated in the occlusal fossae (or equivalent) of the lower teeth, and the lower buccal cusps seated in the occlusal fossae (or equivalent) of the upper teeth. Maximum contact should be at the tips of the cusps and the bottom of the fossa, or at least noticeably deviated toward these areas. There should be no contact on the inclined planes themselves.

Some holding cusps may not be opposed by a suitable holding fossa. The opposing occluding item to such cusps might be one or two adjacent marginal ridges. If a cusp is in contact with one marginal ridge, it will usually occlude with the occlusal inclined plane of that ridge in proximity to the adjacent triangular fossa. If the holding cusp is occluding with two adjacent marginal ridges, the contact should be even on both of them. The cusp tip should be blunt to prevent it from wedging the two marginal ridges apart.

Every cusp in a fossa has an adjacent groove in that fossa. The groove should be wide enough to facilitate the cusp's escape during lateral mandibular movements, without its colliding into adjacent cuspal elements. Cusps occluding with a marginal ridge will have the adjacent embrasures to enable their escape during lateral movements.

The lower anterior teeth should be positively seated in the concavities of upper anterior teeth contacting on the lower's incisal ridges and part of their labial surfaces. Centric contact should be almost even over all holding cuspal elements, i.e., no one area should experience more contact than the other, in terms of magnitude and/or surface area. There should be no occluding contacts on inclined planes, especially on the balancing inclines. Horizontal and vertical overlaps in anterior teeth should be as previously described. Vertical and minimal horizontal overlap of the working cuspal inclines of the buccal cusps in upper teeth should exist over the lower teeth. Also, some overlap of the working inclines of the lingual cusps of lower teeth should occur over the upper teeth.

B. Protrusive occlusion border contact

Such contact usually occurs when the lower anterior teeth are labial to the upper teeth. Often, only incisors are involved in this contact. Sometimes, however, the cuspid is also involved. The contact is usually between the lingual surface of the lower and the labial surface of the upper incisors. In some instances the most border contact anteriorly is an edge-to-edge contact. This situation is most obvious in a cuspid anterior border contact relationship. There will be no contact between posterior teeth at this position of the mandible.

C. Working side lateral border contacts

In this lateral border location usually only the cuspids will be in contact with opposing component(s) through their slopes. Sometimes, however, part of the working inclines of the buccal cusps of the first and second premolars are included.

There should be no occluding contact with the rest of the teeth on the working side.

Also, there should be no tooth contact on the non-working side anteriorly or posteriorly.

II. Dynamic Contact Relationships

During mandibular movements from centric relation to centric occlusion, as the mandible moves in an upward and forward direction, there is a tendency for the distal inclines of the lower cusps to rub against the mesial inclines of the upper cusps until the holding cusps are housed into their fossa or against their indicated marginal ridges. Ideally, there should be no initial contact between these holding (centric) cuspal elements. If such initial contact is present (as usually happens), it is always even, or at least symmetrical on both sides. Also, it should guide the mandible in a pure forward-upward direction, without any deflection laterally or inferiorly.

During mandibular movements from centric to lateral border movements, on the working side, the lower buccal holding cusps may travel for some distance along the working inclines of upper buccal cusps before escaping via the adjacent indicated grooves or embrasures buccally and inferiorly. This movement is dictated by the configuration of these grooves and embrasures, the inclination of the working cuspal incline, and primarily by the nature of the Bennet movement (side shift).

The lower occlusal lingual grooves will travel buccally via the upper lingual cusps fitted into them. The teeth contacts will decline when the mandible (with the teeth) is moved laterally and inferiorly. The nature of the contact will be dictated by the same factors as previously.

On the non-working side, the downward medial movements of the mandible will be accompanied by the initial contact between the balancing inclines of the holding cusps. Ideally this contact should be non-existent as the holding cusp-fossa and/or the cusp-marginal ridge contacts should disengage instantaneously when the orbiting side starts descending and moving medially. In addition, when a functional cusp is in contact with one marginal ridge, during mandibular movement the cusp will travel along either the ridge's mesio-distal inclined planes or its crest. If it is in contact with two marginal ridges, the cusp will glide along the crest of these marginal ridges via the occlusal embrasures.

During mandibular movements from centric to protrusive border positions, as long as the mandible is dropping and moving forward, the lower incisors with their incisal edges and part of their labial surfaces will glide along the lingual concavity of the upper incisors, forward and anteriorly. This gliding path is dictated by the anterior inclination of the upper teeth, their lingual concavities and the condylar eminentia. At the end of this gliding stage, the upper and lower anterior teeth could have an edge-to-edge relationship. The further the mandible is protruded, the more there will be a reverse vertical and horizontal overlap between the upper and lower anterior teeth. This new relation will increase in extent until the lower teeth get to the most protrusive reverse overlap relationship with the uppers. As soon as the protrusive movement is started, there should be no contact between the posterior teeth. If, in fact, there is any contact there, it is usually an initial momentary one. The posterior teeth contact will be between their protrusive cuspal inclines (mesial of the lower and distal of the upper). Ideally, these posterior teeth should disengage as soon as protrusive movements are started. Although the canine is not involved in many of these protrusive mandibular movements, when it is, it always contacts opposing elements with its slopes, and the downward-forward movements of the lower cuspid occupies the mesial part of the lingual surface of upper cuspids.

Modes of Recording and Reproducing Mandibular Movements and/or Their Effects

If one comprehends the brief summary concerning mandibular movements, presented in the previous section, it should be easy to understand that this area in restorative dentistry, namely recording and reproducing mandibular movements and/or their effects, can be accomplished at different levels of detail. Also, it should be clear that all possible mandibular motions and their effects cannot be reproduced by one presently available instrument or technique. In addition, it should be noted that there is no limitation to the number of the techniques used to capture and reproduce these details. The student or clinician should not confine himself to one technique to acquire and reproduce this information, as there is no one technique that can be used for all situations. It is a good idea to recognize one's objectives in the specific case at hand and the available means to fulfill all or some of these. Indeed, one may use *more* than one technique for one case in order to obtain maximum details. In any event, experience and complete comprehension of functional dynamics, as applied to the case at hand, can assure successful results even with the least sophisticated equipment.

I. Physical Manipulation of the Mandible for Occlusion Records

As mentioned before, habitual mandibular movements are always intraborder type movements. To obtain a fixed, reproducible record for mandibular movements it is necessary to move the mandible to one or more of its border locations. This is achieved by guiding, manipulative physical acts. Utilizing these acts might incur resistance and counteraction by the stomato-gnathic system musculature; therefore, the manipulations should have the following characteristics:

A. Patients should be aware of the type, extent, and possible effects of the manipulation.

B. Manipulative pressure should be in the same direction the mandible is moved by the patient's own musculature.

C. The manipulations should be "guiding" in nature, to prevent deviation of the mandible or any of its parts from the required path. The patient should move his (her) own mandible during all procedures, except verification of hinge axis movements.

D. The patient should be trained in the indicated mandibular movements before executing the recordings.

E. There should be complete harmony and synchronization between the movement rate of the operator's hands (fingers) and the rate the mandible is moved. Hand movement speed exceeding that of the mandibular movement speed will introduce external forces in the stomato-gnathic system that are deemed to be spontaneously resisted by its musculature. The reverse can deprive the mandibular movements of the guiding effect of the operator's hand.

F. If noticeable resistance or deviation of mandibular movements occurs during the manipulation, it could be due to TMJ problems or overstrained muscles, or the encounter of an interference. Manipulation should cease temporarily while the reasons for resistance are noted, and their correction can be undertaken.

G. Guiding, manipulative pressure should be applied evenly on both sides of the mandible. This will necessitate holding both sides at the same time while applying pressure centrically at the symphysis area.

The starting point in any occlusion recording is to place the mandible into *centric relation*, i.e., the most superior and sometimes the most anterior location of the mandibular condyle within its glenoid fossa housing or the descending inclines of the eminentia. There are four physico-anatomical facts that can help in obtaining and verifying this position for the mandible:

1. The condyle is in its superior position within the fossa. This can occur by physically guiding the mandible (especially its ascending ramus area) upwards, while manipulating (guiding) it backwards from its habitual location. The act should continue until no further upward movement of the mandible will occur.

2. The mandible at this position will move in pure rotating acts. This can be verified by arcing the mandible up and down in very short arcs, to be sure that the mandible (teeth) is not translating.

3. The muscles at this relationship should be in complete harmony with each other. Clinically the operator should arc the mandible as mentioned in (2), without any resistance.

4. There should not be any tooth contact at this position. It may be at the late stage of arcing the mandible upward which is actually the start of centric occlusion relationship.

To obtain this position there are a number of techniques, all of which are acceptable. As mentioned before, one technique cannot be used for every patient. Whatever technique is used, always modify it to suit the case at hand and to satisfy the characteristics and physio-anatomical facts mentioned in the previous section.

The second stage in the physical manipulation of the mandible is to locate *centric occlusion*. Its attainment is available if we successfully locate centric relation. The patient is asked to bite, while the operator guides and supports the horizontal part of the mandible.

The third stage in the physical manipulation of the mandible is defining *lateral excursions*. These should start from centric occlusion. Supporting pressure should be applied subsequently at the angle of the mandible on the working side to keep the condyle seated within its fossa housing. Guiding hand support may be necessary on the non-working side during the medial drop of the mandible there. The mandible should be guided until the cuspid (or the last tooth to disclude) on the working side is edge-to-edge, ready to disclude. This stage should be done twice, once for each side.

The fourth stage in the physical manipulation of the mandible is *the protrusive movement*. This also starts from centric occlusion and the patient is asked to glide the teeth forward. There should be superio-anterior guiding, light, supporting pressure at the angle of the mandible, while the patient is protruding it. This is to assure the contact of the condyle with the eminentia (condylar guidance). The movement should be exercised until reverse overlap occurs or at least edge-to-edge relation is acquired anteriorly.

II. Non-Transferable Records

Such records are usually used for diagnostic and verifying purposes only. Although there are numerous techniques for this, the coloring ribbon technique is the most widely used. The technique simply introduces a marking ribbon between the dried mandibular and maxillary teeth while manipulating the mandible into one or more of the previously described positions. If more than one position is to be obtained, each should be done with a separate marking ribbon. Different colored ribbons are supplied if a composite picture of more than one movement is needed to be recorded on the occluding surfaces of the teeth.

The following should be observed in using this type of technique:

A. Teeth (restorations) should be carefully dried. For extensive marking procedures (e.g., occlusal equilibration of natural teeth), patients might even require anti-sialogogues.

B. Highly polished (glazed) restorations or extremely smooth enamel surfaces may not be marked with certain ribbons, so contact there can be verified and enhanced by roughening of the surface if possible (restoration surfaces could be temporarily roughened), by pulling the marking ribbon laterally after contact is achieved (to verify positive contact if there is resistance to the pull) or by the use of thick highly colored ribbon.

C. Red markings can be misleading if there is some bleeding from adjacent soft tissues.

D. Some contacts should be marked twice with two different colors in order to verify them by their repetition.

E. Before executing the tooth contact, be sure the marking ribbon is covering all possible occluding surfaces.

F. Before performing the tooth contact while the marking ribbon is in place, be sure no foreign bodies or soft tissues are interfering with any contacts between the teeth.

G. It is preferable to start with gross marking using a thick ribbon, then proceed with final marking using a thin one.

H. One should use marking ribbons that mark in degrees, i.e., heavy contacts are marked darker than light ones.

Application of Non-Transferable Records

These techniques are applied in four main areas of restorative dentistry:

A. Equilibration of natural dentition

Not infrequently, some teeth in the stomato-gnathic system interfere with the normal physiologic motion of the mandible. To avoid these interferences, many components of the system might be placed into hyperfunctional status in an effort to evade the interferences. Such interferences can be caused by any of the following factors:

1. Uneven, non-symmetrical attrition of occluding tooth surfaces.

2. Supereruption, tilting, rotation, or bodily movements of a tooth.

3. Undercontoured (overcarved) occluding restoration leading to occlusal and possibly lateral displacement of opposing cuspal elements.

4. Periodontal diseases facilitating tooth movement, especially laterally.

5. Insufficiently restraining cusp-fossa or cusp-marginal ridge relationships allowing repositioning of teeth.

6. Plunger cusps against marginal ridges separating them, or the same cusp against one side of a tooth tilting it laterally.

There will be no attempt to describe a technique for occlusal equilibration here. However, it might be useful to enumerate the features of a non-pathologic optimum occlusion. These features should be achieved in any natural dentition or in any occluding restoration as part of the stomato-gnathic system.

a. There should be no tooth contact at the early (inferior) stage of centric relation.

b. The mandible should arc along a hinge axis from centric relation to centric occlusion. Any interfering tooth parts with this arcing, creating any translation, should be eliminated.

c. In the early stage of centric occlusion, toward complete intercuspation, there may be forward movements of the mandible. However, there should not be any lateral, medial or backward movements of the mandible (with the teeth) in moving from centric relation to centric occlusion. Any cuspal inclines contributing to this latter "skid" should be eliminated.

d. At centric occlusion, only the occluding items mentioned in the static relation of the mandible should be in contact with each other, i.e., avoid inclined planes in contact as much as possible.

e. At centric occlusion, the holding cusps should be of sufficient height to be in positive contact with their opposing counterparts. This arrangement should be in a way to preserve the vertical dimension of the teeth and the stomato-gnathic system.

f. At centric occlusion, the holding markings should be symmetrical (magnitude and extent) on all holding cuspal elements of both sides.

g. When maximum intercuspation is achieved, there should not be any further movements of the mandible or the teeth by further biting. In other words, markings (extent and magnitude) should be repeated without any skids.

h. Holding cusps occluding with more than one tooth or eccentrically occluding with opposing teeth should not move opposing teeth (tooth) in a non-axial direction. This is accomplished by broadening the contact of the cusps with opposing teeth (tooth) to minimize tipping or wedging.

i. In centric occlusion, the incisal edges of lower incisors should be located at the very gingival end of the lingual concavity of the upper incisors, preferably with a flat horizontal shelf or plane. This plane will enhance the holding capability of the lingual concavity keeping the interrelationship conducive to optimum occlusion.

j. In lateral excursion of the mandible, there should not be any tooth contact on the non-working side of the mandible.

k. In lateral excursion of the mandible, the holding cusps of the working side should have a valley-like space on the opposing teeth (grooves or occlusal embrasures). This is to facilitate their non-interfereing passage during the lateral excursion. These valleys should have the right depth, inclination of their surrounding walls (inclined planes), and directions to allow this passing-by of the holding cusps, and to be symmetrical to and in harmony with the nature of the condylar movements in three dimensions at that side.

l. The disclusive features mentioned previously in this chapter should be fulfilled, especially if group function is involved. The disclusion should start posteriorly and end by the cuspid's disclusion. This mechanism should be such that contacting loads (magnitude and extent) will decrease in a similar pattern.

m. Also, in the disclusion mechanism, the disclusion path should be perfected so that the optimum direction along the lingual surface of the upper cuspid and the working inclines of the non-working cusps is achieved.

n. Marked contacting areas during lateral excursion should be the same going out of centric and back into centric.

o. During protrusive excursions of the mandible there should not be any tooth contact posteriorly.

p. Cuspids should be involved, at least in the initial stage, in the protrusive movement of the mandible.

q. Protrusive contact markings should be evenly distributed and symmetrical on all teeth involved.

r. Protrusive markings should be in straight fashion at the upper incisors' lingual concavity apico-incisally. In other words, it should not cross the lingual surface of upper incisors obliquely or horizontally.

It is a good idea to do an occlusal equilibration of existing dentition before performing extensive restorative procedures, that will involve a change of occluding surfaces of multiple teeth; or if symptoms of facial myofunctional, TMJ dysfunction, or dysfunction of any part of the stomato-gnathic system is exhibited. The first things one might look for, after excluding TMJ structural or pathological changes, are occlusal interferences. If interferences are indeed evident, they should be eliminated. It is preferable to mount upper and lower casts for the patient in an adjustable articulator, to put the articulator through all possible movements, and to remove and record all interferences as they are removed on the study models. This should be done until the teeth on the casts are related, with an absence of any interferences. At this stage, the recorded interferences may be eliminated from the natural dentition as previously planned and executed on the casts.

B. Occlusion adjustment of directly inserted restorative materials

After inserting these types of restorative materials (e.g., amalgam, composite) into the tooth, they should be carved to contact, contour, and correct margins. The first step in occlusal adjustments is to establish the vertical dimension of the restoration. This is achieved by the following steps:

1. Carve the restorative material to grossly coincide with the adjacent and opposing teeth anatomy from the aspect of vertical dimension.

2. Move the mandible from centric relation to centric occlusion while a marking ribbon is between the teeth. Heavy markings on the holding cusp-fossa or cusp-marginal ridge will indicate the necessity to reduce cusp and marginal ridge heights

and to deepen the fossae. This procedure should be repeated until the holding elements meet in the same pattern (extent and magnitude) as the rest of the holding elements in the same and opposing arches.

Then proceed with occlusal adjustment as previously done in occlusal equilibration.

C. Final occlusal adjustment for a cast restoration

As will be seen shortly, no matter how extensive the reproduction of mandibular movements on an articulator, there will still be some adjustment necessary for any cast restoration before it will be ready for cementation. Therefore, the cast restoration should be tried on the tooth and adjusted in the same manner as other restorative materials.

D. Diagnostic occlusion analysis

This is an essential tool not only to detect any interference that may have caused dental or paradental symptoms, which a patient presents, but also to use before building any restoration in the stomato-gnathic system that replaces all or part of an occluding surface.

III. Transferable Records

Occlusal records are usually used for building restorations outside of the mouth. However, sometimes they are used for diagnostic purposes to study patients' casts on a special articulator. These records are mainly fashioned in two steps. The first step involves taking the records intraorally in a fairly non-distortable material. The second step involves transferring the information on this material to a special instrument (articulator) capable of accepting these records. The records enable an articulator to have its parts moved in a way which creates the same effect (occluding surface shapes) on a restoration, as the mandible would. The extraorally fabricated restoration thus becomes a physiological replacement part in the stomato-gnathic system. As may be expected, such transferable records might be for either static or dynamic relations of the mandible.

A. Static relationship transferable records

These records capture the relationship of the maxillary and mandibular teeth at border locations of the mandibular movement path. They are only transferable to a semi-adjustable articulator which is capable of moving from one captured border location to another, with a standard path in-between (Fig. 6 A, B, and C). These records are also used to correlate upper and lower casts at centric relation or centric occlusion in any

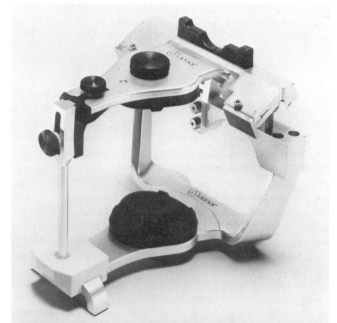

A cont'd

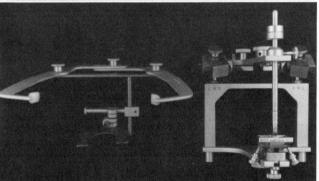

B

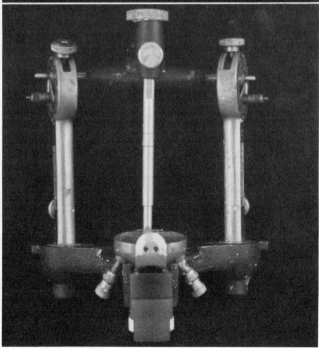

C

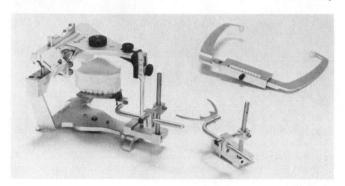

Fig. 16-6. A, Denar semiadjustable articulator and its facebow. **B,** Whip-mix semiadjustable articulator with its facebow. **C,** Hanau semiadjustable articulator.

type of articulator (hinge, semi-adjustable or fully-adjustable). There are an infinite number of materials and techniques that can be used to make this type of transferable records. They may be classified as follows:

a. Interocclusal records

1. Centric relation records should be made in the absence of any occlusal contacts. The mandible should be manipulated, as described before, until there is a definite hinge-axis mandibular arcing. An acrylic (sometimes hard wax) jig is built at the lingual surface of upper incisors with an extension labially that hooks over the labial surface. This jig should have a lingual "braking" concavity that prevents occlusal movements of the teeth. The jig thickness should not exceed the free-way space, and it should allow a 1-2 mm spacing between posterior teeth. The purpose of such a jig is to keep the mandible in centric relation while taking the record of that position in a transferable material. This material can be hard solidifying wax, modified ZOE paste (carried in a mesh), tray (metal sheet)—carried elastomeric impression materials or plaster, etc.

While the material is in a moldable state, and after seating the anterior jig on the upper incisors, it is inserted between the upper and lower teeth. The mandible is then guided to centric relation as predetermined by the lingual slope of the jig. After the material hardens, it is removed and all flanges and excesses if present are trimmed, leaving only the indentations of the cusp tips.

2. Lateral excursion records are taken in pairs, both on the non-working side, i.e., one for the right and the other for the left. The patient's mandible is guided and manipulated so that cuspids (the last discluding tooth) on the working side come to an edge-to-edge relation. This is done while one of the transfering materials (or combination of materials) is between the teeth on the non-working side. The process is repeated for the other side.

3. Protrusive excursion records, the mandible is manipulated and guided to an edge-to-edge incisor relationship. This relationship is maintained while recording material is between the posterior teeth.

The last two types of records are trimmed in the same way as the first, i.e., removing all but the cusp tip indentations.

b. Facial records (Fig. 7)

These are used only for centric occlusion, when interocclusal recordings might create errors. Modified ZOE, plaster, silicon rubber base or auto-polymerizing acrylic resin can be used to make the recording. The patient's mandible is guided and manipulated to centric relation and then to centric occlusion, where the patient is asked to close his teeth forcibly. Then, a paste of the recording material is flowed over the facial surface, covering the canine and, then, the premolars, and sometimes the mesial buccal cusps of the first molars. It should be flowed into the facial embrasures to temporarily lock in them.

After setting, the material is removed in a facial direction and trimmed without impinging on the embrasure extensions.

1. Use of hinge articulators (Fig. 7)

The only situation allowing the use of a hinge articulator is when the occlusion is stable and is not to be changed, and the restorations are few with adequate holding cuspal elements on both sides of the restoration. The only record needed for a hinge articulator is the facial centric occlusion record. The lower or upper cast is mounted on the articulator. The opposing

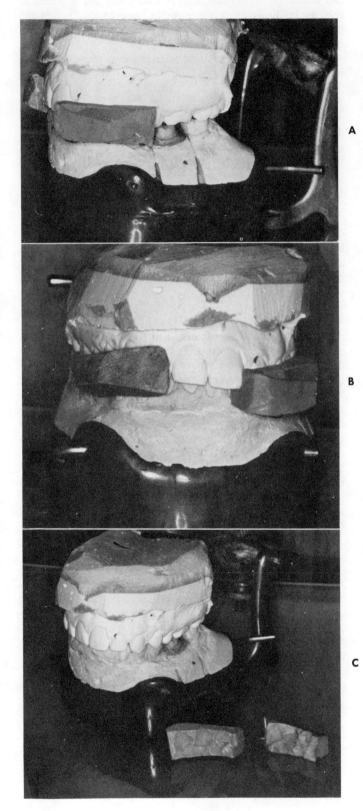

Fig. 16-7. A, Hinge articulator with mounted working models and dies. **B,** Hinge articulator with facial records assembling upper and lower casts in centric occlusion. **C,** Hinge articulator with mounted working casts and assembling facial records.

cast is occluded to the mounted one via this facial record, and then the cast attached to the articulator. Hand mounting, with no occlusal records, will often suffice; instead, in situations with full complements of unprepared teeth.

2. Use of semi-adjustable articulators

A necessary step before using semi- or fully-adjustable articulators is to take a facebow record (Fig. 6, A and B). This is a record capturing the relationship of the maxilla (and maxillary teeth) to the bony cranium. This recorded relationship is transfered to the adjustable articulator when the upper casts will relate to the upper arm of the articulator the same way the maxilla (maxillary teeth) relates to the cranium. To take these records, three reference points are necessary—one in each direction at the cranium part of the stomato-gnathic system. Joining these three chosen points should create a plane, preferably crossing or close to the hinge axis (for mandibular movements). This plane then represents the cranium.

A wax (compound or ZOE) carried on a special bite-fork is indented with the maxillary teeth and this represents the maxilla (maxillary teeth). Creating the assembly having these four point (area) contacts with the stomato-gnathic system will formulate the entire facebow record. The assembly is attached to the adjustable articulator with the three point areas coinciding with the reciprocating points in the upper part of the articulator (representing the cranium). The fourth area (bite-fork with the teeth indentations) will accommodate the upper cast (Fig. 6A).

After fitting the upper cusps of the cast into the indentations, the cast is attached to the arms of the articulator with a non-expanding gypsum. The facebow is removed and the upper cast is ready to be correlated with the lower cast, using the following steps:

a. A centric relation record is used to join the lower with the upper casts.

b. Held at this relationship, the lower cast is attached to the lower arm of the articulator with a non-expanding gypsum.

c. After setting of the attaching gypsum, the left condylar-path controlling screws (knobs) are loosened.

d. The right excursive records are put between the casts and the left condylar path components of the articulator are moved until they are steady and in contact with each other.

e. The same procedure is done for the right condylar-path controls, using the left excursive records.

f. The protrusive excursive records are next placed between the posterior teeth to establish the edge-to-edge relationship between anterior teeth. The protrusive inclines of the articulator's condylar path are adjusted accordingly.

g. Holding this relationship, the incisal guidance part of the articulator is adjusted according to the cast's anterior teeth overjet, over-bite, and lateral disclusion capability. At this stage the articulator will be ready for use in fabricating restorations or for diagnosing purposes.

B. Dynamic relationship transferable records

1. *Functionally generated path*

These techniques capture the effect of the dynamics of mandibular movements as they are performed. The stereographic record thus created is transferred to a "verticulator" (or similar device) where it will impart its configuration on the opposing restoration (see chapters on cast restorations).

2. *Pantograph and fully adjustable articulator*
(Fig. 8, A, B, C, and D)

Although it is not in the domain of this text to present the armamentarium and procedures to use the pantographs and fully adjustable articulators, it is necessary to alert the reader to the availability, capability, and indications of these procedures. The pantograph, in addition to recording the border location of the mandible (in three dimensions), also accurately locates the exact path the mandible travels from one terminal location to another. These paths are recorded in three dimensions on three separate planes (Saggital, horizontal, and coronal). Therefore, it enables recording of such paths of the mandibular movements as immediate side shifts, progressive side shifts, superior-trusion, retrotrusion, etc., i.e., paths that cannot be traced by check-bite procedures. That is why pantographic records are "dynamic" in nature. They give not only the starting and ending points of mandibular movement, but also the path the mandible takes between these points.

The pantographic tracing occurs on recording tables which are attached to either the mandible or maxilla. The marking styli are also attached to either the mandible or maxilla, i.e., to the component that does not have the table. Six to eight tables, with a corresponding number of styli should be attached to either the mandible or maxilla. The intraoral attachment will be through an autopolymerizing resin splint (clutches). From this clutch, antero-posterior and lateral arms extend, one set each for both the maxilla and the mandible. This splint (clutch) is built at centric relation with no teeth contact, but with a thickness not to exceed the intermaxillary free-way space. The upper arm assembly is related to the cranium and the maxilla in the same was as a facebow. On each side there are recording tables in the following arrangement: two in the horizontal plane (one posteriorly and one anteriorly), one in the saggital plane (posteriorly located), and sometimes one in the coronal (frontal) plane (posteriorly located).

In most situations of single tooth restorations it is not necessary to locate the exact hinge axis of the mandibular movements. However, in situations where the vertical dimension of the teeth is to be changed by restorations or complete mouth rehabilitation, the hinge axis should be located and marked (tatooed) on the side of the face. Each pantographic tracer has a specific side arm to be attached to the maxillary splint (clutch), with special styli to be attached to the mandibular one. With this last arrangement, in a sequence of mandibular manipulations from centric relation to centric occlusion, through trial and error procedures, the hinge axis is captured and marked on the face. When marked, it may be used as a posterior reference point in a facebow maxillary pantograph assembly.

With the resin splint (clutch) attached to the corresponding teeth, the upper clutch holds the arms assembly representing the immovable maxilla. This upper splint is in true fixed relationship to the cranium through the four points (areas) of contacts, as with the facebow. The lower splint (clutch) is attached to the corresponding teeth and holds the arm assembly representing the mandible. Each part of the assembly is free to move independently from the other. By activating the styli to be in contact with the recording tables and by moving the mandible in lateral excursions and in protrusive excursions movements, the styli inscribe all possible movements in the

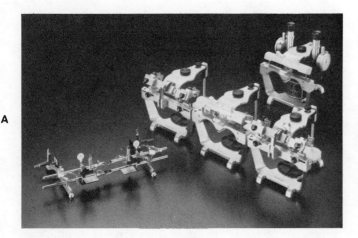

Fig. 16-8. A

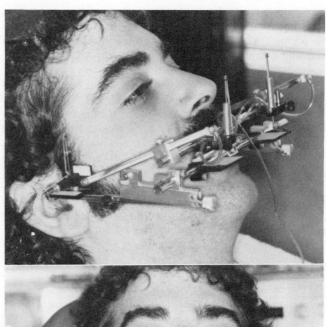

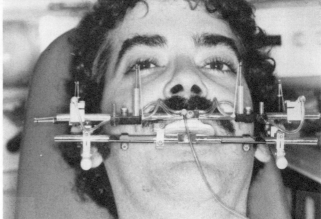

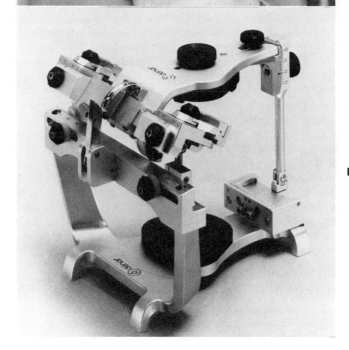

six to eight tables representing the possible spatial planes (Fig. 3, 4, and 5). Next, the tracings on the recording tables are fixed (covered). The entire pantograph assembly is immobilized at centric relation and transfered to the fully adjustable articulator. Once on the fully adjustable articulator, every single tracing is retraced in a non-marking fashion. While doing so, different controls of the adjustable articulators are made to coincide with those tracings. By this adjustment, the articulator can be ready to impart these patterns in the way the restoration is shaped.

3. Stereographic tracing and fully adjustable articulators

Two intraoral clutches are built and adjusted, one for each arch. The lower clutch carries a stabilizing central bearing point. The upper clutch carries three to four indentors. Opposite these indentors in the lower clutch moldable self-curing acrylic knobs are placed. The mandible is guided into centric relation, then moved over the central bearing point to border locations laterally (right and left) and anteriorly, allowing the indentor in the upper clutch to shape the acrylic while setting. When the acrylic sets, it can be transferred to the fully adjustable articulator. When the upper clutch with its cast is attached via a facebow, the upper and lower clutches are related to each other in centric relation. A moldable mix of acrylic resin is placed in the fossa box on each side of the articulator, and the instrument arms are moved through the paths in the acrylic knobs in the lower clutch, molding the acrylic in the fossa box to the exact shape of the fossa. When the shaped acrylic in the fossa sets, it will simulate the original fossa that imparted the paths in the acrylic knobs, and it can dictate the occluding shapes of the restorations accordingly.

For all adjustable articulators, the anterior guidance can be established by a deformable setting acrylic resin mix on the incisal table of the articulator. After mounting the upper and lower casts, using the incisal pin as an indentor, move the upper component of the articulator antero-posteriorly to edge relation and back to centric occlusion. Then laterally right, back to CO, then laterally left, then back to CO. When the acrylic resin sets, the created path is the anterior guidance.

In most of the adjustable articulators the components of the anterior guidance can be mechanically imitated by parts of the articulator. After mounting the upper and lower casts, bring them to CO, move the upper arm posteriorly, until the upper

Fig. 16-8. A, Fully adjustable Denar articulator and pantograph. **B** and **C,** Assembled and mounted pantograph ready for dynamic mandibular movement tracings. **D,** Denar fully adjustable articulator.

and lower anterior teeth touch, then adjust the amount of overjet. Move the upper arm posteriorly and upwards to an edge-to-edge relation, then adjust the overbite. Move the upper arm laterally and on the working side adjust the lateral wing of the anterior guidance to touch the pin at the most lateral border location. Repeat for the other lateral location.

The choice between the different types of occlusal records is a matter of experience and training, but the following table can give a guideline as to when each may be utilized to its best advantage.

Occluding Restoration	Location	Indicated Mandibular Position	Facebow	Articulator	Occlusion Record
1-2	Not including terminal holding teeth	CO	No	Hinge or verticulator	Facial occlusion records or FGP
3-4 posterior	Not including terminal holding teeth	CO	No	Hinge or verticulator	Facial occlusion records or FGP
Not forming a complete quadrant	Including terminal holding teeth	CR	Yes	Semi-adjustable	CR, lateral and protrusive excursion, interocclusal records or FGP
3-4 anterior	Not including cuspid	CO	No	Hinge or verticulator	Facial occlusion records or FGP
	Including cuspid	CR	Yes	Semi-adjustable	CR, lateral and protrusive excursion, interocclusal records or FGP
4 posterior	A posterior quadrant	CR	Yes	Pantograph or stereograph and fully adjustable articulator	Arbitrary hinge axis, pantographic or stereographic tracing, CR to mount lower cast or FG
6	All anteriors	CR	Yes	Pantograph or stereograph and fully adjustable articulator	Arbitrary hinge axis, pantographic or stereographic tracing, CR to mount lower cast or FGP
6 or more	Anywhere	CR	Yes	Pantograph or stereograph and fully adjustable articulator	Exact hinge axis, pantographic or stereographic tracing, CR to mount lower cast or FGP
All posterior teeth	One or both arches contemplating changes in occluding dimensions, especially vertical ones	CR	Yes	Pantograph or stereograph and fully adjustable articulator	Exact hinge axis, pantographic or stereographic tracing, CR to mount lower casts

BIBLIOGRAPHY

Anneroth, G.: The functionally generated path technique for the construction of inlays, crowns, and bridges. Odontol. Revy **19**(2):211-23, 1968.

Balshi, T.J., Mingledorff, E.B., Olbrys, B.H., and Cantor, S.J.: Restorative occlusion utilizing a custom incisal guide table. J. Prosthet. Dent. **36**(4):468-471, Oct. 76.

Bellanti, N.D., and Martin, K.R.: The significance of articulator capability. Part II: The prevalence of immediate side shift. J. Prosthet. Dent. **42**(3):255-256, Sep. 1979.

Blanco Dalmau, L.: The use of the functional generated path concepts in occlusal rehabilitation. Rev. Odontol. PR **11**(2):14-18, Aug.-Dec. 1973.

Braly, B.V.: Occlusal analysis and treatment planning for restorative dentistry. J. Prosthet. Dent. **27**(2):168-171, Feb. 1972.

Branstad, W.: Report of the Committee on Scientific Investigation of the American Academy of Restorative Dentistry. J. Prosthet. Dent. **22**(1):88-98, July 1969.

Broderson, S.P.: Anterior guidance—the key to successful occlusal treatment. J. Prosthet. Dent. **39**(4):396-400, April 1978.

Celenza, F.V.: The occlusal index technique. Quintessence Dent. Technol. **1**(1):27-33, Jan. 1976.

Celenza, F.V., and Litvak, H.: Occlusal management in conformative dentistry. J. Prosthet. Dent. **36**(2):164-170, Aug. 1976.

Dubin, N.L.: Current concepts of functional occlusal rehabilitation. J. Conn. State Dent. Assn. **49**(4):257-261, Oct. 1975.

Erdmann, G.E.: The relationship of occlusion to restorative dentistry. Dent. Stud. **52**(3):34-35, Dec. 1973.

Gilmore, H.W., Carbeneau, G.T., Eames, W.B., Jendresen, M., Phillips, R.W., Ramfjord, S.P., and Roberts D.L.: Report of the Committee on Scientific Investigation of the American Academy of Restorative Dentistry. J. Prosthet. Dent. **40**(2):192-215, Aug. 1978.

Greene, A.R.: Maintaining the physiologic equilibrium of the patient in relation to the temporomandibular joint. Quintessence Int. **9**(11):9-13, Nov. 1978.

Guichet, N.F.: Biologic laws governing functions of muscles that move the mandible. Part IV. Degree of jaw separation and potential for maximum jaw separation. J. Prosthet. Dent. **38**(3):301-310, Sep. 1977.

Guichet, N.F.: The Denar System and its application in everyday dentistry. Dent. Clin. North Am. **23**(2):243-257, April 1979.

Guichet, N.F.: Specifications for the occlusal aspects of dental restorations. J. Prosthet. Dent. **35**(1):101-102, Jan. 1976.

Hughes, H.J., and Meyers, G.E.: Practical aspects of occlusion in restorative dentistry. Aust. Dent. J. **17**(4):284-292, Aug. 1972.

Hughes, H.J., and Meyers, G.E.: Practical aspects of occlusion in restorative dentistry. 3. Guidelines in the diagnosis of complex restorative case. Aust. Dent. J. **17**(6):469-470, Dec. 1972.

Jendresen, M.D., Charbeneau, G.T., Hamilton, A.I., Phillips, R.W., and Ramfjord, S.P.: Report of the Committee On Scientific Investigation of the American Academy of Restorative Dentistry. J. Prosthet. Dent. **41**(6):671-695, June 1979.

Kobes, L.W.: Reproduction of the static and dynamic relationships of the stomatognathic system in crown and bridge prostheses. Rev. Belge. Med. Dent. **31**(4):315-330, 1976.

Lucia, V.O.: Principles of articulation. Dent. Clin. North Am. **23**(2):199-211, April 1979.

Mosteller, J.H.: Occlusion of the natural dentition, Part I. J. Ala. Dent. Assoc. **64**(4):36-45, Fall 1980.

Mosteller, J.H.: Occlusion of the natural dentition. Part II. J. Ala. Dent. Assoc. **65**(1):30-42. Winter 1981.

Rapuano, J.A.: Equilibrating the single crown. J. Acad. Gen. Dent. **21**(6):40, Nov.-Dec. 1973.

Rearden, L: Why gnathology? (I). Quintessence Int. **8**(12):33-7, Dec. 1977.

Sorscher, Y.A.: A simplified procedure to end guesswork when checking occlusion. Dent. Surv. **49**(6):47-48, June 1973.

Stern, N., and Brayer, L.: Collapse of the occlusion—aetiology, symptomatology and treatment. J. Oral Rehabil. **2**(1):1-19, Jan. 1975.

Sullivan, M.M.: Restoration of occlusal defects. II. Guiding principles in the design of restorative procedures. Ann. Aust. Coll. Dent. Surg. **2**:128-143, Oct. 1969.

Taylor, R.L.: Restoration of occlusal defects. I. The influence of occlusion on the plan of treatment. Ann. Aust. Coll. Dent. Surg. **2**:114-127, Oct. 1969.

Wiland, L.: Carving dental restorations. J. Prosthet. Dent. **33**(5):582-586, May 1978.

Wise, M.D.: Occlusion and restorative dentistry. Br. Dent. J. **143**(2):45-52, July 19, 1977.

cast alloy materials
class I - gold alloys
   " II - economy gold alloys
   " III   silver palladium all
   " IV - nickel-chromium
          based all.
   V - cast ceramic allo.

CHAPTER 17

Cast restorations

Taggart permanently changed the practice of restorative dentistry by introducing his technique for cast gold dental restorations, such that, today, cast dental restorations and appliances have become basic treatment modalities in dentistry. Cast restorations for single teeth have several advantages over other types of restorations, namely:

A. Yield, compressive, tensile and shear strengths of alloys and ceramics used for cast dental restorations are far greater than those of any other materials used intraorally, e.g., some cast alloys have five times the ultimate strengths of amalgam. That is why cast restorations are used to replace areas of stress concentration within a tooth, as well as to reinforce weakened tooth structure. They are one of the types of restorations that are free of mechanical failure. One of the main uses of cast restorations in operative dentistry is in situations when a restorative material is needed to impart resistance to the tooth, rather than depending on tooth structure to provide resistance form to the restoration.

B. Casting techniques and materials are capable of reproducing precise form and minute detail. Additionally, these materials will maintain this detail under functional stresses.

C. Any of the metal alloys used for cast restorations contain as one or more of their component metals, a noble or passivated metal, i.e., they are not significantly affected by tarnish and corrosion processes in the oral environment. Cast ceramics are completely inert intraorally. This property is lacking in amalgam. This major advantage improves the longevity, esthetics and biologic qualities of the cast restoration.

D. The very nature of building a metallic or ceramic restoration instantaneously with a casting procedure, as opposed to an incremental build-up in amalgam, imparts advantages to the final structures, e.g., fewer voids, no layering effect, less internal stresses, fairly even stress patterns of the entire structure (at least as compared to amalgam) and maximum bonding between the component phases. All this leads to a strong structure, which is less susceptible to corrosion.

E. Cast restorations can be finished, polished or glazed outside the oral cavity, thereby producing surfaces with maximum biological acceptance without regard to the heat and pressure that would endanger the P-D organ.

However, as with any restorative material and technique, there are some disadvantages.

1. Being a cemented restoration, several interphases will be created at the tooth-cement-casting junction. These interphases, and the leakage accompanying them, will become more significant due to the fact that cast fabrications involve a number of reproductions using different materials (impressions, models, etc.), each of which possesses inherent discrepancies. This produces a restoration which is microscopically ill-fitting and which incompletely obliterates the details of the tooth preparation. Leakage around and under a cast restoration is the most complicated and has the highest dimension among all restorative materials. This leakage will be more pronounced gingivally than at other parts of the restoration.

2. Cast restorations necessitate extensive tooth involvement in the preparation, which creates possible hazards for the vital dental tissues.

3. The cathodic nature of cast dental alloys toward other metals used in the same mouth may lead to galvanic deterioration. Because of their nobility, partial nobility and/or passivity, if cast alloys are involved in a cell of dissimilar metals in the oral cavity (e.g., amalgam), the amalgam will undergo rapid deterioration and failure. As a by-product of this dissimilar metal cell-corrosion, the cast alloy itself will be contaminated by the freed mercury. The created galvanic current may create undesirable effects in the invested and investing vital dental tissues.

4. The procedure for cast restoration fabrication is lengthy, requiring more than one visit, with temporary coverage between visits. Also, cast alloys are much more expensive than other restorative materials, due to the inherent expense of the alloy.

5. Occlusal surface attrition of the natural dentition is a normal physiologic process, occurring throughout the life of the teeth. Some cast alloys and ceramics have a very high abrasive resistance, much more than that of tooth enamel. So if a single restoration or sporadically located restorations are made for a patient replacing the occluding surfaces and opposing natural teeth during functional mandibular relations, there may be an abrasive differential between natural dentition and cast restoration, with the teeth being abraded much more easily. Such an abrasion differential will lead to an imbalance in occlusion resulting in teeth shifting, tilting or rotating, and leading to occlusal interferences during mandibular movements. Such patients may require periodic occlusal equilibration, or even building all the occlusal surfaces in cast restorations, including the opposing dentition.

307

I. Indications for Cast Restorations

A. Extensive tooth involvement

Amalgam is limited in its ability to replace tooth structure; beyond this limit it can act only as a foundation for a reinforcing cast restoration. Cast restorations are the ultimate in both efficiently replacing lost tooth structure and supporting remaining tooth structure.

B. As an adjunct to successful periodontal therapy by correction of tooth anomalies which predispose to periodontal problems

Cast restorations can do this by:
1. Physiologically restoring and permanently maintaining the dimensions of the contact contour, marginal ridges, and embrasures, which are vital for the health of the periodontium.
2. Splinting teeth loosened by periodontitis to a better bone-supported tooth or teeth. The rigid connection of several cast restorations assures the distribution of applied forces to the best supported teeth while minimizing forces on the disable teeth.

C. Correction of occlusion

If any drastic change is planned for the occlusal table or occluding parts of a tooth, cast restorations are ideal. This is very essential for a sound periodontium and a pathology-free, functional stomato-gnathic system.

D. Restoration of endodontically treated teeth

When teeth undergo endodontic therapy they lose structure and become brittle. Almost always the clinical crown portion of these teeth will need a reinforcing restoration, i.e., a cast restoration.

E. Support for and preparatory to partial or complete dentures

Whether they are a clasp type, overdenture type, precision attachment or bar attachment type, most removable prostheses will need cast restorations on or in the abutment teeth to hold or accommodate the retainers for the denture.

F. Retainers for fixed prostheses

For the abutment tooth in a fixed bridge there is no alternative to a cast restoration as a retainer.

G. Partially subgingival restorations

With the exception of high fused porcelain, cast ceramics, and cohesive gold foil, properly finished and polished cast alloys are the restorative materials most compatible with the periodontium. Therefore, these restorations are considered the most practical for subgingival lesions, especially if a rubber dam cannot be applied.

H. Low incidences of plaque accumulation or decay

Patients to receive a cast restoration should have their plaque accumulation under rigid control to avoid problems at and due to the weak link of the tooth structure-cement-cast complex.

I. Functionally sound stomato-gnathic system with complete freedom of the mandible to move without any premature contacts

Patients having their teeth restored by cast restorations should be checked and analyzed stomato-gnathically to be sure of the soundness and function of the system. If any pathology is discovered, the causes should be diagnosed and treated, and if any malfunction is not going to be corrected by the contemplated cast restorations, it should be treated prior to the cast restoration procedure. If this is not done, the cast restoration and procedures may seriously complicate the treatment.

J. Cracked teeth (vertically, horizontally, or diagonally)

Cast restorations are the most rigid and subsequently the most efficient way of restoring and splinting, the cracked, separated segments of a tooth. This prevents further propagation of the crack and occasionally promotes healing of some cracks.

K. Esthetics

Of all metallic restorations (with the exception of direct gold restorations), properly fitted cast restorations are the most pleasant esthetically. Cast alloys will have no tendency to discolor the remaining tooth structures. Naturally cast ceramics can, be tooth colored.

L. Dissimilar metals

Whenever cast restorations are prevalent in a mouth, it is logical to fabricate new restorations in similar materials. This will minimize galvanism, premature abrasion, anodic dissolution of any other less noble materials, or mechanical failure of other less qualified restorative materials. Approximating dissimilar material, continuously or momentarily, can enhance diffusion of restorative materials with high diffusion indices (e.g., amalgam) to the cast alloy, which has very low diffusion indices at mouth temperature. This will lead to vacancy porosities in the former material and alloying of the latter materials, which may weaken them.

People allergic to some restorative materials seldom have any reaction to gold alloy cast restorations and no reaction to cast ceramic restorations.

II. Contraindications for Cast Restorations

Physiologically young dentition with large pulp chambers and incompletely mineralized dentin are poor candidates for cast restorations, as the extensiveness of the tooth preparation and the variables encountered during the multi-step procedures may traumatize these vulnerable tissues.

A. Developing and deciduous teeth

Growth or resorption may be affected by the comparatively traumatic nature of the procedures for cast restorations.

B. High plaque/caries indices

Patients with uncontrollable plaque and high caries and periodontal indices are not candidates for such restorations, even if the tooth involvement indicates their use. Using them, there is too great a possibility for recurrent decay and acceleration of periodontal deterioration initiated at the tooth-cement-cast joint complex.

C. Occlusal disharmony

Cast restorations should not be used in patients with occlusal interference or other defects in the stomato-gnathic system, if there is any doubt that the cast restoration will correct the ailment.

C. Dissimilar metals

Preferably cast alloy restorations are not to be used in proximal contact or in occlusion with an amalgam restoration as this will be detrimental to the amalgam as well as to the cast alloy itself.

III. Materials for Cast Restorations

Until recently gold based alloys have been the only ones used for cast dental restorations. The ADA specification # 5 still requires 75% of gold and platinum group metals to be present in alloys for a cast restoration. At the present time, however, gold and most of the platinum group metals are becoming rare and expensive commodities. Alloy manufacturers buy these metals from the same market as speculators, a situation that has boosted the prices of these metals more than ten times in recent history. Fortunately, gold based alloys are not the only available material for single tooth cast restorations. There are a number of other materials available to the profession. Some have been in clinical use for several years, others are still in the developmental stages, and still other recent materials have dropped out of use due to certain clinical or procedural drawbacks.

An attempt to classify and group these castable materials under a standardized system is futile at this stage of constant change in these restorative casting materials. Nevertheless, a very broad classification that can encompass most or all the trends and thoughts in this continuously changing field will help in describing and understanding the basic ideas of the subject, and facilitate acceptance and use of the techniques and materials that will definitely be introduced to the profession during the 1980's and 1990's.

For the purpose of this discussion materials for cast dental restorations will be classified into the following:

Class I

These are gold and platinum-group-based alloys in accordance with the ADA specification # 5. They are type I, II, III, IV gold alloys.

Class II

These are low gold alloys, with gold content less than 50%. Some may contain as little as 5% gold.

Class III

These are non-gold palladium-based alloys.

Class IV

Nickel-chromium based alloys.

Class V

Castable, moldable ceramics.

A. Composition and effects

Class I

These are the baseline of cast dental alloys. They have stood the test of time, and any new alloy is compared to them for

evaluation. According to the ADA specification # 5, these alloys should have at least 70-75% gold or one of its platinum group substitutes, i.e., platinum, palladium, rhodium, osmium, irridium, and ruthenium. Usually, the required 70-75% is primarily gold, with 1-5% platinum and/or palladium. A large portion of the remaining 25-30% is silver, and, to a lesser extent, copper (which plays a vitally important role in hardening the alloy). The remainder consists of traces of zinc and/or indium.

There are four types of these alloys, each having a range of properties and specific composition. Type I, being the most plastic, has the highest content of gold. Type IV is the least deformable with the lowest content of gold. For a single tooth restoration, type III, or, infrequently, type II is used.

Each constituent metal will impart certain properties on the final alloy, according to its percentage composition, its alloying nature and the environment of fabricating and casting. It should be very obvious that the product alloy is a very complex one, knowing that gold can alloy in different fashions with each of the previously mentioned metals in forming the alloy. Palladium and platinum, in addition to disorderly alloying with gold, can produce several ordered alloys with copper with different constituents and effects. Silver, in addition to substitutional and ordered alloying with gold, can readily alloy with copper, producing several types of alloys, ranging from ordered to eutectic. Silver can also alloy with palladium producing a solid solution alloy. Copper is very influential in the alloy as it can make a solid solution with gold, palladium, platinum and silver. In the amount of gold and copper used in type III and IV gold alloy, copper and gold solid solution alloys can undergo ordered solid state changes producing different intermetallic compounds that are precipitated within the solid mass. These solid state changes affect the hardness, plasticity, and strength properties of the solid mass. Zinc can readily alloy with gold. Indium also alloys with gold, producing some intermetallic compounds that are very influential in shaping the final microstructure of the alloy.

Thus, the properties of the cast solid alloy in the form of a restoration are easily controlled by the extent, nature, and types of the above mentioned, complex combinations. However, generally speaking, gold is primarily responsible for the deformability, strength, characteristic yellow color and density (19.3 g/cm^3) of the alloy. Platinum or palladium are responsible for the rigidity, nobility, strength, hardness and whitening of the alloy, if they are present in sufficient amount. Silver mimics gold in its deformability effect, but adversely affects the nobility. A precipitated silver-gold intermetallic compound in a solid state can enter the hardening process like copper-gold compounds. Copper, in a small percentage, is extremely important in governing the behavior of the gold in solid state. Although it increases the hardness and strength, it also decreases the nobility of the alloy. Zinc in small quantities is essential as a deoxidizer during casting and it should be replaced if the alloy is to be recast. Indium in trace amounts is very efficient in refining the grains of the final alloy, i.e., facilitating smaller, comparable sized, evenly distributed grains in the final product. This produces a more predictable behavior of the restoration. Indium can also act as a scavenger for the alloy during the cast procedure.

nobility is ... tolerates against environment like oxidation. Sulfuration

310   *Operative dentistry*

Class II

Although there is no ADA specification for such type of alloys (sometimes called "economy gold alloys"), the gold content is much lower than Class I. Palladium is usually used as a gold substitute. Copper, silver, and zinc again comprise 25-30% of the alloy composition. Some of these alloys contain up to 60% palladium and as little as 5% gold.

As can be expected, the final products of casting Class II alloys will be different from those of Class I. Even though gold will still impart the same properties as in Class I alloys, they will be much more limited. Palladium will be responsible for most of the desirable physical properties, imparting strength, nobility, hardness, and the plasticity of the mass (expect less plasticity the more the palladium). The low density of palladium (as compared to gold) will show up in the final product. Copper reacts with palladium as it does with gold, forming different types and constitutions of alloys with possible solid state precipitation of certain ordered alloys. This leads to a strengthening-hardening-brittling effect. Silver will form a continuous substitutional solid solution alloy with the palladium and the traces of gold. Zinc has the same reaction and effects as in Class I alloys.

Class III

These are composed mainly of palladium and silver with indium, copper, tin and/or zinc constituting not more than 10%. As in Class II alloys, palladium is the most influential constituent in dictating the properties of the alloy, especially its color (white), density (very light-average 11 g/cm^3), strength, hardness, plasticity and nobility. Understandably, the greater the percentage of palladium is, the more will be its influence on the alloy.

Silver, as mentioned before, can make substitutional alloys with palladium but the greater the amount of silver is, the less will be the nobility of the alloy, the more the plasticity, and the less the strength. Copper, as mentioned before, is very influential in the solid state of the alloy as it will react with palladium in the same way it reacts with gold. Besides, it lowers the fusing temperature of the alloy and increases its resistance to tarnish and corrosion. Zinc is used for the same reasons as in the previous two alloys. Indium and tin can alloy with both silver and palladium. In small amounts they can substantially harden the alloy. Also, indium can be a scavenger during melting, as well as serve to increase resistance to tarnish and corrosion.

Class IV

These are not new to the profession as they are used extensively for partial dentures. However, their introduction for single tooth restorations is still very controversial. The basic nickel and chromium combination requires numerous additions to procure the final alloy. Nickel and chromium can alloy together forming a solid solution which is the base for these alloys. For practical casting procedures, the chromium content should not exceed 30%. Both metals impart the apparent nobility (which is actually passivity), strength, density (8 g/cm^3), plasticity (very little), hardness and color of the alloy.

Low percentages of molybdenum, tungsten and aluminum are added to increase the strength and hardness of the alloy, as all can precipitate intermetallic compounds with chromium and nickel. Berrylium can be added to lower the fusion temperature and improve castability, but its use is not advised, due to potential health hazards, especially for the technicians fabricating the castings. Gallium is the current substitute for berrylium.

Silicone and iron are used in some alloys to increase their strength. They occur in trace amounts, not exceeding 2%. Most of the component metals of these alloys are carbide formers. Although carbide in trace amounts (0.2-0.4%) is essential for the potential strengthening of the alloys, more than this minimal amount will create a very brittle, dentally unusable alloy. Carbon can make complex carbides with both nickel and chromium (MC, M_6C and $M_{23}C_6$) [M − metal (carbide former)]. Boron can also be added in trace amounts at grain boundaries, markedly reducing the solubility of carbon, and thereby stabilizing those carbides. Boron and silica are also used as deoxidizers and flowing agents to improve the castability of the alloy. So the properties of the final alloy are mostly dependent on the techniques used in fabricating them, as carbon is present in the alloy and surrounding atmosphere and can be incorporated in different ways forming carbides at any stage in the melting and casting of the alloy. Some alloying elements include niobium, which is helpful in open air melting of these alloys. Tin and some rare earth elements can control oxidation of the alloy during porcelain firing. Titanium and cobalt are added for strength.

Class V

The fabricated product of these materials is a complex ceramic monolithic structure formed of 70 to 90% (by weight) crystalline material, mostly magnesium aluminate spinel and alumina, with one predominant type of space lattice arrangement. This is not the way the material begins. The original components of the material are aluminum trioxide (Al_2O_2), which forms the maximum percentage of the mass, at least 50%, magnesium oxide (MgO), at least 15%. The ratio of aluminum trioxide (Al_2O_3) to magnesium oxide is 7 to 1. From 5 to 25% glass frit should be compounded to react with silica to form silicate glasses. All are in a fine particle form and are joined in a workable mass with a silicon polymer. To this mass some lubricant not exceeding 0.5% is added to improve the moldability. It is usually a stearate or a wax. The bonding between these ingredients is absolutely secondary. When the material in this form is heated to and above the glass transition temperature of the polymer binder (30-150°), it becomes plastic, deformable and moldable. It is at this stage that it is introduced into a gypsum mold in a place of a lost wax pattern in the desirable form. Cooling the material to room temperature (below the glass transition temperature of the silicone polymer binder) will retain the original rigidity of the material. The formed mass is then subjected to thermal treatment for a prolonged period of time (10 to 18 hours), where the alumina and magnesia react together to the full consumption of the magnesia forming the magnesium aluminate spinel ($MgAl_2O_4$). Because of the larger volume of the spinel (compared to the forming MgO and Al_2O_3), there will be substantial expansion.

The silicon polymer

Dicarus Transport

$$-O-Si-O-Si-,$$

with R groups attached above each Si,

which should have at least 60% of SiO group, will change to silicate (SiO_4) with its classical tetrahedron unit cells. Therefore

nickel chromium is very technique sensitive and using the torch with high carbon increase carbon in them so increase brittleness of the...

the first stage of heating should be done slowly and in an oxidizing atmosphere to eliminate the organic radicals. Because of the electron deficiencies of the corner oxygen ion in the tetrahedron the tetrahedra are able to join cations from the glass frit and Al_2O_3 in an ionic bonding, forming metal silicate glasses, which will be the continuous phase between the aluminate spinel and Al_2O_3 masses.

In other words, the thermal processing will change a composite material with at least four components, weakly physically attached to each other to a solid ceramic body containing crystalline material in an amount from 70% to 90% with the rest in the form of interstitial glasses. The crystalline material is about 70% aluminum trioxide and $MgAl_2O_4$ and the remainder is crystalline aluminum silicate. The bonding within this monolithic structure is a strong primary one. A lack of slips from this type of bonding will make the material extremely strong, rigid, hard, and brittle.

During thermal processing, the spinel and other crystals and glasses undergo allotropic changes and dimensional changes occur which are due to changes in the atomic packing, with shrinkage compensating for expansion and vice-versa. The end result is almost zero dimensional change. Consequently, there is no need to expand or shrink the investing gypsum or dies to compensate for the dimensional changes that can occur during the thermal processing of this material.

The preferred procedure schedule should be done in the following fashion. Bring from room temperature to 500° C at about 160° C per hour, and hold at 500° C for 16 hours (vaporization of silicone radicals and lubricants, silicate formation). Then bring from 500 to 600° C in one hour, and hold at 650° C for 8 hours (complete silicate formation). Then bring from 650° to 1350° C in about 420°/hour, during which the spinel is formed. Stop at 1350°.

B. Physical and mechanical properties

Comparison between the Dentally Applied Physical and
Mechanical Properties of the Five Classes of Materials for Cast Restorations

Types of Cast Materials	Density gm/cm³	Melting Range °F	Tensile Strength PSI	Yield Strength 0.2% PSI	Elongation	M.E. PSI	Hardness VHN	Rate of Tarnish and Corrosion
Class I	15-16	1800-2000	80,000	40,000	20-25%	10-12 million	150-170	almost 0%
Class II	11-12	2200	100,000	47,000	20%	12 million	200	2-3%
Class III	10-11	2250	140,000	65,000	15-18%	15 million	250	5-10%
Class IV	8	3500	160,000	80,000	3-11%	30 million	315	0%
Class V	2.7	3300	19,000	—	0%	60 million	350	0%

a. Density

As you can see in the accompanying table, Class I cast materials have the highest density and Class V is the lowest, Class IV is almost half that of Class I. The lower density necessitates more force in centrifugal casting to compensate for the lower weight/unit volume. However, lower density will allow more restorations per unit weight which can be economical to some extent.

b. Range of melting and firing temperatures

For metallic alloys, Class IV has the highest melting range and Class I the lowest. Practically speaking, Class I and, to some extent, Class II alloys can be cast using regular gas-air fuel, calcium sulfate dihydrate bonded investments, and low heat technique.

For Class IV and, to some extent Class III, we have to use phosphate and silicate bonded investments, acetylene-oxygen, gas oxygen, electric resistance or electric induction melting; and a high heat technique, if silicate is the bonding material for the investment used. Compared to Class I and II alloys, the casting environment for Class III and IV alloys must be much more controlled and devoid of any possible contamination that may adversely change the properties of the alloy (e.g., carbon, oxygen, etc.).

Cast ceramics have two fusing temperatures. The lower temperature is a thermoplastic temperature, required for casting. The higher temperature represents the fusing temperature after completion of the thermal processing. Open flame heating cannot be used for either thermoplasticity or thermal processing. The energy for melting and fusing should be either transmitted or induced heat.

c. Ultimate strength

The strength of these cast materials is more than sufficient for use in the oral environment. Very seldom will they fail mechanically, unless they have a defect in their structure. In regards to tensile and shear strength, metallic alloys are far superior to cast ceramics, but ceramics are stronger under compression. Failure in metallic alloys is in the form of ductile (plastic) failure. For cast ceramics the failure is brittle fracture. For all cast materials the failure is not a catostrophic one. Class IV alloys have almost double the tensile strength of Class I alloys, and Class II alloys are very close to Class I alloys, with Class III alloys in between.

d. Modulus of elasticity

This measures the rigidity of the alloy. It is very obvious that Class V cast materials are the most rigid. They are almost six times as rigid as Class I alloys. Rigidity is a factor in the abrasion resistance of the material.

e. Elongation and yield strength

These are measures of the deformability (burnishability) of the material and the forces needed to achieve that deformability, respectively. It is clear from the table that Class I alloys have the highest deformability under the least amount of forces. Class II alloys still have acceptable figures for conventional dental procedures. Class IV alloys have the lowest deformability and require maximum forces (80,000 PSI yield strength) to accomplish it, a situation that cannot be achieved at all or requires special equipment yet to be designed. Class III alloys, although having measurable elongation, need substantial forces to achieve it. Class V materials, after complete processing, have virtually zero elongation, with a yield strength that almost coincides with the breaking point (brittle fracture).

f. Hardness

It is obvious that Class V cast materials have the highest hardness. However, the hardness of all these materials is more than adequate for oral use, far exceeding that of tooth enamel. This, together with other factors, results in high abrasive resistance.

g. Tarnish and corrosion

Cast ceramics, due to the type of chemical bonding in the final material, are absolutely chemically inert in the oral environment. The resistance of Class I and IV materials to tarnish and corrosion is superior to Class II and III: Class I because of its nobility, Class IV because of its passivity.

Class III alloys are the least resistant to tarnish and corrosion. The greater their silver content is, the higher the corrosion rate will be, especially in a sulfurous environment. Class II alloys are more resistant to corrosion than Class III alloys. However, if their gold content is very low (less than 10%), restorations fabricated from these alloys may demonstrate some surface and marginal deterioration. Therefore, Class II and especially Class III alloys should not be used in patients with high sulfur diets or in areas of the mouth where stagnation of plaque and food substrates for long periods may occur. In Class II and III, the alloy with the highest palladium content should be chosen for questionable cases.

h. Castability-moldability

Palladium has a high affinity for hydrogen gases at the melting stage. Silver has a similar affinity for oxygen. If either or both gases are incorporated during melting, they can be released during solidification, producing proosities and surface roughness. Class III and IV alloys can produce castings with very rough surfaces, mainly due to the types of investment used for these alloys. As mentioned before, nickel-chromium based alloys are very sensitive to the environment of casting. It is advisable to use closed furnaces and electric conduction melting with Class II, III, and IV alloys to obtain the same surface and maximum density as produced by Class I alloys. Because of their density and low fusing temperature, Class I alloys can overcome the gas pressure within the investment mold, forcing their way to reproduce all details of that mold. This condition is not readily achieved with the rest of the metallic alloys, especially Class IV alloys, because of their lower density, higher melting temperature, and the low fluidity of their melt. All four classes of metallic alloys shrink on solidification, necessitating compensating expansion within the investment.

Reproduction of fine details is difficult to attain in Class III and IV alloys, as compared to Class I. The investments used with these alloys do not help in overcoming these problems, but rather complicate the problem even more. With the exception of berylium-containing alloys, Class IV alloys reproduce the least details, necessitating modifications in cavity and tooth preparations, especially in the marginal anatomy of these preparations. The reproduction of the wax pattern into the final restoration is done in two processes (stages) for cast ceramics, with one of the processes done on the original die (compared to only one process, in most cases, for Class I through IV, which is also done off the original die). Because of the comparatively high density of the thermoplastic mass, it can wet all the details of the mold and reproduce the wax pattern without any shrinkage. Therefore, there is no requirement for expansion of the investment for cast ceramics.

i. Finishing and polishing

Understandably, Class IV alloys require high speed equipment, more abrasive tools, and much more time to attain biologic surfaces as compared with the first three classes of metallic alloys, which can be finished and polished with the same armamentarium. Class III alloys will require more time and effort than Class I or II. Cast ceramics can be initially finished after retrieval from the investment prior to thermal processing. During and after thermal processing they can be glazed creating an extremely biologic surface.

j. Soldering

Soldering of Class I alloys and most Class II alloys, using one of the different types of gold solders, is a predictable and easy process with few failures. Soldering Class III alloys can be done using silver solders, with fairly predictable results. However, this requires the use of the correct zone of the flame (the reducing zone), a solder with the appropriate melting temperature (150° C lower than the melting temperature of the mother alloy), and the proper timing and atmosphere for soldering. For Class IV alloys, soldering requires a consistently inert environment (oven soldering), and a specific solder for each alloy. However, there is a persistent risk of both solder failure and, infrequently, change in the composition of the adjacent mother alloy.

There, currently, is no solder available for cast ceramics. Multiple attached units (e.g., a fixed bridge or splint) must be cast in one piece. Adding to the contact or contour is achieved by baking on aluminous porcelain.

IV. Mouth Preparation Prior to Cast Restorations

For a single tooth a cast restoration should be the ultimate and final restoration. Every precaution should be taken to insure the longevity of such a restoration. Following are some of the measures to be taken before preparing a tooth to receive a cast restoration.

A. Control of plaque

Due to the vulnerability of the cast/cement/tooth structure junction, patients to receive a cast restoration should exhibit the ability, willingness and practice of control measures for their plaque. As a rule, patients should show a 10% or less plaque index prior to fabricating cast restorations for their teeth, or the result will be a futile restorative attempt.

B. Control of caries

Understandably, before planning a cast restoration, which may be more durable from the physical and mechanical aspects, but not so from the cariogenic aspect, rampant or uncontrolled carious processes should be halted. Indirect pulp capping and/or amalgam-composite resin restorative procedures should be employed until the patient demonstrates the ability to control plaque, and, subsequently, demonstrates little or no incidence of decay recurrence.

C. Control of periodontal problems

Although cast restorations can be one of the mechanotherapies for the periodontium affected by periodontal diseases, the very nature of the clinical procedures involved in cast restorations as well as some of the final properties of the restorations themselves may be detrimental to an already pathologically affected periodontium. It is ideal to start cast restoration fabrication with a sound periodontium, unless, of course, these restorations are part of the periodontal therapy and maintenance. In the latter case, the peridontal disease should be under control. The pockets should be eradicated, bone resorption arrested, defects corrected, exposed roots and crown surfaces free from deposits, gingival tissues healed, and apparent clinical crown dimensions stable.

D. Proper foundation

As discussed in the chapter on restoration of badly broken down teeth, some teeth will need a substructure or a foundation before preparing them for a cast restoration. The need for such a foundation should be diagnosed and proper material and techniques should be employed before preparing the tooth for a cast restoration. Nothing is more frustrating than attempting to build up a tooth in a foundation form *after* unsuccessfully attempting to prepare the tooth for a cast restoration.

E. Control of the pulpal condition of the tooth

Cast restorations are used for teeth with extensive defects, teeth that usually have been previously restored one or more times with amalgam or other materials. The pulp-dentin/root-canal complex of these teeth has been subjected to numerous traumas which invariably affects their physiology. In many instances, these teeth, after being subjected to the additional trauma of cast restoration procedures, will undergo irreversible pathologic changes necessitating endodontic therapy. Therefore a proper preoperative evaluation of the condition of the pulp-dentin/root-canal system is essential. If irreversible pathologic pulpal changes are present, endodontic therapy should be part of the mouth preparation prior to the cast fabrication.

F. Occlusal equilibration

As cast restorations will maintain the tooth shape and dimensions, any premature occluding contacts built into the res-

toration will create greater and longer standing disturbances in the stomato-gnathic system than if the condition were to remain in natural dentition. That is why, prior to preparing teeth for cast restorations, it is vitally important to equilibrate the natural dentition. There must be no interfering or premature contacts, and there should be a pattern of a reliable protective mechanism for mandibular disclusion.

G. Diagnostic wax-ups and temporary restorations

Occasionally, cast restorations are part of the overall therapy to create a physiologically functioning stomato-gnathic system. This may involve certain changes in the anatomy of occluding surfaces, increasing the vertical dimension, or changing the axial contour of the tooth. In these cases one or both of the following procedures should be performed.

Full arch study models should be made, and properly mounted on a semi- or fully-adjustable articulator. The involved teeth should be reduced and diagnostic wax-ups made in the desired occlusal shape and relationship. Duplicate stone models are then fabricated to serve as an aid in the construction of both temporary and final restorations.

The teeth are roughly prepared and restored with temporary restorations that create the desired features that will be incorporated in the final cast restorations. These temporary restorations are usually made of reinforced resinous materials. Patients should wear these temporaries and be examined periodically. Changes can then be made in the temporaries to achieve the utmost compatibility between the stomato-gnathic system and these restorations. When this is achieved and verified, the teeth are finally prepared, and cast restorations are fabricated as replicas of the temporaries, which proved to be physiologic and therapeutic to the stomato-gnathic system.

Because of the permanency of cast restorations, it is mandatory to plan the restorative treatment for the entire mouth prior to fabrication of cast restorations. Treatment may include full dentures, partial dentures, fixed bridges, etc. So it is necessary to know in advance the location of the contemplated cast restoration, so that modifications may be made in the tooth preparation, restoration dimension and shape, etc., to satisfy the required role of the cast restoration in the restorative treatment for the entire stomato-gnathic system.

V. Principles of Cavity–Tooth Preparation for Cast Restorations

Unlike amalgam, cast alloys and ceramics can restore teeth via intra- and extracoronal preparations. Intracoronal preparations are mortise-shaped, having definite walls and floors joined at line and point angles. Extracoronal preparations are created by occlusal and axial surface reduction, in many cases ending gingivally with no definite flat floor. Most single-tooth restorations are combinations of these intra- and extracoronal types.

The general principles of cavity–tooth preparation may be applied without deviation to cast alloy and ceramic use. In preparations for a cast restoration there is greater surface extension in the outline form than in the case of amalgam. This facilitates support for the tooth and efficient marginal manipulation. Also, there is more extensive surface involvement for cast restorations compared to amalgam to compensate for the cariogenically weak joints of the cast/cement/tooth structure complex. This is done by placing these joints in areas of maximum self-cleansability and/or protection.

Besides applying all the general principles of cavity and tooth preparations, cast restoration preparations should have the following features.

A. Preparation path

The preparation will have a single insertion path, opposite to the direction of the occlusal loading (Fig. 1). All reductions in tooth structure, whether intra- or extra-coronal, should be oriented towards one path, the path of withdrawal and insertion of the future wax pattern and restoration. This path is usually parallel to the long axis of the tooth crown. Adhering to this feature will help the restoration's retention and decrease its micromovements during function. This path should be (as practically as possible) opposite to the direction of occlusal loading, so that function will seat restoration rather than displace it.

B. Apico-occlusal taper of a preparation

Understandably, preparations for cast restorations cannot be prepared in an inverted cone shape or with any undercuts. Several materials are going to be inserted and withdrawn from the preparation. Some of these materials are not elastic, and even elastic materials can be permanently deformed if subjected to such acts, leading to an impractical technique and/or misfitting restorations. Therefore, for maximum retention in a cast restoration, opposing walls and opposing axial surfaces of a tooth preparation should be perfectly parallel to each other. Since exact parallelism can create technical problems in processing and in getting final materials into and out of the preparation, a slight divergence of opposing walls intracoronally (Fig. 1A) and a slight convergence of opposing axial surfaces extracoronally (Fig. 1B) are essential to facilitate cast fabrication with minimum errors.

This taper should be on an average of 2-5° from the path of the preparation. It can be decreased or increased according to the following factors:

1. Length of the preparation wall and/or axial surfaces

The greater the wall length is, the more taper will be necessary, although it should not exceed 10°. The less the wall length is, the less the taper will be, approaching 0° (parallelism), but it should not be less in extremely short walls.

2. Dimensions and details of surface involvement and internal anatomy in the preparation

The greater that the surface involvement is and the more detailed that the internal anatomy is, the greater will be the frictional component between the preparation and the materials contacting it (e.g., impression materials). The energy of this friction could produce distortion in any of the materials used in cast fabrication. To diminish friction, the taper is increased, but not to exceed 10°.

3. The need for retention

The greater that the need for retention is, the more will be the need to approach exact parallelism, i.e., less taper. For example, preparations for non-noble alloys or cast ceramics require greater occlusal reduction and rounded internal and external anatomy. To compensate for this loss of retention, these preparations must be less tapered, approaching parallelism.

It is most favorable for the taper to be done equally at the expense of two opposing walls or axial surfaces to completely insure one path for the preparation (Fig. 2A). However, tapering can be done solely at the expense of one side only, if the opposing side is absolutely parallel to the insertion path (Fig. 2B). Under no circumstances, however, the preparation should be made with one side having more taper than the other (Fig. 2C), as this makes it possible for the preparation to have more than one insertion path, resulting in micromovements of the final restoration. If cariogenic and anatomical conditions dictate two different tapers for opposing walls, it is preferable to create two planes for each involved wall or axial surface; i.e., inner planes parallel to each other (or at least of equal taper) and outer planes, satisfying the needs compelling the different tapers. The inner plane will assure the single insertion path of the preparation (Fig. 2D).

The decision to choose between these three acceptable design features depends on cariogenic and anatomical considerations, different lengths of opposing parts of the preparation (the longer side should have its outer planes tapered more), the need for reciprocal retention (the side to accommodate this retention should be parallel to the insertion path) and the presence of

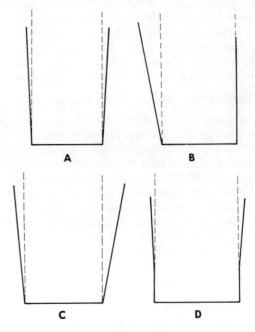

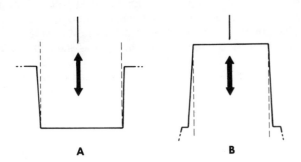

Fig. 17-1

Fig. 17-2

more surrounding walls (axial surfaces) on one side than the other (the side having more surrounding walls and axial surfaces should have its outer component tapered more).

C. Preparation features of the circumferential tie

As discussed before, the weakest link in any cast restoration is the tooth/cement/cast joint complex. Special attention should be paid to the marginal peripheries of the preparation, and every effort should be made to design and prepare these marginal peripheries to create the most favorable relationship with the restoring casting and luting cement. This peripheral marginal anatomy of the preparation is called "circumferential tie", and it should have the following features. If the margin ends on enamel, enamel walls should fulfill all requirements advocated by Noy for an ideal cavity wall, namely: enamel must be supported by sound dentin; enamel rods forming the cavosurface margin should be continuous with sound dentin; enamel rods forming the cavosurface margin should be covered with the restorative material; and angular cavosurface angles should be trimmed. Cast restorations are the only restorations that can fulfill these requirements, for the simple reason that they are stronger than tooth structure.

For the occlusal and gingival walls in intracoronal cavity preparations the tooth circumferential tie will be in the form of a bevel, which is a plane of a cavity wall or floor directed away from the cavity preparation.

Types and Design Features of Occlusal and Gingival Bevels

According to their shapes and types of tissue involvement there are six types of bevels:

a. Partial bevel (Fig. 3A)

This involves part of the enamel wall, not exceeding two-thirds of its dimension. This is usually not used in cast res-

torations, except to trim weak enamel rods from margin peripheries.

b. Short bevel (Fig. 3B) *enamel bevel*

This includes the entire enamel wall, but not dentin. This bevel is used mostly with Class I alloys specially for type 1 and 2.

c. Long bevel (Fig. 3C)

This includes all of the enamel wall and up to one-half of the dentinal wall. This is the most frequently used bevel for the first three classes of cast materials. Its major advantage is that it preserves the internal "boxed-up" resistance and retention features of the preparation.

d. Full bevel (Fig. 3D)

This includes all of the dentinal and enamel walls of the cavity wall or floor. Although it is well reproduced by all four classes of cast alloys, it deprives the preparation of its internal resistance and retention. Its use should be avoided except in cases where it is impossible to use any other form of bevel.

e. Counterbevel (Fig. 3E)

When capping cusps to protect and support them, this type of bevel is used, opposite to an axial cavity wall, on the facial or lingual surface of the tooth, and it will have a gingival inclination facially or lingually.

f. Hollow ground (concave) bevel (Fig. 3F)

All of the aforementioned types of bevels are in the form of a flat plane, but any of them, especially the last three, can be prepared in a concave form. This allows more space for cast material bulk, a design feature needed in special preparations to improve material's castability retention and better resistance to stresses. These bevels are ideal for Class IV and V cast materials.

The bevel portion of the circumferential tie must have a specific angulation relative to the remaining portion of the wall (floor), the long axis of the crown, or a specific landmark. Also, they should extend to certain limits. Both bevel angulation and extent are dictated by a myriad of factors that will be discussed and described with the different designs of preparations for cast restorations.

Function of Occlusal and Gingival Bevels

Besides satisfying the requirements of Noy for ideal cavity walls, bevels create obtuse-angled marginal tooth structure, which is the bulkiest and the strongest configuration of any marginal tooth anatomy, and produce an acute-angled marginal cast alloy substance which, in this configuration, will be the most amenable to burnishing for that alloy. This makes it possible to decrease or eliminate the cement line by bringing the cast alloy closer to tooth structure (Fig. 4).

Marginal bevels reduce the error factors (space between cast and tooth substances) three or more fold at the margins, as compared to their internal dimensions, depending on the bevel's angulation (Fig. 5). Bevels, being part of the circumferential tie, are one of the major retention forms for a cast restoration, as it is only at the circumferential tie that there is the

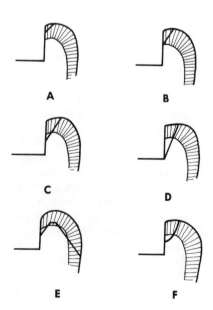

Fig. 17-3

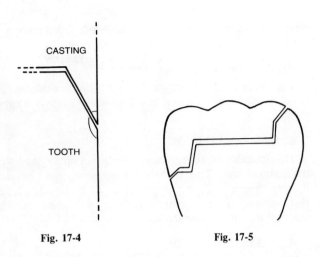

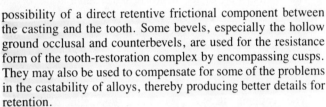

Fig. 17-4   **Fig. 17-5**

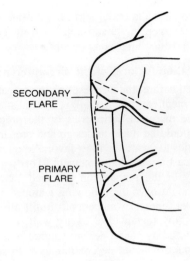

Fig. 17-6

possibility of a direct retentive frictional component between the casting and the tooth. Some bevels, especially the hollow ground occlusal and counterbevels, are used for the resistance form of the tooth-restoration complex by encompassing cusps. They may also be used to compensate for some of the problems in the castability of alloys, thereby producing better details for retention.

Bevels are the "flexible extensions" of a cavity preparation, allowing the inclusion of surface defects, supplementary grooves, or other areas on the tooth surface. Bevels require minimum tooth involvement, and do not sacrifice the resistance and retention for the restoration. Gingival bevels, for example, can bring the gingival margins to cleansable or protected areas.

For the facial and lingual proximal walls in intracoronal cavity preparations for castings, flares are used, which are the flat or concave peripheral portions of the facial and lingual walls.

Types and Design Features of Facial and Lingual Flares

There are two types of flares.

a. The primary flare (Fig. 6) is the conventional and basic part of the circumferential tie facially and lingually for an intracoronal preparation. It is very similar to a long bevel formed of enamel and part of the dentin on the facial or lingual wall. Primary flares always have a specific angulation, i.e., 45° to the inner dentinal wall proper. They may be hollow ground if they are part of the circumferential tie and the preparation is for a non-noble alloy or cast ceramics.

Functions and indications for primary flares

These design features perform the same functions as bevels. In addition, they can bring the facial and lingual margins of the cavity preparation to cleansable-finishable areas. They are indicated for any facial or lingual proximal wall of an intracoronal cavity preparation. If they fulfill the objectives of a preparation circumferential tie they will be the most peripheral part of the proximal preparation; if not, a secondary flare must be placed peripheral to them.

b. The secondary flare (Fig. 6) is almost always a flat plane superimposed peripherally to a primary flare. Sometimes it is prepared in a hollow ground form to accommodate materials with low castability. Usually it is prepared solely in enamel, but sometimes it may contain some dentin in all or parts of its surfaces. Unlike primary flares, secondary flares may have different angulations, involvement and extent, depending on their function.

Functions and indications of secondary flares

In addition to performing the functions mentioned for bevels, secondary flares have other specific indications. In very widely extended lesions bucco-lingually, the buccal and lingual tooth structure will be badly thinned; the primary flare will end with acute-angled marginal tooth structure, occasionally with unsupported enamel. A secondary superimposed flare (Fig. 7A) at the correct angulation can create the needed obtuse angulation of the marginal tooth structure. This is done without any sacrifice in the preparation resistance and retention, because the wall proper and primary flare are maintained at their proper locations and angulations.

In very broad contact areas or malposed contact areas, the primary flare will not bring the facial and/or lingual margins to finishable-cleansable areas. However, a secondary flare placed peripheral to that primary flare (Fig. 7B) will accomplish this without changing the fixed 45° angulation of the primary flare necessary for resistance and retention.

In ovoid teeth peripheral marginal undercuts are especially apt to be present occluso-apically on the facial and/or lingual peripheries of the cavity preparation (Fig. 7C). A cast restoration fabricated in an indirect technique for this preparation will definitely end with marginal failure (misfit). Elimination of these undercuts via wall proper or primary flare extension will unnecessarily involve and weaken tooth structure. However, a secondary flare superimposed on a primary flare in the correct angulation and extent can eliminate these undercuts with minimal sacrifice of tooth structure (Fig. 7, C and D). Surface defects or decalcifications, etc., facial or lingual to the primary flare's facial or lingual margin respectively, can be involved in the preparation with a secondary flare without the need to extend or angulate the primary flare more than indicated.

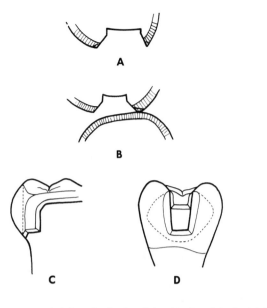

--------- extent of secondary flare to eradicate peripheral marginal undercuts in C.

Fig. 17-7

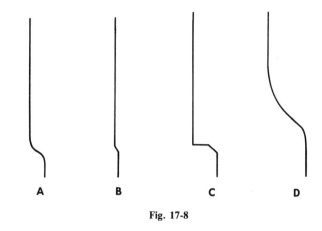

Fig. 17-8

Circumferential Tie Constituents for Extracoronal Preparations

For extracoronal preparations, the circumferential tie constituents will be in one of the following forms:

a. The chamfer finishing line (Fig. 8A) is the most universally used design for Class I, II, and III cast materials. It assures bulk and definite termination for the preparation marginally, with little tooth involvement (0.5 mm maximal depth). Its only disadvantages are the limited burnishability of the marginal cast alloy and the liability of transitional continuation of a circumferential tie and adjacent bevel ties. Chamfers can be placed gingivally on any involved axial surface provided the area is finishable-cleansable or protected. It is the most practical type of finishing line for subgingival extracoronal preparations if anatomical considerations preclude gingival floor preparations. It is contraindicated, however, for Class IV and V cast materials due to their poor castability.

b. The knife edge (feather edge) finishing line (Fig. 8B) is the circumferential tie constituent with the least tooth structure involvement. If the margin is on enamel, it involves part of the enamel only. It should only be used to accommodate a very castable-burnishable type of alloy (gold alloys, preferably type II). Also, it should be located on accessible areas of the tooth surface for proper finishing. It is most indicated when minimal axial depth is required for biologic or anatomic purposes. It blends easily and efficiently with bevelled constituents of the tooth circumferential tie. One of its disadvantages is the possibility of indefinite termination for the casting (technical difficulty). There is a chance of the margin not being covered with a casting made of certain alloys due to lack of bulk space to accommodate the less wetting alloys. There is also the possibility of fracturing the alloy part of the circumferential tie during burnishing-finishing-polishing, because of its very thin cross-section and the ease of over-strain-hardening it at that

dimension. It is definitely contraindicated for Class III, IV, and V cast materials.

c. The bevelled shoulder finishing line (Fig. 8C) is the circumferential tie constituent with the most tooth structure involvement. It is exactly like a gingival floor of an intracoronal preparation, but on a smaller scale. It is indicated when a definite gingival floor, with all its components (wall proper and bevel), is needed for resistance-retention purposes. Also, it is indicated when maximum bulk of the cast is needed marginally for materials that are limited in their castability and/or are difficult or impossible to burnish. It blends very easily with bevelled constitutents of the circumferential tie. Of all the finishing lines for extracoronal preparation it is the one that maximally reduces marginal problems of internal spacing. It is the ideal design for subgingivally located margins, because of the maximum predictability of the casting termination gingivally. The bevel portion extent and angulation are governed by the same factors governing gingival bevels in intracoronal preparations. It can be used for any class of cast materials. Its bevel portion could be hollow ground as this configuration is most suitable for Class IV and V cast materials.

d. The hollow ground (concave) bevel (Fig. 8D) is actually an exaggerated chamfer or a concave bevelled shoulder. Its tooth involvement is greater than a chamfer and less than a bevelled shoulder. Its termination is not as predictable as a bevelled shoulder, but it is mechanically comparable to a bevelled shoulder and superior to a chamfer. Care must be taken to insure there is no residual frail enamel or thinned tooth structure at the periphery of this finishing design. There is good transitional continuity with the bevelled portion of the circumferential tie when using this design as part of the tie. This bevel helps the casting to seat preferentially, aids in stabilizing the casting, and is the ideal finishing line for Class IV and V cast materials. It can be used successfully for materials with limited castability.

Circumferential tie constituents for extracoronal tooth preparation perform the same functions as efficiently as bevels and, to some extent, gingival floors in an intracoronal cavity preparation, with the exception of minimizing symptoms of internal spacing marginally. This is especially true with chamfer and hollow ground bevels. Different combinations of the aforementioned finishing lines could be used to satisfy both the anatomic and cariogenic needs of the same tooth as well as the castability and finishability of the restorative material. The junctions between the different parts of the circumferential tie, which usually occur at the gingival and occlusal corners, should be prepared without sharp angles or interruptions, thereby avoiding stress concentration, noncoverage of the margin by the casting, or possible minor undercuts. The best way to achieve this continuity is to round these junctions, but only at the level of the circumferential tie, i.e., not internally.

The tooth circumferential tie should have its maximal depth at its junction with the component of the preparation proper (wall, floor, or axial surface) to assure complete reproduction and coverage of its details in the casting and to best resist stresses at that location. No element of the circumferential tie should be in occlusal contact during either centric or excursive movements. The peripheral margin of the circumferential tie should be as linear as possible, paralleling the periphery or curvature of the anatomy of the tooth, thereby insuring accurate waxing and casting margination.

Of all the constituents of the preparation, the circumferential tie portion should be the smoothest. Maximum time and effort should be spent to guarantee this smoothness and continuity between its parts, so that impression materials, die materials, waxes, investments, and alloy and ceramic melts can wet its details to the maximum of their ability for precise reproduction.

D. Mechanical problems for cast restorations and preparation design solutions in general

Cast restorations are usually used for compound and complex tooth involvement. The possible loading and displacing forces, their fulcra and their effects on restorations together with their effect on remaining tooth structure, have been fully described in the discussions of the different cavity preparations for amalgam and in the general principles of preparation design. The formability of casting materials enables us to use myriad retention and resistance means that are impossible to use with any other materials.

In addition to the principal retention forms previously described (parallelism, dovetails, surface area frictional retention, circumferential tie, and masticatory loads directed to seat the restoration), there are numerous auxillary means of retention for cast restorations:

a. Luting cements

Their action is primarily mechanical, locking the cast to tooth structure by filling the space between them, wetting the details of both the casting and tooth preparation and filling in these vacancies or irregularities. Cements remain in one solid mass, immobilizing the cast to the tooth. Some cements can create a physico-chemical bonding with parts of the tooth substance. Others can do the same thing with some tooth components and a treated tooth surface of the casting. Some can etch enamel to allow the enamel surface to be wetted with the cement. These ways can work together to retain the casting in or on the tooth. However, all of them are still considered auxillary means since none of them can substitute for frictional retention. All cements are susceptible to dissolution by oral fluids. In addition, they are far weaker than the casting or the tooth structure.

Cements should only fill the space between the casting and the tooth substance, thereby furthering the principal frictional means of retention. The less the thickness of the luting cement, the less the possibility of a clinically recognizable failure at the tooth-cement-casting interface.

b. Grooves (Fig. 9)

All types of grooves should be located completely in dentin. They can be internal in an intracoronal preparation (Fig. 9A), cut at the expense of the dentinal portion of the facial or lingual walls or the gingival floors proximally. They may also be located at the mesial and distal wall or the gingival floors of the facial or lingual portion of a cavity preparation. In any case, internal grooves should be located as internally as possible, adjacent to the axial wall. In addition to providing auxillary retention, grooves help prevent lateral displacement of the mesial, distal, facial and/or lingual parts of a restoration. Grooves can be stepped to preserve certain anatomical landmarks and to increase the locking capabilities of the preparation. Generally, internal grooves are indicated when the dimensions of the walls are fairly limited and a locking mechanism for the restoration is needed proximally (facially and lingually) in addition to an occlusal dovetail. Internal grooves are contraindicated if there is any danger of impinging on the pulp chamber or root canal system, undermining or involving an axial angle of the tooth or undermining adjacent enamel.

Grooves also can be externally located in extracoronal preparations (Fig. 9B), being indicated for preparations lacking retention (due to shortness, severe taper or extreme width). In this case they are placed anywhere where there is sufficient dentin bulk to accommodate them without impinging on the pulp chamber, root canal system, or other important anatomy. External grooves can be placed at the very periphery of a surface extension to prevent its displacement and to guide it to its location. External grooves may be cut in a stepped form, inwards or outwards (according to the preparation's configuration). Such a design feature will increase locking tremendously. Grooves also can be used as a reciprocal means of retention. They improve the seating of a restoration, and minimize marginal discrepancies. Grooves are prepared using a standardized size tapered fissure bur (168 or 699). They should not exceed 2 mm in depth and should be at the expense of the

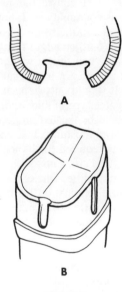

Fig. 17-9

side walls or axial surfaces of the preparation. A groove may be accentuated, using a Wedelstaedt or a hatchet to define its walls and intervening angles, thereby improving its locking capabilities. Grooves, both internal and external, can be used with all types of cast materials. When used with cast ceramics, they should not have definite internal line angles.

c. Reverse bevel (Fig. 10)

This is placed at the expense of the gingival floor, creating an internal dentinal plane inclining gingivally-axially, locking the restoration and preventing proximal displacement. It always has a flat dentinal transition between it and the proximal gingival bevel. It can only be used when the gingival floor has sufficient dimension to accommodate it without decreasing the resistance form of the restoration (flat portion of gingival floor). Ideally, reverse bevels are prepared using gingival margin trimmers. This bevel is indicated for use with Class I, II, and III cast materials, and infrequently with Class IV. It is not used with cast ceramics.

d. Internal box (Fig. 11)

This is one of the most efficient immobilizing retention resistance means. It is prepared in dentin with four vertical surrounding walls joining a floor at definite line and point angles. It can impart four to twelve times the retention of an external box of the same dimensions. It can be located next to a marginal ridge, with the intact proximal wall as one of its walls and at any location in a floor of a cavity preparation where dentin bulk will allow.

Because of its high locking power, it is always advisable to place internal boxes at the very peripheries of a cavity preparation. If placed at the middle of the cavity preparation, there will be uneven immobilization of the casting, with the ends less retained than the middle part. This situation can lead to possible micromovement of the restoration. Similarly, internal boxes must be reciprocated at the opposite ends of a preparation by an equally retaining mode, or the restoration will be extremely micromobile at that opposite end. Internal boxes are indicated for shallow cavities or short tooth preparations, when an occlusal dovetail cannot be prepared because of cavity involvement of the occlusal surface or restricted anatomy. An internal box should have a minimum size of 2 mm in three dimensions, but should not have equal length, width, and depth. It can be stepped apically or occlusally, having different levels in its pulpal floor to improve retention and avoid pulpal anatomy. Internal boxes are initially prepared using a 168 or 699 bur to a dimension compatible with the size of the restoration. The surrounding walls and floors are then shaved to

be parallel and to have definite angles using a small hatchet, a monangle chisel, and an angle former. Internal boxes are contraindicated for Class IV and V cast materials, but can be used for the others.

e. External boxes (Fig. 12)

These are box-shaped preparations opening to the axial tooth surface with three, four, or five surrounding walls and floors. They can be proximal, facial or lingual. They can be stepped (Fig. 12A), occlusally or gingivally, or not stepped (Fig. 12B). Understandably, the stepped boxes will be more retentive than the non-stepped ones, as they contain an axial wall providing more surface area and locking. These boxes can accommodate grooves in one or more of their surrounding walls. Their peripheral portion should be flared (primarily or secondarily) or bevelled (gingivally only).

External boxes are prepared with the same instruments used to prepare proximal intracoronal cavity preparation, i.e., a tapered fissure bur, then a hatchet or chisel to create the proper angulation and interrelationship of their details. In this form, they are contraindicated for cast ceramics, but can be used with other cast materials.

d. Slot (Fig. 13)

This is an internal cavity within a floor of the preparation having a continuous surrounding wall (non-defined angles) and floor. The junction between the floor and the surrounding walls is very rounded. Although it is less locking than an internal box, it is more readily reproduced in a casting. It has the same indications as an internal box, especially for replacing an occlusal dovetail, when anatomical or caries considerations prevent creation of an adequate dovetail. Slots are prepared using a suitable size round bur followed by a tapered fissure bur. They should have a 2-3 mm depth and their dimension should be compatible with the size of the restorations they help retain. They are indicated for all five classes of cast materials.

g. Pins

Pins can be cemented and threaded, parallel and non-parallel, vertical and horizontal, cast and wrought. All these different types of pins and their use will be described in the discussion of pin-lay designs of a tooth preparation for cast restorations.

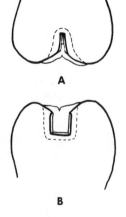

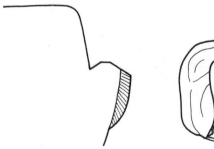 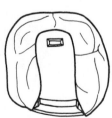 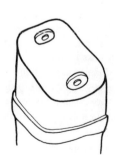

Fig. 17-10 **Fig. 17-11** **Fig. 17-12** **Fig. 17-13**

h. Collar

This is a surface extension completely surrounding a cusp or a surface of a tooth. It will be described in the designs for surface extension cast restorations.

i. Skirts

This is a specific extension involving a part of the axial angle of a tooth. It, too, will be described in the discussion of surface extension designs for cast restorations.

j. Capping of cusps

The method of encompassing a cusp with a casting for resistance and/or retention is very efficient, provided the cusps are not shortened to the extent they will not be effective in locking the restoration. The embracing mechanism may be a combination of hollow-ground bevel-hollow ground bevel or hollow ground bevel-collar. These will be described in detail in the discussion of onlay restorations.

k. Capping of the marginal ridge (Fig. 14)

If a marginal ridge is intact, the adjacent proximal surface sound, and the occlusal embrasure very pronounced, that marginal ridge may be capped, creating a finishing line that is still finishable and cleansable. If there is no adjacent tooth (e.g., the distal marginal ridges of a terminal tooth in the arch), the marginal ridge can be capped by the cast restoration for added retention and resistance. Capping a marginal ridge will be very similar to capping a cusp, but on a lesser scale.

Collars, skirts and caps can be used for all five classes of cast materials, but each material requires specific anatomy in the tooth preparation. These will be discussed in the chapter on preparation.

l. Posts

For reasons mentioned in the chapter on restoration of badly broken down teeth, posts should not be used as a retention means for a final cast restoration. They can be used very efficiently as retaining modes for a cast core foundation (substructure) to be covered with a cast restoration.

m. Grossly roughening, irregularizing or multiple levelling the surface of the preparation (Figs. 15 and 16)

At specific areas of the tooth preparation, especially the pulpal floor or occlusal surface, this irregularity may be in the form of preserving present irregularities (Fig. 16) or creating intentional irregularities (Fig. 15). This is done when the preparation needs to be more retentive and laterally locking. The irregularity or roughness should be of adequate dimension, leaving bulky tooth structure between them to be self-resistant, especially under shear loading. Irregularities should have no undercuts, be fairly smooth surfaced, and have no frail or undermined enamel. Creating different levels out of flat, dished up, (Fig. 15A) or sloped (Fig. 15B) gingival, or, pulpal floors could change a mechanically negative situation to a positive one. Fissure burs followed by chisels are very effective in refining and/or establishing these features. They are indicated for all cast materials.

n. Reciprocal retention

In a cavity or tooth preparation to accommodate a cemented type of restoration, every retention mode must have an opposite retention mode to completely immobilize the restoration. If one end of the restoration is locked and the opposite one is not, movement of the loose end will induce substantial stresses in the locked side, involving both the restoration and the tooth, especially at their interface where the movement will be ex-

aggerated. Placing retention modes at every end of the preparation or parts of the preparation is called reciprocal retention, a basic principle in designing preparations for cast restoration. They can be any form, e.g., opposite grooves or internal box to oppose an internal box, a dovetail to oppose a proximal external box, etc.

o. Capping the occluso-proximo-facial or lingual corners of a preparation (Fig. 17)

This is done for the dual purpose of protecting thinned corners, due to overpreparation or wide preparation in an ovoid tooth, and adding to the restoration retention by locking it. Over a facial and/or lingual corner, a bevel extension facially or lingually at these corners is added to the preparation ending in a knife edge or chamfer finishing line. They are easily

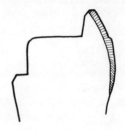

Fig. 17-14

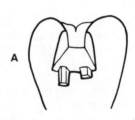 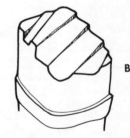

Fig. 17-15. A, Different levelled gingival floor. **B,** different levelled pulpal floor. Both add to retention.

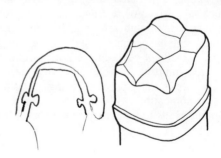

Fig. 17-16

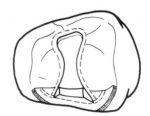

Fig. 17-17

prepared using a filamentous diamond stone. This procedure is not indicated for Class IV and V materials.

p. Precementation grooving of the casting and the adjacent tooth surface or walls (see class V preparations)

To add to the retaining capability of the luting agent, after the casting is ready for cementation, an inverted truncated cone groove is cut on one or more of the sides of the casting, and opposite it on the preparation, a similar groove is cut. If they are not opposite one another, the retaining effect will be minimized. Both should be of sufficient dimension to accommodate a bulky amount of the cementing agent. Several of these grooves can be prepared, provided they do not arrive to the casting or preparation margins. A sufficient amount of cement should be mixed and flown into the grooves when cementing the casting. It has been proven that this technique will enhance the retaining effect of the cement several fold, and it is most effective for Class V cavity preparations where there is very little frictional retention form in the surrounding walls.

q. Electrolytic etching of tooth surface of the casting

The internal (tooth) surface of a Class IV cast material restoration can be subjected to electrolytic etching. The margins and external surface of the restoration are covered with sticky wax, and the restoration is used as an anodic electrode in an electrolytic cell composed of 0.5 N nitric acid and a cathode of another non-noble alloy higher in the electromotive force table (e.g., 316 stainless steel).

A low voltage current is passed into the cell, leading to selective etching of the non-noble alloy, via dissolution of grain boundaries and the less noble elements. This leaves microscopic irregularities, many of which are undercuts, very similar to those irregularities produced in an enamel surface by phosphoric acid application. The etching process will take 10-15 minutes, to create suitable dimensions of the irregularities. A cementing agent capable of wetting these irregularities and similar irregularities on the tooth surface can increase the retention of the cast restoration several fold. In certain selective situations this type of retention can be used as a principal mean of retention if the microscopic retaining irregularities on the alloy are reciprocated with similar ones on the tooth. This requires a tooth preparation that is confined to enamel. There are several techniques that use this phenomenon as a sole retaining device for fixed prosthesis and cast restorations. Although these techniques differ in their clinical application, they share the following principles:

1. The luting-bonding agent is always a composite resin.

2. The tooth should have adequate enamel thickness to be etched with phosphoric acid.

3. The cast alloy is a Class IV cast material (for better selective etching).

4. The tooth preparation is minimal, requiring only enough reduction to accommodate the metal. There is no attempt to create mortise, cone, or box-shaped preparations.

5. The cast alloy should be in contact with the maximum surface area of available enamel.

6. If the casting is an attachment for a fixed prosthesis, the pontic should not be an indexing tooth for lateral movement of the mandible.

Most of the failures occur cohesively in the composite bonding (luting agent), so a minimum thickness of the material should be used. The procedure is generally as follows:

i. The tooth surface is reduced to allow for 1-1.1 mm cast thickness. Frequently this reduction is unnecessary if the tooth is intact and there is sufficient intermaxillary space in centric and excursive locations of the mandible to allow for the cast thickness.

ii. A casting is fabricated in the conventional way.

iii. The casting is tried in the mouth.

iv. The internal (tooth) surface of the casting is etched.

v. The involved enamel surface is etched (see chapter 10).

vi. The composite is flowed into both the enamel and the casting and allowed to cure under pressure. (Different consistencies of the resin can be used as dictated in chapter 11.)

vii. Excess composite is flaked off.

viii. The exposed surface of the composite resin is polished.

A very similar procedure can be done for cast ceramic restorations. The only difference is that the etching of the internal (tooth) surface of the casting is going to be done using hydrofluoric acid 5-10% for 15 min. that will be sufficient to create a very similar type of irregularity. Then the same procedure as for Class IV alloys is followed.

The other preparation features that will help solve the mechanical problems of cast restorations are as follows:

All the line and point angles should be definite, but not angular, so they can be easily reproduced in a casting and to avoid stress concentration in the casting and the tooth structure. The roundness must be substantial for Class V materials.

The axial wall should slant toward the pulpal floor, as part of the taper. This, together with rounding of the axio-pulpal line angle, can reduce stresses at the isthmus area.

Reduction of tooth structure should follow the original anatomy of the tooth, to create even reduction, with minimum tooth involvement, and even physiologic distribution of forces applied on the restoraton and remaining tooth structure.

Maximum reduction should be at the occluding surfaces, especially the parts of the tooth surfaces that are in contact during static and dynamic relations of the mandible. An average of 1 mm should be cleared for metallic casting in the inclined planes of the cusps. This reduction should be 1.5 mm for cast ceramics. The reduction of the occluding inclined planes should be cut in a concave form, to accommodate maximal bulk of the casting where stresses are at their maximum.

The internal parts of the cavity preparation should be mortised to preserve the resistance and retention features of the preparation (and to assure one path for the preparation). The internal boxed-up portion should occupy the maximum dimensions of the cavity preparation as practically as possible. This will necessitate making the cavity wall in different planes. At least, the internal planes are fixed in their angulation (almost right angle) with the adjacent floors or walls.

The rest of the mechanical principles will be described with each design of cavity-tooth preparation.

BIBLIOGRAPHY

Bassett, R.W., Ingraham, R., and Koser, J.R.: An atlas of cast gold procedures. ed. 1. Buena Park, California, West Orange County Pub. Co., 1964.

Bauer, R.W.: Survey on the use of casting alloys in commercial dental laboratories. II: Ceramic alloys NADL J. **24**(8):8-15, Sept. 1977.

Bugugnani, R.: Use of nickel-chromium alloys in conventionally cast restorations. Rev. Odontostomatol (Paris) **6**(4):286-291, July-Aug. 1977.

Burse, A.B., Swartz, M.L., Phillips, R.W., and Dykema, R.W.: Comparison of the in vitro and in vivo tarnish of three gold alloys. J. Biomed. Mater. Res. **6**:267-277, 1972.

Christensen, G.J.: Marginal fit of gold inlay castings. J. Prosth. Dent. **16**:297, March-April, 1966.

Espevik, S.: Correlation between strength and hardness of dental casting gold alloys. Scand. J. Dent. Res. **85**(6):496-499, Sept. 1977.

Gourley, J.M.: Current status of semiprecious and conventional gold alloys in restorative dentistry. J. Canad. Dent. Assn. No. 8, 1975.

Howard, W.S., Newman, S.M., and Nunez, L.J.: Castability of low gold content alloys. J. Dent. Res. **59**(5):824-830, May 1980.

Jorgenson, K.D.: The relationship between retention and convergence angle in cemented veneer crowns. Acta Odontol. Scand. **13**:35, June 1955.

Lewis, A.J.: The effect of aluminum on the metallography of a nickel base removable partial denture casting alloy. Aust. Dent. J. **23**(6):488-491, Dec. 1978.

Lloyd, C.H., and Baxter, G.R.: The effect of mercury on the fatigue life of a dental gold alloy. J. Oral Rehabil. **8**(2):183-190, March 1981.

Lorey, R.E., and Myers, G.E.: The retentive qualities of bridge retainers, JADA **76**:568 March 1968.

Mack P.J.: A theoretical and clinical investigation into the taper achieved on crown and inlay preparations. J. Oral Rehabil. **7**(3):255-265, May 1980.

Moffa J.P., and Jenkins, W.A.: Status report on base-metal crown and bridge alloys. JADA **89**:652-655, 1974.

Mohamed F.A., Sabet, E.M., and Ramadan, F.A.: Spectrographic study on the effect of remelting on the ingredients of some dental alloys Egypt Dent. JADA. **24**(4):453-469 Oct. 1978.

Nielsen J.P., and Tuccillo, J.J.: Grain size in cast gold alloys. J. Dent. Res. **45**:964-969, 1966.

Nitkin, D.A., and Asgar, K.: Evaluation of alternative alloys to type III gold for use in fixed prosthodontics. JADA. **93**:622-629, 1976.

Ohm, E., and Silness, J.: The convergence angle in teeth prepared for artificial crowns. J. Oral Rehabil. **5**(4):371-375, Oct. 1978.

Riley, E.J., Sozio, R.B., Shaklar, G., and Krech, K.: Shrinkage-free ceramic crown versus ceramometal: A comparative study in dogs. J.D.P. **49**(6):766-771, June 1983.

Rosner, David: Function, placement and reproduction of bevels for gold castings. J. Prosth. Dent. **13**:1160, Nov.-Dec. 1963.

Saleh, L.A., Marzouk, M.A., Diemer, R.M.: Clinical behavior of seminoble casting alloys, IADR abstracts, March 1984.

Sarkar, N.K., Fuys, R.A., Jr., and Stanford, J.W.: The chloride corrosion of low-gold casting alloys. J. Dent. Res. **58**(2):568-575, Feb. 1979.

Sarkar, N.K., and Greener, E.H.: In vitro corrosion resistance of new dental alloys. Biomat. Med. Dev. Art. Org. **1**:121-129, 1973.

Sipple, C.H.: Dental casting alloys (I). Quintessence Dent. Technol. **5**(2):179-184, Feb. 1981.

Sipple, C.H.: Dental casting alloys (II). Quintessence Dent. Technol. **5**(3):269-276, March 1981

Sozio, R.B., and Riley, E.J.: The shrinkage-free ceramic crown, J.P.P. **49**(6):182-186, Jan. 1983.

Starling, L.B., et al.: Shrinkage-free ceramic, U.S. patent #4, 265, 669, May 1981.

Stevens, L.: Some aspects of non-precious metal alloys for ceramic restorations. Aust. Dent. J. **22**(1):11-13, Feb. 1977.

Taggart, W.H.: A new and accurate method of making gold inlays. Dent. Cosmos. **49**:1117-1121, 1907.

Tjan, A.H., Miller, G.D., Whang, S.B., and Sarkissian, R.: The effect of thermal stress on the marginal seal of cast gold full crowns. JADA **100**(1):48-51, Jan. 1980.

Tuccillo, J.J., and Nielson, J.P.: Observations of onset of sulfide tarnish on gold-base alloys. J. Prosth. Dent. **25**:629-637, 1971.

Vincent, P.F., Stevens, L., and Basford, K.E.: A comparison of the casting ability of precious and non-precious alloys for porcelain veneering. J. Prosth. Dent. **37**(5):527-536, May 1977.

Willey, R.L.: Retention on the preparation of teeth for cast restorations. J. Prosth. Dent. **35**:526, 1976.

Wise, E.M.: Cast gold dental alloys. ASM Handbook, 1120, 1948.

Woody, R.D., Huget, E.F., and Horton, J.E.: Apparent cytotoxicity of base metal casting alloys. J. Dent. Res. **56**(7):39-43, July 1977.

Woolsey, G.D., and Matich, J.A.: The effect of axial grooves on the resistance form of cast restorations. JADA **97**(6):978-980, Dec. 1978.

CHAPTER 18

Designs of cavity and tooth preparations for cast restorations

There are five general designs of tooth preparations to accommodate a cast restoration, namely:

I. Inlays
II. Onlays
III. Cast restorations with surface extensions
IV. Pin-lays
V. Full veneer cast or cast based restorations

Although each will be described separately, in actual practice, tooth preparation can and usually does combine several features from each of these general designs.

I. Tooth Preparations for Inlay Cast Restorations

A. Indications

These are purely intracoronal restorations, which have limited indications. These are:

1. A cavity's width does not exceed one-third the intercuspal distance.

2. Strong, self-resistant cusps remain.

3. Indicated teeth have minimal or no occlusal facets and, if present, are confined to the occlusal surfaces.

4. The tooth is not to be an abutment for a fixed or removable prosthesis.

5. Occlusion or occluding surfaces are not to be changed by the restorative procedure.

The following is a description of inlay preparations to be used for Classes I, II, and, sometimes, Class III casting materials.

B. General shape (Fig. 1)

The outline of the occlusal portion of this preparation is dove-tailed. The proximal portion is usually boxed in shape.

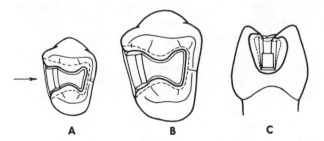

Fig. 18-1. Maxillary bicuspid. Do inlay preparation (indirect).

C. Location of margins

In the occlusal portion (Fig. 1, A and B), the facial, lingual, and, sometimes, proximal margins are located on the inclined planes of the corresponding cusps, triangular ridges or the marginal ridges (crossing ridges). This is designed so that the bucco-lingual width of the cavity preparation (distance measured between the buccal and lingual wall proper), especially at the isthmus portion, does not exceed one-third the intercuspal distance. The most peripheral margins of the preparation are located away from contact with the opposing tooth surfaces during centric closure and excursive movements of the mandible. All adjacent wear facets, supplementary grooves and areas of decalcifications, or any defect in the adjacent parts of the occlusal surface, should be included in the bevelled portion of the cavity preparation only. The margins of this design fulfill all requirements of extension for prevention.

In the proximal portion (Fig. 1C) the facial and lingual margins are each in the corresponding embrasure. This is designed so that the full length of an explorer can be passed freely in the occluso-gingival direction, and so that all undermined enamel, surface defects, and peripheral marginal undercuts are eliminated. The more inaccessible this portion of the tooth preparation is, the more should be this proximal extension, but it should always stop short of the axial angle of the tooth. Extensions should be made in and with the flared portion, not with the wall proper.

Gingival margins should be similar to others, previously described, but in addition, they should be extended to include any surface defects and concavities and to eradicate marginal undercuts. As in the facial and lingual margins, extension gingivally should be accomplished with the bevel and not with the wall proper.

D. Internal anatomy (Figs. 2 and 3)

In the occlusal portion, the facial and lingual walls and sometimes the proximal walls (if marginal ridge is intact) walls, will be formed of two parts:

1. The wall proper, constituting about the pulpal two-thirds of the facial or lingual (proximal) walls, is formed completely of dentin. These walls should taper from each other on the average of 2-5°, or be parallel to each other, if necessary. Each wall should make a right angle or slightly obtuse angle with the pulpal floor. Preferably, each of these "walls proper" should be parallel to the long axis of the crown.

2. The occlusal bevel, which is a long bevel, constituting

almost one-third of the facial and lingual (proximal) walls. This bevelled outer plane of the walls will have an average angulation of 30-45° to the long axis of the crown (or the wall proper). This angulation should increase as the width of the cavity preparation increases (Fig. 3), in order to accommodate more bulk of cast alloy, and to be able to resist increased stresses near the cusps on the inclined planes. Also, this increased angulation is necessary to bevel enamel rods, which are inclined toward the cusps (Fig. 3), in the occlusal one-third of the inclined planes.

The angulation of the bevel should decrease with increased steepness of the cusps. Sometimes, bevels are not needed at all in very steep cusps (especially in a very narrow preparation), as occlusal extension and enamel involvement of the "wall proper" will automatically bevel enamel rods in the inner one-third of the inclined planes (Fig. 4).

An increased bevel angulation is necessary, also, for a direct wax pattern as compared to cavity preparations for an indirect pattern. This is because more marginal bulk is required for the direct wax pattern technique (Fig. 2). In addition, the bevel angulation should be increased to include remotely located defects, supplementary grooves, or decalcifications on the occlusal surface.

The "bevel" part of the facial and lingual, and, sometimes, the proximal walls of the inlay cavity preparation will usually be half that of the cavity "wall proper". This bevel is extended to include wear facets and occlusal defects or decalcifications, if they are confined to the occlusal surface. They are also extended to include supplementary grooves and to move the margin away from occlusal contacts. In wider cavities, and in deeper ones, they are extended to improve the taper and reduce frictional components for easier material manipulation.

3. In the inlay cavity preparation, the pulpal floor (Fig. 5D) should be flat over most of its extent. If this is not possible, at least the peripheral portions should be flat. (The pulpal floor may have different levels according to the number of caries cones and their invasive activities.) The conventional pulpal depth of the inlay cavity preparation is a little more than that for amalgam in order to create more length for surrounding walls. Generally speaking, this depth should be 1-1.5 mm from the DEJ. The pulpal floor should meet all surrounding walls in a definite line angle, except its junction with the axial wall, where the joint should be very rounded.

4. In the proximal portion (Fig. 5C) of the inlay cavity preparation, the axial wall (Fig. 5B) should be either flat or slightly rounded in the bucco-lingual direction, and either vertical or slightly divergent (5-10°) towards the pulpal floor in the gingivo-occlusal direction. Divergence here is important only insofar as it imparts some taper on the preparation, facilitating the procedural steps for the restoration. Creating bulk may be necessitated in small size restorations at stress concentration areas. As previously stated, the axial wall should meet the pulpal floor in an extremely rounded junction as in amalgam. This prevents stress concentration in the tooth and the casting. Furthermore, the depth, axially, should ideally be 1-1.5 mm from the DEJ. However, different depths may be necessary according to the cariogenic pattern of the dentinal lesion proximally.

5. Proximally, facial and lingual walls (Fig. 5, B and C) are comprised of two planes. In the axial half (i.e., the facial or lingual "wall proper") it is formed completely of dentin

Maxillary Bicuspid

Inlay preparation for indirect technique

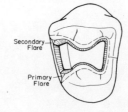

Inlay preparation for direct technique

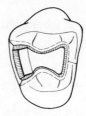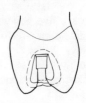

No secondary flare
Steeper occlusal bevel (50°-60°)

Fig. 18-2

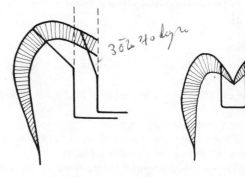

Fig. 18-3   **Fig. 18-4**

and meets the axial wall at a right angle relationship (tangent of the axial wall there). This is the main resistance and retention feature of that part of the cavity preparation. The proximal half of the facial and lingual walls is formed of a primary flare, comprised of enamel and dentin with an unchanged 45° angle to the "wall proper".

6. Sometimes it is necessary to impose a third plane in the form of a secondary flare, placed on enamel peripherally. This serves to simplify impressions and wax patter manipulations and for the other reasons previously mentioned. Secondary flares should not be used if a direct wax pattern technique is to be used. The secondary flare can have variable angulation and extent to achieve its objectives.

7. The gingival floor (Fig. 5, C and D), proximally should be flat in the bucco-lingual direction, making a slightly obtuse angle with the buccal and lingual walls.

In the axio-proximal direction, it is formed of two planes. The axial half consists of gingival wall (floor) proper, being perfectly flat, formed of dentin, and making either a right angle or a slightly obtuse angle with the axial wall. The proximal

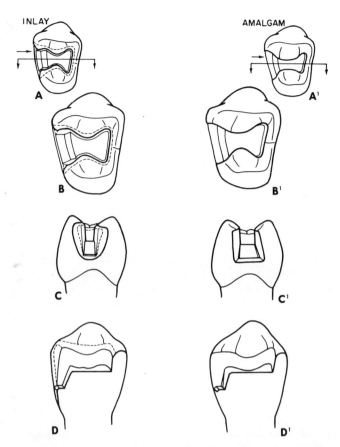

Fig. 18-5. Maxillary biscuspid. Do inlay and DO amalgam preparation compared.

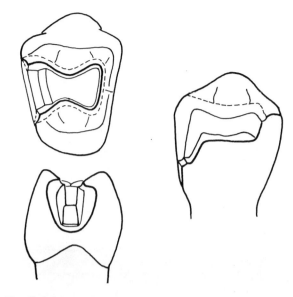

Fig. 18-6. Inlay cavity preparation for Class III and IV cast materials.

half should be bevelled in the form of a long bevel inclining gingivally. This bevel is usually angulated on the average of 30-45° to the wall proper. However, this angulation can be increased by an increase in the gingival extent and length of the surrounding walls. This will serve to minimize marginal discrepancy. Marginal symptoms of internal spacing are inversely proportional to this bevel's angulation.

The bevel's angulation may also be increased with the need to include surface defects, a proximal surface (root) concavity, or peripheral marginal undercuts. Also, in cases where there is a limited axio-proximal dimension of the gingival floor, increasing the angulation of the bevel can minimize the part of the floor used up by the bevel.

Although this bevel is usually equal in extent to the "wall proper", it can be increased to include notches or surface defects, or decreased if the margin ends on cementum rather than enamel. This leaves sufficient flat "wall proper" to resist stresses and to avoid being entangled in unexpected root anatomies. The extent of the bevel may also be decreased if the cavity is increased in length occluso-apically. This creates more room for the flat "wall proper".

8. The junction between the occlusal bevel and the secondary or primary flare proximally, and also, the junction between the primary or secondary flares proximally and the gingival bevel should be very rounded and smooth.

9. Some of the retention means previously mentioned can be used in this design, in addition to or in lieu of other means, to be described (e.g., facial, lingual and gingival grooves prox-

imally, internal boxes or slots occlusally, capping corners of cusps, etc.).

E. Modifications for Class IV and some Class III materials

Although the general shape, location of margins, and most of the internal anatomy of preparations for cast alloys in the Class IV (and sometimes Class III) category are similar to those to be described for Class I and II alloys, certain specific modifications must be enumerated (Fig. 6):

1. Although the preparation will still contain internal boxed portions (buccal, lingual, and proximal "wall proper") occlusally and proximally, the internal line and point angles should be more rounded.

2. Surrounding walls should be more parallel to one another, i.e., less taper. This compensates for the loss of retention resulting from the rounding of internal line angles.

3. All circumferential tie constituents (primary or secondary flares, occlusal or gingival bevels) should be hollow-ground to improve the capability of these alloys to replicate marginal details during casting.

4. Tooth preparation should be deeper axially and pulpally to compensate for the loss of retention that results from the relatively poor castability of these alloys.

5. Extent and angulation of circumferential tie constituents should be dictated by the same factors that influenced them for Class I and II cast alloy cavity preparations.

F. Modifications for Class V cast materials

Use of these cast materials for cast restorations dictates making the same modifications listed above for Class IV alloys. However, the internal anatomy of cavity preparations for these alloys will include the following additional changes (Fig. 7):

1. Definitely flat (at least peripherally) pulpal and axial walls meet surrounding walls in very rounded line angles.

2. There is no decisive differentiation between surrounding walls and the circumferential tie. Both can be in the form of concave surrounding walls (i.e., exaggerated hollow-ground bevels or very rounded shoulders).

(handwritten at top of page) welen etch insil of castable ceramic as denten adhesin.

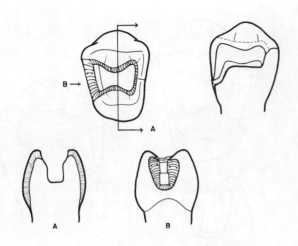

(arrows indicate concavity)

Fig. 18-7. Inlay cavity preparations for cast ceramics.

3. To improve retention, the preparation should be relatively deeper and with minimal or no taper (compared to that for Class I, II, or III alloy). Furthermore, auxillary retention means should be used heavily.

4. The angulation of the marginal termination of the circumferential tie hollow-ground bevel (the actual wall in most cases) is dictated by the same factors that govern the angulation of the bevels and flares in cavity preparations for Class I and II alloys.

5. The gingival floor, if its margins end on cementum (dentin) or at the occlusal or middle third of the anatomical crown may be made a flat, one-planed floor completely formed of dentin (after cementum removal), or enamel and dentin terminating in a 90° cavosurface margin. Although this might reduce the negating effect of bevels on internal discrepancies shown marginally, the exactness of the fit of cast ceramics would counteract this problem.

6. The same could be applied to the surrounding walls proximally and occlusally if the width of the preparation is very limited and the retention resistance is deficient and could be reduced further by the regular hollow ground surrounding walls.

This could simply be done by preparing these surrounding walls in a purely wall proper configuration with no bevel or flare components. This simplified cavity preparation could be done provided that:

—No undermined enamel is left marginally.

—The margins are placed in finishable, cleansable areas (narrow contact areas).

—Joint angles are prepared extremely rounded and the cavosurface ones are made right angles.

—Naturally, the taper and several other correlated features in this simplified preparation could be similar to those in cavity preparations for Class I or II alloy inlays.

II. Tooth Preparations for Onlay Cast Restorations

Onlays are the most indicated and universally used cast restorations for individual teeth. It is a partly intracoronal and partly extracoronal type of a restoration, which has cuspal protection as the main feature (anatomy described later).

A. Indications

Besides the general indication for cast restoration, the following are specific indications for onlay-type cast restorations:

1. In the cast restoration, cuspal protection is to be considered, if the lesion width is one-third to one-half the intercuspal distance.

2. In the cast restoration, cuspal protection is mandatory, if the width of the lesion exceeds one-half the intercuspal distance.

3. In the tooth preparation, if the length:width ratio of the cusp is more than 1:1, but not exceeding 2:1, cuspal protection is to be considered.

4. In a cast restoration tooth preparation, if the length:width ratio of a cusp is more than 2:1, cuspal protection is mandated.

5. Whenever there is a need to change the dimension, shape, and interrelationship of the occluding tooth surfaces, onlay cast restorations are the ideal, most conservative restorations.

6. Onlays are ideal restorations for abutment teeth for a removable partial denture or fixed prosthesis.

7. Onlays are the ideal supporting restorations for remaining tooth structure, combined with conservative tooth involvement.

8. Onlays are indicated when it is necessary to include wear facets that exceeded the cusp tips and triangular ridge crests facially and/or lingually.

The following description will be for preparations to accommodate Class I, II, and some Class III alloys.

B. General shape (Figs. 8 and 9)

Occlusally, onlays are dovetailed internally and follow cuspal anatomy externally. Proximally they appear either box- or cone-shaped. The main features of these designs of tooth preparations are capping of the functional (and sometimes the nonfunctional) cusps, and the shoeing of the non-functional cusps.

C. Location of margins _(handwritten: margin parallett cuspal anatomy.)_

a. Occluso-facio-lingual portion:

1. on the capped cusp side, which is usually the functional side, cusps are capped for the purpose of additional retention and protection. Therefore, the facial or lingual margins will be located on the facial or lingual surface. They must be located far enough gingivally to be away from contact with the opposing tooth surface in either centric occlusion or at any boundary location of the mandible. The margins should be far enough gingivally to properly encompass the facial or lingual cuspal elements. Normally this will involve one-fourth to one-third the facial or lingual surfaces (Fig. 10).

2. Gingivally, margins should include all facial or lingual grooves there (Fig. 10). Margins should parallel the contour of the cusp tips and crests of the adjacent ridges. This will add to retention by increasing the surface area and the interlocking from uneven marginal termination. It also conserves tooth structure (Fig. 9).

3. On the shoed side (Figs. 8 and 9), which is always the nonfunctional side, the facial or lingual margin will be located just gingival to the tip and ridge crests of the involved cusps and away from occlusal contact (static and functional). Again,

(handwritten at bottom) onlay is less retentive than inlay and is 1/2 or 1/3 the inlay

Tubile a cusp as Resistence from is as important as gingival floor. and also increase Surface area and also improves lating capability of resporation

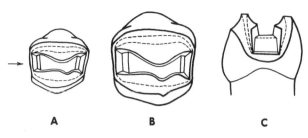

Fig. 18-8. Mandibular premolar–MOD onlay.

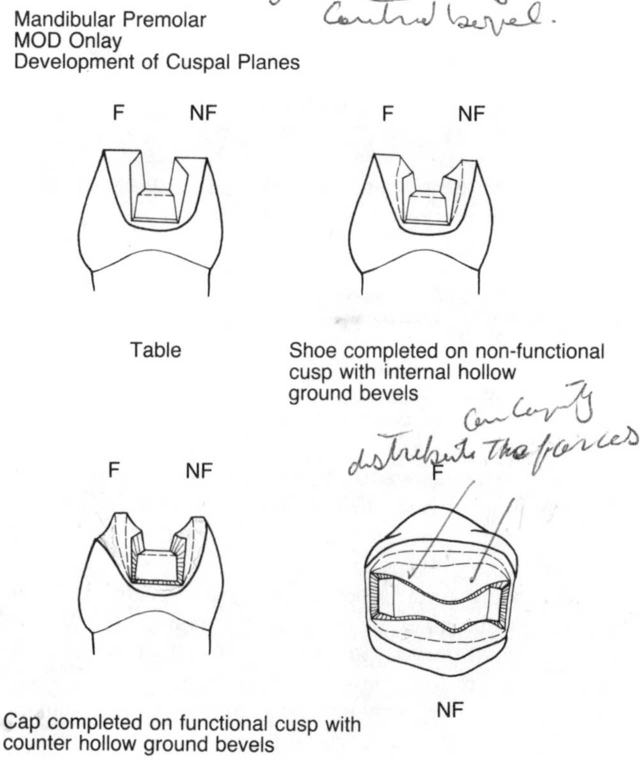

embrasure angle: between long axis and Central bevel.

Mandibular Premolar
MOD Onlay
Development of Cuspal Planes

F NF   F NF

Table   Shoe completed on non-functional cusp with internal hollow ground bevels

F NF   F NF

On cavity distribute The forces

Cap completed on functional cusp with counter hollow ground bevels

Fig. 18-9

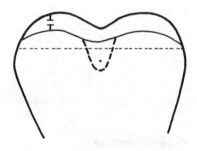

- - - - - - Extensive involvement, wrong outline
———— Conservative & retentive outline
- – – – A dip to include facial groove
⊣ ⊢ ¼ to ⅓ clinical crown length

Fig. 18-10

margins should follow the contour of the cusp tips and ridge crests.

b. Proximal portion (Figs. 8 and 9)

Proximal margins will be in the exact location as in cavity preparations for inlays with the same modifications. The only difference here is that the secondary flares are used in all situations, a condition dictated by the cavity width and the impossibility (in most cases) of joining a counter- or short-bevel facially or lingually with primary flares proximally.

D. Internal anatomy

a. In the occluso-facio-lingual portion (Figs. 8, 9, and 11).

The pulpal floor is like that described for an inlay, but is deeper and usually has different levels. On the capped side, the facial or lingual wall will be formed by four planes:

1. **The wall proper** (Figs. 8, 9, and 11) is an intracoronal portion of the wall which constitutes at least half of the vertical height of the total wall. It is completely in dentin and slightly tapered from the opposing "wall proper" by 2-5°, making a definite angle with the pulpal floor (peripheral part of the pulpal floor).

2. **The occlusal bevel** (Figs. 8, 9, and 11C) is an intracoronal portion of the wall, which constitutes at least ⅓ of the total wall height. It takes the form of a hollow-ground long bevel with a standard angulation paralleling the cusp's occlusal inclined planes. On the average it is 30-45° from the long axis of the tooth crown and approximately the same angulation from its "wall proper". It should be relieved at least 1 mm from the opposing cuspal elements in static and functional occluding contacts. For each cusp, there should be two hollow-ground bevels occlusally: one is directed occluso-distally, and the other occluso-mesially, following the direction of the corresponding occlusal inclined planes (Fig. 12). The hollow-ground dual directional features of the bevel on each cusp are extremely advantageous in giving bulk for the restoration at its inclined planes, areas of imminent stresses. Also, they increase the surface area of contact between the tooth surface and cast, helping to distribute forces physiologically on underlying tooth structures (following removed tooth anatomy). In addition they help to guide the cast to one specific relation with the preparation surface, and substantially increase the immobilization of the restoration.

3. The "table" (Figs. 8, 9, and 11) is the transitional area between the intracoronal and extracoronal parts of the preparation. Usually, it is partly in dentin and partly in enamel, although it can be in either, provided it is relieved from opposing cusps by at least 1.5 mm in both static and functional contacts. The "table" is one of the major resistance forms of the entire structure, and in that aspect it is no less important than a gingival or pulpal floor. At any location, the table should be flat, following the cuspal anatomy in the mesio-distal directions (i.e., three tables for each cusp, each with different directions). This will increase the preparation surface area, provide more locking retention, and conserve tooth structure while helping to physiologically distribute occlusal loads.

4. The "counterbevel" (Figs. 8, 9, and 11) is the extracoronal feature of this part of the preparation. Usually, it is formed in areas of enamel and dentin, or it may be completely in either. It should be relieved from opposing cuspal elements by at least 1 mm in both static and functional occlusal contact.

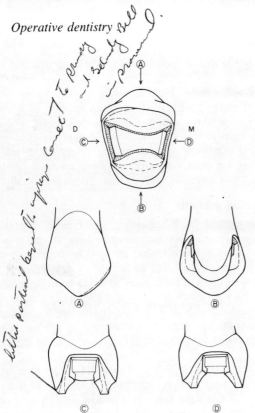

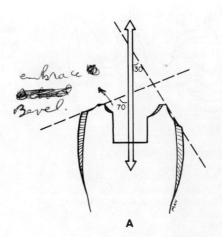

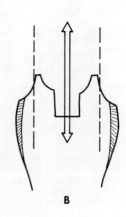

Fig. 18-13.

Fig. 18-11. Maxillary premolar–MOD onlay. (Note absence of partial bevel on mesial slope of shoed cusp).

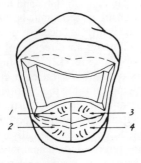

Fig. 18-12. Four hollow ground bevels, for each cusp on the capped side. Bevels have same direction as replaced inclined planes.

It is hollow-ground, inclined away from the intracoronal parts of the preparation gingivally-facially or lingually, and follows the cuspal anatomy (i.e., each of the facial or lingual inclined planes for the cusp will have a hollow-ground bevel). So each cusp on the capped side will have four different hollow-ground bevels, each corresponding to an inclined plane of the cusp (Fig. 12). In addition to the advantages of those features mentioned with the occlusal bevel, the counterbevel will embrace the cuspal elements for retention and/or support.

The angulation of the counterbevel (Fig. 13A) is not as standard as that for the occlusal bevel. It is measured by the embracing angle, i.e., the angle between the bevel and the long axis of the crown. On the average, this angulation is from 30-70°, but it varies according to:

a. The amount of indicated involvement for the facial or lingual surface. The more the desirable involvement there is, the less will be the embracing angle to preserve tooth structure.

b. The amount of needed retention.

The shorter the preparation walls (axial surfaces) are, the less will be the embracing angle with the long axis of the tooth. In some situations, the counterbevel will almost be parallel to the intracoronal wall proper, which will add substantially to the retention of the restoration (Fig. 13B).

c. The type of cast alloy.

The less the castability of the alloy is, the greater will be the embracing angle, to allow for bulk of material marginally.

The extent of the counterbevel is least standardized in this part of the preparation. The same factors that dictate the angulation of the counterbevel will also affect its extent; besides:

a. Location of occluding contacts during static and functional relation of the teeth, as these contacts should be away from the margins

b. Surface defects, grooves, pits, wear facets, decalcification, etc., to be involved in the preparation (Fig. 10)

c. Degree of needed embracing of cuspal elements, according to the future function of the restoration

d. The need for changing the facial or lingual contour of the tooth, especially its occlusal part

e. The need for retention, especially with shortened axial items in the preparation

f. The relation of preparation margins to the height of contour

If, for any reason, the gingival margin exceeds the surface maximum convexity gingivally, we will extend the gingival margin apically according to the same rules dictating the location of the gingival margins proximally.

The junction between these four different parts of the capped side should be definite, but slightly rounded, to improve reproducibility and to prevent stress concentration.

The shoed part (Fig. 9) of the preparation the facial, or, lingual, wall will be formed of three parts:

1. The "wall proper"

This is similar to and reciprocating with the "wall proper" on the capped side.

2. The occlusal bevel

This, too, is similar to and reciprocating with its counterpart on the capped side. However, it can be relieved less from opposing teeth, and it usually has more extent than its counterpart on the capped side (functional side). On the shoed side, the occlusal bevel performs the same function as on the capped side.

[handwritten note at top: "if esthetic is important we don't ... with top of Buccal cusp, just ridges."]

3. The "shoe"

This may be likened to the table on the capped side, but it is relieved in less dimension than the table, and most of the time it is in enamel. It performs the same functions as the table. In some situations the shoe will end facially or lingually with acute-angled marginal tooth structure, leaving frail enamel. In this situation, a fourth plane is placed, in the form of a partial bevel. This should incline away from the cavity preparation facially or lingually-gingivally, and follow cuspal anatomy (Fig. 11C). This peripheral partial bevel is also indicated when there is difficulty in making a proper continuation between a shoe and a primary or secondary flare proximally. On the other hand, in some locations, e.g., mesio-buccal segments of the upper first or second premolars and first molars, the shoe will end with margins facially that might be unacceptable for esthetic reasons. In this situation, the occlusal bevel (the second plane) should be the terminal circumferential tie constituent at the mesio-occlusal inclined planes of the buccal or mesio-buccal cusps of these teeth (Fig. 11D).

Just as on the capped side, the junction between these two, three or four constituents should be definite, but rounded.

b. Proximal portion

The internal anatomy of tooth preparation for onlay proximally is very similar to the proximal part in cavity preparations for inlays, i.e., with standard "wall proper" and primary flare. For onlays, however, the secondary flare with its flexible angulation and extent, is an integral feature of the cavity preparation.

E. Modifications for Class IV and some Class III alloys

For these classes of alloys, the preparation parameters and details are similar to what has been described for Class I and II alloys. However, the following modifications in preparation design may be indicated (Fig. 14):

1. The occlusal reduction (tables and occlusal hollow-ground bevels) must be greater, in order to accommodate bulkier cast material.

2. All circumferential tie constituents must be hollow-ground (i.e., all secondary flares or involved primary flares, gingival bevels and counterbevels). Extent and angulation of the tie are dictated by the same factors as in Class I and II alloys.

3. All cusps must be capped rather than shoed, as a means of cuspal protection.

4. Because of the possibility of shortening the cavity walls occluso-apically and axio-proximally (facially or lingually) due to modifications 1-3, maximum parallelism (i.e., minimum taper) should be strived for.

5. The preparations should not feature any small, complicated internal or external details (e.g., internal boxes, reverse secondary flares).

6. The concavity of hollow-ground bevels should include enamel and dentin. Thus, secondary flares will be deeper and more extensive than described for the other classes of alloys.

F. Modifications for Class V cast materials

Again, most of the parameters and details described for the preparations for Class I and II alloys will be applicable to Class V cast materials. However, there must be certain modifications in preparation design, as follows (Fig. 15):

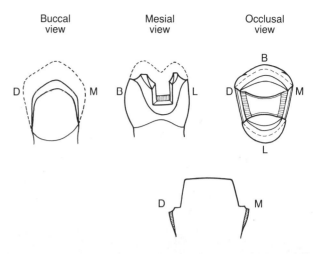

Fig. 18-14. MOD onlay preparation for Class III and IV cast alloys (#29).

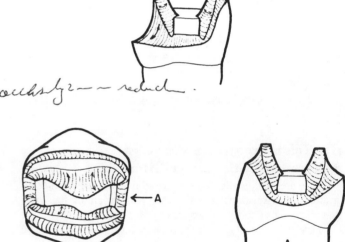

[handwritten note: "occlusly — — reduce."]

Fig. 18-15. Onlay preparation for cast ceramics (arrows indicate concavity).

1. Cuspal protection must take the form of capping, rather than shoeing.

2. In most cases, capped cusps consist of three distinct planes: an exaggerated hollow-ground bevel extending from the pulpal floor to the table; a table, as described for onlays made of Class I and II cast materials; and an exaggerated (both in surface extension and depth) hollow-ground counterbevel, extending from the table to the facial and lingual termination of the preparation. This counterbevel should extend more gingivally, to improve retention. The embracing angle of this counterbevel should also be more acute than that described for Class I and Class II alloys.

3. There is more occlusal reduction for the table and counterbevel to accommodate sufficient bulk of cast ceramic (i.e., 1.5-2 mm).

4. The gingival, buccal, and lingual walls, proximally, should be similar to those for inlay cast ceramics, including

the possible configurations of preparations with very limited dimensions proximally.

5. Because of the frequent absence of "boxed-up" internal portions of the preparatoin, and of shortened walls, the preparation should be deeper than that for Class I and II cast alloys.

6. No taper should be exhibited by any wall; rather parallelism should be strived for to compensate for loss of retention due to design modifications 2, 3, and 4.

7. In cases of extreme occlusal involvement bucco-lingually, where making three planes of a capped cusp will leave minimal self-resistance, it is advisable to make a preparation similar to Class II, design six for amalgam, wherein the cap will be formed of two planes—a wall proper and a flat table terminating in a right-angled cavosurface margin. This modification may be accomplished, provided:

a. The junctions between the walls and pulpal floor and table are very rounded.

b. The facial or lingual margin ends in the middle or the occlusal ⅓ of that surface (to avoid unsupported enamel that would necessitate a two-planed table), or on dentin.

c. The margins will not end in a concavity (e.g., groove).

d. The internal walls of the cavity proper are sizeable and reciprocating enough to guarantee retention of the casting (there will be no cuspal embracing).

e. Remaining cuspal elements will not need reinforcing.

This type of cap preparation usually accompanies totally boxed-up facial and lingual walls and shouldered gingival walls proximally.

8. There will be no reverse secondary flares in these preparations.

III. Tooth Preparations for Cast Restorations with Surface Extensions

These are modifications for basic onlay and inlay tooth preparations, and restorations involving part or all of the axial surface(s), but short of a veneer crown preparation.

There are three types of surface extensions that may be superimposed on any type of tooth or cavity preparation.

A. Reverse secondary flare (Fig. 16)

This is a surface extension of the basic intracoronal inlay or onlay cavity preparation.

1. Indications:

a. Surface extensions are required to include facial or lingual defects beyond the axial angle of the tooth.

b. A surface extension is needed to eradicate severe peripheral marginal undercuts which have not been removed by the maximum angulation and extent of a secondary flare.

c. A surface extension is necessary to encompass an axial angle for reinforcing and supporting reasons.

d. A surface extension is needed to add to the retentive capability of the restoration proximally, especially with shortened facial and lingual walls or as a reciprocal means of retention.

e. More surface extension is required to fulfill the objectives of secondary flares in extremely wide cavities or contact areas.

This type of surface extension is contraindicated for Class IV and Class V cast materials.

2. Features (Fig. 16)

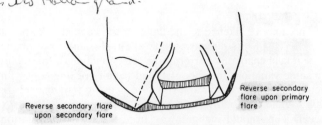

Reverse secondary flare upon secondary flare

Reverse secondary flare upon primary flare

Fig. 18-16

Reverse secondary flares can be added to a cavity (tooth) preparation in lieu of a secondary flare, i.e., superimposed directly over a primary flare, if the secondary flare cannot satisfy its designated objectives. This may be due to extreme facio-lingual width of the lesion or the contact area, or to rotation of the tooth, etc.

It can also be placed in a cavity (tooth) preparation upon a secondary flare, if the secondary flare can fulfill only parts of its own objectives, e.g., open the contact area. The reverse secondary flare can fulfill the rest of the objectives, e.g., provide obtuse angle marginal tooth structure (Fig. 16).

Usually, the reverse secondary flare is in the form of a partial bevel. It involves enamel only, with its maximum depth at its junction with the main cavity preparation. It ends on the facial or lingual surface with a knife-edge finishing line, and its extent should not exceed the height of contour of the facial or lingual surface in the mesio-distal direction, nor should it include the tip of the cusp.

The reverse secondary flare, like the secondary flare, may not include the entire periphery of the preparation occluso-apically. Rather, it could include only the middle part of the periphery, so as to fulfill its objectives there. The reverse angulation of this flare has no limitation, so long as it does not create any undercuts in the occluso-apical path of the cavity or tooth preparation.

B. Skirt (Fig. 17)

This is a more extensive surface extension than the reverse secondary flare, also superimposed on the basic intracoronal inlay or onlay cavity preparation facially and/or lingually.

1. Indications

a. Skirting is required to involve defects with more dimensions (especially depth) than those that can be involved in a reverse secondary flare.

b. A skirt is required to impart resistance and retention on a cast restoration in lieu of missing or shortened opposing facial or lingual walls.

c. Skirting is necessary when the contact areas and contour of the proximal surface(s) are to be changed in the contemplated restorations. They are necessary (facial and lingual to the proximal part of the cavity preparation) to house such a modifying restoration. They allow sufficient cast material to be accommodated without sacrifice of the facial or lingual walls.

d. Skirts are essential facially and lingually for tilted teeth, in order to restore the occlusal plane. They will allow for the bulk, resistance, and retention of the additional occlusal cast material required in building the occlusal table. When so indicated, skirts should be prepared at the side towards which the tooth is tilted.

sheylly of PFC is better but esthetics of castelle ceramic is better.

i first of mette is better, we use castelle ceramics becaus moldelld desn't produce good color.

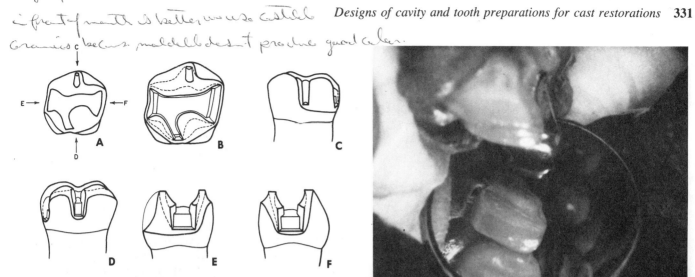

Fig. 18-17, A-F. Maxillary molar. MODBL onlay cavity preparation skirting DB axial angle, and capping L cusps. Preparation has lingual external box, and a buccal skirt-terminating groove.

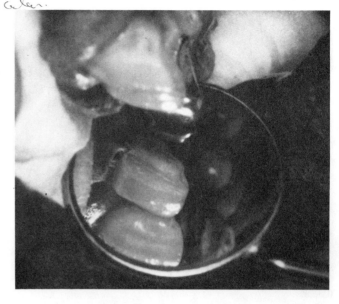

Fig. 18-17, cont'd. G. A facial skirt terminating groove.

2. Features (Fig. 17)

Skirts include part of the facial and lingual surfaces near the axial angles (Fig. 17, C and E) to a depth of 0.5-1 mm in preparations for Class I and II alloys, and to a depth of 1.5-2 mm for some Class III, and all Class IV and Class V cast materials. The maximum depth of all skirts should be at the junction of the surface extension with the cavity preparation proper. For Class I, II, and III casting materials, the skirt ends mesially or distally in a chamfer line. For Class IV and V materials, the skirt ends either in a hollow-ground bevel or a rounded shoulder.

It is sometimes preferable to terminate the skirt mesially or distally in a vertical groove (Fig. 17, C and G), which will not only accommodate bulky cast material, but will also act as a seating guide for the casting at this peripheral area. The axial depth of this groove should be 1-2 mm for Classes I-IV alloys, and 2 mm or more for cast ceramics. This groove should have definite surrounding walls for cast alloys, but be completely rounded in the mesio-distal direction for cast ceramics. The groove should include most of the occluso-apical dimension of the skirt, but be just shy of the gingival finishing line.

Because the skirt is a surface extension that usually includes some convexities of the facial or lingual surface, there are enhanced possibilities of undercuts when it is utilized. Every effort should be made to have the axial reduction of the skirt parallel to the rest of the cavity preparation. Sometimes, the skirt may even be tapered relative to the remainder of the preparation.

The mesial and/or distal extent of the skirt should be sufficient to include those defects it is used to encompass. If it is used as a reciprocal means of retention, it should include an area of the facial or lingual surface equal in dimension to the area in the preparation it is going to reciprocate with. Any intervening cusp, between the cavity preparation proper and a skirt, should be prepared the same way as a capped cusp except with the skirt replacing the counterbevel.

For Class I, II, III, and IV cast alloys, the intervening facial or lingual wall proximally, between the cavity preparation proper and the skirt extension, should have, the boxed portion

and a primary flare. For cast ceramic preparations, however, this intervening wall should have an exaggerated hollow-ground configuration. These features will minimize tooth structure loss and assure a locking property for the restoration. These intervening cusps or walls may be formed completely of dentin, and they should have sufficient bulk (2 mm) to be self-resistant. By no means, should a skirt end on the facial or lingual surfaces in line with the tip of the cusp. Rather it should terminate shy of that cusp tip or past it, with a mesio-distal angulation that is almost standard, i.e., paralleling the proximal "wall proper".

If the skirt is to be used to change the contact and contour of the tooth, it should be extended far enough on the facial and lingual surfaces of the tooth to create sufficient retention (e.g., surface area) for the cast material, and to avoid marginal overhangs and overcontouring. Likewise, if the skirt is to be used to create a regular occlusal plane for a tilted tooth, it should be extended far enough on the facial or lingual surfaces proximally, away from the direction of tilting. This will minimize the effect of displacing forces in the tilted direction and facilitate the accommodation of enough cast material occlusally to establish the desired occlusal plane.

C. Collar

This type of surface extension is the most involving surfacewise and depthwise. It may be one of two types: cuspal collars (Fig. 18A), which involve the facial or lingual surfaces of one cusp only in a multicusped tooth, or tooth collars (Fig. 18, B and C), which involve the entire facial or lingual surface of the tooth. Either type can surround the cuspal elements (Fig. 18B) or be apical to an already lost cuspal element (Fig. 18, A and C).

1. Indications

a. They help in retention and resistance when an entire cusp is lost prior to the tooth preparation or when it is necessary to remove it due to excessive undermining.

b. They help retention in shortened teeth.

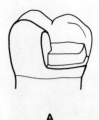 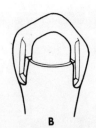 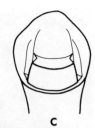

A   **B**   **C**

Fig. 18-18. Collars.

c. They help resistance and to enhance support for the tooth that is endodontically treated.

d. They are used in situations where pins are contraindicated for retention purposes.

e. They are used in teeth with large foundations replacing cuspal elements, where it is necessary to place margins on tooth structure apical to the gingival margins of these foundations.

f. They are used for cast materials with low castability.

g. They are used for areas in a cast alloy restoration to be veneered by fused porcelain. A collar can accommodate both alloy and porcelain bulk and facilitate marginal seating of the casting's circumferential tie.

2. Features

With an axial depth of 1.5-2 mm, collar surface extensions end gingivally in a bevelled shoulder finishing line, making it the most reproduceable surface extension. For Class IV cast material, the bevelled portion of the shoulder should be hollow-ground. In preparations for cast ceramic materials, the shoulder can be bevelled in a rounded and exaggerated fashion, or can have no bevel. The choice is dictated by the same factors that influence the gingival floors of inlays and onlays.

When using a collar surface extension, any intervening cusp or proximal, facial or lingual walls, should be preserved in the same way as with a skirt surface extension. In preparations for cast alloy, there should be a definite line angle gingivally, at the junction of the bevelled shoulder with the axial collar. Also, if tapering is necessary, collars should have less taper toward the cavity preparation than skirts. This improves retention in these shortened teeth or cusp preparations. The shoulder portion of the collar should be perpendicular to the long axis of the crown, paralleling any floor or table in the preparation (gingival, pulpal or occlusal).

The peripheral bevelled portion of the collar will have its angulation and extent dictated by the same features as those governing the angulation and extent of the gingival bevels in inlay and onlay preparations. It should be emphasized that the more bevel angulation there is relative to the shoulder, the better will be the marginal seating of the cast restoration.

IV. Tooth Preparations for Pinlay Cast Restorations

Pin-retained cast restorations differ from pin-retained amalgam and direct tooth-colored restorations in that the latter are a form of composite structure, in which pins are one of the phases and in which there are definite macroscopic interfaces between them and the restorative material, and with no adhe-

sion between them. In pin-retained cast restorations, on the other hand, the pins completely adhere to the cast material, with no macroscopically evident interface. This feature alone prevents any possible failure at the juncture of the pin with the cast material. Pin-retained cast restorations can be any type of a cast restoration which contains one or more pins for retention or other reasons. It should again be emphasized, that pins are *auxillary* means of retention. Under no circumstances should pins be the sole retention means.

A. Indications

1. Pinlay involvement should be considered for shallow and wide cavity (tooth) preparations, when it is impossible or contraindicated to use surface extensions for retention purposes.

2. They are used for short teeth occluso-gingivally (e.g., due to attrition, fracture or decay processes), necessitating the use of the root dentin to accommodate pin retention modes.

3. Pins are used when there is incompatibility in length between two (or sets of two) opposing axial walls, e.g., one proximal preparation having very short surrounding walls opposed to another proximal preparation with very long surrounding walls occluso-gingivally. To assure proper reciprocation between the retention of the opposite sides, with minimal micromovements of the cast restoration, a gingival pin is used at the shorter side to achieve an axial retaining length compatible to that of the long side.

4. When proximal axial walls are unusually long in a proximo-occlusal preparation. To prevent proximal deflection of the proximal part of the restoration during function, and to guide the restoration to its exact gingival seat, a short gingival pin is incorporated in the cast alloy restoration proximo-gingivally.

5. A tooth preparation with very tapered axial walls or surfaces, negating or minimizing its retentive abilities, requires using pins in the restoration to immobilize it.

6. In teeth with completely lost cusp(s), pins can be used in place of a cusp as a reciprocating measure opposite to another mode(s) of retention (Fig. 19).

7. In occluso-proximal cavity preparations where the occlusal outline form is not conducive to a dove-tail locking, a pulpal pin at the intact marginal ridge end of the preparation can function like a dove-tail.

8. In proximo-occlusal or proximo-occluso-proximal preparations where the axial wall(s) is (are) not present or very short, limiting the locking ability of the proximal portion of the preparation, a gingival pin(s) can internally increase the axial length of the preparations proximally to assure the immobilization of the restoration.

9. In cases of high pulp horns and/or large pulp chambers limiting the depth and extent of the preparation, pins with their minimal tooth involvement can be used to retain a cast restoration without interfering with or endangering the P-D organ physiology.

10. In thin and delicate teeth, e.g., anterior teeth, where bulky boxes and extensive cavity preparation can be detrimental, pins are ideal to retain a cast restoration (Fig. 27).

11. Accidental or unavoidable loss of gingival floor, which can be detrimental to the resistance-retention form of a cavity preparation, can be compensated for by use of a pin.

12. In rounded preparations and lateral to a root canal post

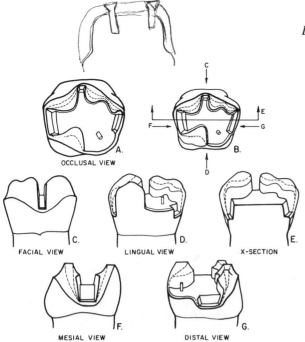

Fig. 18-19. Mandibular molar—MODBL pin onlay.

(dowel), pins act as antirotational devices, immobilizing the restoration(s) laterally.

13. For esthetic reasons, especially in premolar and anterior teeth, pins can be used instead of surface tooth involvement in order to secure retention and resistance.

14. Pins can be used to seal venting orifices in a cast restoration after cementation.

15. Pins can be used to retain a repair type of restoration, marginal to an already serviceable cast restoration.

B. Types

According to the modes incorporating them in a casting, pins for cast restorations can be classified into the following:

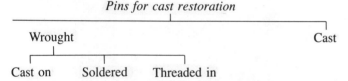

According to their relationship to the long axis of the tooth, the above pins can be:

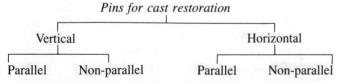

Wrought pins for cast restorations can be made of iridio-platinum or rhodium-gold alloys to be used with cast gold alloy restorations. For silver-palladium or nickel-chromium cast alloy or cast moldable ceramic restorations, the same type of pins can be used. In addition, chromium based or stainless steel alloys can be used for pins in Class III, IV, and V cast material restorations.

Wrought metal pins are prefabricated, cold worked pins that come in different diameters and surface configurations. They

are cut to the desired length and engage the casting in one of three ways:

1. It is fitted into the pin channel of the tooth and/or its die followed by the wax pattern being built over it. It is then invested, and the cast material is cast on it (cast on pins). There will be true adhesion between the pin and the cast material of the restoration if these are properly handled. Of course, the melting point for the pin alloy should be higher than that of the casting material.

2. The cast is fabricated without the pin, then, the pins are fitted in their pin channel on the tooth, keyed, and attached to the fabricated casting with a suitable agent (resin). The assembly is solder invested, and the pins are then soldered to the main restoration. (This is not indicated for ceramics.)

The two above mentioned types are cemented pins, subject to all the principles and effects mentioned in the chapter on pin- and post-retained restorations.

3. The casting is fabricated without the pins, then pin holes are drilled into the casting to coincide with pin channels already prepared in the tooth dentin, or both pin channels and holes are prepared together after the casting is fitted. Threaded pins, slightly larger in diameter than the pin hole and channel, are threaded in to hold the casting to the underlying tooth dentin. In some situations, the surface end of the pin is no different than any other cross-section of the pin. In others, the surface end of the pin will be bevel shaped to fit a bevel prepared with a special tool in the casting around its pin hole. To minimize marginal discrepancies in the latter, the length of the pin to be used must be predetermined, so the two bevels will coincide.

The major advantages of wrought pins are their strength, which is much higher than that of cast pins, and the ability to adjust them directly in the cavity preparation before incorporating them in the casting. The major disadvantages include possible overheating during casting or during soldering of these pins to the main restoration. This may invite grain growth of the pin alloy, which will weaken it. Secondly, overheating may lead to alloying between the metal components of the pin and the casting alloy, with unpredictable properties may occur. Thirdly, the attachment of threaded pins to the casting is mainly mechanical, and, as such, it is subject to all the variables mentioned with pin- and post-retained restoration. Fourthly, as a result of heating the pin and the casting alloy while in contact, the pins will share the nobility and passivity with that of the cast alloy, and vice versa.

Cast pins can be fabricated as part of the restoration in an evaporating wax casting technique. They have the major advantage of structural continuity between the restoration proper and the pin.

Parallel pins can be used parallel to the long axis of the tooth crown or at another angulation to that axis if the casting path necessitates it (Class IV and V). In any event, parallel pins should be parallel to each other as well as to the direction of the casting path. They are always the cemented type and either made with or attached to the casting before cementation. Non-parallel pins are usually inserted into the casting and the tooth dentin after cementing the casting. They can be wrought cemented or wrought threaded, though threaded types can be more mechanically advantageous.

The same principles and features of tooth pin channel preparation to receive a pin for casting, as was mentioned in the chapter on pin- and post-retained restorations, are applicable. However, for cast pins, the occlusal end (outer end) of the pin channel will be surrounded by a struss compartment or countersink to accommodate cast material bulk at this area of massive shear stress concentration (Fig. 20). For wrought pins it is not necessary to prepare such a compartment, as their strengths are very accommodating (Fig. 19).

The armamentarium for pin channel preparation for cast alloy restoration is not too different from that described for the amalgam restoration. The only differences are:

a. In the parallel pin technique, plain, unaided visual orientation of the twist drill, so as to prepare parallel pin channels, may be sufficient for a limited number of pins. With multiple pins, however, or if the pins must be parallel to numerous details in the same preparation, or if the pin must be parallel to pins and other details in adjacent preparations (so as to have a splint or bridge), a parallelometer is needed to insure parallelism (Fig. 21). This is a device with a fixed platform that is stabilized on the vault of the palate or across the lower molar teeth with certain attachments and adhesives (compound or resin). From this immobilized platform, an arm extends which is movable in three dimensions. The end of the arm has holes for the handpiece. As soon as the path of the preparation or preparations is determined, the twist drill placed in the hole in the movable arm is oriented with the pin channel (or other preparation part) at different locations in the same tooth, or in different teeth. They can thus be prepared with complete assurance of their parallelism.

b. For cast restorations there are different sizes and types (final and intermediaries) of pins. To perfect the match between the diameter of the pin channel, their restoration's pins, temporary restoration's pins, and burnable pins for the wax pattern, color coding is used (Fig. 22A).

c. To prepare pin channel for threaded pins (Fig. 22B) in the cast restoration, a special type of drill is used that can cut metal.

d. To prepare the struss compartment around the outer end of the pin channel, a tapered fissure bur is adequate, followed by a monangle chisel or a small hatchet.

V. Tooth Preparations for Full Veneer Cast or Cast Alloy Based Restorations

These are restorations necessitating preparation of the entire clinical crown portion of a tooth to receive a cast restoration or a cast substrate (substructure) that will be partially or totally veneered with fusing porcelain.

A. Indications

Besides the general indications, full veneer castings are indicated in the following situations:

1. They are required where extensive involvement of the tooth precludes the use of other forms of cast restorations due to resistance-retention problems.

2. These restorations, when completely made of cast ceramic or veneered with porcelain or tooth-colored resin, can be the most esthetic type of single-tooth restoration. For this reason, the porcelain-fused-to-metal crown is presently the most used single-tooth restoration for badly broken down or otherwise disfigured anterior teeth.

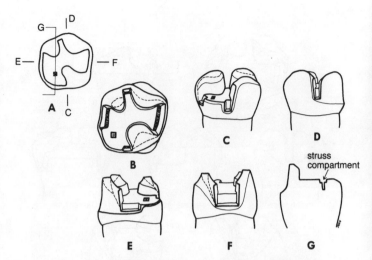

Fig. 18-20. Maxillary molar MODBL pin onlay with a skirt extension. Pin channel is for cast pin.

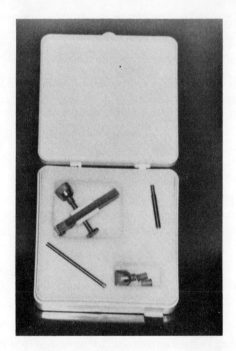

Fig. 18-21

3. Full veneer restorations are indicated when substantial changes in the contact, contour, or occluding anatomy of the tooth is to be created by a cast restoration, beyond the capabilities of onlays, even with surface extensions.

4. Full veneer castings are indicated as a superstructure on a tooth with an amalgam or cast alloy foundation to reinforce it and/or change its alignment.

5. The full veneer casting is the most resistant type of extracoronal cast restoration to displacing forces. Therefore, it is the last resort for restoring a single tooth.

6. Teeth preparation, precementation and post-cementation adjustment for such type of cast restorations (cast based) are the easiest and most feasible. Therefore it is the restoration of choice in areas with difficult access.

Despite (maybe because of) these advantages, this type of cast restoration is the most abused in clinical practice, because of the tremendous involvement of tooth structure in the preparation, the inconspicuousness of the margins (gingival margins only) for inspection and adjustment, and the definite creation of new contacts, contours, and occluding anatomy in the final restoration.

B. Features (Figs. 23, 24)

The full veneer restoration preparation has only one set of circumferential tie constituents, i.e., gingival. Therefore, locating the preparation margins is subject to all rules governing the positioning of gingival margins relative to the tooth surface, periodontium, resistance, retention, esthetics, etc. This margin can be any of the four previously described types of finishing lines. The chamfer finish line is the most frequently used for Classes I, II, and, sometimes, III cast alloy full veneer restorations (Fig. 23). The hollow-ground bevel is the most universal for alloys with low castability (i.e., Class IV and some Class III alloys). The bevelled shoulder is regularly used for cast-based porcelain (tooth-colored resin) restorations. The bevelled portion of the shoulder should be hollow-ground (Fig. 24) if the alloy for the substructure is Class III or IV. For cast ceramics, whenever possible the finishing line should be a very rounded shoulder (exaggerated hollow-ground bevel); an unbevelled shoulder may be used as a finishing line when the preparation is deficient in resistance (flat floors) and generally has short axial length. But these shouldered margins should end on the occlusal ⅔ of the anatomical crown or on the anatomical root surface.

The following are general features for these types of preparations.

1. The vertical reduction for posterior teeth preparation should follow the cuspal anatomy, preparing a concavity in place of each cuspal inclined plane.

2. Vertical reduction for anterior teeth preparation should follow the configuration of the incisal ridge (incisors) or the mesial and distal slopes (canine).

3. Horizontal (axial) reduction for posterior teeth should create axial surfaces with reasonable parallelism to the preparation path with the indicated taper (Fig. 23). Horizontal (axial) reduction for anterior is the same as that for posterior teeth, except that in place of the lingual concavity, reduction should create an axial surface with a concavity in the same shape, dimension and extent of the replaced surface (Fig. 24).

4. Labial reduction should be in two planes: a gingival plane, involving most of the labial surface (⅔) and parallel to a reciprocating plane on the lingual surface, and another plane, sloping inciso-lingually and involving about one-third of the reduced surface.

5. Vertical and horizontal reduction should be of sufficient magnitude to create a space for the replacing cast material or cast material and veneering tooth-colored material, without compromising the integrity of the involved tissues. Class V cast materials will require a preparation with greater overall reduction, while Class I materials demand a preparation with less reduction.

6. Horizontal (axial) reduction should create axial surfaces following the same configuration of the replaced surface mesio-distally and bucco-lingually, but not occluso-gingivally, i.e.,

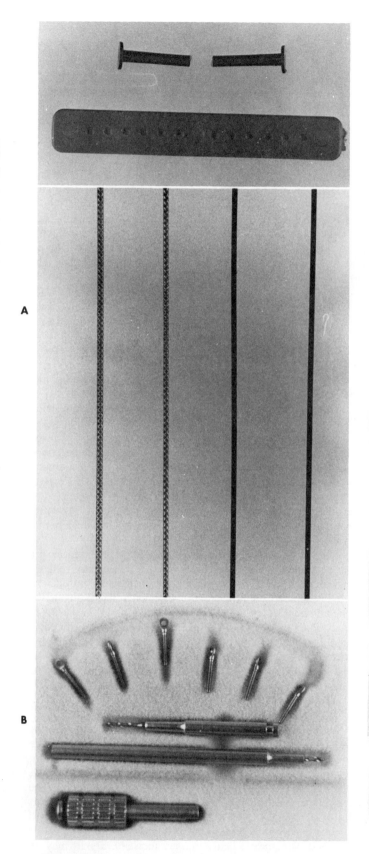

Fig. 18-22. A, top, burnable resin pins to be incorporated in the wax pattern. **A,** bottom, premade pins for cast on or soldering. **B,** Threaded pins for post-cementation casting-tooth attachment.

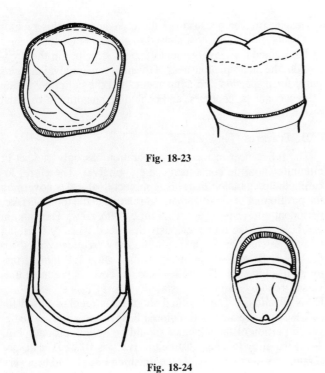

Fig. 18-23

Fig. 18-24

the reduced axial surfaces should have the same grooved, fluted and flattened areas of the original axial tooth structure (Fig. 23).

7. All created preparation surfaces should be definable and distinguishable from each other, and the junction between them should be very definite, but rounded.

8. If the preparation should have more than one type of circumferential tie, as is the case in tooth preparation for porcelain fused to cast alloy veneering restoration, the transition between these should be rounded and gradual.

9. All types of auxillary and reciprocal means of retention, even intracoronal ones, that were described in detail with the general features for cast restorations, can be used with this preparation for a full veneer type restoration.

The present discussion would be incomplete without mentioning cavity preparations for Class III, IV, and V restorations. This is especially true since the introduction of cast ceramics as a viable material for cast restorations.

Because of their unique location and special anatomical considerations, the paths of Class III, IV, and V restorations are usually not parallel to the long axis of the tooth crown. Furthermore, they are frequently pinlays due to the very limited available tooth structure.

Class III cavity preparations for cast alloys are usually indicated for the distal of the cuspid when a strong, durable tooth structure replacement is needed. The design of choice is a box cavity preparation with a lingual or inciso-lingual insertion path, and with definite gingival, labial, axial, and incisal walls. For cast alloys, each of these walls should have its own flare or bevel. If the preparation is designed with a lingual insertion path, it will have no lingual wall. If it is designed with an inciso-lingual insertion path, it will have a partial lingual wall and a very inciso-labially deviated incisal wall. For cast ce-

ramics, the preparation, due to its very limited dimensions, will have no flares or bevels. The boxed walls, however, should be deeper. Retentive grooves are placed at the expense of the incisal and gingival walls, and sometimes on the labial or lingual wall (rarely), following the insertion path of the preparation.

Class IV cavity preparations for cast restorations may have several designs:

1. Proximally grooved box with gingival pins (Fig. 25)

This design may be used for any type of cast material. If the facial and lingual walls are sufficiently intact to accommodate dentinal grooves, this is the ideal design for use on the distal of the cuspid. The cavity preparation is basically box-shaped, having an incisal insertion path, and definite gingival, facial, and lingual walls. For cast alloys, the circumferential tie constituents consist of a gingival bevel, facial and lingual flares, and, sometimes, an incisal bevel. For cast ceramics, the preparation should have no bevels or flares; rather, the boxed up walls continue axio-proximally to the surface. If this leads to unsupported enamel, hollow-ground surrounding walls should be prepared instead. The gingival floor of this design may accommodate a dentinal groove and/or pin(s). The facial and lingual walls should also accommodate a dentinal groove (Fig. 25).

2. Class IV cavity preparation with incisal shoulder (Fig. 26)

This design is used only for cast ceramics, and is usually indicated when the proximal portion is not sufficiently retentive, and the preparation is short, inciso-gingivally. The proximal part could be similar to the previous designs described for cast ceramics, but with less dimension of the surrounding walls. Usually, there will be no facial, lingual or gingival grooves. In most cases, the proximal part will be prepared as an exaggerated groove, having its axial wall flat and in dentin, with surrounding walls in enamel and dentin, forming a partial circle.

The incisal portion of this design should take the form of a very rounded shoulder circumscribing a sufficiently reduced incisal ridge (to accommodate 1.5 mm ceramic bulk). The labial shoulder should be more gingivally located than the lingual shoulder on lower teeth, and vice versa on the upper teeth. The stump of dentin between these surrounding shoulders has all the features of a full veneer preparation. The preparation should have a labially inclining incisal surface for the lower and lingually inclining one for the upper, both in the gingival direction. This design of restoration is the most mechanically locked design of all.

3. Proximal box with incisal step (Fig. 27)

In this design, which is also indicated for cast ceramics, the proximal part will be very similar to the previous design. The incisal part is in the form of a grooved cavity preparation, within the incisal ridge. It has definite pulpal, labial, lingual, and intact proximal walls, if the restoration is unilateral. The incisal part will be continuous with the opposing proximal part if it is a bilateral Class IV. The surrounding walls incisally will be like an occlusal portion of an inlay cavity preparation. If the tooth structure is badly thinned incisally, a skirt may be placed labially and/or lingually. To minimize proximal displacement of the restoration, in unilateral lesions, a pin channel is placed pulpally, at the very proximal end of the incisal

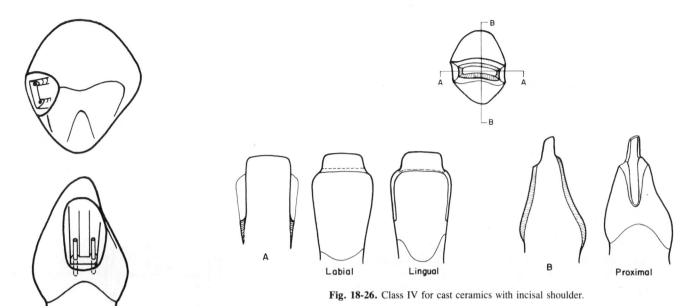

Fig. 18-25. Mandibular cuspid–DI inlay preparation with pin channels.

Fig. 18-26. Class IV for cast ceramics with incisal shoulder.

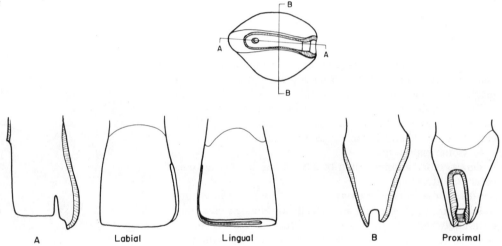

Fig. 18-27. Class IV for cast ceramics with incisal step.

preparation, closer to the intact proximal surface. This design is indicated when the incisal end of the tooth is bulky enough to accommodate such a grooved cavity preparation, without undermining the labial and/or lingual enamel plates. It is usually used after sizable incisal attrition has relocated the incisal edge at a bulky part of the anterior tooth.

4. Proximal box with a lingual skirt (Fig. 28)

This design is indicated for all types of cast materials. The proximal part(s) will be very similar to the first design, except that the lingual wall is lost. Most of the lingual surface will be reduced in the form of a skirt, ending in a groove at the intact proximal surface (in case of a unilateral Class IV). If the lesion is bilateral, the lingual skirt will be between two proximal boxes. To increase the retention of the casting and especially the skirt portion, pins can be located parallel to the insertion path (inciso-lingual), at the expense of the lingual bulk of the tooth (as pin-ledge). The ledges should be prepared

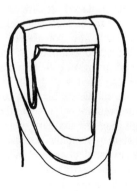

Fig. 18-28

first, then a pin channel can be drilled through them. Circumferential tie constituents will be as mentioned for each type of cast material.

5. Pin-ledge cavity and tooth preparation (Fig. 29)

This design is indicated for cast alloys only. It is in the form of full veneer axial reduction of the lingual surface, short of the incisal ridge and the lingual proximal axial angles. Proximally, the lingual reduction could join a proximal box or a plane proximal reduction, ending gingivally like the lingual reduction, i.e. in a chamfer or hollow-ground bevel. At least three steps (ledges), each accommodating a pin channel, should be prepared in the lingually reduced area, paralleling the incisal or inciso-lingual insertion path and strategically located to avoid the pulp, and to be reciprocally retentive.

6. Three quarter crown (Fig. 30)

This design is indicated for all types of cast materials. The proximal parts may be in a groove or box form. The lingual reduction should be similar to a preparation for a full veneer restoration, following the lingual surface anatomy. The incisal ridge should be minimally reduced, with a little bevel (skirt for cast ceramics) inclining labially and paralleling the incisal ridge or slopes. The circumferential tie constituents of the tooth preparation for cast alloys are composed of proximal labial flares and gingival chamfers proximally and lingually. They can be shoulders only for cast ceramics (see Section on inlays).

7. Class IV with a lingual dovetail

This design is indicated only for upper teeth with an inciso-lingual or pure lingual insertion path. It is a design to be avoided for the same reasons mentioned in the discussion of amalgam for the distal of the cuspid. The lingual dovetail involves most of the incisal two-thirds of the lingual surface, and the proximal box has all surrounding walls except the lingual walls.

8. Combination design

This may be a compilation of any of the first six designs described herein.

Class V cavity preparations for cast alloy restorations are usually indicated for lesions in teeth already having a cast alloy restoration and contraindicated for direct gold restorations. Also, it can be used when there is minimal tooth structure, surrounding an extensive lesion, preventing creation of compatible size walls and retentive grooves, and in the absence of enamel for etching retention.

The cavity preparation is basically a pinlay (Fig. 31A). It can be prepared in infinite shapes according to the extent of tooth structure to be replaced. If anatomical and cariogenic conditions allow, as many surrounding walls as possible should be made, no matter how short or uneven they may be. Each wall should have an appropriate bevel. The preparation has a pure facial or lingual insertion path. Pin channels are prepared at the expense of the axial wall tooth structure at the very proximal peripheries of the preparation, at least one at each side, paralleling the preparation path and the adjacent proximal surfaces. Although they are auxillary means of retention, pins play a very important part in the retention of these types of restorations. It is advisable, when cementing these types of restorations, to cut grooves in the cavity side of the casting and in the surrounding cavity walls to be filled with the cement medium to lock the restoration further (Fig. 31, A and B), as mentioned previously.

In extensive cases of Class V cavity preparation, when no

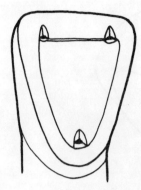

Fig. 18-29

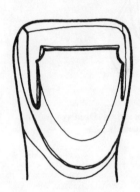

Fig. 18-30

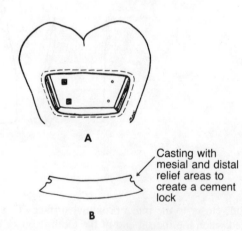

A

B

Casting with mesial and distal relief areas to create a cement lock

Fig. 18-31

surrounding walls can be prepared, a cast alloy restoration can be prepared with only a finishing line (chamfer or knife edge) cut at the periphery of the defect. The restoration is held into the tooth mainly by pins. Although this is not a very serviceable restoration, it can satisfy immediate needs.

The facial or lingual Class V cavity preparation may have a proximal boxed extension, necessitated by cariogenic reasons. If these proximal boxes are extended proximally enough, and their occlusal and gingival walls can accommodate dentinal grooves, continuous with the facial and lingual surfaces, pins may not be needed at all. Unilateral pins can reciprocate with a boxed proximal extension.

Instrumentation for Tooth Preparations for Cast Restorations

Prior to any cutting of tooth structure in the restorative phase, procedures should be planned and executed in a disciplined and systematic way. This rule should be especially applied in preparing teeth to receive a cast restoration, as abusing and misusing the armamentarium for those preparations is, unfortunately, the usual occurrence. The possibility of overcutting tooth structures, traumatizing the P-D organ, and misangulating preparation details, necessitating drastic corrective measures, is great.

The following steps provide a general scheme for preparing a tooth for a cast restoration:

A. Removal of undermined enamel and gaining access

Undermined enamel is easily removed with hand-cutting instrumentation, e.g., chisel, hatchet and/or Wedelstaedt. These instruments are self-limiting in cutting undermined enamel only, causing it to flake off in large chunks. Rotary instruments, in the form of carbide fissure burs, are seldom used for this purpose except for very thick undermined enamel. Eliminating this enamel may, in and of itself, facilitate the access. If it does not, the operator may proceed with one of the two previously described techniques (see Class II cavity preparation for amalgam).

B. Removal of carious dentin and placing intermediary basing

Decayed dentin is always removed using excavators, especially spoon-shaped excavators, and as soon as the cavity is cleared of these diseased tissues and double checked for its complete elimination, the proper intermediary base is applied and locked in place.

C. Defining the facial and lingual marginal and axial parameters of the extra-coronal portion of the preparation

At this stage, the operator should have some knowledge about the dimensions and condition of the remaining tooth structure, so the tooth preparation design can be positively identified. Using a # 3, 4, or 5 round bur or a ball-shaped diamond stone, gouge out the axial surface near the contemplated circumferential tie. This drilling should be to a depth that approximates the contemplated axial depth of the preparation. Several of these gougings may be made within the parameters of the extra-coronal preparation. They will serve as guides in the overall axial reduction.

D. Proximal reduction

If proximal reduction is needed extracoronally, it should be accomplished now. Use # 168 or 699 carbide burs in bucco-lingual actions, terminating shy of the gingival facial and lingual peripheries, but almost to the contemplated axial periphery of the preparation.

E. Gross removal of tooth structure

Using bullet-shaped cylindrical diamond stones on enamel and # 555, 556 or 701 carbide on dentin, grossly remove bulky areas of tooth structure, following the contemplated design configuration. However, this removal should stop distinctly short of the final location of preparation anatomy. Apply the same procedure to occlusal reduction to gain clearance of opposing contacts.

F. Preliminary shaping

Guided by the peripheral termination and the axial depth of the previous facial and lingual gouging, use tapered fissure burs or diamond stones, with or without rounded ends, to reduce the axial surface to the depth of the gouges. Cutting strokes should be preplanned in their starting and ending points, their angulations, and their direction of pressure. Rotary tools should be chosen, not only to create the reduction, but also to establish the planned preparation's configuration. At this stage, the periphery of the preparation should be established. Also, the axial (horizontal) and occlusal (vertical) reduction should be complete.

G. Boxing up

If the preparation is to have intracoronal features, now is the time to work on them. Using a tapered fissure bur, establish the walls proper, e.g., for cast alloy onlay, the inner (pulpal) half to two-thirds of the facial or lingual wall occlusally, the axial half of the facial and lingual walls proximally, and the axial half to two-thirds of the gingival floor proximally. If there will be any external boxes other than the proximal, this is the time to create the internal boxed-up dentin portion. Remember that this step establishes the most resistant and retentive feature of the preparation, so the angulation of the cutting tool is very influential in fulfilling the objectives of these features.

H. Formulation of cap and shoe anatomy

The rest of the details of the cap and shoe, if they are features in the preparation not created by the previous step, should be done now. Prepare occlusal bevels, counterbevels, tables and shoes, in that order. First use cylindrical diamond stones or tapered fissure burs; then the bevels and counterbevels are hollow-ground with a suitable size round carbide bur or ball-shaped diamond stone. In any cutting, follow cuspal and inclined plane anatomy.

I. Merging walls and bevels

At this stage, for cast ceramics (if indicated), merge the "wall proper" and occlusal bevels in one continuous concave plane, using a round or hour-glass shaped diamond stone.

J. Preparing auxiliary and reciprocal means of retention

At this point, the preparation exhibits most of its basic anatomy. Comprehensive evaluation of the mechanical problems of the future restoration should now be done. The most feasible auxiliary and reciprocal retention means should be decided upon. These may, in fact, differ from what was anticipated for use before this stage. These features, whether they be pin channels, boxes, skirts, reverse secondary flare, etc., should be added to the preparation now.

K. Establishing circumferential tie constituents

This step is accomplished first with the most gingival constituents, and then, proceeding occlusally establishing each constituent individually. Gingival bevels are best created with gingival margin trimmers. Primary and secondary flares are easily made with chisels or hatchets. Occlusal bevels are conveniently prepared by a cone-shaped aluminum oxide stone. A feather-edged finishing line is prepared with filamentous stone. A bevelled shoulder is conveniently prepared with a tapered fissure bur and a gingival margin trimmer or Wedelstaedt chisel.

A hollow-ground bevel can be prepared either with a torpedo-shaped stone or a bullet-shaped stone, followed by a round bur or ball-shaped stone. For the reverse secondary flare, the preparation can be done using a tapered-end diamond stone followed by hand instrumentation with a hatchet or binangle chisel.

L. Merging and establishing circumferential tie concavities

For preparations to accommodate cast ceramics, the merging of the circumferential tie and adjacent wall anatomy, forming a concave plane (if indicated), is done using an hour-glass shaped stone or a round diamond stone. The terminal concavity of the circumferential tie for Class IV and some Class III alloys is done using a round diamond stone. All concave and hollow-ground circumferential ties, should be further instrumented with lateral cutting hand instruments to eliminate remnants of frail enamel.

M. Final shaping

Final shaping is mainly done by hand instrumentation. As all the preparatin details are now present, it is time to give each of them its utmost shape without interfering with the configuration of the other details. For axial walls and surfaces, chisels, hatchets, and Wedelstaedts, in the proper angulation, can accomplish this. For floors, tables and shoes, and non-marginal bevels, Wedelstaedts or hatchets are very efficient. As each detail is being shaped properly, the junction between them is established in the most well defined, non stressing fashion, using angle formers, gingival margin trimmers and Wedelstaedt chisels.

N. Finishing and establishing the continuity between the circumferential tie constituents

As mentioned before, the results of this step are very influential for the success or failure of the cast restoration. Therefore, much time and effort should be spent here. In many instances this step is done after retracting the gingiva, if it is covering some or all of these constituents, for this improves access and prevents unnecessary traumas for the periodontium.

Smoothing of the tie can be done with the same hand instruments and finer-grit rotating tools as used to establish them in the first place. 12-fluted and sometimes 40-fluted carbide burs are useful. Also, fine-grit sand-paper discs, if access allows, can be used effectively. Establishing continuity between the circumferential tie constituents is best done by a Wedelstaedt chisel, binangle chisel, or any other sharp chisel. It should be accomplished meticulously, in the best possible configuration with the least amount of tooth structure reduction.

BIBLIOGRAPHY

Amorim, A., De Lima Navarro, M.F., Mondelli, J., and Lopes, E.S.: Influence of axiopulpal line angle and proximal retention on fracture strength of amalgam restorations. J. Prosth. Dent. **40**(2):169-173, Aug. 1978.

Baum, L., and Contino, R.M.: Ten years of experience with cast pin restorations, Dent. Clin. N. Amer. **14**:81, 1970.

Beheshti, N.: Fabricating a post and core to fit an existing crown. J. Prosth. Dent. **42**(2):236-239, Aug. 1979.

Chan, K.C., and Boyer, D.B.: Auxiliary retention for intracoronal cast gold restorations. J. Prosth. Dent. **44**(2):187-189, Aug. 1980.

Chan, K.C., Boyer, D.B., and Reinhardt, J.W.: Comparison of the retentive strength of two cast gold pin techniques. J. Prosth. Dent. **42**(5):527-529, Nov. 1979.

Chan, K.C., Khera, S.C., and Torney, D.L.: Cast gold restoration with self-threading pins. J. Prosth. Dent. **41**(3):296-298, March 1979.

Courtade, G.L., Sanell, C., and Mann, A.W.: Use of pins in restorative dentistry. Part II. Paralleling instruments. J. Prosth. Dent. **15**:691, 1965.

Courtade, G.L., and Timmermans, J.J.: Pins in restorative dentistry. St. Louis, 1971, The C.V. Mosby Co.

Goransson, P., and Embrell, A.: Parallel pins in gold restorations, Int. Coll. Dent. Bull. 3, 1970.

Goransson, P., and Parmlid, A.: A new paralleling instrument, Parmax II and the Kodex drills. J.P.D. 34, p. 34, July 1971.

Johnston, J.F., Phillips, R.W., and Dykema, R.W.: Modern practice in crown and bridge prosthodontics, ed. 3, Philadelphia, W.B. Saunders Co., 1971, p. 68.

Lovdahl, P.E., and Nicholls, J.I.: Pin-retained amalgam cores vs. cast-gold dowel-cores. J. Prosth. Dent. **38**(5):507-514, Nov. 1977.

Mann, A.W., Courtade, G.L., and Sanell, C.: Use of pins in restorative dentistry. Part I. Parallel pin retention obtained without using paralleling devices. J. Prosth. Dent. **15**:502, 1965.

Sanell, C.: Vertical parallel pins in occlusal rehabilitation. Dent. Clin. N. Amer., p. 755, 1963.

Sanell, C., Mann, A.W., and Courtade, G.L.: Use of pins in restorative dentistry. Part III. The use of paralleling instruments. J. Prosth. Dent. **16**:286, 1966.

Tylman, S.D.: Theory and practice of crown and fixed partial prosthodontics, ed. 6. St. Louis, The C.V. Mosby Co., 1970, p. 220.

CHAPTER 19

The biologic form and choice of materials for cast restorations

I. The Biologic Form

In evaluating cast restorations biologically, certain questions should be asked. The first: Are the restorations and the procedures to fabricate those restorations irritating to the P-D organ? The answer is definitely "yes". The irritating ingredients and characteristics, in addition to the cavity and tooth preparation and instrumentation, are the following:

A. Chemicals from some impression and temporary restorative materials—the unreacted chemicals (monomer) of temporary restorative materials and by-products of the hardening reaction of some impression materials (alcohol and ether) can be irritating to the P-D organ, especially at minimal effective depths.

B. Pressure used with certain impression materials, which, in addition to mechanically irritating the P-D organ (aspiration of odontoblastic elements), can drive superficially located microorganisms or chemicals into the P-D organ, if sufficient magnitude of force with penetrable effective depth is present.

C. Heat energy from certain impression materials or temporary restorative materials (e.g., the temperature of reversible hydrocolloid, exothermic heat from some impression materials and acrylic temporary materials), if transmitted to the pulp tissues, can establish some pathology.

D. Heat of electrical energy can be transmitted to the pulp tissues when electrosurgery is used in controlling the periodontium. The energy will irritate the pulp tissues if the electrode accidentally touches tooth structure or a metallic foundation.

E. Thermal conductivity of the cast alloys allows the transmission of temperature fluctuations in the oral environment to the pulp tissues.

F. Galvanism poses a potential for irritation, especially when the cast alloy restoration is statically or dynamically in contact with an amalgam restoration.

G. Hydraulic pressure during cementation of a casting can be of great magnitude, if the axial surface areas of the preparation are sizable. This hydraulic pressure will increase the penetrability of the cementing agents towards the pulp tissues, thus increasing their irritating capability. In addition, this hydraulic pressure can produce areas of energy concentration in vital dentin, precipitating the aspiration of odontoblastic elements in the dentinal tubules.

H. Cements, both for the temporary and for the final restoration, have irritating qualities that will be exaggerated by the hydraulic pressure of cementation.

I. Microleakage, if in sufficient dimensions, can allow irritating agents from the oral environment to permeate towards the pulp tissues.

J. The high abrasive resistance of cast restoratives materials precludes the possibility of occlusal prematurity being abraded back to a functional occlusion (as can happen with amalgam or composite resin). The subsequent occlusal trauma may initiate the strangulation of blood vessels at the tooth apex, leading to pulpal pathology.

K. The procedure of trying-in of several items on the preparation. This would include impressive materials, wax patterns, temporary restoratons as well as the casting itself. These procedures can introduce stresses and pulpal irritants to the P-D organ, both of which can create pulpal degeneration if in sufficient magnitude.

L. Burnishing the casting margin after cementation may require a lot of energy and friction which is expressed in the form of thermal and mechanical stresses in the underlying tooth structure. This may be very detrimental if the margins being burnished are cervical in location with a very limited effective depth from the pulp chamber and root canal system.

M. Pins incorporated in pinlays, with their attendant procedures, will precipitate irritation in the P-D organ.

N. The heat of polishing marginal and adjusted areas in the restoration after cementation can adversely affect the pulpdentin organ.

In addition to the irritants previously mentioned, the new alloys have the following hazards:

Alloys containing nickel are a possible hazard insofar as nickel is the most potent allergen of all metals and is considered to be carcinogenic. However, its presence in a cast alloy is in a combination form, alloyed with chromium and other metals. It is doubtful that a sufficient amount of metal would be able to diffuse to surrounding tissues to create considerable pathology, but allergic reactions from nickel-containing restorations have been reported. It is a good idea prior to fabricating a nickel-containing alloy to have the patient tested for a nickel allergy by means of a skin patch test.

Beryllium, which was used in some base metal alloys to improve castability, is responsible for a chronic beryllium disease which affects the respiratory system. Technicians who would grind the metal were the most susceptible. No cases have been reported with patients wearing dental restorations containing beryllium. At any rate, beryllium is no longer used in cast alloys. Chromium, in a pure state, has also been reported as being responsible for the creation of skin lesions, if in direct contact with the skin.

It should be mentioned that, to the credit of nickel and chromium, they have been used in alloys for partial dentures since the late 40's with great biologic and mechanical success. Also, nickel-based and chromium-based alloys have been used extensively in the general population and in direct contact with body tissues with few problems. Growing numbers of orthopedic surgeons are using nickel and chromium-based alloy implants in bone tissues. It can be stated with confidence that these alloys are applicable and useful for dentistry. Testing for allergy should be performed prior to use to assure safe reactions. As for cast moldable ceramics they are the least toxic of all restorative materials.

The second biologic question should be: What are the effects of cementated castings at different effective depths?

1. Although the irritating variables here are greater than with any other restorative material or procedure, the following figures are drawn from experiments done on intact vital teeth that were prepared for casting. These castings were cemented with zinc phosphate cement without any intermediary basing material. Although the results do not show the exact situation clinically, they provide information that may serve as a guide in prescribing the intermediary basing material and cementing procedure.

2. An effective depth of 3.5 mm or greater usually resulted in a healthy reparative reaction with rare occurrences of unhealthy reparative reactions.

3. An effective depth from 2.5 to 3.5 mm resulted in an unhealthy reparative reaction or, infrequently, destruction.

4. With an effective depth of less than 1.5 mm, there was destruction within the P-D organ.

Intermediary Basing for the Protection of the Pulp-Dentin Organ Against Cast Restorations

Presently the two major cementing agents are zinc phosphate cement and polycarboxylate cement (ASPA may soon become the third). ZOE cements are used for temporary cementation. Our discussion here will be concentrated on the first two, insofar as ZOE is considered non-irritant in any effective depth, and because of its temporary nature. ASPA, although not yet properly tested, can be used in the same circumstances with similar effects as poly-carboxylate cement.

A. Cementing with zinc phosphate cement

1. If the effective depth is 3.5 mm or more, only varnish is used on all enamel and dentinal walls prior to cementation.

2. If the effective depth is 2-3.5 mm, a base of polycarboxylate cement, or varnish and zinc phosphate cement, is required before taking the impression or the direct wax pattern. Both cements should be inserted in a base consistency (thick) and properly locked. Prior to cementation, varnish all dentinal and enamel walls.

3. If the effective depth is less than 2 mm, before taking the impression or direct wax pattern, use a subbase of calcium hydroxide or unmodified ZOE (according to location and condition of the P-D organ), followed by varnish and a base of zinc phosphate cement. A base of polycarboxylate cement can

be used only over a calcium hydroxide subbase with no varnish. Before cementation, use varnish overal all dentin and enamel walls.

B. Cementing with polycarboxylate or A.S.P.A. cement

1. If there is an effective depth of 2 mm or more, cement directly, i.e., use no intervening varnish.

2. If the effective depth is 1-2 mm, before taking the impression or the direct wax pattern, use a base of polycarboxylate cement (ASPA) (base consistency). Then, when the cast is ready, cement directly.

3. If the effective depth is less than 1 mm, before taking the impression or the direct wax pattern, use a subbase of calcium hydroxide or unmodified ZOE. The calcium hydroxide subbase can be covered with P.C.C. (A.S.P.A) base, but the ZOE sub-base has to be covered with varnish and a zinc phosphate cement base. When the cast is ready, cement directly. P.C.C. or A.S.P.A can replace Z.P.C. in situations indicated for its use, but Z.P.C. cannot replace P.C.C. or A.S.P.A. in situations indicated for their use.

The subbases and bases that are placed in the preparation before taking the impression or the direct wax pattern should be properly retained, so as not to be disturbed by the manipulative action of a cast fabrication procedure. That is why a crevice or a small undercut should be prepared in the surrounding walls of the area in the preparation to receive the intermediary base and/or subbase. A small round bur (¼ or ½) is effective in preparing such a locking mechanism.

It is imperative that concavities or deep areas indicated for basing be appropriately treated prior to taking the impression. Under no circumstances should the impression be taken first, with the areas requiring basing being obliterated on the die, allowing the cementing medium to then act as the base at cementation. There are several reasons to avoid this procedure.

a. The cementing consistency of the cementing agent is very thin, containing far more irritating ingredients than the base consistency. So, in conjunction with hydraulic pressure, these ingredients can drastically change the biologic reaction of the P-D organ, enhancing the possibility of pulpal destruction.

b. The presence of concavities or deep areas in the preparation distort the impression, since they are usually undercuts with possibilities of altering the impression materials path of insertion and withdrawal which leads to a misfit final casting.

c. Delicate subbases can be displaced, if placed just prior to casting cementation, allowing the hydraulically driven cementing medium to be the base.

II. Material Choice For a Cast Restoration

Several years ago the choice of an alloy for a cast restoration was simple, insofar as there was no other choice than the four types of gold alloy. At the present time, however, the choice is made difficult not only due to the various alloys available to the profession, but also to the availability of cast ceramics. It is the dentist's duty both to understand the properties of the cast materials used, and to prepare the teeth and manipulate the materials to get the most out of them. It is also our professional responsibility to inform the patient of the advantages and possible drawbacks of the material used and the measures required by the dentist and patient to prevent any shortcomings from making the restoration a failure.

Without doubt, gold alloys maintain several advantages primarily because the technique for fabricating a cast restoration in a gold alloy has been perfected over the years. This does not mean that newer materials are not suitable for oral use. It is fair to say that they still have a long way to go to arrive to the current status of gold alloys. It is a grave mistake to try to apply gold alloy techniques to fabricate restorations from these newer materials, especially Class IV and V materials.

Class I alloys (gold alloys) are usually indicated when the casting has lengthy margins with the possibility of marginal discrepancies, even with the most meticulous technique. The burnishability of these types of gold alloys makes it easy to adjust these margins after fabricating the casting.

When using a Class I alloy for a single tooth restoration, if the casting is going to be subjected to normal and above normal type of loading, type III gold alloys are the ideal alloys to use. Type II gold alloys are used only in smaller castings and in areas of normal and less than normal loading.

Type I gold alloys are seldom used. They are indicated for use in areas with no direct occlusal loading, e.g., Class V and III restorations. The softness of the alloy makes it easy to adapt the margins properly at these locations. Type IV gold alloys are rarely used in single tooth restorations, but may be indicated if the casting will be carrying an attachment for a partial denture, or if it is a part of a long splint, i.e., the casting will be subjected to unusually high loading situations.

In evaluating Class II alloys, present clinical data reveal that there is little different between them and Class I alloys. The major difference is in their tarnish and corrosion resistance, especially when the gold content gets lower than 40%. Therefore, they can be used in lieu of high gold alloys in areas with low corrosion activity, but the patient should be advised of what to expect. The tooth preparation and cast fabrication are no different than those for Class I alloys, and these alloys are definitely much less expensive than Class I alloys.

In selecting Class III and IV alloys, the decision could be difficult to make, and the patient should be consulted. Both are definitely workable and serviceable alloys for use in the mouth, if the tooth condition, oral environment, and the patient as a whole will allow. These alloys can substantially reduce the cost of a cast restoration. With our present technology these two types of alloys can be used for restorations, if:

A. Tooth structure will permit preparing bulky circumferential tie constituents, preferably hollow-ground bevels and bevelled shoulders.

B. The tooth condition will permit more sizable axial reduction than that for gold alloys for extracoronal preparation of the tooth.

C. Very thin cross-section details in the casting can be avoided, such as thin reverse secondary flares, delicate internal boxes or very small cast pins.

D. Margins can be placed in a highly self-cleansable, reachable and reproduceable area, because there is no allowance for post-fabrication cast margin adjustment.

If these four criteria are feasible, there will be no objection to use either of these two types of alloy. However, a patient receiving a Class III cast alloy should be screened to insure that the oral environment has minimum corrosion activity (verified by evaluating any amalgam restorations that are present), that their diet does not contain excessive amounts of sulfurous food, and that the contemplated restoration will not be in contact with an amalgam restoration either statically or dynamically. The patient to receive these silver-palladium alloys should be required to have periodic polishing of the restoration with their routine check-up prophylaxis visit.

For patients receiving Class IV alloys, there is no need for such screening. The only additional instruction would be to tell the patient that they must have their occlusion checked periodically, which may require occasional occlusal equilibration. (This may also be true of Class III alloys, but to a much lesser extent).

If esthetics are important, i.e., the tooth to be restored is an anterior or is conspicuous to the viewer, cast ceramics could be the ideal cast material provided that the remaining tooth structure is bulky enough to accommodate the required depth of axial reduction and pronounced finishing lines, and long enough occluso-apically to allow more surface area for retention which may be deficient due to the roundness of the internal parts of the preparation. Cast ceramics are also indicated for areas in the mouth where plaque control measures are difficult to apply.

BIBLIOGRAPHY

Brannstrom, M.: Dentinal and pulpal response. I. Application of reduced pressure to exposed dentin. Acta Odont. Scand. **18**:1, 1960.

Brannstrom, M.: Cavity preparation and the pulp. Dent. Prog. **2**:4, 1961.

British Dental Journal 144: (11) 345-350. Pulpal response to a glass ionomer cement. Tobias, R.S., et al.

Gettleman, L., Nathanson, D., Shklar, G., Brathwaite, W.J., Jr., Darmiento, L., Levine, P., and Judes, H.: Preliminary evaluation of the histotoxicity and radiopacity of lead-containing elastic impression materials. J. Am. Dent. Assoc. **96**(6):987-993, June 1978.

Hensten-Pettersen, A., and Jacobsen, N.: Nickel corrosion of non-precious casting alloys and the cytotoxic effect of nickel in vitro. J. Bioeng. **2**(5):419-425, 1978.

Johnson, L.B., and Cutler, G.S.: Large quantities of dental alloys by splat cooling. J. Biomed. Mater. Res. **12**(6):939-940, Nov. 1978.

Marx, J.J., Jr., and Burrel, R.: Delayed hypersensitivity to berryllium compounds. J. Immunology **3**:590-598, 1973.

Mitchell, D.F., Shankwalker, G.B., and Shazer, S.: Determing the turmorigenicity of dental materials. J. Dent. Res. **39**:1023-1028, 1960.

Piliero, S.J., Carson, S., Licalzi, M., Pentel, L., Piliero, J.A., and others: Biocompatibility evaluation of casting alloys in hamsters. J. Prosth. Dent. **41**(2):220-223, Feb. 1979.

Sandrik, J.L., Kaminski, E.J., and Greener, E.H.: Biocompatibility of nickel-base dental alloys. Biomater. Med. Devices Artif. Organs **2**:31, 1974.

CHAPTER 20

Techniques and rationale for control of the periodontium preparatory to cast fabrication

Frequently the gingival peripheries of a preparation come close to or in contact with the gingiva. It is essential then, to have the following features present in the gingiva and underlying periodontium, prior to taking the impression or direct wax pattern, or to allow for adequate preparation of the circumferential tie constituents.

A. The crest of the free gingiva is at its normal healthy position relative to the tooth surface with no anticipated recession. This may necessitate cutting of hyperplastic gingival tissues if present.

B. The periodontium should be sound or undergoing healthy healing prior to a tooth preparation.

C. The free gingiva should be temporarily reduced in dimension, to expose the gingival termination of the preparation for final adjustments and proper reproduction of its details. This temporary reduction should be done in a way so that the free gingiva will regain its dimensions after completion of these procedures.

D. Crevicular fluids and bleeding from the gingiva and its crevicular walls should be completely arrested, so as not to interfere with the proper vision, manipulation, and reproduction of the details of the circumferential tie.

E. Consequently, a temporary trough (Fig. 1) in the gingival crevice should be created, which is devoid of any fluid, readily accessible, and which exposes all the details of the circumferential tie as well as a portion of the unprepared tooth surface apical to it.

F. These objectives should be accomplished without any detachment of the apically located epithelium attachment and periodontal ligaments. They should not induce irreversible trauma to the free gingiva, walls of the gingival sulcus, or any part of the periodontium. Any local temporary changes will be resolved by healthy healing via primary intention.

G. These objectives will also not generate hazards or undesirable effect on distant tissues or organs, orally, para-orally or systemically.

There are four means of accomplishing these objectives, and they are frequently used in combination.

I. Physico-Mechanical Means

This constitutes mechanically forcing the gingiva away from the tooth surface, laterally and apically. It is most frequently indicated for absolutely healthy gingivae which will have a

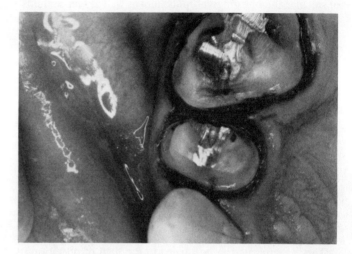

Fig. 20-1

very good vascular supply and a definite zone of attached gingivae apical to the free gingivae to be displaced. Bone support should be of adequate dimension with no signs of resorption. Usually one of three general techniques is used:

A. The use of a custom temporary restoration, with its gingival ends blunted and covered with bulky temporary cements like ZOE or non-eugenol periodontal pack, has results which cannot be observed for at least 24 hours.

B. The use of rolled cotton or synthetic cords which are forcibly introduced into the gingival sulcus has results which are achieved in 30 min. or less.

C. The use of heavy weight rubber dam with proper interceptal dimensions, which necessitate multiple tooth isolation, has an effect which is immediate. Procedures should be done while the dam is on, not after removal. Full arch impressions are difficult. Single tooth or quadrant impressions only are feasible with this technique.

II. Chemical Means

These constitute the most universally used technique. A variety of chemicals are available, but each will fall under one of three categories:

A. Vasoconstrictors physiologically restrict the blood supply to the area by decreasing the size of the blood capillaries, thus decreasing hemorrhage, tissue fluid seepage, and consequently the size of the free gingiva. The agents most frequently used are racemic epinepherine and non-epinepherine. Their use should be very limited because of their systemic effects on patients with potential middle and old age diseases (e.g., cardiovascular disease, diabetes, etc.). These patients are the predominate candidates for cast restorations.

B. Biologic fluid coagulants coagulate blood and tissue fluids locally, creating surface layer that is an efficient sealant against blood and crevicular fluid seepage. These are very safe agents, insofar as they induce no systemic effects. Examples of the agents producing these effects are: 100% alum, 15-25% aluminum chloride, 10% aluminum potassium sulfate and 15-25% tannic acid.

C. Surface layer tissue coagulants coagulate surface layer of sulcular and free gingival epithelium as well as seeped fluids, thus creating temporarily impenetrable film for underlying fluids (including blood). There are some local hazards when using these chemicals, e.g., ulceration, local necrosis, and changes in the dimension and location of the free gingiva. This can happen as a result of an excessive amount and/or concentration or excessive time in application of the agents. Examples of these chemicals are 8% zinc chloride and silver nitrate.

There are numerous commercial products available that have combinations of these basic chemicals. Before using them you should know the ingredients and under what category they fall. Then evaluate the local conditions of the periodontium, systemic conditions of the patient, and the goals you want from these chemicals. Generally speaking, these agents should be procurred in their generic structure. They then may be used individually, in combination prior to use, or in combination in the gingival sulcus, as conditions dictate.

These chemicals can be carried to the field of operation in one of three ways.

1. Cords

These are ready-made cotton or synthetic woven cords, some have a metallic or resin wire wrapped around them to assure their compactness, immobility, and non-shredding. They come in different sizes, arbitrarily numbered by their manufacturers. They may be supplied already impregnated with the chemical, or the chemical may be added before insertion of the cord or after insertion while the cord is within the sulcus. The main advantage of this type of carrier is that it is fairly non-adhesive to the affected tissues because of its compactness. The main disadvantage is the possible difficulty in inserting them into the sulcus.

2. Drawn cotton rolls (Fig 2)

Soft loose cotton rolls can be readily rolled to a desired diameter. They are then introduced in the sulcus, already impregnated or to be impregnated with the chemical. The advantage of this type of carrier is that because of its looseness, it can be compacted in the sulcus easier than the cords. Its disadvantage is that part of the coagulated sealing layer on the sulcus wall may be deeply incorporated in the cotton. When the cotton is removed, the coagulated sealing membrane may be peeled off, initiating bleeding and fluid seepage which can be more vigorous than before. Drawn cotton rolls are always used subsequent to cords after the treated cords create this coagulated sealing membrane. They are very efficient in widening the trough and generating more shrinkage within the free gingiva, because they can accommodate more chemicals than the cords.

3. Cotton pellets (Fig 2)

Cotton pellets are used to carry the chemical to the already compacted inserted cord or drawn cotton rolls. If allowed to remain on top of the inserted items, they provide a continuous source of the chemical.

In inserting the cords or drawn cotton rolls there are certain rules:

a. Start with a well-compacted, completely-woven cord or a drawn cotton roll.

b. The exact length to be incorpoated in the sulcus should be precut. An excess may lead to displacement of already packed portions, and it is very difficult to add lengths in inaccessible areas. It is a good idea to measure the tooth diameter before cutting the cord.

c. If using several inserts in the sulcus, start with the smallest diameter followed by larger ones, until the sulcus is filled and brought to the desired dimensions.

d. Always start packing at one end of the cord, systematically going to the other end, being sure that the packed part of the cord (drawn cotton roll) is stable in place before packing the next part.

e. Avoid putting the ends of the cord (drawn cotton roll) interproximally. The ideal location is at the axial angles of the tooth, where the interdental col has its maximal height, creating better gripping and stabilization of the packed cord.

f. The packing instrument should be blunt, with definite corners, hatchet or hoe-shaped, preferably with serrations. You should have different sizes to accommodate different locations within the same sulcus (the deeper parts require a smaller packer than the superficial parts) and different sizes of sulci.

g. Always use steady static loading directed apically and angulated slightly towards the tooth surface. The amount of force applied is a matter of judgement. Every area of the periodontium, every tooth, and every individual require different packing forces, so as not to strip the tooth out of its periodontal attachment or injure the periodontium.

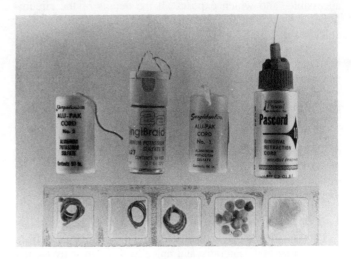

Fig. 20-2

h. In shallow sulci or thin, unfirm free gingiva (e.g., adjacent to bony eminentia), there may be difficulty keeping the items being packed in place. In this case, after inserting one end of the cord (drawn cotton roll), stabilize it with a blunt instrument which the assistant may keep holding during packing the remainder of the cord.

i. When removing the packed material, it should always be done in a hydrous field, so that the moisture will act as a lubricant between the cord and the sealing film. Disturbing this film or peeling it off will start profuse bleeding. The packed material should be removed very slowly and gently.

j. It is a good idea to flush the created trough with the chemical solution via a blunt hypodermic syringe, provided the solution is a non-vasoconstrictor or does not possess systemic effects.

k. If the packed material does not interfere with the reproduction of the circumferential tie and the tooth surface immediately apical to it, and if it is immobile in its location, it can be allowed to remain during the impression or direct wax pattern.

l. After reproducing the details in an impression or direct wax pattern, remove any remaining packed items, curette the field, removing films of coagulated materials, and create a healthy blood clot.

m. For healthy healing of the peridontium a favorable environment should be provided through the fabrication of an adequate temporary restoration and efficient plaque control measures.

III. Electrosurgical Means (Fig. 3, A and B)

It is not within the domain of this book to give complete details of electrosurgery and its techniques. Suffice it to say, however, that it is becoming a very popular and applicable procedure given our greater understanding of its mechanisms, actions, and its effects on the periodontal tissues.

Generally speaking, ordinary alternating current electric energy is passed through a certain apparatus (Fig. 3A) to substantially increase its frequency (from 60 to 120 to a million and more per second). The current at this extremely high velocity will pass through human bodies without inducing shocks. The idea is to concentrate this energy at tiny electrodes, producing extremely localized changes in the tissues, changes which can be confined to as little as 2-3 cell layers.

Four types of actions can be produced at the electrode end:

A. Cutting

This is extremely precise, bloodless, with minimal tissue involvement and after-effects, if properly controlled and executed.

B. Coagulation

This creates surface coagulation of tissues, their fluids and oozed blood; the effect is due to the thermal energy introduced. If overdone, it will be accompanied by carbonization.

C. Fulgeration

Because of the greater energy used, fulgeration has deeper tissue involvement. It is always accompanied by carbonization, and is less limited in its after-effect than cutting and coagulation.

D. Desiccation

It includes massive tissue involvement both in terms of depth and surface area. It is the most unlimited and uncontrolled of all four actions. Tissue reactions are unpredictable most of the time.

For fulgeration and dessication bi-polar electrodes are required, while cutting and coagulation require a uni-polar electrode.

The type of electrosurgery is dictated by the electric variables involved, i.e., frequency, conduction, size and shape of the electrode, electricity input and output, etc. At any rate, for our purposes, cutting and, very rarely, coagulation are employed.

There are certain general rules to be followed in using electrosurgery for creating a sulcular trough and controlling moisture and blood contents.

1. The tooth and the adjacent area are to be properly isolated, with only minimal moisture content. Avoid complete

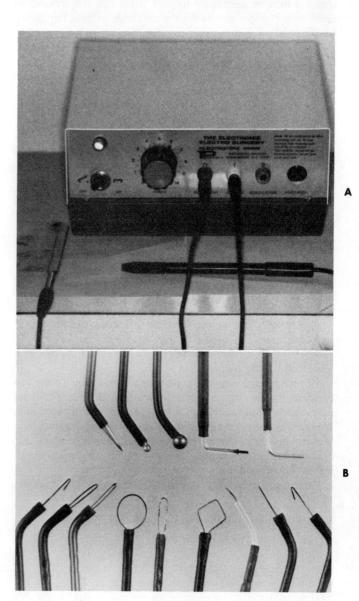

Fig. 20-3

drying of the area as electrosurgery current applied on highly dried tissues can be very detrimental.

2. The patient should be adequately conducting to avoid using hazardous excessive electric energy.

3. Use only fully rectified, undampened, filtered current with the minimum energy output required for the desired purpose. Logically, the output is proportional to the dimensions of the tissues to be removed, the type of action employed (e.g., coagulation needs more energy than cutting), and the proximity of critical anatomy.

4. For cutting, extremely shallow involvement of the sulcular epithelium should be observed. Use light touches and rapid intermittent strokes until the desired size of sulcular trough is created. Never involve the crest of the free gingiva in the cutting line of the electrode. Always keep the cutting in the internal walls of the sulcus, as involving the crest will definitely lead to loss of gingival height, i.e., recession. Sometimes it may be necessary to pack a cord in the crevice, in order to get proper access for the electrode without impinging on the crest.

Probe type of electrodes and occasionally J- or loop-shapes (Fig. 3B) are suitable for this. For the removal of hypertrophied hyperplastic gingival tissues, the cutting line is estimated and the electrode is passed in the same manner, as mentioned above, through that estimated line until the tissues are released. Cutting is usually associated with surface hemostasis.

5. For coagulation, specially shaped bulky electrodes (Fig. 3B) are used with a partially rectified, partially damped output from the apparatus. The electrodes are brought very close to, barely in contact with the tissues to be hemostasized. Immediate surface coagulation will occur, mostly in the oozing fluids, with several areas of localized carbonization, creating a sealing film on the tissues.

6. The tooth metallic restorations should not be touched. This can create a short circuit through structures not intended for involvement.

7. Never approach the attaching epithelium or periodontal ligament with the electrodes. The separation that may occur will be permanent.

8. Always clean debris from the electrodes using alcohol soaked gauze.

9. If sparks appear, this means that the electricity output is too much for the purpose.

10. After adjusting and capturing all the details of the circumferential tie, the involved tissues should be curetted, removing any films that have formed creating a fresh blood clot. If bone has been exposed or any of the attaching apparatus has been involved, a suture and a perio pack should be applied to enhance healing. Create as favorable an environment for healing of the periodontium as possible.

Electrosurgery is a very valid technique which produces amazingly good results if performed with a good understanding of its scientific basis.

IV. Surgical Means

Use a sharp, cold knife, which is not different from the regular periodontal or oral surgery. It is needed only in cases of interfering and unneeded gingival tissues to be surgically removed. Also, it is used for apical repositioning of the whole periodontal attaching apparatus to create a healthy, safely manipulated, easily retracted free gingiva, etc. Understandably, after healing of the surgical wound, the gingiva is going to be handled in one or combinations of more than one of the previously mentioned ways to arrive to the objectives mentioned at the beginning of this section.

BIBLIOGRAPHY

Anneroth, G., and Nordenram, A.: Reaction of the gingiva to the application of threads in the gingival pocket for taking impressions with elastic material. Odontol. Revy **20**:301, 1969.

Barkmeier, W.W., and Williams H.J.: Surgical methods of gingival retraction for restorative dentistry. J. Am. Dent. Assn. **96**(6):1002-1007, June 1978.

Bejamin, S.D., and Colman, H.L.: Periodontal considerations in gingival retraction procedures. J. South Calif. State Dent. Assn. **38**(9):823-826, Sept. 1970.

Bull, A.W., and Brinsden, G.I.: Gingival tissue retraction for the elastic impression materials. Aust. Dent. J. **12**(4):310-313, Aug. 1967.

Dilts, W.E.: Comparisons of clinical techniques in tissue retraction. J. Okla. State Dent. Assn. **64**(4):11-13, April 1974.

Donaldson, D.: Gingival recession associated with temporary crowns. J. Periodont. **44**:691, 1973.

Eisenmann, D., Malone, W.F., and Kusek, J.: Electron microscopic evaluation of electrosurgery. Oral Surg. **29**:660, 1970.

Harrison, J.D.: Effect of retraction materials on the gingival sulcus epithelium. J. Prosth. Dent. **11**:514, 1961.

Klug, R.G.: Gingival tissue regeneration following electrical retraction. J. Prosth. Dent. **16**(5):955-962, Sept.-Oct. 1966.

Loe, H., and Silness, J.: Tissue reactions to string packs used in fixed restorations. J. Prosth. Dent. **13**:318, 1963.

Nixon, K.C., Adkins, K.F., and Keys, D.W.: Histological evaluation of effects produced in alveolar bone following gingival incision with an electrosurgical scalpel. J. Peridontol. **46**:40, 1975.

Pelzner, R.B., Kempler, D., Start, M.M., Lum, L.B., Nicholson, R.J., and Soelberg, K.B.: Human blood presure and pulse rate response to racemic epinephrine retraction cord. J. Prosthet. Dent. **39**(3):287-292, March 1978.

Pope, J.W., Gargiulo, A.W., Staffileno, H., and Levy, S.: Effects of electrosurgery on wound healing in dogs. Periodontics **6**:30, 1968.

Shaw, D.H., Krejci, R.F., and Cohen, D.M.: Retraction cords with aluminum chloride: Effect on the gingiva. Oper. Dent. **5**(4):138-141, Autumn 1980.

Stark, M.M., Nicholson, D.J., Soelberg, K.B., Kempler, D., and Pelzner, R.B.: The effects of retraction cords and electrosurgery upon blood pressure and tissue regeneration in rhesus monkeys. J. Dent. Res. **56**(8):881-888, Aug. 1977.

Wilson, C.A., and Tay, W.M.: Alum solution as an adjunct to gingival retraction. A clinical evaluation. Br. Dent. J. **142**(5):155-158, March 1, 1977.

Woychesin, F.F.: An evaluation of the drugs used for gingival retraction. J. Prosthet. Dent. **14**:769, 1964.

Xhonga, F.A.: Gingival retraction techniques and their healing effect on the gingiva. J. Prosthet. Dent. **26**(6):640-648, Dec. 1971.

CHAPTER 21

Impressions for cast fabrications

The indirect technique for fabricating cast restorations is the most common technique now in use. This is due to the vast improvement in impression materials in the past thirty years. The main purpose of this procedure is to capture in a suitable material all details necessary to build an accurate model of the prepared tooth and intraoral tissues. Impressions for indirect fabrication of cast restorations should have the following objectives:

1. They should record the most finite details of the tooth preparation in the impression material.

2. They should duplicate unprepared surface areas beyond the peripheries of the preparation. These duplicated areas should be of sufficient dimension to help in creating the proper contour of the future restoration.

3. They should duplicate the surface anatomy of the adjacent and opposing teeth, preferably in a whole arch to insure reasonable and workable contacting anatomy of the future restoration.

4. They should duplicate the surface anatomy of adjacent soft tissues, especially the gingiva (attached and free), facial and lingual sulci, and interdental col, so as to build a restoration morphologically compatible with them.

5. They should be able to maintain these details unchanged during the subsequent steps and waiting periods until the details are reproduced in the working model (cast) and die.

6. They should perform all these objectives, while employing the least amount of time, equipment and untowards effects on the vital dental tissues, future die, model materials, and operator.

To fulfill these objectives, there are six types of materials from which to choose. They are:

a. Reversible agar hydrocolloid
b. Irreversible alginate hydrocolloid
c. Polysulfide rubber base
d. Condensation polymerization silicone rubber base
e. Additional polymerization silicone rubber base
f. Polyether rubber bases.

Prior to using them clinically, the operator should have a comprehensive grasp of their advantages and liabilities. The following is a brief comparison between these materials.

I. Composition and Setting Reaction

A. Reversible agar-agar hydrocolloid materials are formed mostly of water (80-87%), which is the dispersion phase of the colloidal system of the material. The dispersed phase is agar-agar. This occurs naturally as metabolite of sea weed; chemically, it is a sulfuric acid ester of a linear polymer of the polysaccharide galactose. It comprises 8-15%.

A sol state of the material is produced by heating. It occurs as a result of thermally vibrating the polymer molecules of the agar, increasing their kinking activity and breaking the weak secondary bonding holding them together. A gel state is produced by cooling, which creates a fairly solid mass. In the gel state the poorly joined agar molecules will create a fairly porous mesh-work, into which the dispersion phase (water) will be absorbed. This is the set mass. The material is introduced and brought in contact with the details to be duplicated in a sol state, then gelled by cooling. After a specified period of time, it is removed in the gel state. The agar and water relation plays the major role in dictating the behavior of the material. To these two basic ingredients several additives may be incorporated to improve the material's properties.

1. Borax is added to improve the quality and strength of the secondary bonding between the agar macromolecules.

2. Potassium sulfate: Borax, water and agar are retarders for the setting of gypsum. Since gypsum (in the form of dental stone) is necessary to fill the impression to create a die or model, potassium sulfate is added to counteract this retardation by accelerating the setting of the gypsum.

3. Some bactericidal and antifungal agents are added to interfere with the growth of those microorganisms in the agar-agar medium.

4. Flavoring and coloring agents are added to improve the workability, patient's acceptability, and use of the materials.

5. The material in the above described form can be injected, but for use in a tray it must have more bulk and viscosity. To achieve this, fillers are added according to the consistency desired. They may be diatomacious earth or silica.

B. Irreversible alginate hydrocolloid in the form of a powder and a liquid

1. Powder

The reacting ingredients are: sodium (potassium or ammonium) alginate (12-18%); calcium sulfate dihydrate (12-15%); and sodium phosphate (2-3%).

2. The liquid is water.

When the liquid is mixed with the powder, a sodium alginate sol is formed, as it is soluble in water. It soon reacts with calcium sulfate dihydrate, precipitating the gel structure of calcium alginate, which has the same morphology as the agar-

agar gel. However, the bonding here is primary and strong.

Since the reaction can occur very fast, sodium phosphate is incorporated to retard the reaction. This is because calcium sulfate dihydrate has a greater preference to sodium phosphate than to the sodium alginate. The time used to consume the sodium phosphate translates as additional working time. Also, if the reaction goes to completion, i.e., all the sodium alginate is transformed to calcium alginate, the produced mass will be too solid for dental use. So the remaining calcium sulfate dihydrate, after reacting with sodium phosphate, should be in such an amount to make the gel conversion incomplete. Thus the mass will be reasonably elastic.

To these basic ingredients potassium sulfate is added for the same purposes, as in agar-agar hydrocolloid.

The same types of fillers are used as in reversible hydrocolloid, but they occupy the maximum space in the mass, approximately 60-74%. Because of this high filler content, alginate does not have consistency that allows it to be syringe-injected.

Some coloring and flavoring agents may be added to enhance its workability and use.

C. Polysulfide rubber base materials

The end product of this material is a classical elastomer. It is composed of highly kinking long coiled macromolecules with intermolecular secondary bonding. The intramolecular bonding is covalent. The basic ingredients responsible for the reaction are a polyfunctional mercaptane polymer, sulfur, and lead peroxide. The reaction has a liquid polyfunctional sulfur containing mercaptane polymer, undergoing condensation polymerization when it encounters lead peroxide. The condensation polymerizaton reaction leads to lengthening of the original macromolecules and periodic (but not complete) cross-linkage, giving a rubbery elastomeric mass with water as a by-product of the reaction.

To these basic ingredients, fillers, in the form of zinc oxide, colloidal silica, titanium dioxide (whitener), etc, are added to create the paste or the putty form in which they are supplied. Some retardants for the reaction are added (oleic or stearic acid) which interfere with lengthening and/or cross-linkage.

The material is supplied in four forms, according to its viscosity (consistency). The difference is dictated by the amount, shape, and type of fillers. These four forms are: light-injectable, regular, heavy-tray, and putty forming, which is the thickest of them all. Every form has a specific use as will be mentioned later. The material is always supplied in a two-paste system: one is called the base paste (lighter color) and it contains the liquid polymer, fillers, retardants, and some sulfur; the other is called the catalyst or reactant paste (darker color), and it contains lead peroxide fillers, flavoring, and deodorizing agents.

D. Additional polymerization silicone rubber base materials

The product is also an elastomer, but the bonding is different than the polysulfide rubber base as it is ionic. The base ingredient is a polysiloxane, which is a liquid polymer with silane terminal groups. This small size, low molecular weight polymer can undergo additional polymerization with no by-products when catalyzed by a chloroplatinic acid catalyst in the presence of a liquid polymer containing available terminal vinyl groups.

The original macromolecules will lengthen and cross-link producing the rubbery elastomeric material.

To these basic ingredients there are added fillers and coloring agents. The size, shape, and surface treatment of these fillers are very critical in the behavior of the material, since the affinity of the formed macromolecules to each other is not as strong as with polysulfide rubber base. So the fillers or any additive should be as wettable and compatible with the macromolecules as possible.

According to their consistencies, the material is supplied in four forms, as the polysulfide rubber base. The only difference between one form and another is in the amount, type, and shape of the fillers. The base paste always contains the polysiloxane and fillers. The catalyst (accelerator) paste contains the vinyl polymer, the chloroplatinic acid catalyst, fillers, and coloring agents.

E. Condensation-polymerization silicone rubber base materials

The main ingredient here is a liquid polymer of dimethylpolysiloxane, whose reactive terminal is a hydroxyl group. The polymer macromolecules undergo lengthening and cross-linkage by a condensation-polymerization process, when brought in contact with a catalyst of tin-octoate in the presence of an alkyle silicate (ethyl silicate), forming a rubbery elastomer. As a result of the condensation polymerization, an alcohol will be a by-product (ethyl alcohol). This material, like the previous two, is supplied in four different consistencies. The base paste contains the dimethyl-polysiloxane and fillers. The catalyst paste contains the ethyl silicate, tin-octeate, fillers, and coloring agents.

As with the additional polymerization silicone rubber bases, the filler shape, size, type and surface treatment are very critical for the cohesion and behavior of the mass. Sometimes the material is supplied in a base paste. The catalyst and ethyl silicate are supplied in separate tubes (bottles) or combined together to be added to the base paste in drops, then mixed to facilitate the reaction.

F. Polyether rubber bases

Its final product is also an elastomer, but with less coiling and more bonding between its polymer macromolecules. The basic ingredient is a liquid polyether polymer, with a small molecular weight and size. The polymer macromolecules have imine rings terminal groups. A condensation-polymerization will start (cationic polymerication) when the base polymer is incorporated with a dichlorobenzine sulfonate catalyst, forming a more rigid elastomer than those previously described. The by-product is a very complex alcohol. To improve the plasticity of the end product, a plasticizer is always included in the form of glyco-ether phthalate. The material is supplied in one form only, regular consistency. The base paste contains the base polyether liquid polymer, fillers, and plasticizers. The catalyst paste contains the catalyst, plasticizer, fillers and coloring agents.

II. Dimensional and Shape Stability

A. Setting shrinkage

All six materials shrink slightly during the change from the liquid to the rubbery status. This is understandable, due to the increased proximity and bonding between the formed macro-molecules. At the time of removal of any of these materials from the mouth, the setting reaction is still not complete. As a matter of fact, it can continue indefinitely in some materials. Further shrinkage, although on a much lesser scale, can be expected after removal. Therefore, the impressions should be poured immediately to avoid loss and distortion of the captured details.

B. Evaporation of vaporizable ingredients in the impression mass

The water present in both hydrocolloid materials can evaporate, a phenomenon more obvious with the reversible than irreversible type. To a much lesser degree, the water of the polysulfide and the alcohols of the condensation-polymerization silicone and polyether rubber bases may undergo vaporization in a fairly hot and dry environment. In addition, low molecular weight ingredients of these materials may undergo evaporation if subjected to a hot, rapidly changed atmosphere. Understandably, the vaporization of these ingredients will create shrinkage and distortion of the impression, a situation most obvious with reversible hydrocolloid, least obvious with polyether but *not* present at all with additional polymerization silicone rubber base material. These materials, susceptible to the evaporation process, should not be subjected to drafts of air or dried with compressed air before pouring an impression made of them.

C. Synersis

The phenomenon of exuding water is characteristic only for hydrocolloid materials. Reversible hydrocolloids exhibit this phenomenon much more than irreversible hydrocolloids, but it can happen for both in a dry atmosphere or in any environment with less than 100% humidity. The result is shrinkage and distortion of the impression details.

D. Imbibition

The phenomenon of absorbing water from the environment is a characteristic property of hydrocolloid materials only. The reversible hydrocolloids exhibit a memory for the amount of water lost from synersis at a specific temperature and at a certain composition. They may regain it under the same temperature and composition, if the water is available. Irreversible hydrocolloids do not possess this memory. This feature cannot be used to compensate for the water lost during synersis, insofar as the fixed temperature and composition at which synersis occurred cannot be determined and reproduced. The result of this imbibition is swelling of the impression materials and uneven increase in size, leading to obliteration, loss, and warpage of some details. Synersis and imbibition can be minimized by increasing the percentage of the dispersed phase, by storing the impression in 100% humidity for the minimal time possible and, most importantly, pour the impression immediately after removal from the mouth.

E. Release of stresses

From the composition of the hardened products, it is obvious that all these materials are amorphouse. Although they are flexible to some extent, some induced stresses, if at a sufficient rate, amount, and direction, can be released after the material is removed from the mouth, creating changes in the shape of the preparation and tooth details. The only guard against these anticipated discrepancies is to pour the model immediately. The longer the time lapse between removing the impression and pouring the model, the greater the possibility of stress release with loss or distortion of detail.

F. Set

This is a measure of the resistance of the materials to permanent deformation, i.e., the flexibility of the material. According to the ADA test, set is the percentage of permanent deformation after a specimen of the material is compressed 10% for 30 seconds. Examination of the microstructure of these materials reveals that they are all classical visco-elastic materials, with the characteristic time-dependent strain-stress relationship, i.e., the faster the rate of applying the stressing forces, the less the set will be, and vice versa. Using the ADA test, the set exhibited by the agar reversible hydrocolloid is 1.5%, and for alginate hydrocolloid it is 3%. Regarding the elastomeric impression materials, additional polymerization silicone rubber bases exhibited the least set, 0.2%, this is followed by condensation polymerization silicone rubber bases; 0.6%; polyether rubber base; 1.1% and polysulfide rubber bases, 2.5-4%.

To guard against permanent deformation, especially if the induced deformation is more than 10%, remove the impression from the mouth in a very fast snap (rate), so as to minimize the effective permanent deformation. Also, the more complete the setting reaction is, whether it is polymerization or gelation, the more the elastic component in the mass will be and the less the viscuous component will be, thereby enhancing more complete recovery.

G. Coefficient of thermal expansion

Hydrocolloid impression materials exhibit the lowest coefficient of thermal expansion of all these materials. The value is of no clinical significance. Polysulfide rubber bases have a coefficient of thermal expansion of 150 PPM/1°C. Both silicone rubber base materials have 200 PPM/1° C. Polyether has 220 PPM/1°C. So, with the elastomeric impression materials, it is best to use the minimal thickness of the material to minimize the discrepancies that may occur going from the mouth temperature to the room temperature at which the impression is going to be poured.

H. Dissolution of ingredients of the impression materials in water or fluids during subsequent manipulation

Many of the components of the set products of the impression material are soluble in water, e.g., many of the modifying salts and by-products. If any of these components were lost in the period prior to pouring or during pouring and setting of the gypsum, they could eliminate some details and distort others. Extreme care should be taken to use a minimal amount of water with the gypsum used to fill the impression, especially the hydrophilic ones (hydrocolloids and polyether rubber base materials).

I. Tray material variables

As impression materials are carried in trays, any change in the dimension of the tray will be imparted to the dimensions of the impression. The warpage and sorption that may come from the acrylic tray or thermal expansion of the metal tray, etc., can drastically affect the shape and dimension of the impression.

J. Non-bonding

Detachment of the material from the tray, or non-bonding between the syringe and tray material, may occur due to improper technique. Either occurrence will lead to excessive stressing of the detached material with subsequent distortion of detail.

III. Strength Properties

Again, by examination of their microstructure, we can predict weak visco-elastic materials. Although the materials are not subjected to too much loading, possible failure can occur at thin cross-sections in the sulcular area (trough), at severe undercuts, or with second pours of impressions. As can be expected, the faster the rate of loading is, the more resistant these materials will be to strength failure. The tear strength, as designated by MacPherson, Craig, and Payton, is more indicative of the strength properties of the material than any other strength measurement. It shows the strength of the material in cross-sectional areas, similar to the sulcular area where most of the strength failures occur.

The tear strength for alginate is from 350 to 700 gr/cm; for agar-agar it is 700 gr/cm; for polysulfide rubber bases it is 6300 gr/cm; for additional polymerization silicone rubber bases it is 4700 gr/cm; for condensation polymerization silicone rubber base it is 4500 gr/cm; for polyether rubber bases it is 3600-3800 gr/cm. In hydrocolloid materials, strength is the product of the relative dimension, density, bonding and configuration of the dispersed phase. Strength is the product of the length and degree of cross-linkage of the polymer macromolecules in elastomeric impression materials. Also, strength is greatly influenced by the size, amount, shape, and relative configuration of the filler particles and their types and degree of attachment to the mass within the same material. The more fillers there are, the better will be the strength properties, provided they are all attached.

IV. Reproduction of Details

This is a product of multiple factors, mainly the factors dictating the wetting ability of the material to the details of the preparation. An example of these factors is viscosity, to which the reproduction of detail is inversely proportional. Therefore light body materials are more reproducing than heavier consistencies. Other factors are: the affinity of the material for dental tissues, forces used to introduce the material and hold it while the material is setting (hardening), confinement of the material, and cleanliness of the preparation surface, i.e., the elimination of moisture, debris, blood, or saliva, etc.

Generally speaking the agar-agar hydrocolloid, the oldest of these materials, is still the best reproducer of details. It can reproduce grooves of a width of 0.01 mm. The smallest dimension of a groove irreversible hydrocolloid can reproduce is 0.075 mm. For elastomeric rubber impression material the smallest they can reproduce is a groove diameter average of 0.020 mm.

V. Compatibility with Gypsum and Resin Die Materials During Setting

With the exception of hydrocolloid impression materials, all previously mentioned impression materials have no effect on the setting of gypsum or resin die materials used for the pour. Hydrocolloid materials tend to retard the setting of the adjacent hemihydrate of calcium sulfate to a dihydrated one, resulting in a stone surface that is soft, chalky, easily abraded and does not replicate all the details of the impression. This should be obvious recalling that colloidal materials in general are retarders to gypsum setting. Additionally, the presence of borax in the mass aggravates the situation. Also, water in the mass tends to dilute the gypsum, thus locally delaying its setting and weakening the product. To counteract this, immersing the impression for 5-10 min. in 3% solution of potassium sulfate can accelerate the setting of the gypsum sufficiently to neutralize the retarding effect of hydrocolloid and its contents.

Also, proper washing of the impression of saliva and blood will enhance the hardening of the contacting gypsum. If the impression has been stored temporarily in a humidor, it should be thoroughly washed to remove any exuding solutions. It must be emphasized that not all gypsum dental stone and hydrocolloid impression materials are mutually compatible. Compatibility differs because of the different compositions, additives, and environment of composing these materials. Therefore, materials should be carefully selected that are compatible with each other to insure predictable, consistent results. Resin die materials do not set at all in contact with hydrocolloid impression material. So if a resin die is essential for a technic, use other impression materials or pour the hydrocolloid one in gypsum, then take an impression for created model in any of the other impression materials.

It should be mentioned here that even with the elastomeric impression materials, incomplete details or an unworkable die surface may be produced if excessive moisture in the form of saliva, blood, or water is present in the impression during pouring, or if the die material is not vibrated sufficiently into the impression to counteract the hydrophobic nature of rubber base materials. If treated and handled properly, all impression materials will produce a workable die surface and detail.

VI. Workability

Using these materials necessitates the following steps:
A. Choosing the material
B. Constructing or customizing a tray
C. Preparing the mouth, the teeth, and the preparation
D. Preparing the material
E. Loading the syringe and tray
F. Introducing the material to the tooth preparation and the mouth
G. Establishing and controlling the environment for material hardening
H. Removing the tray rapidly from the preparation and the mouth
I. Preparing the impression for the pouring of die-working model material

A. Choosing the material

This is a personal preference. Reversible hydrocolloid requires the utmost discipline and exact timing in its handling.

Office personnel must be well trained. In addition, it involves the purchase of a conditioner. However, the results are always consistent and the best of all the materials.

Although new brands of irreversible hydrocolloid have been promoted as being capable of producing an impression that is adequate for fabricating dies and working models, irreversible hydrocolloid should be used only for opposing arch impressions to create articulating models, for study models, or for models preparatory to temporary restoration fabrication. That is because of the variety of shortcomings in the material, especially its inability to reproduce details. Recently, new brands of irreversible hydrocolloids have been introduced that are used as the tray material for injected reversible hydrocolloid. These irreversible hydrocolloids are similar in composition to those previously described, except that the alginate polymer can physically adhere to the agar-agar polymer. Polysulfide rubber base, although it has undergone many improvements, still possesses a most unpleasant odor and is the messiest material to use. It is the most sensitive to temperature changes of all materials in its setting and the one with the highest set of all elastomeric impression materials.

Silicone rubber base materials have the shortest shelf life, especially the condensation-polymerization silicone rubber base. Polyether rubber bases are the hardest and toughest of all the impression materials but are limited by being supplied in only one consistency. Therefore, selection is dependent upon weighing your facilities and capabilities with your needs. In terms of expense, reversible hydrocolloids are the most economic in the long run. The newest additional polymerization silicone rubber base materials are the most expensive of them all.

B. Constructing or customizing a tray

Since these materials are intiially in a pasty, highly deformable form when inserted in the mouth, they necessitate a tray to carry them. Any tray should have the following requirements:

1. Confinement

The tray should be able to keep the impression material mass within it under the seating and holding pressure of the operator. This is essential to regulate dimension changes during setting and to keep sufficient bulk of the material to reproduce the details.

2. Retention

It is mandatory for the tray to retain the impression material after setting during the forceful removal from the mouth. Retentive features in a tray could be in the form of locking rims at the peripheries of the tray, perforations, and/or adhesives.

3. Stabilization-immobilization

The relationship of the tray to the structures to be reproduced in the impression material should be predetermined in three dimensions. This is to insure proper thickness of the impression materials and the preservation of that thickness during the material's setting. Even more importantly, this is done to prevent the induction of unnecessary stresses on the impression material due to unavoidable movements. Immobilization is done by occlusal and lateral stops. The stops can be built in the special tray from the tray's own material. For the customized tray they should be added to the tray in the form of compound, acrylic, or wax stops. The idea of the stop is to

have only one contacting relationship with the teeth and the arch, a position in which the tray will not move further occlusally, apically, or be displaced laterally.

4. Uniform thickness of the impression material in the tray

A tray should be built or customized to allow even thickness of the material in three dimensions to insure an even stress pattern in the impression material. At least one-eighth of an inch of space should be left for the impression material to surround the surfaces to be duplicated. The thickness should be greater for hydrocolloid materials, since the greater the bulk of this material, the less the potential for distortion. This is opposite to elastomeric impression materials where the less the bulk (but not less than ⅛″), the less the potential for distortion.

5. Choice of special trays for certain techniques

For example, with reversible hydrocolloid, metal trays with cooling tubing should be chosen. When using a wash technique, a sufficiently large tray should be chosen for the fabrication of the customized putty tray.

6. Adhesives

For elastomeric impression materials an adhesive should be painted over all inner surfaces and edges of the tray to insure holding of the material in the tray. For rubber base material the adhesive is a butyl rubber cement; for silicone it is always part of the catalyst; for polyether it is always a fraction of the base material.

C. Preparing the mouth, the teeth, and the preparation

Presumably, the preparation has been completed and the periodontium has been controlled. Now the cavity and the preparation should be washed, clearing it of debris, blood, and saliva. The area to be duplicated should be isolated with cotton rolls. Saliva should be completely evacuated from the mouth just prior to inserting the impression material. It is preferable to keep the saliva ejector in place if possible. All teeth should be dried with maximum emphasis on completely drying the prepared tooth, especially the preparation details. If hydrocolloid is to be used, the isolating cotton rolls should be slightly moistened with water just prior to the insertion of the impression material to avoid them absorbing water from the colloidal material.

If the preparation contains a pin channel for a cast pin, a proper size nylon bristle is tried and adjusted. With a hot spatula, touch the cavity end of the bristle to form a holding button to be engaged in the impression material. Some bristles are supplied with a ready-made button. If the pin channel is for a wrought pin, the proper dimension of the pin is cut from a wire of the material and tried in, adjusted and left in the pin channel to be picked up by the impression material. The surface roughness of the pin will hold it in the impression material. Some pins are supplied with a custom sleeve that is to be incorporated into the die. After the impression is removed from the mouth, the pin is verified to be in the proper position within the impression. The custom sleeve is slipped over the pin and the model is poured.

Occasionally, the teeth and preparation details are painted with a wetting agent, usually a modified soap. This will decrease surface tension and improve the wettability of the impression material, enhancing the capturing of maximum details in the final impression.

D. Preparing the material

Reversible hydrocolloid materials should be prepared in a thermally controlled conditioner which has three compartments (Fig. 1).

1. The boiling compartment has water at the boiling temperature. The material is kept there in the form of tubes filled with the tray material and carpules or syringes filled with the injectable material. They should be kept there for at least 15 minutes to insure the liquification to the sol state. (Fig. 1B)

2. The storage compartment is at a temperature of 145-150°F. The liquified materials from the boiling compartment may be stored there indefinitely. (Fig. 1B)

3. After the tray is filled, it is placed in the tempering compartment for at least four minutes to bring it to a physiologically tolerable temperature for the patient's involved tissues. The syringe material is moved directly from the storage compartment to the preparation. The latter step is justified to insure the maximum wetting ability of the material to the preparation details, and because the bulk of the material used for that purpose does not carry sufficient thermal energy to harm the involved tissues.

For irreversible hydrocolloids, the prescribed amount of cold water and powder are dispersed in a rubber bowl, then mixed together until the water is absorbed by the powder. At this time, with a stiff wide-bladed spatula, the material is mixed vigorously against the walls of the bowl until a hemogeneous putty mix is obtained. To retard the setting, in addition to the use of cold water, a sprinkle of sodium phosphate can facilitate effective retardation. To accelerate the setting warm water or a sprinkle of gypsum powder will suffice.

For elastomeric impression material, dispense equal lengths of the base and the catalyst paste on a thick stable paper pad. The catalyst paste is incorporated in the base paste with rotary strokes, then with padding and folding strokes, using the entire surface of the pad. The mixing is continued until a completely homogeneous paste with no streaks is obtained. If using tray and syringe material, start by mixing the tray material, then the syringe material.

A recent innovation is to supply the elastomeric impression pastes in a two-tube assembly attached together. One tube contains the catalyst paste and the other contains the base paste. The two tubes lead to a single tube which has a fixed spiral inner configuration. The original tubes have a piston that can force equal amounts of each paste into the terminal combining tube. By going through the spiral arrangements, the pastes are mixed in a closed compartment, resulting in less possibility of air bubble entrapment. From the single terminal tube, mixed material can be injected directly into the preparation or a tray (Fig. 2).

If using the wash technique, the putty consistency paste is loaded in a tray and placed over the tissues and teeth, sometimes prior to starting the tooth preparation, then placed aside until the preparation is completed. The putty impression surfaces are trimmed, with the exception of the stop areas, using a sharp knife.

Some of the silicone rubber base materials are supplied in a one-paste form only. The prescribed amount of the paste is dispensed in the hand. The indicated number of drops of the catalyst is added, then kneaded in the palm of the hand until the catalyst disappears. The process can be done on a paper

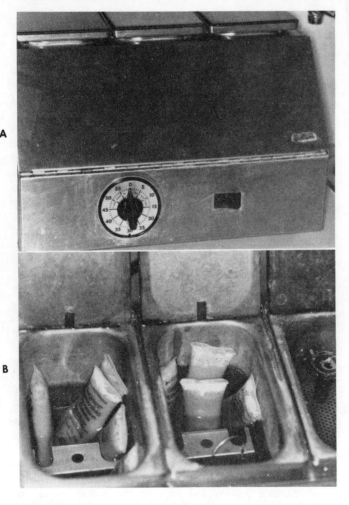

Fig. 21-1

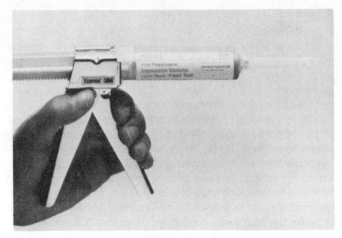

Fig. 21-2

pad if the consistency is too thin to warrant using the palm of the hand.

To delay the setting of polysulfide rubber bases, oleic or stearic acids can be added. To delay the setting of any other elastomeric impression materials, less catalyst paste is used than base paste. To accelerate the setting of any of the elastomeric impression materials, a drop of water can be added to the mix.

E. Loading the syringe and tray

For reversible hydrocolloid materials, the syringe material is already in a carpule or already loaded in a syringe before the boiling liquification process. It is only the tray that has to be loaded. A tube from the storage compartment is squeezed into the tray, and the tray then placed in the tempering compartment.

For irreversible hydrocolloid materials, there is no syringe material. The tray is loaded by scopping the paste from the bowl and loading the tray with it. Then with moistened fingers mold the material into the tray, gently smoothing its surface, making it more wettable.

To load a syringe with elastomeric impression material, the mixed mass is heaped in the middle of the paper pad. Using the back of the syringe drag it from the peripheries of the pad into the mixed mass, forcing the material into the syringe barrel. When completely filled, the piston is inserted, and visible air bubbles are injected out. The tray is lined gently with the tray material or the wash material, taking care to maintain a uniform thickness of material.

F. Introducing the material to the tooth preparation and the mouth

The syringe material is introduced first. Place the syringe tip at the least accessible portion of the preparation, begin injecting, and gradually move to more accessible areas of the preparation until it is completely filled and covered. During the injection stage, the syringe tip should, at all times, remain in the material already injected. This avoids trapping air bubbles, which may obliterate impression details or weaken the impression. The loaded tray is immediately inserted over the injected syringe material. When using reversible hydrocolloid, the surface of the tray material should be dabbed with a piece of gauze to remove excess water that is present from the tempering compartment. The tray is forced to its predetermined position and immobilized.

G. Establishing and controlling the environment for material hardening

When using reversible hydrocolloid, a connecting tubing should be attached to the tray at one end and to a source of cold water (regular tap water) at the other end. This facilitates circulation of cold water in the tray, causing gelation of the sol hydrocolloid. At least five minutes should be allowed for the water to circulate, so that reasonable gel strength can be established. Extremely cold water should not be used insofar as it can create abrupt gelation of certain areas of the material in contact with the tray, thus inducing stresses at its junction with the rest of the hydrocolloid material.

In all situations the tray should be held rigidly without move-ment. Any movement at this stage will induce stresses between the newly formed phases in the material leading to subsequent impression distortion. Saliva should be evacuated from the mouth, and the patient asked to partially close his mouth so that the jaws will assume normal dimensions.

The tray should be kept in place until the material reaches a stage in its setting reaction which will insure its removal without possibility of distortion. This stage is exhibited in hydrocolloid material by brittle fracturing of unused pieces or recovery of protruding portions from the tray when pressed by the finger. For polysulfide rubber bases, it is indicated by loss of surface gloss and recovery when indented with a blunt instrument. For silicone rubber bases and polyether rubber bases, it is indicated by tough fracturing of remaining unused pieces.

H. Removing the tray rapidly from the preparation and the mouth

In a predetermined outward movement from the tooth and the mouth, the tray is held firmly, then snapped off and out of the tooth and the mouth. This is more easily facilitated with custom trays.

I. Preparing the impression for the pouring of die-working model material (Fig. 3)

For hydrocolloid impression materials containing potassium sulfate, it is advisable to start mixing the gypsum material two minutes before the hydrocolloid hardens, while the impression is still in the mouth. This is to facilitate pouring it immediately after withdrawing it from the mouth. For those impressions to be soaked in a 3% potassium sulfate solution for five min., the stone should be mixed 2 min. prior to removal from the solution.

All impressions should be properly washed, excesses trimmed and properly inspected for debris. Mislocated or torn items in the impression should be relocated in their position. If this is not possible, the impression should be retaken. Vaseline or petroleum jelly should be applied on pins and bristles engaged in the impression to prevent them from adhering to the die material.

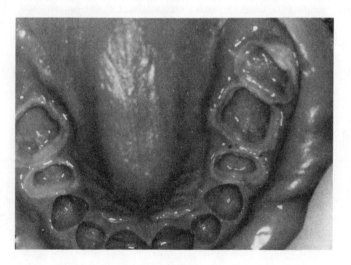

Fig. 21-3

BIBLIOGRAPHY

Asgar, K.: Elastic impression materials. Dent. Clin. North Am. **15:**81, 1971.

Bergman, Olsson, S., and Bergman, B.: Elastomeric impression materials. Dimensional stability and surface detail sharpness following treatment with disinfection solutions. Swed. Dent. J. **4**(4):161-167, 1980.

Brown, D.: An update on elastomeric impression materials. Br. Dent. J. **150**(2):35-40, Jan. 20, 1981.

Ciesco, J.N., Malone, W.F., Sandrik, J.L., and Mazur, B.: Comparison of elastomeric impression materials used in fixed prosthodontics. J. Prosthet. Dent. **45**(1):89-94, Jan. 1981.

Combe, E.C., and Moser, J.B.: The rheological characteristics of elastomeric impression materials. J. Dent. Res. **57**(2):221-226, 1978.

Craig, R.G.: A review of properties of rubber impression materials. J. Mich. Dent. Assoc. **58**:254, 1977.

Craig, R.G.: Status report on polyether impression materials. Council on dental materials and devices. J. Am. Dent. Assoc. **95**(1):126-130, 1977.

Craig, R.G., and Peyton, F.A.: Physical properties of elastic duplicating materials. J. Dent. Res. **39**:391-404, 1960.

Eames, W.B., Rogers, L.B., Wallace, S.W., and Suway, N.B.: Compatibility of gypsum products with hydrocolloid impression materials. Oper. Dent. **3**:108, 1978.

Eames, W.B., and Sieweke, J.C.: Seven acrylic resins for custom trays and five putty-wash systems compared. Oper. Dent. **5**(4):162-167, 1980.

Eames, W.B., and Sieweke, J.C., Wallace, S.W., and Rogers, L.B.: Elastomeric impression materials: Effect of bulk on accuracy. J. Prosth. Dent. **41**(3):304-307, 1979.

Eames, W.B., Wallace, S.W., Suway, N.B., and Rogers, L.B.: Accuracy and dimensional stability of elastomeric impression materials. J. Prosth. Dent. **42**:159, 1979.

Farah, J.W., Clark, A.E., and Ainpour, P.R.: Elastomeric impression materials. Oper. Dent. **6**(1):15-19, 1981.

Gilmore, H.W., Phillips, R.W., and Swartz, M.L.: The effect of residual stress and water change on the deformation of hydrocolloid impression materials. J. Dent. Res. **37**:816-823, 1958.

Herfort, T.W., Gerberich, W.W., Macosko, C.W., and Goodkind, R.J.: Tear strength of elastomeric impression materials. J. Prosth. Dent. **39**(1):59-62, 1978.

Indue, K., and Wilson, H.J.: Viscoelastic properties of elastomeric impression materials. II: Variation of rheological properties with time, temperature and mixing proportions. J. Oral Rehabil. **5**(3):261-267, 1978.

Indue, K., and Wilson, H.J.: Viscoelastic properties of elastomeric impression materials. III. The elastic recovery after removal of strains applied at the setting time. J. Oral Rehabil. **5**(4):323-327, 1978.

Jarvis, R.G., and Earnshaw, R.: The effect of alginate impressions on the surface of cast gypsum. II. The role of sodium sulphate in incompatibility. Aust. Dent. J. **26**(1):12-17, 1981.

Krug, R.: Multiple uses of a plastic template in fixed prosthodontics. J. Pros. Dent. **30**:838-842, 1973.

Lacy, A.M., Bellman, T., Fukui, H., and Jendresen, M.D.: Time dependent accuracy of elastomer impression materials. Part I: Condensation silicones. J. Pros. Dent. **45**(2):209-215, 1981.

Lacy, A.M., Fukui, H., Bellman, T., and Jendresen, M.D.: Time dependent accuracy of elastomer impression materials. Part II: Polyether, polysulfides, and polyvinylsiloxane. J. Pros. Dent. **45**(3):329-333, 1981.

Lacy, A., Treleaven, S., and Jendresen, M.: The effect of selected surfactants on the wetting behavior of gypsum die stone on impression materials. CDA J. 36-40, 1977.

Luebke, R.J., Scandrett, F.R., Kerber, P.E.: The effect of delayed and second pours on elastomeric impression material accuracy. J. Pros. Dent. **41**(5):517-521, 1979.

Marcinak, C.F., Young, F.A., Draughn, R.A., and Flemming, W.R.: Linear Dimensional changes in elastic impression materials. J. Dent. Res. **59**(7):1152-1155, 1980.

McCabe, J.F., and Storer, R.: Elastomeric impression materials. The measurement of some properties relevant to clinical practice. Br. Dent. J. **149**(3):73-79, 1980.

Nishiyama, M., Ono, M., Hirose, H., Yamaguchi, M., Akimoto, S., and Isaji, M.: Physical properties of vinyl silicone impression materials compared with other elastomeric impression materials. J. Nihon Univ. Sch. Dent. **19**(3):134-140, 1977.

Nogawa, I.: Factors influencing dimensional accuracy of indirect working model. The method by the use of thiokol rubber base and silicone rubber impression materials. Odontol (Tokyo) **56**:396, 1968.

Phillips, R.W.: Factors influencing the accuracy of reversible hydrocolloid impressions. J. Amer. Dent. Assn. **43**:1-17, 1951.

Phillips, R.W.: Physical properties and manipulation of rubber base impression materials. J. Ohio Dent. Assoc. **45**:236, 1968.

Podshadley, A.G., and others: Accuracy of a mercaptan rubber impression technique using a stock tray. DADA **83**:1303, 1971.

Rehberg, H.J.: The impression tray—an important factor in impression precision. Int. Dent. J. **27**(2):146-153, 1977.

Reisbick M.H., and Matyas, J.: The accuracy of highly filled elastomeric impression materials. J. Prosth. Dent. **33**:67, 1975.

Sandrik, J.L., and Sarna, T.: Temperature of elastomeric impression materials while setting in the mouth. J. Dent. Res. **59**(11):1985-1986, 1980.

Sawyer, H., Birtles, J., Neiman, R., and Podshadley, A.G.: Accuracy of casts produced from seven rubber impression materials. JADA Vol 87, July 1973.

Skinner, E.W., and Kern, W.R.: Colloidal impression materials. JADA and the Dental Cosmos **25**:578-584, 1938.

Smith, D.C., and Fairhurst, C.W.: Effect of hydrocolloid impression materials on the surface of the dental stone. J. Dent. Res. **41**:1103, 1962.

Stannard, J.G., and Craig, R.G.: Modifying the setting rate of an addition type silicone impression material. J. Dent. Res. **58**(4):1377-1382, 1979.

Swartz, M.L., Norman, R.D., Gilmore, H.W., and Phillips, R.W.: Studies on syneresis and imbibition in reversible hydrocolloid. J. Dent. Res. **36**:472-478, 1957.

Thompson, M.J.: Hydrocolloid: its role in restorative dentistry. Dent. Clin. North Am. **12**:101, 1959.

Tolley, L.G., and Craig, R.G.: Viscoelastic properties of elastomeric impression materials: Polysulfide, silicone and polyether rubbers. J. Oral Rehabil. **5**(2):121-128, 1978.

CHAPTER 22

Working die and model construction

Working die and model construction, like all steps in the sequence of casting fabrication, require attention to detail and precise manipulation of materials to insure a mechanically successful restoration. The die and working model should fulfill several objectives.

The die should replicate the tooth preparation in the most minute detail as well as all accessible unprepared areas of the tooth. The die should have a fixed location, in three dimensions, in the working model. This location will exactly represent the location of the tooth in the arch. The die can be removable from the model, but when replaced, should occupy the correct position and be immobile.

The die should be trimmed to reveal all marginal elements as well as adjacent unprepared tooth structure. The die and model material should be compatible with the impression material, and should have a smooth, non-abradable surface. The die should be able to accommodate premade means of auxiliary restoration retention (e.g., pins). The die will, on selected areas, receive a spacer to create room for the luting agent of the casting.

I. Gypsum for Die and Working Model Construction

The materials used to fabricate the die and working models are usually gypsum products. There are a number of variables that can affect the behavior of these gypsum products. In their powder form they are primarily calcium sulfate hemihydrate in the alpha form. This signifies only that their crystals are very regular and have smooth surfaces that can be readily wetted with the least amount of water, as compared to the other types of hemihydrates (beta hemihydrate). Some contain silica (for divesting investment). When mixed with distilled water, the setting reaction starts. The setting reaction is a process of dissolution and hydration followed by supersaturation and precipitation of dihydrate crystals of the calcium sulfate. When the aforementioned crystals are in sufficient number and dimensions, they intermesh, collide, and harden the mass. The collision of these formed and growing crystals, if in sufficient impact, can create stresses at their interfaces. If conditions allow (nonconfinement), the outward release of these stresses will be in the form of expansion of the plastic mass. This situation is not desirable at this stage of the cast fabrication.

A. Dimensional Stability

a. Setting expansion

Any physical manipulation that accelerates the setting time increases setting expansion, which is understandable from the brief description of the setting reaction. Accordingly, setting time variables should be controlled to create a reasonable time for setting, so that the rate of the crystal growth can be compatible with their intermeshing, resulting in minimum stresses and consequently minimum expansion. Generally, chemical accelerators and retarders reduce the setting expansion. Also, increasing the water : powder ratio decreases the expansion, but it is not to be used to control the expansion, insofar as it drastically decreases the strength and hardness properties of the material.

b. Hygroscopic expansion

This is a modification of the setting expansion. Basically, it is the deconfinement of the crystal growth by the addition of water. It should be avoided in die and model construction, i.e., no water should be added or brought in contact with the setting gypsum.

c. Abrasive resistance

During wax carving, some die details may be lost due to the low abrasive resistance of the die material. Abrasive resistance is governed by many factors, especially strength and hardness properties. It is directly proportional to these two factors. Every effort should be made to increase the surface abrasive resistance of the die material.

B. Strength

This is governed mainly by the water content during the mix and after setting. The strength properties are inversely proportional to both of them. That is why type I stone is less strong than type II stone, the former requiring more water than the latter to create a workable wetting mix. Type II stone should be used for die and working model construction. Type I stone can be used for opposing articulating models. Drying the gypsum to lower its residual water content will dramatically increase its strength (more than double). That is why dies should not be manipulated immediately after removing them from the impressions. They should be dried and left in open air to lose some of this water before carving. Occasionally, they are oven-dried for that purpose. Decreasing the porosity of the set material could substantially increase its strength. This could be done by incorporating amalgam powder in the mix, vacuum

C. Hardness

Hardness is governed by the same factors as strength, especially the water content. The hardness of gypsum material is decreased when it sets in contact with hydrocolloid, if the setting of the gypsum is not accelerated or hydration of the system is not retarded.

Certain water substitutes can dramatically increase the strength and hardness properties of gypsum, e.g., an aqueous solution of colloidal silica or soluble resin solutions. They do this by increasing the friction between the dihydrate crystals. Applying talcum powder or oil on the die surface will increase the smoothness, decreasing the possibilities of die surface injury during carving because the instruments will glide rather than bite into the gypsum.

D. Reproduction of details

The smallest dimension that a dihydrate gypsum product can reproduce is a groove in the width of 0.050 mm, which is greater than that reproduced by elastomeric impression materials and reversible hydrocolloid. Reproduction of details can be enhanced by:

1. Insuring the compatibility of the gypsum with the impression materials.
2. Introduction of small increments of the material into the impression at a time.
3. Proper vibrating energy to force the material mix into the details.
4. Elimination of any intervening moisture or debris between the impression material and the gypsum.
5. Use of wetting agents on the impression material surfaces prior to gypsum pouring.
6. Acceleration of the setting of gypsum at the surface in contact with the impression material.
7. Fine particle size and dimension of the gypsum.
8. Plastic mix of the gypsum (high water : powder ratio; this may, however, interfere with the strength properties).

Setting time can be accelerated by the operator by use of fine-particle gypsum, low water : powder ratio, long and fast mixing, use of 3% potassium sulfate solution, or the use of slurry water. The last method of acceleration is the most practical, and is due to the incorporation of more nuclei of calcium sulfate di-hihydrates in the mix. Use of borax or more than 5% sodium chloride can retard the setting, as can coarse particle gypsum, a high water to powder ratio, or a short and slow mixing time.

II. Resin Die Materials

These are basically epoxy resin. They are supplied in two or three parts that are mixed before insertion into the impression. The first part contains 50-60% epoxy novolac polymer, 30-50% vinyl, #3 Cyclo-hexene diepoxyde and from 0-20% 3,4 epoxy cyclohexyle methyl 3,4 epoxy cyclohexane carboxylate. The second part consists of a partially hydrolyzed 3,4 benzophenene tetracarboxylic acid dianhydride not to exceed 20% and a partially hydrolyzed pyromelletic acid dianhydride, not less than 50% and preferably 90% or more.

When mixing these two components, in a ratio of 20 to 50 parts of the second component for each hundred parts of the first component (by weight), a condensation polymerization and cross-linkage reaction will occur, creating a solid mass.

To encourage this polymerization, especially when the second part is 100% partially hydrolyzed pyromelletic acid dianhydride, a third part, a tertiary amine catalyst, should be added in the amount of 0.03 part (by weight) for each part of combined components. Each compound is supplied separately. They are mixed just before using the material. The mixing should be completed in a vacuum and the material poured into any type of impression with the exception of hydrocolloid impressions. If the impressions are taken in hydrocolloid, they have to be duplicated in an elastomeric impression material before pouring epoxy resin die materials into them. The poured impression is then left, for the resin to cure, for 8 hours at room temperature. During this curing the material shrinks on the average of 0.02-0.6% depending on the configuration and bulk of the die. To compensate for this shrinkage and to create more expansion if needed for the future fabrication of the cast, the cured resin model or die is subjected to thermal treatment in an oven where the temperature is increased from room temperature to 160° C at the rate of 10° per minute and then held at 160° C for 1 hour. Do not exceed 200° C. It is then rapidly cooled to room temperature. The created expansion will be permanent as the material does not shrink on cooling. The exact reason for the expansion is not known, but it is hypothesized that during the heating there is further cross-linking of the polymer, which generates water that causes the expansion. Because the expansion is gradual, further heating during the fabrication of a ceramic casting, which will be cast on a die formed of the material, will not create any further expansion because of the fast heating during casting. This material was specifically formulated for mouldable ceramics since the die will form one of the walls of the mold during molding of the ceramics. However, it can be used for any other cast materials.

The abrasive resistance and strength properties of this die material are far superior to gypsum die materials. Reproduction of details is much better than that of gypsum and can be controlled and improved by the same factors as gypsum products. The setting time can be accelerated by increasing the amount of the catalyst or increasing the amount of hydrolyzed anhydrides in second component, namely, the tetracarboxylic acid.

III. Construction of the Die and the Working Model

The fabrication of the die and working model has no limit in types and techniques other than the imagination of the operator. However, these techniques can generally be classified into two main categories:

A. Techniques necessitating two sets of pours (casts) from the same impression (elastomeric impression materials), or two separate impressions (reversible hydrocolloids)

B. Techniques that require only one set of pours (casts)

A. Techniques necessitating two sets of pours (casts)

The dies will be prepared from the first pour. These dies will be separate and not incorporated in a working model (Fig. 1). They are reserved for final margination, detail adjustments, surface treatment and sprueing of the wax pattern. The latter procedures are done after building the wax pattern contacts, contours, and occluding morphology on the second cast. The second cast will be mounted on an articulator with

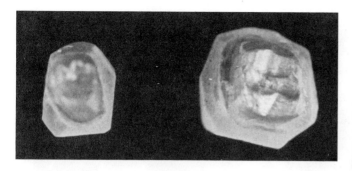

Fig. 22-1

the opposing models. The preparation replicas are inseparable from the second casts.

The main advantages of this class of techniques are that:

1. There is a complete immobilization of the prepared tooth replica, when building the occluding anatomy, contact and contour of the wax pattern.

2. The mounted casts are not subjected to sawing and mechanical removal and insertion of the die which might stress them and could slightly interfere with their interrelationship.

3. If two impressions are taken, the one with the best marginal and detailed reproduction is selected for the die fabrication.

4. This procedure does not require the tools and equipment that are needed for the other techniques.

The disadvantages of this technique are:

1. Moving the wax pattern from the working model (second cast) to the die and vice versa will be done several times, a manipulative procedure that can induce stresses in the wax.

2. The two replicas of the prepared tooth may not have the same exact dimension and shape, especially internally, a situation that may aggravate the stress pattern in the wax.

Although, there are several ways to do this technique, the following is a basic general outline when using gypsum.

a. The impressions are boxed up with boxing utility wax. For a lower impression, the tongue space is obliterated with blocking compound, alginate, wet paper towels, or plasticine.

b. Dispense the proper ratio of the die stone and distilled water. It is preferable to use preweighed packages of the die stone and measure the distilled water in CC's.

c. The powder and water are mechanically mixed, preferably under vacuum.

d. Starting at one end of the boxed impression, carry small increments of the die stone material on a wax spatula and vibrate it gently and slowly in the impression. From that same end, add subsequent increments and vibrate them into the details of the impression. The vibrated stone should fill the occlusal portions prior to the gingival ones, and so on, until the tooth impression is filled. At this point, increase the increments, until the impression is filled completely. It should be emphasized that the smaller the preparation is and the more complicated that the details are, the smaller the increment of gypsum that should be introduced. This may require introducing beads of gypsum, using a small painting brush.

e. The stone is left to harden for at least one hour. If poured in hydrocolloid material, it should be kept in a humidor (100% humidity) during setting, but not in direct contact with water.

For elastomeric impression material it is acceptable to allow it to set in the open air.

f. The impression material with the tray is removed from the hardened stone and any remaining impression material is peeled off the replicated details.

g. For the opposing articulating model one can use die stone. Although regular stone is quite acceptable.

h. The details of the preparation and involved tooth surfaces may now be covered with slurry water or any other protective film, and the model trimmed to remove gross peripheral excesses.

i. Of the two fabricated models for the same arch, one model is mounted with opposing arch and the other model is sawed interproximally to separate the replica of the prepared tooth from the adjacent teeth.

j. The resulting die (Fig. 1) is cleared of any overhanging stone, exposing all peripheries of the preparation. It is a good idea to taper the die to a cone shape with a flat base. Also, it may be helpful to cut a groove in the die 2 mm. peripheral to the circumferential tie, especially its gingival elements.

B. Techniques utilizing one pour (cast)

In these techniques, the die will be part of the working articulated model, where it can be used to build occluding, contacting, and contouring anatomies of the wax pattern. The die can be removed from the working cast to marginate, adjust, and surface the wax pattern. When the die is seated in the working model, it should be completely immobile in three dimensions. To establish this fixed-removable relationship between the die and the working model, two things are necessary: a bed and a locking mechanism for the die.

1. Fabricating a bed for the die in the working model (Fig. 2A)

There are several ways to do this. Examples might be:

a. The bed can be in the form of a stone or plaster base (Fig. 2A). The stone which forms the bed is poured over the die material that fills the crown portion of the impression after covering the die material with a separating medium.

b. The stone bed may be located in a resin or metal tray (Fig. 2B). The working model is trimmed to loosely fit in the tray. The tray has multiple keying retention irregularities inside. A separating medium is applied on the inner surface of the tray. A stone mix is poured into the tray and the trimmed model is seated within.

c. Some trays of this type have, additionally, horizontal removable pins that enhance immobilization and keying of the die. The pins are placed through holes in the tray into the stone bed before it is set. Both types of pre-formed trays have attachments for mounting to virtually any type of articulator.

d. In any of these methods, after the bed material sets, the prepared tooth replica is sawed and separated. It is very important to maintain the mesio-distal dimension of the die and working model to avoid incorporating errors into the wax pattern.

2. Locking mechanisms for the die (Figs. 2 and 3)

a. A dowel pin may be incorporated in the die material mix after it fills the crown portion of the prepared tooth. This necessitates marking the proximal limits of the preparation in the impression on the facial and lingual borders of the impressions to insure proper placement of the dowel pin (Fig. 3).

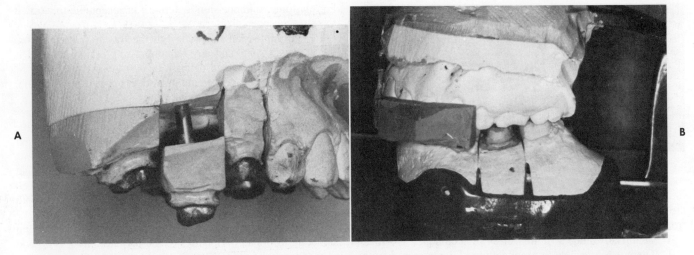

Fig. 22-2

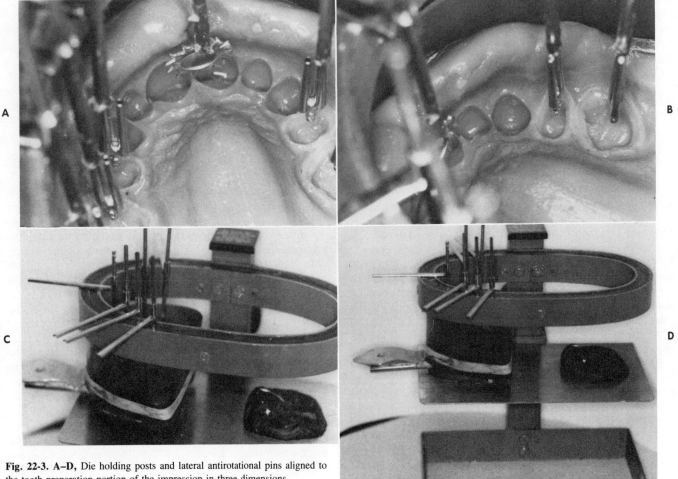

Fig. 22-3. A–D, Die holding posts and lateral antirotational pins aligned to the tooth preparation portion of the impression in three dimensions.

Courtesy of Dr. Ronald H. Pflueger.

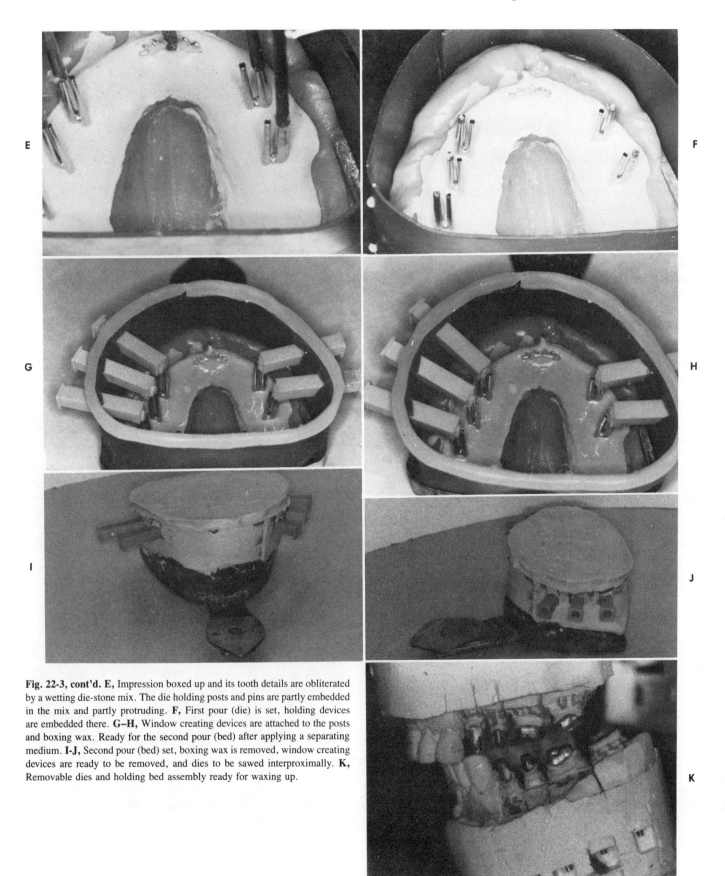

Fig. 22-3, cont'd. E, Impression boxed up and its tooth details are obliterated by a wetting die-stone mix. The die holding posts and pins are partly embedded in the mix and partly protruding. **F,** First pour (die) is set, holding devices are embedded there. **G–H,** Window creating devices are attached to the posts and boxing wax. Ready for the second pour (bed) after applying a separating medium. **I-J,** Second pour (bed) set, boxing wax is removed, window creating devices are ready to be removed, and dies to be sawed interproximally. **K,** Removable dies and holding bed assembly ready for waxing up.

mixing and pouring with vibration and soaking set model in a resin monomer, to be heat or auto-cured.

b. Dowel pins are not completely resistant to rotary movement of the die, especially if a sizable amount of the proximal gypsum is lost during sawing. Lateral antirotational pins can be incorporated in the die material mix next to the dowel pins (Fig. 3). Frequently little concavities or V-shaped grooves etc. are prepared in the base of the die to be reproduced as convexities or V-shaped protuberances in the bed, etc.

c. The immobilizing irregularities of the locking tray, if reproduced in the working model and the bed (Fig. 2), will prevent any movement of the die or the adjacent parts of the working model. To allow the die to be removed, the sides of the tray can be detached by a releasing hatch lock, thereby facilitating removal of the die.

d. There is another technique (Fig. 4) that necessitates the use of an apparatus to drill dowel-pin receptor channels in the working model for a dowel and an antirotational lateral pin. Both can then be attached to the working model. They are often supplied with sleeves which are incorporated in the bed. In this way, you assure proper reproducibility of the die from the impression before possible disturbances from post incorporation.

The main advantages of the techniques that can use one pour (cast) are:

a. They save time and effort by using one cast only.

b. They eliminate dimensional discrepancies between dies.

c. There is less distortion to the wax pattern since it is not moved from one die to another.

The disadvantages of this technique are:

a. Mobility in one or more direction is not completely prohibited, especially with the loss of the interproximal gypsum of adjacent teeth.

b. The use of different additional materials, as compared to the first technique, can introduce additional variables in the cast fabrication with more possibility for error.

c. Necessity for additional tools and equipment.

IV. Preparing the Die for the Wax Pattern

The following are the preparatory steps for the die to receive the wax in the process to make the wax pattern.

A. Die trimming

The margin and the details of the circumferential tie should be readable and recognizable. This can be done in several ways, but the simplest is to create (leave) a flat or convex surface peripheral to them. Preferably, the replica of an unprepared tooth surface, to be followed by a groove or a troughing in the die, which can be done using a round or inverted cone bur.

B. Die spacing (Fig. 5)

1. The main objective of a die spacer is to create room for the final casting-cementing medium. By creating that room, hydraulic pressure during seating is minimized.

2. Also, it is done to insure complete seating of the casting for the following reasons:

a. The investment surface of the mold will reproduce the wax pattern in a rougher fashion than presented. This roughness will be in the form of excesses rather than deficiencies. A space is created by die spacing for these excesses, thereby preventing

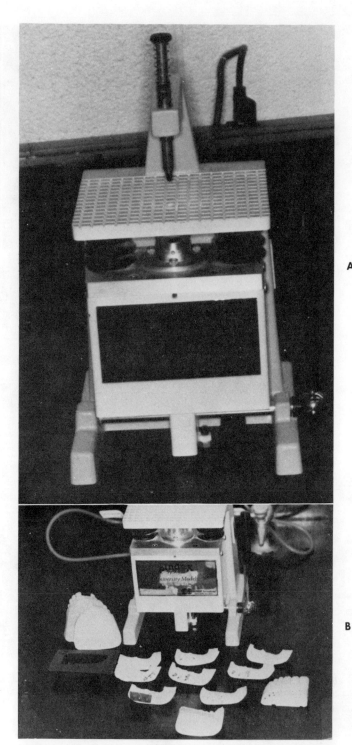

Fig. 22-4

them from interfering in the seating of the casting. If a space is not established for these rough excesses and the casting is forced onto the tooth, it can "bounce back" due to these isolated multiple non-accommodable contact areas (tips of the excesses).

b. In addition, it has been proven that die spacing can increase the casting retention (25% estimated increase) as a result

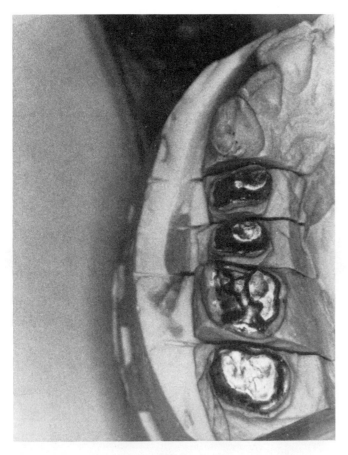

Fig. 22-5

of more intimate contact between the casting and tooth structure.

3. Die spacing can be done using insoluble paints (model airplane paints are very adequate). It should be applied on the die so as to cover the axial walls, cavity floor, and preparation surfaces short of the circumferential tie constitutents. The paint should be in a contrasting color from that of the die to insure its location.

It should have a film thickness of at least 25 microns, which may necessitate several applications (4-5). Always wait until the previous layer dries before applying another layer. It is a good idea to use a different color for each layer in order to be sure that no locations were missed and that there is an even thickness. With a paint remover (organic solvent) remove any paint that comes in contact with or close to the circumferential tie. The longer the surrounding walls are, the greater is the thickness of the die spacing that should be placed.

C. Pin preparation

Incorporated wrought pins or nylon bristles should be readily removable from their pin channels in the die or the metal sleeves that are incorporated in the die. Previously applied separating medium greatly aids this. Avoid pin channels, internal boxes and slots when placing the spacer.

As soon as the die spacing paint dries, a separating medium in the form of a thin film-forming oil (mineral or vegetable) is applied with a soft sable brush in a minimum amount as possible to coat all of the die surfaces. Any excess should be driven away with a light stream of air.

The aforementioned procedures can be done, using either gypsum-based or resin-based die and model materials. For resin-based materials, it is usually sufficient to only replicate the prepared tooth in resin, and the model base, unprepared teeth and the bed can be made in gypsum-based material.

BIBLIOGRAPHY

Beck, D.B.: Precision technique for trimming dies using a magnification device. J. Prosth. Dent. **43**(5):590-591, 1980.

DeLuca, R.: Personal communication.

Dilts, W.E., and others: Accuracy of four removable die techniques. JADA **83**:1081, 1971.

Dilts, W.E., and others: Accuracy of a removable die-dowel pin technique. J. Dent. Res. **50**:1249, 1971.

Eames, W.B., Edwards, Jr., C.R., and Buck, W.H., Jr.: Scraping resistance of dental die materials: A comparison of brands. Oper. Dent. **3**:66, 1978.

Finger, W.: Effect of the setting expansion of dental stone upon the die precision. Scand. J. Dent. Res. **88**(2):159-160, 1980.

Fukui, H., Lacy, A.M., and Jendresen, M.D.: Effectiveness of hardening films on die stone. J. Prosth. Dent. **44**(1):57-63, 1980.

Fusyama, T., and others: Relief of resistance of cement of full cast crowns. J. Prosth. Dent. **14**:95, 1964.

Harrison, J.D.: Prevention of failures in making impressions and dies. Dent. Clin. North Am. **23**(1):13-20, Jan. 1979.

Hembree, J.H., Jr., and Cooper, E.W., Jr.: Effect of die relief on retention of cast crowns and inlays. Oper. Dent. **4**(3):104-107, Summer 1979.

Hosoda, H., and Ohsawa, M.: Evaluating dimensional accuracy of stone models. J. Dent. Res. **58**(4):1352-1357, 1979.

Jorgensen, K.D.: Studies on the setting of plaster of paris. Odont. T. **61**:305-346, 1953.

Karesh, S.H.: An alternative impression and die technique for full crowns. Quintessence Int. **10**(8):17-20, 1979.

Khera, S.C., Girsch, W.J., Jr., and Thayer, K.E.: Fabrication of dies using typadon trays. Gen. Dent. **26**(6):55-60, 1978.

Mahler, D.B.: Hardness and flow properties of gypsum materials. J. Prosth. Dent. **1**:188-195, 1951.

Moghadam, B.K., Drennon, D.G., Thayer, K.E.: A die transfer technique. J. Prosth. Dent. **37**(2):226-230, Feb. 1977.

Nicholson, R.J., Soelberg, K.B., Stark, M.M., Kempler, D., and Leung, R.L.: Accuracy and smoothness of gypsum die stones with reversible hydrocolloid impression material. Oper. Dent. **2**(1):17-20, 1977.

Nomura, G.T., Reisbick, M.H., and Preston, J.D.: An investigation of epoxy resin dies. J. Prosth. Dent. **44**(1)45-50, 1980.

Peyton, F.A., Leibold, J.P., and Ridgley, C.V.: Surface hardness, compressive strength and abrasion resistance of indirect die stones. J. Prosth. Dent. **2**:381-389, 1952.

Picichelli, J., Mondelli, J., Galan, J., Jr., and Ishikiriama, A.: Fit of casting obtained from three different die materials. Oper. Dent. **2**(2):50-54, Spring 1977.

Schwartz, H.B., Leopold, R.J., and Thompson, V.P.: Linear dimensional accuracy of epoxy resin and stone dies. J. Prosth. Dent. **45**(6):621-625, 1981.

Smith, C.D., Nayyar, A., and Koth, D.L.: Fabrication of removable stone dies using cemented dowel pins. J. Prosth. Dent. **41**(5):579-581, 1979.

Stephan, J.E., Boduch, P.A., Elverun, J.N.: Method for making cast epoxy resin bodies and epoxy formulation. U.S. patent 4374076, Feb. 1983.

Stone, T.E., and Welker, W.A.: A method for lacting dowel pins in artificial stone casts. J. Prosth. Dent. **44**(3):345-346, 1980.

Sweeney, W.T., and Taylor, D.F.: Dimensional changes in dental stone and plaster. J. Dent. Res. **29**:749-755, 1950.

Vermilyea, S.G., and others: Evaluation of resin die materials. J. Prosth. Dent. **42**(3):304-307, 1979.

CHAPTER 23

Temporary restorations, occlusion records and transfer

Temporary Restorations

In almost all situations, a cast restoration cannot be completed in one visit. This necessitates that the prepared tooth be restored temporarily (Fig. 1) until the casting is fabricated. Besides, it is an advisable procedure to allow the pulp-dentin organ and periodontium to recover before permanently cementing the restoration. A good temporary restoration has several objectives. From a biological and physiological standpoint, the temporary restoration should cover, protect, and sedate the P-D organ or the periodontium. This necessitates the use of inert or sedative materials and cements. The temporary should be smooth and free from marginal discrepancies that might encourage plaque accumulation. It should create an adequate seal for the preparation to prevent the ingress of irritating fluids to the P-D organ.

Functionally, the temporary should maintain, in three dimensions, the position of the tooth in the arch. Its occlusal and axial contours should harmonize with the stomato-gnathic system and adjacent supportive structures. Mechanically, the temporary should be easily removed and replaced without damage to itself or irritation to the tooth or periodontium. It should be easily fabricated and adjusted chair-side with minimal laboratory procedures. The materials used for fabricating temporary restorations are usually either unfilled acrylic and composite acrylic (or BIS-GMA) resins, or premade polycarbonate, celluloid and metallic (aluminum) crown forms that are adjusted and customized for the prepared tooth.

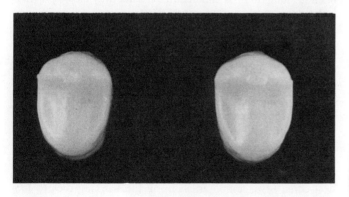

Fig. 23-1

The cements used are usually various types of modified ZOE cements. As with the die and working model construction there are limitless numbers of techniques used for fabricating temporary restorations. The following will not be a description of all the techniques used, but only an attempt to categorize them.

I. Temporary Cements

These are usually ZOE modified with fillers, rosin, and orthoethoxy benzoic acid. Temporary restorations completely made of these cements are indicated for small inlay cavity preparations, in areas of minimal loading when the cavity walls are well preserved. If more than the occlusal surface is involved, a matrix, as for amalgam restorations, is adapted to the tooth, and a thick mix of the cement is inserted into the cavity with a water-moistened cotton pellet. Water will accelerate its setting. The material is then carved with a suitable plastic instrument. The matrix can be removed and the carving is completed. This technique produces the weakest of all types of temporary restorations which sometimes necessitates reinforcing the ZOE with cotton fibers, amalgam alloy powder, etc.

II. Customized Preformed Crown Forms

These are fabricated of cellulose, polycarbonate, acrylic, or metal. The metal crowns, which are indicated only for posterior teeth are usually made of aluminum, but similar soft alloys may be used.

A suitable size of crown form that conforms with the tooth dimensions is selected. It is trimmed using a pair of scissors. Excesses and areas of the crown form corresponding to unprepared tooth surfaces are removed. The crown's gingival margins are festooned to the gingival architecture of the preparation and the edges are smoothed.

If the adjusted crown form fits the tooth fairly snugly, it can be cemented as is with modified ZOE cement. If the adjusted crown form fits loosely, it must be customized. A separating medium (vaseline or petroleum jelly) is painted over the preparation. The crown form is vented at one or more points, then filled with an unfilled acrylic resin mix. The crown form containing the acrylic mix is pressed over the prepared tooth with the bulk of the excess expressed out the vent. This insures minimal voids. Any marginal excesses of the mix are wiped off. The material is allowed to set until the rubbery stage, when it is removed and allowed to polymerize on the bench (setting can be accelerated by putting it in hot water). The acrylic relined crown form is trimmed marginally, relieved on the inside to create space for the cement and tried on the tooth. All adjustments are made, and the temporary is now polished on a lathe with pumice. The tooth is washed from the separating medium. Any minute auxillary retention mean not reproduced in the temporary should be filled with a passive material, e.g., a paper point in pin channels, cotton pellets in internal boxes and slots, etc.

Line the temporary restoration with the temporary cement and seat under pressure. Higher temperature, saliva, and water in the oral environment will accelerate the setting of the cement. When the cement medium is set, flake off excesses from both the tooth and temporary surfaces, and curette the remnants of the cement from the gingival crevice.

This technique is ideal for preparations with axial surface reductions and for teeth with no or minimal undercuts in their occluso-apical curvature. This technique cannot be used for purely intracoronal preparations or for preparations involving less than three surfaces. It is fast and lends itself to any modifications deemed necessary for the situation at hand. It produces the strongest type of all temporaries because of the premade component.

III. Temporaries Formed Completely of Polymerizable Resins

There are many ways to fabricate the entire temporary restoration from a monomer-polymer mix of the resin. Examples are:

A. The matrix technique

A matrix is adapted to the tooth in the same way as for amalgam insertion. The preparation surface is lubricated, and in a brush-bead technique the resin mixes are introduced in the preparation until it is overfilled. The resin material is removed with the matrix while still in the rubbery stage, and is allowed to complete polymerization on the bench. It is trimmed, adjusted, polished, and cemented as in the previous technique.

This technique is suitable when the proximal and occlusal reductions of the preparation are minimal or not present. It cannot be used when there is any facial or lingual axial reduction. The technique is usually workable where there are adequate retentive intracoronal walls.

B. The initial gross mass technique

The tooth is lubricated. A dough mix of the resin is prepared. A sufficient amount is pressed onto the preparation. The patient is asked to move his mandible functionally while the mass is soft. When sufficiently rigid, the mass is removed and allowed to complete polymerization on the bench. The hardened resin is carved to the proper shape, dimensions and margins, using lab carbide burs, stones and sand paper discs. The carved restoration is tried on, relieved from inside, finished, polished, and cemented as other techniques.

This technique can be used for any situation. It is very time consuming and the resulting temporary can be weak due to porosity and residual monomer. However, in the hands of a trained operator, excellent results can be achieved by this technique.

C. Techniques producing temporary restorations that replicate the original or modified tooth morphology

Any defect in the tooth before preparation is restored in wax. This can be done in the mouth or on the study models. If done in the mouth, a quadrant alginate, elastomeric, or plaster impression (confined to portions occlusal to the height of contour) is taken. Any flange excesses are trimmed. The impression, if in alginate, is kept in a humidor during preparation of the tooth, that is not necessary for elastomeric or plaster ones. If done on study models, an alginate or elastomeric impression can be taken as in the mouth, or a sheet of temporary splinting material (resinous or celluloid) can be thermoplastically molded to the shape of the tooth crowns, using a special apparatus incorporating heat and a vacuum. After preparing the tooth, the preparation and surrounding unprepared surfaces are lubricated as usual. The crown portion of the impression or the molded splinting sheet is filled with the resin mix and seated on the tooth intraorally. The unprepared teeth will act as guides for seating and as stops to prevent further seating.

While the resin mix is in the late rubbery stage, the impression or the splint sheet is removed. Usually the temporary will stick to the tooth. It is gently removed, using plastic instruments or towel clamps. It is imperative that temporaries done in this way be removed before they are rigid insofar as a considerable amount of the resin will flow into undercuts. Since these areas are inaccessible for removing the resin while soft, the only way to remove the temporary is during the rubbery stage while it is still elastic. The molded resin is left to cure on the bench and treated as in the previous techniques.

Sometimes these procedures are done completely out of the mouth. A second quadrant impression is taken after tooth preparation is complete. This impression is poured in die stone mixed with slurry water to accelerate its setting. The resulting model is lubricated and the temporaries are fabricated on this model rather than intraorally. This allows the temporary to completely cure on the replicated preparation. A modification of this technique involves a heat cured resin being used to fill the plaster impression of the unprepared teeth. This filled impression is seated on the post-preparation model and wrapped tightly with wire. It is then placed in a pressure cooker to cure the acrylic in a short time. In either case, the cured resinous temporary is handled in the same way as the previous techniques.

These are very fast techniques if the pre-preparation morphology is adequate and properly captured in the impression. The main disadvantage is the intraoral difficulty or impossibility of removing the temporaries if the teeth have severe surface undercuts. Also if the temporary requires an anatomy different than that of the pre-preparation tooth, those morphological changes are usually in wax with its possible distortion. But with some care, very successful results can be obtained.

Many restorative cases require the use of long-range temporaries. In these instances it is advisable to fabricate custom heat-cured resin temporaries, using the working dies to fabricate the patterns for the temporaries. These patterns should then be flasked and replicated in the appropriate resin using conventional procedures.

Occlusion Records and Transfer

Since cast restorations are fabricated outside the mouth, their construction should involve a way to duplicate the mandibular movements and/or their anticipated configurative effects on the future restoration. This is to insure that the restoration is compatible with and conducive to a sound and functional stomatognathic system.

The objectives for these duplications are to facilitate the means to build a restoration with the following specifications: The restoration must have the appropriate configuration, dimensions, and anatomy. This requires that the occluding components are in a stable, non-deflecting relationship with the opposing occluding components. This relationship must not change the vertical dimension. The non-functional (balancing) cuspal elements will be in a non-contact relationship with their opposing reciprocating cuspal elements, especially in excursive mandibular movements.

In addition, the occluding surfaces of the restorations must participate in the mandibular movements as dictated by the posterior (condylar) and anterior (incisal guidance) determinants, i.e., they will not interfere in any way with the physiologic predetermined pattern of movement. During mandibular movements from centric relation to centric occlusion and from centric relation to the border positions the restoration should not have any interfering or deflecting elements in its occluding surfaces.

If the tooth receiving the restoration takes part in a disclusion mechanism, the restoration must have a cusp height and cuspal inclinations to fit in the exact sequence, timing, and contact location angulation and extent during the disclusion mechanism. A restoration capable of fulfilling all the above mentioned criteria should be loadable not to exceed tolerable stresses in the underlying tooth structure, periodontium or any other components of the gnatho-stomatic system.

To build a restoration with such detail, the mandibular movements, jaw relations (static and dynamic) and occlusal determinants must be recorded in a transferable manner. The minimum occlusion information to build a restoration in the above mentioned specifications requires:

A. Static relationship recording in the form of

1. The vertical (occluso-apical) and horizontal (mesio-distal and bucco-lingual) dimensions of the tooth as determined by occlusion factors.

2. Tooth components and surface areas of contacts that meet (or should meet) in centric occlusion (maximal intercuspation).

3. The nature of condylar fossae relation in centric relation.

4. Tooth components and surface area of contacts that meet (or should meet) at the very border limits of the lateral and protrusive excursion.

B. A dynamic relationship recording in the form of

1. The pathway for the occluding elements of the lower teeth along their reciprocating counterparts in the upper teeth from centric relation to centric occlusion. The pathway record should reflect the type of tooth components and their surface areas of contact at different stages of movement as well as the directions of these movements in three dimensions.

2. The occluding tooth parts and their surface area of contact at different stages of mandibular movements from centric occlusion to border limits (laterally and anteriorly), as well as the directions of these paths at different contact areas in three dimensions.

3. The disclusion mechanism components, pattern and pathways including the location and number of teeth involved, the specific anatomical elements involved, and the location and extent of the surface area of contact at different disclusion stages. The recording should also reveal the sequence of disengagement of occluding elements and the direction of the path in three dimensions.

There are two major classes of techniques that will obtain and record the aforementioned data.

I. Instrumental Techniques

These are techniques that are dependent upon identifying and duplicating the determinants for mandibular movements and for the interrelationship between the upper and lower jaws and, consequently, the teeth. Duplication is done through specific clinical records that are transferred to an anticulator where the determinant's duplicates are established. The restoration is built on this anticulator, which is capable of movements and relations dictated by the transferred determinant replicas. The techniques and their procedures are described in detail in the chapter on single tooth restorations and the stomato-gnathic system.

II. Conformative Techniques or the Functionally Generated Path Techniques

These are techniques that are dependent upon the creation of an intra-oral three dimensional stereo-pattern for the shape and paths of, and, within the occluding elements of the tooth to be restored, resulting from all possible movements of the mandible. The three-dimensional stereo pattern should be created and duplicated in a material that has minimal distortion during its use. This class of techniques is basically indicated for cases with the following prerequisites:

1. Teeth to be restored are upper molars or premolars where the posterior anatomical and anterior incisal guidance determinants are physiologic and well established.

2. Opposing lower teeth have normal pronounced and physiologic occluding anatomy capable of functionally deforming the material used for the stereo path pattern.

3. The involved teeth (both upper and lower) should be immobile in their housing periodontium. This is essential to prevent the tooth from being moved or jarred during the formation of the stereo-occlusion pattern.

4. The teeth to be restored will accommodate the stereo pattern material with sufficient retaining capability for that material, so that the material does not move separately from the tooth during the formulation of the stereo pattern. If this is not a certainty, then the teeth adjacent to the prepared teeth should be stable and have components for retention of the stereo pattern material.

5. The teeth to be restored should at least have an unprepared tooth anterior and another one posterior to them, to act as a reference surface in checking the complete seating of the recorded stereo path on the working model, and to insure complete stabilization of the recording material during its functional deformation.

This technique does not allow for altering the original occlusion, dimensions of the occlusal table, or the vertical dimension. If the prerequisites cannot be met, this technique must be modified or a different technique employed.

A. The basic functionally generated path technique for a single non-terminal upper posterior tooth

After completing the tooth preparation or, preferably just after the occlusal reduction, softened compound is adapted over the tooth and allowed to harden under pressure. Any excess compound occlusally should be trimmed to insure that the compound is not touching opposing occluding surfaces at any location. This should be checked visually and by using articulating paper. The compound should accommodate some retention modes for the wax that will be applied, e.g., undercuts or roughening.

Functionally generated path wax is flowed over the compound with buccal-lingual dimensions comparable to adjacent teeth. The wax should be deformably soft just above mouth temperature, but should harden at mouth temperature and have a very narrow melting range. When it hardens, it should be brittle and fracture rather than deform.

While the wax is soft, the mandible is guided to centric relationship. It is then guided slowly forward to centric occlusion, then gradually guided from centric occlusion to the furthest lateral border limits and back to centric occlusion. Finally, it should be gradually guided to the most anterior limit of the frontal border movement, then back to the centric occlusion.

The patient is then asked to move the mandible laterally and forward in a slow motion to deform the wax in the way the teeth relate in their intraborder movements, completing the stereo path pattern. The wax should be hardened by now. Trim any gross lateral excesses that may invite pattern displacement by adjacent musculature. Also, trim excesses that are not carrying any path for the opposing teeth. These are usually the wax that has been moved aside as a result of the deformation along the cuspal component path.

A creamy mix of functionally generated path plaster (fast setting plaster) is made and carried in small beads to the details of the created stereo path pattern and the occluding anatomy of adjacent teeth (one tooth on each side minimally). When these details are completely filled, a sufficient amount of the plaster is carried in a functionally generated path tray or a wooden tongue depressor and brought into contact with the rest of the inserted plaster. Be sure that the plaster does not go apical to the height of contour of the involved teeth, especially the intact teeth. Also, the plaster should not go apical to the contact areas in the embrasures. The plaster is allowed to harden.

The hardened plaster impression of the three-dimensional occlusion pattern is removed gently. It is trimmed laterally, removing any unnecessary details, and the wax pattern is discarded. This plaster impression is called the *functional core*

and should be placed aside until the preparation is completed and working models and dies are available.

The functional core is tried on the working model, which can be a quadrant model. A space between the functional core and the unprepared anterior or posterior keying teeth on the working model may represent an interference, preventing the complete seating of the functional core. Any interference should be detected and removed. The functional core is then checked for any lateral movement or rocking. If present, and if the causes cannot be recognized and/or corrected, a new core must be made. The functional core should fit the working model as it fits the teeth intraorally in a stable three-dimensional relationship.

The functional core is seated on the working model and attached to it with sticky wax or wooden sticks held in place with compound, creating a non-mobile assembly. This assembly is then mounted on a simple articulator called a verticulator (Fig. 2, A and B). This is a device which holds the core and working model in a predetermined position and is capable of up and down piston movements only. Its movements are controlled by piston arrangement in its back. While mounting, the two arms of the verticulator should be prevented from separating due to plaster expansion or distortion in the assembly mechanism of the two components. This is done by applying pressure while the mounting gypsum is setting.

After the plaster hardens, the assembly mechanism is detached, the upper model and the functional core are checked

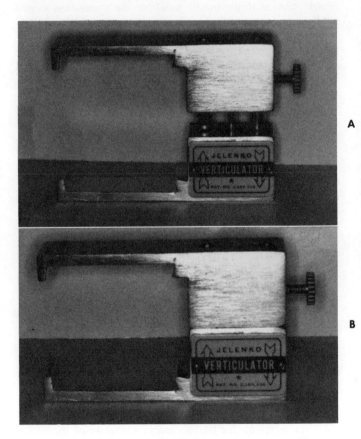

Fig. 23-2

again for complete closure. If verified, the dies are made ready for waxing. Since the configuration of all possible mandibular movements is built into the functional core, there is no need for any lateral or protrusive movements in the articulator.

The casting wax is flowed onto the tooth preparation in excess. The lubricated functional core is brought to its pre-determined relation with the working model (containing the dies) by closing the verticulator. It is kept there until the wax hardens. Upon opening the verticulator the occluding morphology is almost completely established. It should be refined and modified as follows:

1. Establish and accentuate missing or blunted grooves by carving, not by wax addition.

2. Relieve the wax from contacting balancing inclines where there should be no contact. Although recorded as a contact in the functional core, it only represents an unmoved functional path wax pattern area.

3. Since the functional core usually has greater facio-lingual dimensions than the prescribed width of the tooth, the buccal-lingual width of the wax pattern should be reduced to conform to the adjacent teeth.

4. If the occlusal inclines of the buccal cusps are involved in a disclusion mechanism, their length should be arbitrarily reduced relative to that of the tooth anterior to it. This reduction is done to insure that the tooth disengages prior to the tooth anteriorly. The restoration will definitely need intraoral adjustment to refine this relationship.

5. The contact and margins of the wax pattern are established. The dies with wax patterns are checked to see if they can move occlusally while the verticulator is closed. If they can move, this is due to overcarving (missing contacts) occlusally which must be corrected. The wax pattern is then invested and the casting is fabricated.

After fabrication, the casting is seated on its die and checked for the following:

a. Any interference preventing complete closure of the verticulator is identified, using articulating paper, and eliminated.

b. The verticulator is closed—any vertical movement of the die indicates the casting may have been distorted or undergone surface loss during fabrication. Any lateral movement of the die may indicate interferences, distortion or surface loss. If the discrepancies are not correctable in the casting, the casting should be re-done.

B. Basic techniques for several bilaterally distributed upper posterior teeth

In this situation the advantage exists of using cross-arch stabilization and retention. The procedure can be done as follows:

1. On a model for the upper teeth, including the prepared teeth, an occlusal splinting type base is constructed. It is to be purely tooth supported without any contact with the palatal or gingival mucosa. The base can be made of base-plate wax, or auto-polymerizing unfilled resin. It should be as sturdy and rigid as possible which may require reinforcing it with 0.050″ diameter stainless steel wires across the palate.

2. The base should be retained by the lingual surfaces of the unprepared teeth and through complete coverage of the prepared tooth surfaces. The base should not cover the oc-

cluding or facial surfaces of the unprepared teeth.

3. The base is tried in the mouth to insure that it is not touching or interfering with any soft tissue or musculature and that it is stable in three dimensions. The patient is then asked to move the lower jaw in all possible movements and to all possible relations, with articulating paper in position. Any contacts on the base are removed.

4. The base is placed on the working model and the functionally generated path wax is flowed onto the parts of the base covering the prepared teeth. The base is seated back in the mouth, and while the wax is soft, the procedures of guiding the mandible into all possible movements and relations is performed. Then the patient is allowed to make his own mandibular movements. The wax is chilled and excesses are trimmed.

5. The functionally generated path plaster is flowed over the prepared and adjacent teeth as mentioned in (A), being sure to include the occluding surfaces of the cuspid. The plaster is allowed to harden and the base with the functional path pattern and the hardened plaster are removed in one piece.

6. A gypsum base is built for the created functional cores that connects and supports them. After the gypsum base material hardens, the pattern base and the functional path wax patterns are removed from the functional cores which are now joined in one piece with the created base. The gypsum base-joined functional core will act as the opposing model in a mounting assembly using a semi-adjustable articulator with the upper working model attached via a facebow record. The articulator should be used in hinge movements only. All devices for lateral movements in the articulator should be deactivated and locked. The same procedures as previously described are employed in checking the mounting, the patterns, and the post-casting trial of the castings.

C. Modified technique for unilateral terminal upper posterior teeth

A unilateral terminal upper posterior tooth presents the operator two problems. First, the functional path pattern is not sufficiently stable during lateral movements since there is no distal tooth or cross-arch extension to lock the wax during deformation. Second, there are unprepared teeth anteriorly to act as keys, but none posteriorly. This situation creates an additional problem in that the functional path pattern and the core could move apically, distal to the terminal tooth, at the expense of deforming the soft tissues they come in contact with. So there is some possibility of discrepancy in the pattern and core dimensions occluso-apically.

If the other prerequisites for the functionally generated path technique are satisfied, the basic technique can be modified as follows:

1. A putty mix of silicone rubber base is prepared. An oblong length of it is applied on the occlusal surfaces of the quadrant with the prepared tooth, covering at least two unprepared teeth anterior to it. The rubber is pressed against the covered tooth surfaces and tucked interproximally to retain it on the maxillary quadrant.

2. While the material is still moldable, the mandible is guided to centric relation and then forward to centric occlusion. The patient is asked to firmly close the mouth there until the material hardens. The patient then opens, and with the rubber

base in place on the maxillary quadrant, lateral excesses of the set silicone rubber are cut away without interfering with the stability of the centric configuration.

3. Functionally generated path plaster is flowed into the mandibular occlusal details of the set rubber base. Plaster is then carried on a functionally generated path tray and pressed against the previously inserted plaster and allow to set. The functional core is then removed from the rubber centric pattern.

4. The portion of the silicone rubber covering the prepared tooth is cut away. Hard setting wax is applied on the occlusal surface of the functional core in the prepared tooth area, and the functional core is replaced intraorally with the rest of the rubber pattern. Being sure that the wax is in contact with the prepared tooth occlusally, the wax is allowed to harden.

5. The functional core is removed with its keying wax, which has verified and captured the occluso-apical location of the functional core relative to the prepared tooth.

6. The rubber pattern is removed from the mouth and placed on the upper working model. The upper working model is then mounted against the wax-keyed functional core on a verticulator. As soon as the assembly gypsum hardens, the keying wax and rubber pattern are discarded, and the casting is fabricated as mentioned previously.

7. Since the functional core recorded only centric relation and centric occlusion, the resulting casting should be tried on the tooth intraorally, and any lateral interferences should be removed.

D. Modified technique for lower posterior teeth

The functionally generated path technique for lower posterior teeth presents two problems. First, intact lower teeth are excellent deformers for functional wax on upper teeth. However, intact upper teeth are poor deformers for functional wax on lower teeth. This is because the mandible is the moving component in the deformer-deformee relationship, so that not all of the details of the functional path of lower teeth will be reproduced in a stereo-path pattern. The second problem is that the lateral stability of the deformable wax on lower teeth is not as secure as with the upper teeth (e.g., there is no possibility of cross arch connections).

Provided that the rest of the prerequisites are fulfilled, the modified technique for lower posterior teeth, whether single or multiple, uni- or bilateral, terminal or non-terminal tooth is as follows:

1. After completion of the tooth preparation, a temporary restoration for the tooth is fabricated in an auto-polymerizing resin.

2. Occlusal contacts on the temporary are marked using articulating paper while the mandible is guided or moved in all possible ways. The temporary is relieved completely from any opposing tooth contacts.

3. The temporary is seated back on the tooth and, in a brush-bead technique, beads of colored unfilled resin are flowed onto the occlusal surface of the temporary in an over-built-in fashion. A color different than that of the temporary is used.

4. While the colored resin is polymerizing, the patient's mandible is guided to centric relation and then to centric occlusion, and the patient is asked to keep this mandibular relation until the resin sets.

5. The temporary is removed, the lateral excesses are eliminated, and the temporary is returned to the mouth.

6. The patient's mandible is guided from centric occlusion to lateral and anterior border limits with a marking ribbon between the upper and lower teeth.

7. Undesirable contacts are selectively removed. This may require several trials.

8. The temporary is put back in place, and, using articulating paper, the patient is asked to go through different mandibular movements without any guidance. Again, undesirable contacts are selectively removed.

9. Occasionally, desirable contacts are not present due to overgrinding or their failure to be created initially in the resin. For either case, a bead or more of the resin mix is added to the area, missing the contact. The resin is allowed to harden and the occlusion is again checked.

10. If the restoration is to be a part of a disclusion mechanism, the involved portion of the temporary should be over-built. The temporary is then tried intraorally and adjusted to conform to the desired extent, location, angulation and sequence of disengagement as dictated by the disclusion of the mandible.

11. After verifying that the temporary is in functional participation, it may be cemented and left for several days to confirm its configuration. A functional core is then fabricated as previously described. If there is no uncertainty in the configuration of the temporary, the functional core can be made immediately.

E. Modified technique for anterior teeth

The problem of using functionally generated path records for anterior teeth is that the anterior teeth are one of the determinants (i.e., the incisal guidance) of occlusion. Functionally generated recording depends upon them.

However, the following is a procedure for a modified technique to resolve this problem, assuming other pre-requisites are present.

1. If the tooth is to be prepared for an extracoronal preparation, and it still has enamel to be etched, prior to preparation, the tooth could be built up in composite resin to the appropriate configuration asthetically and functionally. On the other hand, if the tooth is to be prepared for intra- or extra-coronal preparation, it can be prepared first and an adequate temporary restoration fabricated.

2. The composite build-up or the temporary is now adjusted according to the lip line, tongue and lip locations, opposing occluding elements, compatible mesio-distal dimension, protrusive and lateral mandibular movements, adjacent periodontium, and soft tissues. Adjustment can require addition or grinding. It is advisable to leave the temporaries in place for a while (a few days to a week). Evaluate them again and make any necessary adjustments.

3. When the composite build-up or temporary is perfected a stock plastic impression tray is tried in the mouth. It should loosely fit the teeth. For the uppers, the labial (buccal) flanges (lingual ones for the lowers) of the tray are eliminated.

4. For the uppers, functionally generated path plaster is flowed over the lingual and incisal (labial and incisal for the lowers) surfaces of the temporarily restored tooth, and then

the tray is filled with the same plaster and seated. Be sure the plaster does not cover any labial (lingual for the lowers) surfaces of the teeth or pronounced undercuts.

5. This technique results in a plaster functional core that will be used as an opposing model for the fabrication of the permanent anterior cast restorations.

F. Modified technique for loose teeth

Conformative occlusal record techniques are usually contraindicated for loose teeth, for the obvious reason that forces used to deform the wax for the functional stereo pattern will be used partly or totally in moving a loosened tooth away from its normal position, resulting in an incorrect functional path record. An attempt should be made to temporarily immobilize the prepared tooth prior to proceeding with the creation of the stereo wax pattern. Methods for immobilization might include etching and splinting the teeth with composite resin. The resin would be placed on the buccal surfaces of the maxillary teeth or the lingual surfaces of the mandibular teeth (provided a normal overbite existed). This would require that the resin be placed prior to the preparation of these axial surface of the involved tooth. If the enamel has already been removed in tooth preparation, wire ligatures or wedges can be placed around or inbetween the teeth interproximally, followed by sticky wax or compound. In any instance, the loose teeth should be attached to as many stable teeth as possible, especially the canines. As soon as the immobilization is achieved any of the previously detailed procedures for conformative records could be used.

If immobilization is not feasible, the functional path can still be used, provided the following criteria are satisfied. First, the loose tooth must not be the terminal one in the arch. Second, the tooth anterior and the tooth posterior to the prepared tooth are intact. Third in these adjacent intact teeth there should be a definite single path for each lateral excursion and another single path for protrusive excursion. These teeth should preferably be more stable than the prepared tooth. Finally, the occluding anatomy of the contemplated restoration should be dictated by the occluding anatomy of these adjacent teeth.

The procedure is as follows:

1. A full arch working model and full arch opposing model are constructed.

2. The wax pattern is constructed on a separate die and placed on the preparation replica in the unsawed working model.

3. Talcum powder or resinous washable paint (with a different color than that of the wax) is applied on the occluding surfaces of the wax pattern for occlusal marking. The upper and lower models are assembled by hand in a position of maximum intercuspation. Wax is selectively removed from locations of undesirable contacts and selectively added to areas where desired occluding contacts are deficient.

4. The occluding surfaces of the wax pattern are covered again with the talcum powder or the paint, and the two models are moved laterally and anteriorally, via paths that are predetermined by the existing occlusion.

5. Again, interferences are selectively removed and deficient contacts are built-up. This procedure is repeated until the proper occlusal configuration is established. The wax pattern is then returned to the original die where it is margined. A casting is then fabricated.

6. The final casting may need further occlusal adjustment upon trying it intraorally. The adjustment will mainly be for the elimination of interferences during lateral and protrusive excursions and for harmonizing any disclusion involvement. Generally speaking, the more teeth there are anterior and posterior to the prepared tooth, and the less the number of the prepared teeth, the better will be the results of this technique.

G. Modification for a quadrant of maxillary teeth

For a quadrant of maxillary posterior teeth, provided there is an intact cuspid, it is advisable to build a temporary resin restoration for the terminal tooth as described in the technique for the lower teeth. The temporary is cemented, and the regular reproduction of the stereo wax pattern is performed for the remaining prepared teeth. A verticulator is satisfactory for mounting the case.

H. Modification for opposing prepared teeth

For opposing prepared teeth, it is advisable to build a temporary restoration for the lower tooth, or, occasionally, to fabricate its permanent restoration to an occlusion as ideal as possible. Cement the perfected lower restoration temporarily and use it to create the stereo wax pattern for the prepared upper tooth.

I. Modification for full mouth restoration

For full mouth restorations the recommended procedure for use of a functionally generated path is to restore the lower anterior teeth (either permanently or temporarily) to as ideal an occlusion, phonetics, and esthetics as possible. Conformative inciso-lingual records are used to restore the upper anteriors. With the upper and lower anterior permanent restorations cemented temporarily, the lower posterior (temporary or permanent) restorations are built with as ideal occluding surfaces as the available parameters will allow. They are temporarily cemented and conformative temporaries for the two terminal upper teeth are built. Conformative records are taken for the remaining prepared teeth, or the technique described in (B) with a cross-arch stabilizing base is used. A facebow and semi-adjustable articulator, with lateral and protrusive movements locked out, should be used in any of these steps.

BIBLIOGRAPHY

Benfield, J.W.: Advantages of functional bit technique in reducing chair time. N.Y. J. of Dent. **32**:296, 1962.

Benfield, J.W.: Di-lok system with functionally generated paths, work simplication in dental practice, Philadelphia, 1964, W.B. Saunders Co., p. 359-370.

Benfield, J.W., Mellana, F.L., Ras, E.M., and Lyons, G.V.: Reproducing occlusal anatomy for crowns and extensive inlays. J. Prosth. Dent. **18**:326-336, 1967.

Berman, M.H.: Reproduction of functional tooth form in full cast crowns. J. Prosth. Dent. **15**:491-496, 1965.

Celenza, F.V.: The centric position. Replacement and character. J. Prosth. Dent. **30**:591, 1973.

Celenza, F.V.: The physiological development of occlusal morphology, ed. 2. Berlin, Chicago, Rio de Janeiro, and Tokyo, 1975, Die Ouintessenz, p. 17.

Celenza, F., and Litvak, H.: Occlusal management in conformative dentistry. J. P. D. Aug. 1976.

Fiasconaro, J., and Sherman, H.: Vacuum-formed prosthesis: A temporary fixed bridge or splint. J. Am. Dent. Assn. **76:**74-78, 1968.

Granger, E.R.: Functional relations of the stomatognathic system. JADA **48:**638, 1954.

Ingervall, B., Helkimo, M., and Carlsson, G.E.: Recording of the retruded position of the mandible with application of varying external pressure to the lower jaw in man. Arch Oral Biol. **16:**1165, 1971.

Kantor, M.E., Silverman, S.I., and Garfinkel, L.: Centric-relation recording techniques—a comparative investigation. J. Prosth. Dent. **28:**593, 1972.

Krug, R.: Temporary resin crown and bridges. Dental Clinics of N. Am. vol. 19, No. 2, April 1975.

Lucia, V.O.: The fundamentals of oral physiology and their practical application in the securing and reproducing of records to be used in restorative dentistry. J. Prosth. Dent. **3:**213, 1953.

Mann, A.W., and Pankey, L.D.: Dental Clinics of N. Am. p. 621, 1963.

Mann, A.W., and Pankey, L.D.: Oral rehabilitation utilizing the Pankey-Mann instrument and a functional bite technique. Dental Clinics of N. Am. p. 215-230, March 1959.

McCollum, B.B.: Fundamentals unsolved in prescribing restorative dental remedies. Dent. Items Int. 48, 1940.

Meyer, F.S.: Can the plain line articulator meet all the demands of balanced and functional occlusion in all restorative work? J. of Colo. State Dent. Assoc. **17:**6-16, 1938.

Meyer, F.S.: The generated path technique in reconstruction dentistry, parts I and II. J. Pros. D. **9:**354-366, 432-440, May 1959.

Moulton, George H.: The importance of centric occlusion in diagnosis and treatment planning. J. Prosth. Dent. **10:**5, 1960.

Pankey, L.D., and Mann, A.W.: Oral rehabilitation, parts I and II. J. Prosth. Dent. **10:**135-162, 1960.

Pankey, L.D., and Mann, A.W.: Oral rehabilitation. II. Reconstruction of the upper teeth using a functioning generated path technique. J. Prosth. Dent. **10:**151-162, 1960.

Schuyler, C.H.: The function and importance of incisal guidance in oral habitation. J. Prosth. Dent. **13:**1011, 1963.

Schweitzer, Jerome M.: Concepts of occlusion: A discussion. Dent. Clin. N. Am. p. 649-671, 1963.

Schweitzer, J.M.: Oral rehabilitation. St. Louis, 1951. The C.V. Mosby Co., p. 1011-1115.

Smith, H.F.: A comparison of empirical centric relation records with location of terminal hinge axis and apex of the Gothic-arch tracing. J. Prosth. Dent. **33:**511, 1975.

Stallard, H., and Stuart, C.E.: Eliminating tooth guidance in natural dentition. J. Prosth. Dent. **11:**474, 1961.

Stuart, C.E., and Stallard, H.: Principles involved in restoring occlusion to natural teeth. J. Prosth. D., March-April, 1960.

CHAPTER 24

Casting fabrication

After perfection of the tooth preparation and, in most cases, the reproduction of its details and surrounding tooth surface in a suitable die mounted on an appropriate articulator, a wax replica of the future restoration is built. The wax replica must be perfected in terms of occlusion, contact, contour, anatomy and marginal adaptation. The information necessary to do this is supplied by the die, the anatomy of the working casts, and the movements or the occlusal registration of the articulator. The wax pattern is invested in the appropriate investment for the restorative cast material. The pattern is then evaporated (through burn-out) and the space created by its loss within the investment is completely filled with the wetting cast material. The resulting casting will be the final restoration.

For most casts, this technique involves five subsequent reproductions of the original details of the tooth preparation. In the procedure for each reproduction, different materials are used. Each material has dissimilar components, properties, behavior and method of manipulation. Despite that, the final product mismatch or discrepancy should not exceed 0.05-0.1%. Therefore, a full comprehension of the behavior of these materials and how to intelligently incorporate possible changes in one material to compensate for or counteract changes in another is basic to arrive at a serviceable restoration.

Given an accurate die attached to a cast (the latter mounted on an articulator) the procedure for the fabrication of the casting will be:

I. Wax Pattern Fabrication
II. Sprueing and Surface Treatment of the Completed Wax Pattern
III. Investment of the Wax Pattern
IV. Thermal Treatment of the Investment-Wax Pattern Complex
V. Casting or Injection Molding
VI. Cleaning the Casting from its Encasing Investment and Surface Deposits
VII. Possible Thermal Treatment of the Casting

I. Wax Pattern Fabrication

This is still the most empirical of all the steps in cast fabrication and the cause of most casting failures. This becomes evident in recalling the following facts about waxes for cast restoration patterns.

A. Composition

The ingredient with the highest percentage in these waxes is paraffin wax (40-60%). It is a basic petroleum hydrocarbon, characterized by non-homogenecity in the size of macromolecules and their spatial arrangement and combinations. This nature leads to ranges in the wax melting temperature and different extents in their coefficient of thermal expansion at different temperatures. Also, having this non-homogeneous microstructure can explain the abrupt changes in strength, plasticity and flow properties according to temperature, molecular weight and molecular arrangement. It can be clear that most of the factors dictating the behavior of this wax are not controllable by the operator. To improve the workability of the base ingredient, certain agents are added.

Carnauba wax (up to 25-30%) is added to increase the melting range and temperature and to decrease the wax's plasticity and increase its strength properties. Being of natural origin, its molecules are of different dimensions, shape and sometimes compositions. In addition, it contains alcohols and acids. Resins (5%) are added to reduce the flakiness and assure smooth surfaces. They are sometimes in the form of a dammer resin (naturally occuring), while in other times polyethylene or vinyl resins (synthetic) are added. The synthetic resins are more predictable in their behavior. Traces of fats are added to improve the plasticity. Coloring agents are also added to make the wax color different from that of the die and tooth structure.

It is obvious from the composition that secondary bonding (Vanderwalls forces) are responsible for most of the workable behavior of these materials. Besides, if it is recognized that the melting temperature of these ingredients is not very far from the working temperatures (range) in fabricating a wax pattern for cast restoration. It is a fair statement to say that temperature, time, and stresses in very minimal amounts can noticeably change the behavior of these waxes.

B. Dimensional stability

From the composition, casting waxes are predictably the least stable dimensionally of all materials used in restorative dentistry. Unstability can be categorized under the following:

1. Coefficient of thermal expansion

They possess the highest coeff. of thermal expansion of all dental materials (up to 400 PPM/1°C.) Thermal expansion is not linearly related to temperature. It varies in amount at different temperatures (unpredictably).

2. Flow and plasticity

According to their flow-temperature relationship, waxes for casting wax patterns are classified into three types—type A having the lowest flow and type C having the highest flow at 37° (mouth temperature). The higher the flow and plasticity are, The more adaptable the wax is to the preparation details; but the less the flow is, the less will be the distortion within a wax pattern. Plasticity and flow are mainly increased by temperature and stresses, both of which are inherent in the wax pattern build-up.

3. Strength properties

The modulus of elasticity, proportional limit, and the various ultimate strengths are affected mainly by temperature. Some strength properties can change ten fold by only increasing the temperature 10°C (between 40 and 55°C). Some waxes are very brittle at a lower temperature (less than 20°C). These properties are understandably due to the secondary bonding forces responsible for the coherence of the mass.

4. Residual stresses—the resulting effects of their attainment and their release

Molecules and macromolecules of the ingredients forming the casting wax are held together with very weak physical forces. Therefore, the relationship of the forming molecules to each other can be changed very readily, with limited forces sometimes moving the molecules away from each other, toward each other, or past each other, thereby changing the dimension and shape of the mass. In many occasions the effect is not immediate with the application of the forces. In other words, induced stresses from the applied forces will not manifest their effects until thermal energy, due to temperature elevation, increases the thermal vibration of the component molecules. The resulting thermal vibrations, together with the already induced, but yet ineffective, stresses can be of sufficient magnitude to break some of these weak bonds precipitating the above mentioned shape and dimensional changes.

A stress-free wax pattern is practically impossible. However, the following are certain manipulative guidelines and precautions to observe in order to obtain a wax pattern with the least and most evenly distributed residual stresses. A wax pattern with this stress arrangement will be minimally distortable and, if subjected to temperature, will change dimensions evenly over the entire mass. This situation may be advantageous in certain techniques. The guidelines are:

Start with stress-free or annealed wax, i.e., completely molten wax or a mass of wax that has been kept in a 55° C. oven for 15 minutes to consume all stresses present. For carving always use warm to hot instruments, so that stresses, if induced, could be consumed immediately with less possibility of subsequent dimensional changes. For wax already hardened, always use sharp instruments, if carving is required. This will minimize stresses in the wax, as minimal energy is needed to operate these sharp instruments and most of the energy will be consumed in the actual carving and cutting.

It is sometimes advisable to stress the pattern evenly if stresses cannot be avoided. Stresses should be to the maximum capacity that the pattern can store. This can be done if the evenly applied and distributed stresses will be released in an expansive fashion for the pattern. This calculated expansion can compensate for some of the various types and levels of shrinkage during cast fabrication, if the plasticity of the investment and temperature of the environment allow. Even stressing can be done by allowing the molten wax introduced in the preparation (die) to solidify under pressure from all directions, e.g., using a matrix or solidifying each area of the pattern separately, under finger pressure or using certain hydraulic devices.

Another way of controlling stresses is to release them by thermal energy as soon as they are introduced or suspected to be introduced. This can be done by passing a hot instrument (blunt explorer) deeply into each increment of wax added to build up the wax pattern, just short of melting it. This can also be done by inserting the wax into the preparation in layers. The added layer must contain the maximum heat energy short of vaporization. The heat will accelerate diffusion in the already solidifed layer when it encounters it, thus releasing stresses and making the dimensional changes while the mass is not in its final shape. Both ways can be used simultaneously.

The previous methods, however, will not give a wax pattern that is totally satisfactory from the view point of stress. The only reliable hedge against these disrupting dimensional changes is to invest the pattern immediately. A second and less reliable measure is to refrigerate the pattern (if immediate investment is not possible within 5 minutes of the completion of the pattern.)

5. Volatile ingredients:

Some ingredients can evaporate if extreme heat is used in manipulating the wax pattern, e.g., alcohols and acids inherent in the wax mass can vaporize and escape leaving voids that may lead to local collapse or dimensional changes. The proper amount of thermal energy should be employed to minimize these possibilities. If voids become apparent, they should be filled with additional wax.

6. Air bubbles incorporated in the pattern

During the build-up of a wax pattern, especially if done in an incremental technique, air bubbles can be trapped. Besides increasing intermolecular stresses, they can expand with temperature elevation leading to additional dimensional changes and internal stresses.

C. Reproduction of details

Contact angles of waxes used in cast fabrication are inversely proportional to heat. Therefore, the wax used to reproduce preparation details should be in the most molten, wetting state prior to and immediately after its insertion. (The ability of wax to reproduce details is much better than gypsum materials and far better than silica-containing investment materials). Besides heat, the separating medium used to prevent adhesion of wax to die stone can influence detail reproduction. If used in thick films, it can interfere with the wetting property of the wax. Film thicknesses of these separating media are proportional to the molecular weight, number of applications and amounts applied. Every effort should be made to minimize the film thickness of the separating medium to the smallest dimension that can prevent adhesion of the wax material to the die.

Debris or foreign bodies in the wax or on the preparation can understandably prevent the intimate contact of the wax to the actual details of the preparation. The capability of casting waxes to reproduce the details is quite adequate, but this requires getting the waxes in close contact with the preparation details and maintaining the captured details without changes until they are reproduced in the investment.

D. General procedures for wax pattern fabrications (Fig. 1A and B)

There are four basic methods for producing wax replicas of cast restorations. One way is to create a wax mass, then carve it to the restoration shape, using hot, sharp instruments. The

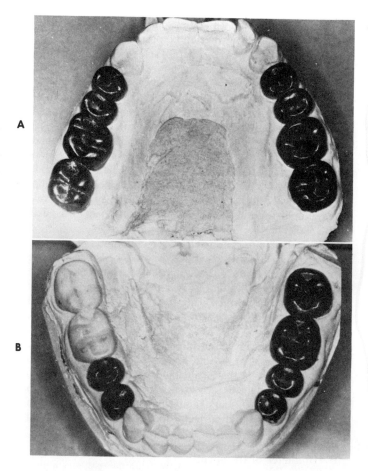

Fig. 24-1

a. Cusps with their tips are built in their exact location and tried in a static and dynamic occlusal contact. Any deficiencies or interferences are corrected.

b. Triangular ridges of cusps are added and the same testing for occlusal deficiencies or interference is done and any correction is performed.

c. Marginal ridges are built up and tried in the same way as the cuspal components.

d. Facial, lingual and proximal contour and anatomy are established by the addition procedure. Their occlusion is checked and corrected.

e. Fossae and grooves occlusally, facially, and lingually are completed if not yet done. Their occluding parts are checked and corrected.

f. The wax pattern is marginated and the surface is polished.

3. The direct wax pattern

a. A matrix is applied on the tooth as applied prior to amalgam insertion, except that no wedges are used. A separating medium is applied on the cavity details and the matrix.

b. An inlay wax stick is softened at its tip. The softened portion should be gently kneaded to assure homogenecity.

c. The softened tip of the wax stick is inserted into the matrixed cavity preparation. It is kept there under pressure until it hardens.

d. Gross excesses of wax are cut off and the occlusal anatomy is carved with warm sharp instruments.

e. The matrix band is released from its retainer and removed. The pattern usually comes out with it.

f. The wax pattern is replaced into the cavity preparation after lubricating it for the second time. Any deficient contouring can be adjusted now. The pattern should be marginated occlusally, facially, and lingually, using a hot tine.

g. While holding the pattern with apical pressure, using a small burnisher, the accessible surfaces can be polished, using the same tools as in previous methods.

h. While still holding it in the same way, pass a dental tape or floss interproximally to assure wax adaptability and the absence of any discrepancy proximally, especially proximo-gingivally.

This technique is indicated for:

i. One or two surface inlays

ii. when an area is readily accessible, especially to the gingival marginal portions

iii. when the preparation has no thin details, like skirts or secondary flares

iv. when the wax pattern can be sprued on the tooth

4. Anatomic core wax pattern

a. This technique is very similar to the functionally generated path technique. Before preparing the teeth for the cast restoration, they are built in hard wax to the desired shape of the future restoration (at least the occlusal two-thirds of each tooth). The patient is asked to go through all mandibular positions and movements, and the wax is adjusted accordingly.

b. In a functionally generated path quadrant tray, a fast setting impression plaster is carried to the wax and adjacent teeth, taking their impression, duplicating at least the surfaces occlusal to the height of contour (to avoid undercuts). Be sure there is an anterior and posterior stop for the impression, so as to have reference points when using it later. The resulting impression is the anatomic core which should be kept aside.

second way is to incrementally build up the restoration, using wax cones, triangles, drops, etc. The third way is to fabricate a wax pattern directly intraorally, and the fourth one depends on a preoperative anatomic core. For each way there are several standard techniques.

1. Formulation of a wax pattern by carving

Generally, the technique involves the following:

a. After lubricating the die, all details are overfilled with wax, covering all margins, in intimate contact with the preparation details and containing no voids.

b. The occlusal, facial, lingual and proximal limits of the pattern are marked and established.

c. The facial and lingual axial anatomy and contour of the pattern are created.

d. The occlusal anatomy is created.

e. The occluding components of the pattern are checked and corrected.

f. The proximal contour and anatomy are carved.

g. All surface anatomical components of the pattern are blended together.

h. The wax components of the circumferential tie are marginated.

i. The pattern is polished using silk cloth and brushes.

j. The occluding components of the pattern are checked during static and functional relations.

2. Incremental build-up of the wax-pattern formulation is carried out as follows:

Proceed with the teeth preparation, the impression, etc. Opposing models or articulators are not required.

c. After constructing the dies and working models and preparing them for the wax pattern, the anatomic core is tried on the quadrant to be sure there is no interference in seating it the way it seats in the mouth. The anterior and posterior stops will help here.

d. One die at a time is filled with molten wax and the lubricated anatomic core is pressed down to the predetermined location and kept there under pressure until the wax solidifies.

e. The anatomic core is removed. There will be little adjustment required in the wax pattern, e.g. some margination.

f. The next die is treated the same way and so on.

The wax pattern can be fabricated in minimal time using this method.

The technique is a modification of the functionally generated path and its occlusal recording technique. It is mainly indicated:

i. When no change in the present occlusion is planned

ii. For small to moderately large restorations with minimum surface extensions

iii. When there is an anterior and posterior stop present to create a workable, reliable anatomic core

iv. When the teeth to be restored are not involved in a lateral or protrusive disclusion mechanism.

II. Sprueing and Surface Treatment of the Completed Wax Pattern

The main objective of sprueing is to create an inlet for the wetting melt into the investment mold created by the wax pattern. This inlet should accommodate the final portion of the restorative material to solidify, in order to allow uninterrupted melt flow into the mold until the mold is completely filled. It also directs the flow and velocity of the cast material so as not to deform any internal details of the mold, that is why, it should be in the most effective and safe direction for filling the mold.

Attachment of the sprue-former to the wax pattern should be done while the wax pattern is on the die or the tooth in order to assure the confinement of the wax pattern, preventing any changes in it due to the possible thermal release and mechanical induction of stresses during sprueing. In most cases this is feasible. The only situation where we cannot sprue directly on the die or the tooth, is the sprueing of a direct wax pattern at its proximal surface. In this case the pattern is removed and sprued freely with the least stress induction and release as possible. Whatever precautions, however, it is not a recommended way of sprueing.

A. Types and desired characteristics in a sprue former

There are three types of sprue formers available, each made of a different material: resin, wax, and metal. Some resin and all wax sprue formers have the advantage of being burnable, so there is no need to remove them like the metal ones. The metal ones have the distinct disadvantage of possibly stressing and deforming the sprue walls or the wax pattern during their removal. The fusion temperature of the resin or wax sprue formers should be lower or at most the same as that of the pattern wax in order to allow for the evaporation of the pattern wax.

Resin and wax sprue formers have very low thermal con-
ductivity. They transmit a minimal amount of heat to the pattern with minimal possible distortion before evaporation.

Metal sprue formers have the advantage of rigidity during investment. This characteristic is not exhibited with wax ones and exhibited only in a limited extent with resin types. The mechanical removal of metal sprue formers assures an inlet for the melt. However, their removal may loosen some investment in the walls of the sprue or roughen its walls.

Metal sprue formers can be supplied in solid or hollow (tube) forms. It is preferable to use tube metal ones as they are more retentive to the pattern and supply minimal heat to the already formulated pattern. It is advisable to fill the tube sprue former with sticky wax to reduce its thermal conductivity and improve its retention in the wax pattern without involvement of the wax pattern bulk.

Sprue former surfaces should be very smooth to prevent any irregular inlet walls. Irregularities in these walls can separate from the main investment and can become incorporated in the stream of the melt, leading to obliteration of some details or creation of internal voids. This risk is very real with metal sprue formers, less so with resin ones, and minimal with wax types.

The sprue former material should not rust or react with any ingredient of the environment, thereby avoiding the formation of product materials that could modify the properties of the restorative materials or act as dislodged pieces or foreign bodies. The sprue formers should be perfectly cylindrical in shape so as to create a perfectly rounded inlet for the mold which is the easiest inlet for the melt ingress.

B. Diameter of the sprue

The diameter of the sprue is the most important factor in dictating the speed with which the melt enters and fills the mold. Melt velocity is directly proportional to the sprue diameter. Basically, for most of the cast materials, the sprue diameter should be greater than the thickest part of the wax pattern.

The velocity of the melt into the mold is also governed by:

1. The density of the cast material. The more its weight per unit volume is, the faster it will be driven into the mold.

2. The melt velocity, which is directly proportional to the energy supplied by the casting machine.

3. The velocity with which the air and gases in the mold can be evacuated. The greater that velocity is, the faster the melt will be sucked and driven into the mold.

4. The viscosity of the melt. The lower the viscosity of the melt is, the faster it can be driven in.

5. The length of the sprue pin former. The shorter the sprue is, the faster the melt will ingress into the mold.

6. Flaring. The more flared the sprue is as it comes close to the mold, the greater the speed of melt ingress will be.

7. The size of the pattern. The larger the formed wax pattern is, the slower the velocity of the ingressing melt will be.

8. The dimensions of the walls surrounding the mold. The greater the thickness of those walls is, the slower the rate of heating will be, the slower the escape of the gases will be, and the less the vacuum, and so the slower the speed of filling the mold with the melt.

In choosing the diameter of the sprue the above mentioned eight items should be considered. Mostly importantly, the speed of filling the mold should not be faster than the speed of evacuation of the gases and air from the mold, since this can create a mixture of cast materials and gases in the mold with a subsequent porous or incomplete casting.

Also, every castable or moldable material has its optimum ingress speed to wet all the details of the mold, besides the driving energy will play a major role in determining the rate of ingress. Generally the sprue former diameter will be between 8-18 gauge, 8 being almost 3 mm in diameter and 18 being 0.8 mm in diameter. The choice is a matter of judgement, according to operator experience and the above mentioned factors.

C. Length of the sprue

The major factor governing the sprue length is the length of the ring. The end of the wax pattern that is away from the sprue should be within ⅛-¼'' from the end of the ring to allow the minimum thickness of investment that can both withstand melt impact and at the same time allow the escape of the mold gases. Understandably, the longer the ring, the longer the sprue will be and, consequently, the wider the sprue will be to compensate for the slowing of the ingress due to the length it must travel. Another factor that affects the length of the sprue is the spatial location of the pattern within the ring. This location is essential in determining the way the wax pattern encounters the differential expansion of the investment around the mold. (This will be discussed later.) This spatial location can be arranged and governed by the sprue length.

D. Number of sprues

It is not the size, but rather the configuration of the wax pattern which dictates the number of sprues to be used. The sprue should be attached to the thickest part of the pattern in a way that will allow the melt to flow uninterrupted from the sprue to the furthest end of the mold, i.e., the pattern should maintain the same dimension or be decreased in dimension going from the sprue end to the other end. If this is the case, whatever the size of the pattern, one sprue is quite sufficient. However, should the wax pattern have a thin area between the sprue and the periphery of the pattern, the melt will solidify at this reduced cross-sectional area, preventing the filling of the furthest parts of the mold. In this case, two or more sprues are essential to completely fill the mold with the melt without any solidifying interruptions.

Deciding the number of sprues is a matter of evaluation and judgement, depending on observation and experience. If multiple sprues are used, after being attached to the wax pattern separately, they should join together at the crucible former level in a reservoir larger in diameter than all sprues combined.

E. Location of sprues

The sprue formers should be attached to the bulkiest part of the wax pattern. First this will minimize the effect of released residual stresses by the heat of attaching the sprue. Secondly, it will insure that the thinner cross-section of the mold will be completely filled. Thirdly, the melt will always be fluid enough and available until all lesser dimension sections are completely filled. (The ratio of the mold wall surface area to the mold dimension in a thick section is much less than the same ratio in thinner sections, a situation that leads to faster solidification in the latter than the former.)

Sprue formers should be attached to the least anatomical area in the wax pattern, i.e., an area of no grooves, cuspal anatomy, fossae or ridges. The proximal surfaces are the ideal location for the sprue attachment. Since the expansion of investment around the mold is not even, cast alloy sprues should be located, as practically as possible, so that areas of the pattern needing maximal and minimal expansion coincide with the areas of the investment capable of providing either.

F. Angulation of the sprue former

The sprue is never directed toward thin, delicate cross sections of the wax pattern. The melt flow should not hit these areas of the mold at 90° to avoid fracture failure, missing details or excesses. It should be directed away from, or at 45°, to these details.

Also, the sprue is never directed at a right angle to a flat portion of a wax pattern as this will create a reverse flow (with turbulence) of the melt, decreasing the melt's ability to fill the mold. Also, a melt ingress at 90° to a flat wall or floor can create a concavity in this wall opposite to the sprue. The mold concavity will be reproduced as a convexity in the restoration, preventing its seating and making the restoration rock.

The sprue angulation should be planned to assure the easiest and most efficient way of flowing the melt.

G. The sprue-wax pattern joint

This should have a smooth and uninterrupted surface. If high velocity ingress of the melt into the mold is required (due to the rapid solidification of the alloy, a large surface area of the mold, etc.), the sprue-wax pattern joint should be flared, with smooth, uninterrupted surfaces. Flaring will make this joint the area of maximum dimension in the sprue-wax pattern complex, thereby insuring a fluid melt and non-obstructed flow.

If low velocity ingress is required (due to high viscosity of the melt, slow escape of gases from the mold, piston-injection used to drive the melt into the mold etc.) A constricted junction should be made where the sprue meets the wax pattern. This configuration will introduce shear stressers in the melt passing at the constriction, thus decreasing the viscosity of the melt and making it more wetting.

To minimize stress release while joining a sprue former to a wax pattern, a drop of sticky wax should be applied to the wax pattern. Then the sprue, also with a bead of sticky wax, is brought into contact with the sticky wax on the wax pattern and held immobile until the sticky wax is solidified. Once the sprue former is attached to the wax pattern, it should not be disturbed with any further manipulation. The flare shape of the junction with the wax pattern also insures the retention of the sprue in the wax pattern.

H. Reservoir

Occasionally, wax is added around the sprue former 1-2 mm from the pattern in order to create an area in the mold (a reservoir) with dimensions far exceeding that of the thickest portion of the pattern. It is always indicated when the sprue is long and/or thin or for any other reason that might cause the flow of the melt to be interrupted before all the mold details are filled.

I. Venting

In some situations, there is some doubt about the speed with which the mold gases will escape relative to the speed the melt is entering. This could be due to; a considerable thickness of the investment walls surrounding the pattern, a high density of the investment, (e.g., a higher binder percentage for strength purposes or a complete gypsum investment), the use of pattern material whose residue may clog the investment pores, or wax pattern with a lot of minute details or thin cross-sectional areas that are difficult for the melt to wet.

These cases require attaching a wax rod to the furthest, or close to the furthest, part of the pattern, which will stop short of the ring (investment) surface. In most cases they are curved toward the sprue. Gases that will not escape fast enough ahead of the ingressing melt will be compressed and trapped in these vents. The number indicated for each pattern is a technical judgment depending upon the evaluation of the path of the mold gases and areas where their escape may be impeded. For the injection molding of cast ceramics venting tubes are built into the investing flasks that connect the mold with the flask surface.

J. Removal of the wax pattern and sprue former from the die or the tooth

There is a definite possibility of stressing the wax pattern while removing it from the die or tooth, so an effort should be made to make these stresses even. The first choice is to use the sprue former in removing the pattern if this will not stress one area more than another. If uneven stressing is anticipated, resort to the second choice. The second choice is to use two fingers (thumb and first finger) on both sides of the pattern and gently remove in the direction of the path with very light pressure. This method is only used on dies and is most applicable when the pattern has two or more sides (onlay and full crowns). If this method does not seem to insure even stressing, resort to the third choice.

The third choice is to formulate a suitable size staple from a paper staple or wire of the alloy to be used for the restoration or one of its metal ingredients. The staple is attached with sticky wax to the furthest two ends of the pattern. Then the wax pattern is removed, using the center of the staple, being sure that removing stresses are applied evenly on both sides of the pattern. The staple can be removed from the pattern by heating a pair of tweezers and holding the staple. The transmitted heat will free the staple from the wax. If the staple is made of the same alloy or one of the component metals of the alloy for the final restoration, it can be left in the pattern and cut off after casting.

K. Forming the crucible and attaching the pattern

The crucible part of the investment will, in most cases, be funnel-shaped and connected to the sprue in the same way as the sprue is attached to the mold, i.e., it should be the bulkiest in cross-section and flared and smooth. The depth of the crucible and the inclination of its walls toward the sprue are dictated by factors similar to those governing the diameter of the sprue (alloy density, casting machine energy, melt viscosity, size of pattern, porosity of investment, etc.). The deeper the crucible is and the more inclined its walls are, the more velocity will be imparted on the melt on its way to the mold.

Most of the time, crucible formers come ready-made (rubber, metal, or plastic), with different sizes, diameters, and wall inclinations. Crucibles for moldable ceramics are metallic and have the exact dimension as the pellets of the raw ceramic which will be injected. The choice of the size is fixed with the ring size, However, the choice of the depth and wall inclination should be the result of a technical judgment after considering all the factors involved. If the proper depth or wall angulation is not available, modifications can be made by adding waxes. After the exact dimension, details, and configuration are established in the crucible former, the wax pattern with its sprue former is attached, usually in a special locking area. The junction between the sprue and the crucible former should now be covered with wax and carved to obtain the proper bulk and flaring. The crucible former surface and its junction with the sprue former are meticulously smoothed to create as smooth a crucible as possible.

L. Surface treatment of wax pattern

Casting waxes are hydrophobic materials that are very difficult to wet with water and investment liquids. For the investment to capture all the wax pattern details these repulsing forces must be counteracted. Surface active agents (soaps) are applied on the pattern before investment. These cleaning and wetting agents facilitate the intimate proximity of the investment mix to the wax pattern by reducing involved fluids surface tension and encouraging solid components surface energy thus precipitating closeness. Also, vibration is used during flowing of the investment over the pattern. The energy supplied by this will help counteract the repulsion forces between the investment and the wax pattern. Vacuum investment will be described later.

III. Investment of the Wax Pattern

The main objective of the investing process is to capture all the wax pattern details in a solid investment material which is capable of maintaining these details after evaporating (washing) the wax pattern at the appropriate casting (molding) temperature of the restorative material. With the introduction of newer material for cast restoration this is the area in the casting procedure which has been and will be subjected to numerous changes.

A. Composition of investment for cast alloys (i.e., silica containing investment)

Basically, any of these investments should have three component ingredients:

1. A refractory, thermally expandable material

These are in one form of silicone dioxide; e.g. quartz, cristobalite, tridymite, or fused quartz. Their two main functions in the investments are:

a. By being very poor thermal conductors and having extremely high heat capacity, they can preserve the attained temperature in the mold and investment mass for a period sufficient for the casting process.

b. By being capable of polymorphism, these silica materials can undergo atomic rearrangement by thermal energy. In most cases this rearrangement decreases its density and consequently increases its volume leading to expansion of the mass which is essential in some casting techniques to compensate for the shrinkage of some of the ingredients in the procedures.

2. Binders

At room temperature silica particles cannot be combined together to create a coherent mass without an intermediate or a binder.

For casting procedures needing a mold temperature of 700°C. or less, gypsum (calcium sulfate dihydrate) binders are the most feasible and durable. They are usually in the form of alpha hemihydrate and when combined with water will form the dihydrate crystal network hydraulically holding silica particles within.

For alloys or casting techniques where the mold temperature must exceed 700°C there is a great possibility of disintegration of the calcium sulfate dihydrate with sulfur gases as a by-product. The latter can contaminate the molten alloy. As a result of its disintegration, the binding effect of the gypsum will be reduced to failure level at these high temperatures. The higher the temperature is, the more certain this possibility becomes. The binder for silica in such a high temperature technique is either a silicate or phosphate.

a. The silicate binder is basically silicic acid or colloidal silica (SiO_2) which can be formed from one of many reactions, e.g., the reaction between ethyl silicate and an aqueous solution of hydrochloric acid, or between Na silicate and an aqueous solution of any active acids. The network of silicic acid or colloidal silica (SiO_2) will form the carrier frame to hold the reinforcing silica particles. By heat, the colloidal silica and silicic acid lose water and are transformed to a three-dimensional silica polymer network which is mechanically very strong and capable of expansion like the originally introduced refractory silica. Over 1000° C, the whole final product is actually silicone dioxide tetra-hedra. Some of these will polmerize in three dimensions with the original silica and polymerization increases as the temperature rises.

b. The phosphate binder is a product of a very complex reaction with multiple solid state changes upon heating. Primarily, the reaction starts by mixing ammonium dihydrogen-phosphate ($NH_4H_2PO_4$) with MgO. The phosphate and oxides should be in excess in this reaction for further reactions to occur. The product is a network of hydrated ammonium-magnesium phosphate ($NH_4MgPO_4 \cdot 6H_2O$), trapping the silica particles and hydraulically holding them within. The excess MgO and ammonium dihydrogen phosphate constitutes the rest of the room temperature mass of the investment. By heating, several complex, not fully explained, reactions will occur through loss of water, giving $NH_4MgPO_4 \cdot H_2O$, degrading to a polymer with the mer $(Mg_2P_2O_7)n$, then crystallizing with a unit cell of $Mg_2P_2O_7$, which can react with magnesium oxide, gives a three-dimensional network of $Mg_3(PO_4)_2$. Also, the excess ammonium dihydrogen phosphate ($HN_4H_2PO_4$) can react at some stage of this heating with the refractory silica (SiO_2), forming strong bonded silico-phosphate crystals. All in all, the product increases in dimension and strength by heat.

3. Modifiers

They can be coloring agents to distinguish investment from other gypsum products, carbon or colloidal copper to create a deoxidizing atmosphere in the mold, and/or oxalates that deteriorate with heat, forming carbon dioxide and carbon monoxide, preventing sulfur contamination of alloys in gypsum bonded investments. These last three modifiers should not be

used with nickel chromium based alloys. Sodium chloride or boric acids are added to retain the water of crystallization of some binders for certain period of time during heating to prevent detrimental shrinkage.

B. Dimensional stability of silica-containing investment

By means of its setting, its effect on a wax pattern, and its reaction to thermal energy, casting investment should make the most adequate extent and direction of dimensional changes. These dimensional changes should be opposite to and compensate for shrinkage, which occurs in the wax pattern; in the binder; in the alloy when it changes from liquidus to solidus; and when it cools from solidus to room temperature. Prior to handling this important link in the cast fabrication, comprehension of the factors affecting the dimensional changes of the casting investment in general, and specifically those affecting the dimensional changes of the investment mold (which are called the effective dimensional changes), is essential.

1. Effective dimensional changes during setting of the silica containing investment

During setting-hardening of the investment, both the investment and the invested wax pattern will undergo changes affecting the final dimension and shape of the mold. The following are the factors and their effects:

a. Exothermic heat of setting reaction of the investment

Hydrolysis of some binders during hardening of the investment is accompanied by release of thermal energy. This heat, if it encounters the wax pattern, will impart energy to it, activating some of its unconsumed stresses. This heat will also produce the normal thermal expansion of the wax. Both activities lead to dimensional changes in the wax pattern depending on the degree and direction of prior stresses in the wax pattern and on confinement of the pattern.

b. Confinement

There are restrictions in the dimensional changes of both the wax pattern and the investment. The wax pattern is confined by the investment and the investment is confined by the wax pattern and the ring. Both of these will limit the amount of possible expansion of the mold.

During setting of the investment there are inherent tendencies and intentional manipulations that cause the investment to expand. The surface expansion of the investment away from the wax pattern surface is confined only by the ring. If this type and direction of expansion is desired, the ring should be very elastic (rubbery) and removed as soon as possible. Another way to counteract the confinement of the ring is to line the ring with a yielding substance, such as asbestos or kaolina. Still another way is to locate the wax pattern within the ring in a way so that there will be no outward confinement (e.g., toward an open end of the ring). Expansion of investment trapped between opposing walls of the wax pattern is confined by these parts of the wax pattern and depends upon their yielding ability to allow the expansion to be effective. This, in turn, is dependent on the flow of the wax at the temperature of the investment expansion—the greater the flow is, the more effective will be the expansion. If this type of expansion is the main method to compensate for shrinkage, the wax pattern should be made from soft type III wax.

On the other hand, the ability of the wax pattern to create effective expansion is dictated by its confinement in the surrounding investment. If this investment is unyielding during the wax expansion and/or does not move fast enough away from the pattern, as a result of its own expansion, the possible expansion of the wax pattern will not be used to its limit. It must be mentioned here that if the wax pattern is tensilely stressed prior to its investment, the dimensional changes will be in the form of contraction rather than expansion.

c. Percentage and fineness of silica

Silicone dioxide particles act as dilutants to the investment mass, delaying the interlocking of the growing binder crystals, thus permitting them to grow further with more expansion. Therefore, the greater that the percentage of silica is and the finer that the silica particles are, the more will be the possible expansion.

d. Water (liquid) : powder ratio

The greater the water (liquid) : powder ratio is, the less will be the formed binder crystals per unit volume so the less will be the possibility of expansion.

e. Rate and energy of spatulation

By their increase, the more delayed will be the interlocking of the binder crystals, and the more will be the possibility of this crystal growth, and consequently the more will be the expansion.

f. Hygroscopic expansion

This can be accomplished in all gypsum and some phosphate bonded silica containing investments. It is actually a magnification and continuation of the setting expansion, facilitated by reducing or eliminating the surface tension confinement for binder crystal growth and feeding the mass with ingredients to precipitate this growth. It is always done by the addition of water to the investment mass undergoing hardening-setting. It is governed by the same factors that govern the regular setting expansion.

Every investment composition has a maximum limit for the amount of water it can accommodate to react with (depending mainly on the possible reactants). So within this limit, the more water that is added, the more will be the expansion. Every investment composition has a time limitation for water to come in contact with and be effective in hygroscopically expanding it, with both starting and ending points. Within this limit, the earlier the water is incorporated, the more will be the expansion.

2. Effective dimensional changes during heating of the silica containing investment

Understandably, the mass of the set-hardened investment will be intentionally heated to evaporate the wax pattern and bring the temperature of the created mold to a degree compatible to that of the melt. During this heating the mass can undergo expansion at one or several stages. If these expansions are directed properly, they can effectivley compensate for the aforementioned types and stages of shrinkage. The following are the factors and their effects:

a. Type of refractory silica

Cristobalite SiO_2 can exhibit the maximum expansion of all silica polymorphs; fused quartz exhibits almost none (it does not undergo polymorphic changes). Quartz and tridymite are in between, with quartz expanding more than tridymite. If thermal expansion of the mold is the main compensating mechanism for the various types of shrinkage, cristobalite is the ideal choice. A calculated blend of these silica polymorphs is usually supplied to get the exact expansion desired in the investment to be used.

b. Temperature

Below the fusion temperature of the refractory silicone dioxide used, the higher the temperature is, the more will be the expansion. Expansion is not even from room temperature to fusion temperature. Generally speaking, most of the expansion will occur just before and at the transformation temperature for the specific refractory silicone dioxide used.

c. Percentage and uniformity of silica

The more refractory silica there is, the more is the possibility of expansion. Also, the less uniform the particle size of silica content is, the better will be the silica packing ability, i.e., adequacy of using space and more density. Therefore, the more the silica/unit volume is, consequently more expansion will occur when heated. Improperly blended powder, non-homogeneous mixes, or excessive vibration may lead to concentration of refractory silica at certain areas around the mold with the possibility that the expansion could be greater at that specific areas than at the others.

d. Water (liquid):powder ratio

The greater this ratio is, the less will be the silica content per volume and, consequently, the less will be the expansion.

e. Thickness of the mold walls

The thicker the walls of the mold are, the more will be the expansion of that specific wall.

f. Confinement

After wax loss, the only confinement for mold expansion will be the external confinement, namely, the ring. If the coefficient of thermal expansion of the ring metal is less than the possible coefficient of thermal expansion of the investment, the mold will not expand. On the contrary, it will undergo reduction in dimension as the investment expansion will be directed inward. An asbestos or kaolina lining of the ring, or no ring at all, can make the investment expansion effective in expanding the mold.

g. Changes in the binder as a result of heating

Every type of binder reacts differently when heated. Gypsum binders undergo contraction as soon as their temperature exceeds 105°C. Part of the bonded silica expansion from the same heat will not be effective as it is going to be consumed in neutralizing the gypsum contraction. Sodium chloride or boric acid can be added to delay this contraction.

Silicate binder will undergo contraction initially but some of the formed silica network will expand in coordination with its refractory polymorphs, i.e., the carried refractory silica. As can be expected, the final expansion far exceeds the gypsum-bonded investment. The phosphate binder will undergo successive contraction and expansion due to loss of water and solid transformation. However, the end result is substantial expansion comparable to and possibly exceeding that of the silica-bonded investments.

h. Differential expansion of parts of the mold as a result of the spatial location of the pattern in the ring or within the investment

From the previous discussion it should be clear that the thermal expansion of the investment mold will not be uniform in each cross-section. This condition is created mainly by the uneven thickness of the surrounding walls and the differences in confinement at different locations. The asymmetrical expansion will be enhanced by a variety of other factors, such as the percentage of silica in each area, different temperatures, the type of wax, etc. The ultimate goal in locating a wax pattern inside a ring is to get as effective and even an expansion as possible.

Generally, the investment bulk is least confined lengthwise within a ring. If the investment segment with the maximum mold wall thickness is in that direction, expansion in length will far exceed width, resulting in mold distortion. Therefore, the least thickness of the mold wall should be in the direction of least confinement. The configuration of the wax pattern is vitally important in deciding what will be the spatial location within the ring and, accordingly, where the sprue will be attached. Also, the need to expand some areas of the mold more than others for easier manipulation of the casting can be a major factor in choosing the location of the pattern within the confines of the ring and the investment. Sometimes most of the needed expansion is done during the setting of the investment, and minimum or no expansion is needed thermally.

Additionally, all the factors dictating the location of the sprue will influence and be influenced by the spatial location of the pattern in the ring. Porosity of the investment (which will be discussed in the next section) will determine, to some extent, the location of the pattern within the investment. The less porous the investment, the closer the pattern periphery should be to the investment surface. In weak investments (those with a gypsum binder), the greater that the energy required to force the melt into the mold is, the more will be the investment bulk needed around the pattern. This again influences the spatial location of the pattern.

The spatial location of the wax pattern within the investment is dictated by many variables. The type, extent and direction of thermal expansion are major factors in determining the location of the pattern in the investment. If these factors are not adequately accounted for, a distorted mold with needless expansion or contraction can be the result.

C. The utilization of porosity in silica-containing investments to facilitate casting

As previously mentioned, the ability of a cast melt to adequately wet and fill the entire mold within the investment is the product of a differential speed with which the mold gases leave and the melt enters the mold space. One of the major factors influencing the escape speed of the mold gases is avenues of porosity within the investment facilitating that escape. In the investment surrounding the mold, the escape speed is enhanced by the number of pores, the interconnectedness of the pores, their size and the distance the mold gases have to travel through them to get to the surface. Many factors affect the porosity pattern of casting investment. These include:

1. The greater that the refractory silica percentage in the investment is, the more will be the investment porosity.

2. The higher the water (liquid):powder ratio of the original investment mix is, the more will be the number, size and interconnection between the pores.

3. Uniform size and shape of the refractory silica particles will definitely increase the potential for pores within the investment mass.

4. Mold wall thickness

Understandably, the thicker these walls, the greater the dis-

tance for the mold gases to travel to the surface and, consequently, the slower their escape.

5. Uneven porosity distribution around the mold can occur due to excessive vibration, inadequately blended powder ingredients, non-homogeneous mixes, or use of more than one mix. The asymmetrical porosity can accelerate or decelerate the escape of mold gases according to pore concentration and distribution.

6. The porosity of phosphate bonded investment is the least of all three types, followed by silica bonded. The most porous is calcium sulfate dihydrate-bonded investment.

D. Strength properties of silica containing investment

Strength properties are the function of the binder. The more that the percentage and interlocking of the binder components are, the more will be the strength properties. Investments are basically brittle materials, with little or no plasticity, which is a very important property to preserve the established dimension of the mold. The investment strength at the casting temperature should be of sufficient magnitude to withstand the driving energy of the melt. From the strength aspect, gypsum-bonded investments are the weakest. Silicate-bonded ones are the strongest, with phosphate-bonded being very close to the silicate-bonded. For gypsum-bonded investments, a compressive strength as low as 356 PSI at 500°C. is still adequate for most casting procedures. Since most of the transformations in the binder during heating are irreversible, strength at a specific temperature is the product of the binder component at that temperature. When an investment is cooled after heating, the original dimension may be regained, but the original binder components will not be regained at this lower temperature. This situation will lead to cracks, which may interconnect and result in a collapse of the total binder system with drastic loss of strength. The resultant investment mass cannot withstand any melt impact, because most of the binders will not be binding any more. An investment mass should be heated just once to its destinated temperature.

E. Reproduction of details

Silica containing investments are the material least capable of reproducing details of any of the materials used during the multiple steps in the cast fabrication. This can be understood if reference is made to the composition, specifically the refractory ingredients. Although the contact angles of these investment are less than that of gypsum, the reproduced details have much more irregularity than those present on either the gypsum or the wax-pattern surface (as a result of silica particles). Surface irregularities of the mold are very extensive in silicate and phosphate bonded investments, but have much lesser extent and degree in gypsum bonded investments. This is one of the weakest points in the silicate and phosphate bonded investments. Reproduction of detail can be improved by:

1. Investing in a vacuum atmosphere, which will eliminate air from the investment, improving its adaptability and enhancing its proximity to the wax patterns.

2. Investing with vibration, which will mechanically force the investment into close contact with the wax pattern.

3. A favorable consistency of the investment—the lower that the viscosity of the investment is, the more wetting it will

be to the wax pattern. So the earlier during its setting that the investment is adapted to wax, the closer the investment will be to wax pattern.

4. Surface treatment of the wax pattern with a wetting agent.

Whatever measures are taken, the details and smoothness of the wax pattern will not all be reproduced in the investment mold. The wax pattern, therefore, should have the maximum detail and surface smoothness to minimize their anticipated loss in the investment mold.

F. Silica-free investments

These are made from pure gypsum, calcium sulfate hemi then di-hydrate. They have the same investment additives as mentioned in the previous section of this chapter to prevent their contraction or deterioration during heating. They are used with the castable moldable ceramics where no compensating expansion is needed (for details of their composition, and, behavior, refer to chapter 22).

G. Principles of investing

1. Choice of the ring

For the hygroscopic expansion technique, a rubber ring is used. For the thermal expansion technique, a metal ring is used. The diameter and length of the ring should be selected to allow for the desired dimension of the mold walls. For the injection molding technique of moldable ceramics, a special two-part flask of standard size is used.

2. Preparation of the ring for non-confinement of the investment expansion. A rubber ring may be used, or a metal ring is either lined with asbestos or kaolina, or a split metal ring is used.

3. Assembling the ring and crucible former

The prepared ring is attached to the crucible former in a way to complete the preparation for the spatial location of the pattern within the investment mass. This step should be coordinated with sprueing and choosing the size of the ring. For moldable ceramics, there is only one specific location for the wax pattern within the investing plaster, since no compensation expansion is required. The wax pattern should be on its epoxy resin die. The part of the die within the wax pattern will be in the top one-half of the flask, and the remainder of the die will be in the bottom one-half of the flask.

For low fusing Class I and II alloys, it is possible to attach the stone die to the wax pattern and invest them together. The preparation surface of the die will become one of the walls of the mold. This requires that the casting technique is a low-heat technique and that the casting is very limited in dimension, e.g., small inlays or onlays. This is called die-vesting. It can be used with other classes of alloy if the dies are poured in a phosphate-type reinforced investment.

4. Preparation of the investment mix

Use distilled water or indicated liquid for the mix. Mechanical vacuum mixing is the most appropriate in order to lessen voids and insure standard predictable behavior of the mix.

5. Adapting the investment mix to the wax pattern and filling the ring (flask) with investment

This can be done simultaneously, if the procedure is done under vacuum and vibration; or in two steps: the mix is adapted to this pattern, using small beads of investment with light

vibration, and the ring is then filled with large increments of investment, also under vibration.

6. Facilitating the desired setting through hygroscopic expansion during hardening of the investment

If maximum hygroscopic expansion is needed, the entire setting investment mass can be immersed in a water bath. If less than the maximum is desired, the amount of water producing the needed expansion (every investment is different and the manufacturer's instructions should be consulted) is added to the setting investment in its container. In either situation the water should be incorporated as early as possible in the hardening process. The investment is then left to harden for at least 45 minutes. (Manufacturer's recommended time should be followed.)

7. Removal of the solid or non-burnable sprue former

The crucible former is detached from the ring if it is still present. The sprue former, if it is not going to be left in the investment wax complex, is warmed to soften the wax that attaches it to the main wax pattern. The sprue former is then removed in a gradual rotary movement. The formed crucible and sprue are checked to insure that they are smooth and free from any loose investment pieces prior to placing the ring in the burn-out oven, or opening the flask for wax washing.

IV. Thermal Treatment of the Investment— Wax Pattern Complex

There are three objectives for this step:

A. Complete elimination of the wax from the future mold and from the investment mass itself

In the case of a plaster-invested wax pattern for cast ceramics, prior to thermally treating the flask—investment assembly, the flask halves are opened and the wax is washed out with boiling water. Any residual wax in the flask pores will be evaporated by the subsequent thermal treatment. For wax patterns invested in silica-containing investments, the thermal treatment is done directly since the wax pattern will be evaporated by this procedure.

B. Elevating the temperature of the mold and its surrounding investment to a degree comparable to that of the fusion temperature of the cast alloy or the glass transition temperature of the cast ceramic.

C. Thermal expansion of the investment and the pattern mold, if thermal expansion is a part or all of the compensation for shrinkage

It should be done in a time-temperature controlled oven. The time the mass takes to arrive at a certain temperature is especially important to the technique. Therefore electric ovens are preferred over ovens using other fuels. Heating should start from a cold oven. The temperature should be gradually and evenly elevated to the designated temperature for three reasons:

1. Investments are very poor conductors of heat. Upon heating, the external part will undergo changes (expansion or contraction) prior to the inner parts. The differential changes will create cracks that may be continuous with the mold, producing a final casting with multiple unpatterned and undesirable extensions.

2. The residual water, the water of hydrolysis, washing wa-

ter, molten wax, or other fluids in the investment that can undergo evaporation by heating should do so and leave the investment mass in a gas form via the investment pores. If the vaporization of this liquid is faster than the rate the produced gasses leave the investment, pressure will build within the mass and inside the mold, leading to explosion, cracks, or at least roughening of the mold walls or loss of details. This imbalance between the rate of producing gases and their escape capacity can be produced by rapid and/or abrupt heating of the investment mass.

3. Gradual heating is essential to insure even expansion of the mold walls with less possibility of mold distortion which can happen with fast, abrupt heating.

Oxygen (air) ventilation within the oven and the mold should be ample and unrestricted to help the combustion of the wax remaining.

The investment mold should not be heated more than that prescribed by the investment manufacturer, in terms of either time or temperature. Overheating can change some of the investment components to gases, which roughens the mold walls due to substance loss and gas pressure and may contaminate the cast materials. At casting stage, the mold temperature should be at least 50-100°F lower than the fusion temperature of the cast material to facilitate material solidification toward the mold walls (casting details). For injection molding, there should not be any difference in temperature. Therefore, for each type of casting material or technique, use the prescribed investment.

Conversely, underheating may lead to incomplete elimination of the wax pattern with the possibility of a deficient casting and/or an explosion of the investment if the melts come in contact with a substantial amount of the wax pattern. Also, unevaporated wax residues will clog the investment pores, contributing to incomplete ventilation with possible back pressure porosity and/or an incomplete casting. And, finally, a substantial difference between the temperature of the melt and that of the mold will precipitate subsurface porosity or generalized porosity in the casting.

The investment should be properly contained in a coherent mass that is transportable to the casting machine when its temperature has arrived at the required degree for casting. Additionally, it should possess enough rigidity and strength to withstand the casting manipulation and forces without deformative or fracture failure.

V. Casting or Injection Molding

The objective of these procedures is to fill the investment mold with the wetting cast material as completely, efficiently and quickly as possible.

The procedure involves three steps and each has certain objectives and goals.

A. Fusing the alloy or thermoplastically softening the ceramic material

This step should create the most fluid, wetting, and least viscous condition of the cast material without the incorporation of contaminating or unreacted gasses that may lead to casting porosity. This should be done at a temperature that is compatible to that of the mold temperature (50-100°F above), and one that does not evaporate the low fusing ingredients of the cast material.

These objectives can be achieved very easily if there is an understanding of the characteristics of the cast material. Fulfilling these objectives requires:

1. A proper energy source

A variety of energy sources can be used but they are basically one of two types:

a. Gas fuels

These are usually produced by one of three mixtures of gases.

i. Natural gases (mainly propane) and air

This supplies the lowest temperature of all sources, and is very efficient for Class I and II cast alloys.

ii. Natural gases and oxygen

This supplies a higher temperature and can be used for Class I, II and III cast alloys.

iii. Acetylene and oxygen mixture

This is the hottest of all gas fuels and can be used for all types of alloys. It may be too hot for Class I and II alloys, leading to overheating with loss of some ingredients through evaporation.

Fusing energy, using gas fuels, necessitates a blow-torch. It should be adjustable as to the amount and percentage of each gas in the mixture. Usually the produced flame has multiple zones, each with a different color. The most reducing, hottest, and non-contaminating zone should be the zone to incorporate and be in direct contact with the alloy to be melted. This zone usually has a blue hue. Extreme caution should be taken not to introduce any of the gas fuels into the melt. This necessitates an adequately adjusted flame and the use of the indicated zone for melting.

b. Electric energy

Heat produced from electric sources is the most controlled, efficient and easily used. It is produced through induction or resistance. Induction heat is the most efficient and popular. They are the only heat sources that can be used for cast ceramics, and Class IV alloys, but they may also be used for any of the other three classes of cast materials.

2. A proper container in which cast material may be fused or softened

It should be unaffected by the necessary heat and should not contaminate the cast material. It should be located in contact with the ring, investment or flask, or as close as possible, to facilitate immediate uncooled transportation of the melt to the mold. It should adequately contain the cast material during the melting (softening) and casting (molding) procedures.

For cast alloys the container is usually in the form of an inert, infusible ceramic crucible attached to the casting machine close to the investment mass (ring). It should be lined with asbestos or kaolin which is discarded after casting to insure non-contamination of the crucible which may be re-used. In some instances of cast alloys and for all cast-mouldable ceramics, the cast material is melted (softened) in the crucible of the investment, which is the most proximal location for the melt to the mold.

3. A proper environment for casting

There should be a controlled, reducing (or at least inert) atmosphere around the cast metal being fused or softened. The most controlled environment is a closed-fusing compartment whose atmosphere is an inert gas (argon) to which the cast material has no affinity at any temperature. The melting device is always electric induction heating. Gas flames can produce a fairly adequate environment if their reducing zone is the only zone in contact with the alloy until it completely fills the mold; i.e., it is a technique-controlled environment.

Applying limited amounts of fluxes, which are in the form of borax glass in borax with some charcoal powder, on the alloy surface during melting can isolate the melt from the surrounding atmosphere. The acquired protective layer prevents oxides from forming, and it can also extract them from the melt if present. The flux and its oxide contents, being much lighter than the melt, will always be on the surface, away from the mold. Fluxes are not effective against sulfides or carbides. Only proper flame use and adjustment can prevent their formation.

B. Transporting the thermally treated investment to the casting machine

In most cases, the investment mass is heated in an oven and has to be carried to the casting machine while it is at its highest temperature. This should be done using forceps, tweezers, or specially designed tongs. The process should be performed gently, swiftly, and quickly, with the extension of the flask for moldable ceramics or the crucible part of the investment facing downwards to allow the gravitational drop of any loose investment particles in the mold or crucible.

C. Forcing the melt into the investment mold

It should be very clear that to properly wet the mold details and to fill the mold with the cast material, a variety of resisting forces must be overcome. Some of these resisting forces are in the investment, others are in the mold, and still others are in the melt itself. To counteract these, positive forces must be imparted to the melt while it is entering the mold. The energy precipitating this pattern for melt entry can be supplied by one or more of the following:

1. Centrifugal pressure

This is the most feasible and commonly used mode. The investment mass is in the center of a revolving arm. Adjacent to the investment mass is the crucible, containing the melt. A revolving arm is activated by a spring or by electric power. The centrifugal forces produced by the revolving arm will drive the melt from the crucible into the mold.

2. Gas pressure

This is introduced over the melt, in a closed compartment. The gas can be carbon dioxide, carbon monoxide or nitrogen. The gas should be chosen so that the cast material has no affinity for it. This technique is usually used when the cast material is melted (softened) in the investment crucible.

3. Vacuum forces

A vacuum is applied to the external surface of the investment mass, drawing out the investment and mold gases, allowing the melt to ingress. It cannot work alone in filling the mold, however, even if gravitational forces are used in the melt driving. Therefore, machines are employed that use a combination of centrifugal pressure and a vacuum, gas pressure and a vacuum, or centrifugal and gas pressure with the vacuum to create the driving energy.

Generally, machines that employ a vacuum, in conjunction with other sources of driving energy, can produce most of the details of the mold.

4. Piston-plunger forces (for moldable ceramics)

The pre-made crucible will be filled with a softened raw ceramic. The plunger piston, which snugly fits the crucible, is driven into the filled crucible driving the softened ceramic into the mold.

The amount of driving energy used is a matter of judgement, but it is dictated by:

a. The density of the cast material: the lower the density, the higher the energy needed

b. The porosity of the investment: the more the porosity, the less the energy needed

c. The number of sprues: the more the number of sprues, the more the driving energy needed to force the melt into these different avenues

d. The size of the sprue: the larger the diameter of the sprue, the less the energy needed

e. The length of the sprue: the longer the sprue, the more the energy needed

f. The size of the pattern (mold): the larger the size, the more the energy needed

g. The amount of the melt: the more the amount of the melt, relative to the mold size, the less the energy needed

h. The angulation and funnelling of the sprue: The more the sprue is oriented toward immediate and fast filling of the mold, the less the energy needed

i. The differential temperature between the melt and the mold: the more the lag between the two temperatures, the less the energy to be used to a certain extent

j. The configuration and the details of the mold (wax pattern): the more details in the mold, especially minute ones, the more the driving energy needed to replicate them in a casting

For the purpose of discussion, the steps for casting are presented separately. In actual practice there may be overlap between them, e.g., melting the alloy can be done while the ring (investment mass) is being transported. It is most important, however, that there should not be a lag of more than 30-60 seconds between getting the ring from the oven and activating the driving energy of the melt into the mold. The induced energy should be applied for at least 120 sec. (preferably more) to insure its effect.

VI. Cleaning the Casting from its Encasing Investment and Surface Deposits

For cast alloys, after solidification of the molten alloy, (as indicated by the hardening and changing of color of its button portion in the investment crucible), the investment mass (ring) is dropped into room temperature water. The water absorbed in the investment pores will undergo immediate vaporization within the hot mass. Steam in large amounts will be produced, cracking the investment into small pieces and, most of the time, peeling it off the casting. The remainder of the attached investment can be mechanically removed, using a brush or sharp explorer.

Frequently, oxides will be present on the casting surface after being cleaned from the investment (with the exception of

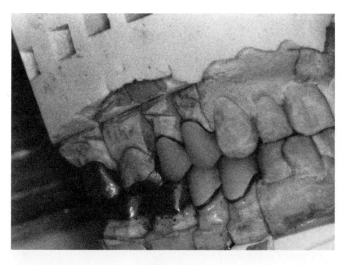

Fig. 24-2

silver-palladium alloys). If so, treating the casting with oxide dissolving agents is indicated. A 50% aqueous solution of sulfuric or hydrochloric acid is used for no more than two minutes. This should remove most of these stains. Stubborn deposits that have not been removed by the chemical treatment are usually sulfides and carbides. They should be removed mechanically, or the entire casting should be done over if their removal will obliterate casting details. For castable ceramics, peeling the investing plaster off the casting is easily achieved using a suitable knife. It should not be quenched in water while hot or the ceramic casting will crack. Any discoloration can be removed with appropriate carbide burs (Fig. 2).

VIII. Thermal Treatment of the Casting

For cast-mouldable ceramics the cleaned formulated cast is subjected to a thermal cycle as detailed in chapter 17 to attain the desired properties. For some cast alloys it may be necessary to harden heat treat the final casting to transform it from its soft-as-cast condition to a tougher, more rigid condition. This can be done by raising the temperature slightly above its re-crystallization temperature keeping it there for the specified time then cooling it slowly to room temperature, allowing the formation and precipitation of the hardening elements (see chapter 17). This process should be done in a time-temperature controlled oven, according to the alloy manufacturer's instructions.

BIBLIOGRAPHY

Barreto, M.T., Goldberg, A.J., Nitkin D.A., and Mumford, G.: Effect of investment on casting high-fusing alloys. J. Prosth. Dent. **44**(5):504-507, Nov. 1980.

Bauer, R.W., and Stewart, S.: Survey on the use of casting alloys in commercial dental laboratories. 1. Classification of equipment, cast partial denture alloys, inlay alloys. NADL J **24**(3):7-11, March 1977.

Consani, S., and Ruhnke, L.A.: An explanation for the water distribution in a hygroscopic expansion technique. J. Dent. Res. **59**(6):1048-1054, June 1959.

Cooney, J.P., Doyle, T.M., and Caputo, A.A.: Surface smoothness and marginal fit with phosphate-bonded investments. J. Prosth. Dent. **41**(4):411-417, April 1979.

Crawford, W.H.: Selection and use of investments, sprues, casting equipment and gold alloys in making small castings. JADA 27:1459, 1940.

Dewald, E.: The relationship of pattern position to the flow of gold and casting completeness. J. Prosth. Dent. **41**(5):531-534, May 1979.

Dootz, E.R.: Fabricating non-precious metal bases. Dent. Clin. N. Am. **241**(1):113-122, Jan. 1980.

Eames, W.: The casting misfit and how to cope. J.P.D. Vol. 45, No. 3, p. 283, March 1981.

Eames, W.: Improving the seatings of castings. Quintessence of Dental Technology. No. 5, May 1981, p. 1.

Eames, W.B., and Macnamara, J.F.: Evaluation of casting machines for ability to cast sharp margins. Oper. Dent. **3**(4):137-141, Autumn 1978.

Eames, W.B., and others: Techniques to improve the seating of castings. JADA Vol. 96, March 1978.

Finger, W., and Jorgensen, K.D.: An improved dental casting investment. Scand. J. Dent. Res. **88**(3):278-284, June 1980.

Finger, W., and Jorgensen, K.D.: Surface roughness of gold alloy castings. Scand. J. Dent. Res. **88**(3):273-277, June 1980.

Ghazala, W.A.: Surface configuration of the cast gold restoration. Egypt Dent. J. **24**(4):373-391, Oct. 1978.

Hagman, H.C.: The evolution of metal castings for dentistry. NY J. Dent. **47**(2):46-51, Feb. 1977.

Howard, W.S., Newman, S.M., and Nonez, L.J.: Castability of low gold content alloys. J. Dent. Res. **59**(5):824-830, May 1980.

Ida, K.: Dental casting technique for preventing casting defects. Kyoto Daigaku Kokukagaku Kiyo **18**:1-15, 1978.

Johnson, M.A.: Finishing procedures that compensate for deficiencies in stone dies. Oper. Dent. **3**(2):57-59, Spring 1978.

Johnston, J.F., Phillips, R.W., and Dykema, R.W.: Modern practice in crown and bridge prosthodontics, ed. 3. Philadelphia, W.B. Saunders Co., 1971, p. 356.

Jones, D.W.: Thermal behavior of silica and its application to dental investments. Part I. Br. Dent. J. **91**:122, 1967.

Jones, D.W., and Wilson, H.J.: Variables affecting the thermal expansion of refractory investments. Br. Dent. J. **125**:249-255, No. 6, Sept. 17, 1968.

Jorgensen, K.D.: Investment materials: Properties and techniques (I). Quintessence Dent. Technol. **4**(5):43-49, May 1980.

Jorgensen, K.D.: Investment materials: Properties and techniques (II). Quintessence Dent. Technol. **4**(6):53-59, June 1980.

Jorgensen, K.D.: Investment materials: Properties and techniques (III). Quintessence Dent. Technol. **4**(7):73-77, July-Aug. 1980.

Lewis, A.J.: The effect of variation in the technique of metal fusion on the development of internal porosity in cast structures. Aust. Dent. J. **22**(5):356-359, Oct. 1977.

Lewis, A.J.: The effect of variation in mould temperature, metal temperature and mould size on the development of internal porosity in cast structures. Aust. Dent. J. **22**(4):243-246, Aug. 1977.

Lewis, A.J.: The influence of the refractory investment on the development of porosity in cast structures. Aust. Dent. J. **22**(6):455-457, Dec. 1977.

Mackert, J.R., Jr., and Moffa, J.P.: A castability test for dental alloys. J. Dent. Res, 54, Special Issue A, Program and Abstracts of Papers, Abstract No. 355, p. 134, 1975.

Neiman, R., and Sarma, A.C.: Setting and thermal reactions of phosphate investments. J. Dent. Res. **59**(9):1478-1485, Sept. 1980.

Phillips, R.W., and Biggs, D.H.: Distortion of wax patterns as influenced by storage time, storage temperature, and temperature of wax manipulation. JADA **41**:28-37, 1950.

Sanad, M.E., Combe, E.C., and Grant, A.A.: Hardening of model and die materials by an epoxy resin. J. Dent. **8**(2):158-162, June 1980.

Sarkar, N.K., Fuys, R.A., Jr., and Stanford, J.W.: The chloride corrosion of low-gold casting alloys. J. Dent. Res. **58**(2):568-575, Feb. 1979.

Sawada, T.: On setting mechanism and hygroscopic expansion of phosphate-bonded investment mixed with colloidal silica solution. The Journal of the Japan Research Society of Dental Materials and Appliances, **32**:6-16, No. 1, 1974.

Schell, R.J., Mumford, G., and Phillips, R.W.: An evaluation of phosphate bonded investments used with a high fusing gold alloy. J. Prosth. Dent. **13**:324-336, March-April, 1963.

Senoussi, J.C., Burdairon, G., and Klapisz, J.: Setting of phosphate-bonded investment materials in relation to wax models. Can. Prosth. **7**(25):143-151, Jan. 1979.

Stackhouse, J.A., Jr.: The accuracy of stone dies made from rubber impression materials. J. Prosth. Dent. **24**:337, Oct. 1970.

Teteruck, W.R., and Mumford, G.: The fit of certain dental castings using different investment materials and techniques. J. Prosth. Dent. **16**:910-927, Sept.-Oct. 1966.

Tuccillo, J.J., and Nielsen, J.P.: Sprue design for gold castings. Dent. Lab. Rev. p. 1-16 (July 1964).

Tunick, G.: How to eliminate miscasts with low gold alloys. Dent. Lab. Rev. **55**(8):26-27, July 1980.

Vaidyanathan, T.K., Schulman, A., Nielsen, J.P., and Shalita, S.: Correlation between macroscopic porosity location and liquid metal pressure in centrifugal casting technique. J. Dent. Res. **60**(1):59-66, Jan. 1981.

Wagner, A.W.: Causes and cures of porosities in dental castings. Quintessence Dent. Technol. **3**(8):57-58, Sept. 1979.

Walsh, J.F.: Neutronographic investigation of was elimination from high temperature investment molds. J. Dent. Res. **56**(4):448-449, April 1977.

Wight, T.A., Grisius, R.J., and Gaugler, R.W.: Evaluation of three variables affecting the casting of base metal alloys. J. Prosth. Dent. **43**(4):415-418, April 1980.

Wirth, C.G.: Accurate relief of the die surface of the wax pattern prior to casting. J. Prosth. Dent. **37**(6):684-685, June 1977.

Metalled abt cements. breakage pan of casting and cementation a bridge and of
casting

worst thing which is when the gagging stays in between the margin in casting so
it dries and shrinks and is best media from microorganism

CHAPTER 25

Casting pre-cementation, cementation, and post-cementation adjustments

If these simple, but extremely important steps are not done properly, all previous time and effort spent in the fabrication of the cast restoration may not lead to a successful result.

I. Pre-Cementation Adjustment, Finishing, Polishing or Glazing

The main objectives of this phase of cast restoration-fabrication are to determine that casting recovered from the investment has reproduced all bulk and surface details that were present in the wax pattern, to detect any discrepancy in the casting and determine whether or not it is correctable, to modify, as necessary, the casting to insure that it fits and covers all details of the preparation internally and marginally. Additionally, superficial scratches and irregularities should be eliminated from the oral surface of the casting, converting the very superficial layer of the oral surface of the casting to the most biologically acceptable inert layer possible.

To attain these objectives, systemized, orderly procedures must be followed. In general, they can be achieved by the following steps:

A. Diagnosis, evaluation and correction of surface and marginal casting discrepancies

The correction of discrepancies should be done in stages starting with gross adjustments and going to finer adjustments. Most of these adjustments should be done on the die if available (indirect technique). Round carbide burs are effective for metallic castings, while diamond stones should be used for ceramic castings.

a. Gross excesses

The tooth surface and circumferential tie constituents of the casting are examined visually and compared to the tooth and cavity preparation surface. Any noticeable excesses detected should be ground away, being careful not to injure, crack, or perforate the circumferential tie constituents of the casting.

b. Fine excesses

The casting is now tried on the die to evaluate its fit. If it does not seat all the way, as revealed by uncovered tooth circumferential tie constituents, the tooth surface and circumferential tie of the casting are examined using a magnifying lens. Pressure indicating pastes or water soluble dyes are available to aid in locating discrepancies.

Fine excesses are usually in the form of veins, small nodules, etc., internally or marginally, which should be removed with extreme care. The casting should be tried again on the die, preferably with the indicator paste or dye, to verify that it is seating better, indicating that the correct excesses are being removed.

Overextended casting circumferential tie constituents should be trimmed very cautiously in small increments. The casting should periodically be tried on the die to verify that the correct area is being trimmed and in the proper direction. Bent circumferential tie constituents should be evaluated for the feasibility of straightening them without fracturing. If not correctable, the casting should be done over.

A distorted casting due to mold, wax pattern, die, or impression warpage, is verified when the casting does not fit, even grossly, after eliminating all possible visible excesses. In these instances the casting should be done over.

c. Rocking

The casting is checked for rocking. If the casting rocks from side to side while on the die, it should be carefully watched while it is rocked in a slow motion and the fulcrum of this rocking should be determined. At this fulcrum, internal or marginal excesses or bent margins may be found, (Again, indicating paste or dye will aid in this detection.) They are handled in the same way as mentioned previously. If this does not eliminate the rocking, it indicates a distorted casting that must be done over.

d. Gross marginal deficiencies

Their presence necessitates that the casting be done over, insofar as they will interfere with the strength, retention and caries prevention capabilities of the restoration.

e. Fine marginal deficiencies

If the deficiencies are internal in the form of blebs, pores, unreproduced details, etc., and they do not involve critical retention areas, they may be allowed to remain, if few in number and isolated. Otherwise, the casting should be re-done.

Excluding restorations made in Class IV and V cast materials, discrepancies in the circumferential tie constituents, either internally or externally, should be evaluated for their correctability. This is done by correlating the elongation and deformability of the alloy with the extent and angulation of the tooth circumferential tie constituents that need to be covered.

use whitestone on gold restoration after cementation at margins and with water
spray to smooth the margins because it can carry the gold particles with it
and it work very smoothly.

387

It should be clear that coverage can only be facilitated by plastically deforming (burnishing) the adjacent section of the restoration. Understandably, the chances for an adequate coverage are enhanced by:

1. The greater the elongation percentage of the alloy.
2. The less the yield strength of the alloy.
3. The less the extent of the defect.
4. The less angulated the uncovered part of the tooth circumferential tie is from the covered part. The best chance of coverage for the uncovered part is a continuation from the covered part, from which the metal will be "dragged."
5. The alloy still being in a softened state, if it is amenable to hardening heat treatment.
6. The less the cross-section of the alloy adjacent to the uncovered part, provided it will not be thinned to a fracture level or create gross underhangs in the restoration by burnishing.
7. Accessibility, insofar as the burnishing will be done intraorally.
8. Terminating on enamel, as burnishing against enamel is more effective and less traumatic than burnishing against dentin.

Burnishing will not be done at this pre-cementation state. It will be done on the tooth during or after cementation. Circumferential tie casting constituents are to be burnished only once, for fear of brittle fracture of these very non-bulky cross-sections.

If it is impractical or impossible to correct the marginal defects, the casting should be done over. If burnishing is deemed possible and will cover the exposed part of the tooth circumferential tie, proceed as described in "B" under the cementation steps. Any circumferential tie discrepancy in a restoration made of a Class IV or V material, however minute, requires that the casting be done over, because these materials are impossible to burnish.

f. Surface pores or deficiencies

If isolated and small in dimension, can be corrected by adding solder (for alloys) or porcelain (for cast ceramics). If they are gross and/or multiple, the casting should be done over.

g. Contacts

The casting should now properly fit the die. The die is reassembled on the working cast and the contact with the adjacent teeth is checked. If an excess is present, the die with the cast will not seat or the cast will loosen from the die. Excesses should be removed carefully in small increments. Marking papers and indicator pastes can help in locating the interfering areas. An open contact is verified by passing dental floss through the contact areas. If present, contact solder can be added for metallic alloys, or aluminous porcelain can be added for cast ceramics.

h. Contour

Any gross excess should be ground away. A casting with any gross deficiency should be done over. If surface porosity discoloration or gross excesses cannot be corrected by grinding and finishing without compromising the casting contour, the casting should be done over. Severe surface porosity is indic-

ative of internal porosity. No attempt should be made to correct this; rather, the casting should be done over.

i. Occluding surfaces

With the casting in place in the working model, the articulator is moved in all possible movements, being sure the casting is immobile. To insure this, the castings may be cemented with a water soluble adhesive, e.g., denture adhesive or luted with sticky wax at their margins. Any prematurities should be removed. There are only limited possibilities of building up occluding surfaces to functional contact (if not present at this stage) using solder for cast alloys. However, cast ceramics can be freely built up with porcelain. If the loss in this dimension is substantial or complicated, the casting should be done over. If functionally generated path records are used, the functional core is seated on the working model with the casting in place. The functional core should fit the unprepared tooth surfaces without any spacing or rocking, and the castings will not move occlusally or laterally. If these criteria are present, the occlusion is correct.

j. Glazing, finishing and polishing

For cast ceramics, after the aforementioned adjustments, the restoration is fired in a porcelain oven according to the manufacturer's recommended time and temperature.

For cast alloys, all circumferential tie constituents of the casting are marked in pencil, especially on the oral surface, to avoid finishing and polishing them at this time. The remainder of the oral surface of the casting will be finished and polished, using rotary instruments. The speed of the instruments (revolutions) differs from one alloy to another, generally increasing, going from Class I to Class IV alloys. This should be done on the die (in a holder if it is a direct wax pattern technique), according to the following sequence:

1. Gross finishing

This should remove roughness imparted on the casting from the investment mold walls, eliminate surface discoloration not removed by pickling, and eliminate fine excesses and obliterate minute defects. This step is always done using abrasive stones and discs, ranging from sand and silicone carbide to alumina, until no surface discrepancies are detected.

2. Removal of scratches and irregularities

This will eliminate undetected fine scratches by removing the alloy substance between these scratches or locally melting the alloy at the surface, obliterating these irregularities. Also, the conversion stage of the finishing process is initiated. This step is done using wire metal brushes, usually brass or steel, to be followed by rubber wheels and cones. There is a large amount of heat produced in this stage, and it may be a factor in fulfilling its objective. The alloy surface should have a satin-like surface by the end of this step.

3. Conversion

Conversion will create the most biologically compatible surface. This step is done using a rubber wheel or cone, followed by brushes carrying extremely fine abrasives, such as tripoli or specifically compounded abrasive pastes. The alloy surface should be shiny by the end of this stage.

4. Final lustre

This creates a reflective, non-adhesive surface.

It is done using rouge on a felt cone or wheel. The alloy surface should be extremely shiny by the end of this stage. The entire oral surface of cast alloys should be finished and polished with the exception of the circumferential tie constituents.

B. Casting try-in and intraoral adjustment

a. Contacts

After removal of the temporary and proper isolation of the tooth, the casting is tried in the mouth. While seating it, any proximal contact interfering with complete seating should be observed visually and relieved incrementally. The contact is checked using unwaxed dental floss for its tightness and dimensions. Again, any excess should be corrected by incremental abrasion, preferably using rubber-bonded abrasives or rubber wheels. Contact adjustment is always needed as a result of positive build-up during the cast fabrication. Rarely at this stage is solder or porcelain added to the contact as a result of an open contact, except due to accidental overabrasion during adjustment.

b. Internal and/or marginal interferences for the complete seating of the casting

These are discrepancies frequently unrecognized during seating on the die. They were not discovered because of yielding potential of the die material not exhibited by tooth structure. The same procedure used on the die in diagnosing and treating this should be used here. It is to be remembered that burnishing of certain areas of the marginal portions of the castings to correct a discrepancy will not be done now.

c. Occluding surfaces

The casting is dried and sometimes roughened on its occluding surfaces (by sand-blasting or alumina abrasive stone grinding) if they will not mark with articulating paper. The casting is checked to insure that it is immobile during mandibular movements. This may require temporary cementation. The patient is guided in moving the mandible from centric relation to centric occlusion with a marking ribbon between the teeth. Excesses deflecting the pathway or interfering with complete intercuspation should be removed. After perfecting their contact, the centric stops are marked with colored ribbon. Another color of marking ribbon is placed between the teeth, and the mandible is moved from centric to lateral and protrusive border limits. Laterally interfering excesses should be removed. These last two steps are repeated. The markings on the castings are compared with the markings on adjacent and opposing teeth, and any prematurities or interferences should be removed. Removal of interfering excesses should also be done using incremental removal, with periodic trials with the two-colored marking ribbons, until a physiologically occluding casting is produced.

d. Final evaluation and preparation of the circumferential tie constituents of the casting

At this stage it is a good idea to control the periodontium to expose the preparation parts of the circumferential tie as was done prior to taking the impression. The casting is then seated, being sure that it is at its most intimate contact with the tooth internally. The circumferential tie and how it relates to the tooth should be closely examined, prefereably using magnifying loops and/or mirrors. Four potential relationships exist between the circumferential tie of the casting and the tooth:

1. The casting adequately covers the tooth circumferential tie in a dimension coinciding with the tooth contour counterpart.

2. The casting adequately covers the tooth circumferential tie, but is too thick and does not coincide with the tooth contour.

3. The casting adequately covers the tooth circumferential tie, but overextends slightly onto unprepared tooth surfaces (overhang).

4. The casting does not cover all of the tooth circumferential tie, but can be corrected by burnishing.

For (1) and (4), nothing will be done until the cementation stage. However, for (2) and (3), the alloy should be shaved very gently, in minute increments, with frequent trials on the tooth to insure that circumferential tie portions of the tooth are not exposed. Shaving in (2) reduces bulk while shaving in (3) reduces length. Fine sand paper discs or gold foil files can be used for these shaving actions, preferably on the tooth in the mouth. If impossible, it can be done partly on the die, partly on the tooth.

e. Evaluating the luting cement space and creating additional cement space if necessary

The use of die spacer is the most practical way to insure the complete seating of the casting during cementaiton, especially if the casting has long surrounding walls with good frictional retention. If, however, the cement space does not seem sufficient, it is advisable to do one of two things to insure the complete seating of the casting, i.e., to minimize hydraulic pressure and to create room for the cementing medium.

1. Stippling (stripping) requires that all the casting circumferential tie constituents and oral surface are covered with wax. The casting is then immersed in an aqua-regia solution (for cast alloys) or hydro-fluoric acid (for cast ceramics) for 5-15 minutes. The tooth surface of the casting will be stripped creating sufficient space for the cement. For metallic restorations, the procedure can be done electrochemically by placing the wax-treated casting at the anodic side of a cell containing an appropriate electrolyte and cathode.

2. The casting can be perforated at an area of minimum stress concentration just prior to cementation. The perforation will relieve the hydraulic pressure, facilitating complete seating of the casting. For cast alloy restorations, the perforation is then restored with gold foil or with specially premade threaded pins, coinciding in diameter to the drill that was used to perforate the casting. For cast ceramics the perforation is restored with composite resin. In both situations, avoid using zinc phosphate cement as a luting agent insofar as it can create the highest hydraulic pressure between the casting and tooth.

f. Glazing or finishing and polishing

The same procedure as in finishing and polishing is repeated for these areas that have been adjusted intraorally with the exception of the circumferential tie for cast alloy.

II. Cast Cementation

The main objective of cementation is to bring the preparation surface of the casting, especially its circumferential tie constituents, as intimately close as possible to the tooth substance. Cementation should obliterate residual space between the casting and the preparation. The cement should intimately wet both the casting and tooth, it should have the least possible solubility and possess a strength comparable to both tooth structure and casting materials. Cementation should create a marginal environment that will encourage healthy repair of the periodontium while discouraging cariogenic activity. It should correct minor marginal discrepancies between the casting and tooth, and enhance immobilization of the restoration, without producing any additional irritation to the P-D organ and periodontium.

A. Cementation procedure

The temporary is removed usually using a scaler or a towel clamp, without injuring the tooth or investing tissues. The preparation is cleaned of any remaining temporary cementing medium, and passive fillers in any auxiliary means of retention are removed. Any remaining cement is dissolved using a biologically safe solvent-cleaner such as hydrogen-peroxide, soluble detergent, liquid of polycarboxylate, or ASPA cement, if using any of them for cementation.

At a safe effective depth (3 mm or more), weak citric acid (3-5% solution) can be used to clean the preparation surface. Washing the preparation with copious amounts of water for 30 seconds will help eliminate cleaning agents, their reaction products, and any residual debris. A tooth surface free from debris, especially temporary cement, will be in the most adherent form. In addition, ZOE cement must be removed to insure the proper setting of PCC and ASPA luting cements. The tooth is isolated and dried, but not to a desiccation level. Varnish is applied on all preparation surfaces of vital teeth if zinc phosphate cement is the cementing medium.

If zinc phosphate cement is to be used, the cement is mixed on a cool glass slab in the same way as mentioned previously in the chapter on intermediary basing, but to a luting consistency, i.e., creamy consistency (secondary consistency). If polycarboxylate cement (PCC) is to be used for cementation, on a paper pad or preferably a cool glass slab it is mixed to a creamy luting (secondary) consistency. If ASPA cement is the cementing medium, a cool glass slab is used with very limited surface mixing to a secondary consistency, i.e., luting consistency. The choice between the three types of permanent cements is a clinical judgement and should be decided upon after considering and compromising between the biological needs of the tooth and the mechanical needs of the restoration.

Zinc phosphate cement is definitely the most adhesive of all three. It has the lowest film thickness and creates enamel etching producing a more locking enamel surface. It has the highest mechanical properties of all three in this consistency, but it is the most irritating to the P-D organ. It is ideally indicated for endodontically treated teeth, or vital teeth whose preparations are deficient in retention but have a minimum effective depth of 3 mm.

PCC is the most inert and least irritating to the P-D organ. Under certain conditions it has an ability to chemico-physically combine with some parts of the tooth structure and treated casting surface. It is indicated for almost all situations.

ASPA is mainly advantageous for its fluoride-ion leaching ability to tooth structure with the consequent anticariogenecity. Under certain prerequisites, chemico-physical adhesion can occur to some components of the tooth and sometimes to the treated preparation side of the casting. It is comparable in its effect on the P-D organ to that of polycarboxylate cement, but it possesses a higher film thickness. It should be used when its anti-cariogenic capability is needed.

ZOE is used only for temporary cementation of the casting for trial periods when the castings are part of an occlusal treatment, or for teeth with possible endodontic interference, to prevent having to go through the restoration for endodontic treatment; or if there is concern of a potential allergic reaction to the restoration material.

After obtaining the proper cement mix, the casting should be lined first as follows. Part of the cement is evenly applied, lining the preparation side of the casting. A fine explorer is used to drive cement into minute details of the casting. Second, the tooth preparation is lined with the cement, special effort being made to introduce the cement into auxiliary retention forms, e.g., pin channels, grooves' internal boxes, etc., using fine explorers or a rotary carrier (lentulo-spiral).

The casting is seated following the path of insertion. For metallic or metallic-based castings, vibrating condenser with a suitable shape is applied on the casting. Forces are delivered in high intensity vibrations to insure the seating of the casting to its proper location.

For cast ceramics finger pressure or occluding pressure is quite sufficient. Pressure is applied statically continuously on the casting during setting of the cement. For that purpose any available devices are used, ranging from orange wood sticks to 2''x2'' gauze pads, to specially designed seaters.

B. Burnishing for Class I, II, and certain Class III alloy castings

Burnishing should bring the restoration portions of the circumferential tie into direct contact with the tooth portions of the circumferential tie. This will minimize or eliminate the cement line, improving retention by the direct coupling and frictional component between the cast alloy and tooth substances, while decreasing the dissolution rate of the cement.

Burnishing should also plastically elongate and mould the marginal alloy to cover uncovered portions of the tooth circumferential tie. It should also strain-harden the alloy at this critical area, increasing its rigidity.

Burnishing is always done from the restoration surface to the tooth surface. It should be performed at all peripheries of the casting, with special emphasis on the uncovered burnishable areas. Hand burnishers may be used. Sometimes rotary burnishers are necessary for alloys with fairly high yield strengths. If ZPC is the cementing medium, burnishing should be done during the setting of the cement. This cannot be done with PCC and ASPA, as the setting polymeric material when burnished tends to be dragged from beneath the casting, removing substantial amounts from the main part of the preparation. Burnishing should be continued until no apparent interruption can be detected with an explorer passed from the casting to the tooth surface and vice versa.

There are several advantages to burnishing the casting intraorally. For one, the casting is permanently fixed on the tooth and will not move. Second, the alloy is adapted marginally to the tooth proper, rather than the replica (die). Third, brittle fracture of delicate areas of the circumferential tie are less likely to happen if the casting is not repeatedly manipulated onto and off the tooth. However, there are several instances where burnishing intra-orally is impossible. With some Class III and all Class IV alloys, for example, it is impossible to burnish on the tooth. Additionally, any casting may have areas that require burnishing but are inaccessible intraorally. In these cases, adjustment and polishing of the circumferential tie constituents must be done on the die.

III. Post-Cementation Adjustments of the Casting

Excess set cement adhering to the surface of the tooth and casting is removed and any remnant cement is curetted from the gingival crevice using curettes or scalers. The restoration is dried and centric stops and lateral pathways are marked. Any contacting areas additional to what was perfected before cementation should be eliminated now. The adjusted areas should be finely polished using small aluminium oxide stones and rubber points.

For metallic castings, load a white polystone with the same alloy of which the restoration is made. This can be done by running it in a button of the cast alloy until the space between its abrasive particles is filled with the alloy material. Use the loaded stone with a very light touch and moderately high speed, keeping it either revolving from the restoration to the tooth surface or partly on the tooth and partly on the restoration revolving laterally. This is virtually a process of burnishing where the burnishing tool is made primarily of the same alloy as the restoration. There should be absolutely no interruption when an explorer is passed from the casting to the tooth and vice versa after this step is performed. It is a step to insure the marginal continuity of the casting and the tooth surface.

With a rubber cup carrying precipitated chalk or tin oxide, a final polish is given to the circumferential tie casting constituents or adjusted areas. Sodium or stannous fluoride solution (8-30%) is applied to the enamel and dentin surfaces peripheral to the casting to protect any injured area. Also, tincture of iodine or merthiolate is applied on the adjacent gingiva to control any possible infection to these injured tissues.

Maintenance and Care of Cast Restorations

No restoration or available restorative material can replace lost tooth structure mechanically, biologically, and anticariogenically. Periodic follow-up maintenance and the interception of problems are the principal measures to compensate for these shortcomings.

When the cast restoration has extensive margins adjacent to the gingiva, the gingiva may undergo varying degrees of traumatization during a cast restoration construction. After cementation and removal of all cements from the gingival crevice, the patient should be advised of this trauma and advised to rinse with warm saline rinses. A post-cementation visit is advisable to detect and remove any remaining cement that may become obvious after the gingiva has reached its normal dimensions. The weakness and possible break-down of the tooth structure-cement-cast joint complex is well established and the patient should be educated how to control plaque at this critical area.

Teeth, especially those that have been subjected to previous restorative procedures, should have their P-D organ monitored after being restored with a cast restoration. The patient should be advised that a slight thermal sensitivity is expected for varying periods (one to six months) after cementation. If this sensitivity exceeds this interval, or is severe in nature, or painful symptoms arise spontaneously, the patient should report immediately for proper therapy to be initiated.

Any change in the location of the free gingiva relative to tooth or restoration surfaces, or any symptoms of pocketing or bone loss around the restored tooth should be observed, and the tooth should be examined for trauma from occlusion. Any interferences should be eliminated, and necessary periodontal corrections should be performed. If the free gingiva has receded permanently, exposing bifurcations or root structure surfaces, recontouring of the cast restorations may be necessary if possible without replacement.

Minute occlusal interferences may not be discovered at the cementation visit, mainly due to strained musculature. Shortly after the casting is in function, they can be recognized by the patient. A post-cementation visit is advisable to discover these and correct them. Periodic occlusal analysis is recommended, especially for patients receiving castings with high abrasive resistance. Also, the patient should be aware of the signs and symptoms of gnatho-stomatic disturbance in order that they may be diagnosed and corrected.

Signs and symptoms of tarnish and corrosion should be explained to patients and if any is exhibited, it should be reported. Any restorations made of Class II and III cast alloys should be polished periodically. Care should be taken not to cause overheating during this periodic polishing if the teeth are vital.

Signs and symptoms of allergic reaction toward these restorations should be explained to the patient and if any appear, it should be reported and a full investigation for any correlation between these symptoms and the cast alloy should be done. (Of course, allergic tests are preferable before planning to use any of these materials.) If the casting is proven to be allergenic, the restoration should be replaced with another proven nonallergenic alloy.

If marginal break-down is discovered with recurrent decay, the best measure is to replace the casting. If the break-down is created from traumatic incidents without any decay and the original restoration is well retained, an adjacent restoration can be built in direct gold (if access will allow), small casting, preferably with a pin (if anatomy allows), or composite resin (if away from the gingivae, and loading is minimal).

BIBLIOGRAPHY

Beech, D.R.: Improvement in the adhesion of polyacrylate cements to human dentin. British Dental Journal **135**:442-445.

Beech, D.R.: A spectroscopic study of the interaction between human tooth enamel and polyacrylic acid (polycarboxylate cement). Arch. Oral Biol. **17**:907, 1972.

Buonocore, M.G.: Principles of adhesive retention and adhesive restorative materials. JADA **67**:382, 1963.

Eames, W., and Little R.: Movement of gold at cavosurface margins with finishing instruments. JADA Vol. 75, July 1967.

Eames, W.B., Monroe, S.D., Roan, J.D., Jr., and O'Neal, S.J.: Proportioning and mixing of cements: A comparison of working times. Oper. Dent. **2**:97, 1977.

Eick, J.D., Wilko, R.A., Anderson, C.H., and Sorensen, S.E.: Scanning electron microscopy of cut tooth surfaces and identification of debris by use of the electron microprobe. Journal of Dental Research **49**:1359-1368, 1970.

Engelman, M.A., and Blechner, C.: Nickel-chromium alloy: A technique to produce clinically acceptable castings. N.Y. J. Dent. **48**(2):41-48, Feb. 1978.

Finger, W., and Jorgensen, K.D.: Surface roughness of gold alloy castings. Scand. J. Dent. Res. **88**(3):273-277, June 1980.

Hollenback, G.M., (editor): Science and technique of the cast restoration. St. Louis, 1964, C.V. Mosby, p. 171-185.

Jorgenson, K.D., and Esbensen, A.L.: The relationship between the film thickness of zinc phosphate cement and the retention of veneer crowns. Acta Odontol. Scand. **26**:169, No. 3, 1968.

Kaufman, E.G., Coelho, D.H., and Colin, L.: Factors influencing retention of cemented gold castings. J. Prosth. Dent. **11**:487, 1961.

Kidd, E.A., and McLean, J.W.: The cavity sealing ability of cemented cast gold restorations assessed in vitro by an acidified gel artificial caries technique. Br. Dent. J. **147**(2):39-41, July 17, 1979.

Krug, R.S., and Markley, M.R.: Cast restorations with gold foil-like margins. J. Prosth. Dent. **22**:54, July 1969.

Lund, M.R.: Finishing and cementation. In Hollenback, G.M., (editor: Science and technique of the cast restoration. St. Louis, 1964, C.V. Mosby, p. 207-218.

McCune, R.J., and others: The effect of occlusal venting and film thickness on the cementation of full cast crowns. J. S. Calif. Dent. Assn. **39**:361, Jan. 1971.

McEwen, R.A.: Efficient restorative procedures. Dent. Clin. North Am. p. 343-354, July, 1965.

McLean, J.: A new method of bonding dental cements and porcelain to metal surfaces. Operative Dentistry, Vol. 2, No. 4, 1977.

Mizrahi, E., and Smith, D.C.: The bond strength of a zinc polycarboxylate cement. Investigation into the behaviour under varying conditions. Br. Dent. J. **127**:410, 1969.

Nishimura, F.: Influence of vibration on the thickness of cement. J. Jap. Res. Soc. p. 29-34, 1971.

Norman, R.D., Swartz, M.L., and Phillips, R.W.: Studies on film thickness, solubility and marginal leakage of dental cements. J. Dent. Res. **42**:950, 1963.

Oliveira, J.F., Ishikiriama, A., Vieira, D.F., and Mondelli, J.: Influence of pressure and vibration during cementation. J. Prosth. Dent. **41**:173, 1979.

Phillips, R.W.: Skinner's Science of Dental Materials. 7th edition, chap. 29. Philadelphia, W.B. Saunders, 1979.

Skinner, E.W., and Phillips, R.W.: The science of dental materials. Ed. 6, Philadelphia, 1967, W.B. Saunders.

Van Nortwick, W.T., and Gettleman, L.: Effect of internal relief, vibration, and venting on the vertical seating of cemented crowns. J. Prosth. Dent. **45**(4):395-399, April, 1981.

CHAPTER 26

Direct gold restorations

Undeniably, direct gold materials and restorations are the most permanent type of restorative modality. However, among the objections to their use are the color of the restorations, (especially when they are in conspicuous locations), the length of the restorative operation (especially for beginners), and the need for extra training to achieve adequate skills to produce these restorations. Unfortunately, there is also a historical association of these materials and restorations with Board examinations, and this has created a real fear or awe of the material and procedures.

Direct gold restorations are the only type of restorations that use pure metal, namely gold, with the exception of one type of direct gold, i.e., electralloy. Direct gold materials can be classified into two main categories: precipitated gold and gold foil (Fig. 1).

A. Precipitated gold

Gold is precipitated through a process of atomization; i.e., the gold is melted and sprayed into cold compartments within an inert atmosphere. This causes the gold melt to precipitate in the form of spherical particles. After the atomization process, the gold particles are passed through different layers of sieves. Larger holes of the sieves are at the top and smaller holes are at the bottom of the compartment. Thus, smaller particles will be precipitated at the bottom of the compartment and the larger particles will be deposited at the top of the compartment. The particle diameters will range, then, from 5 to 75 microns.

Another way of precipitating gold is through electro-deposition; i.e., cathodic deposition of gold from an electrolyte via a suitable anode. Gold particles precipitated through such a process will not have the regular shape produced by atomization, although they will range in diameter very closely to those produced by atomization.

Precipitated gold materials can be supplied in one of three forms:

1. Powdered gold (e.g., Goldent) (Fig. 1, third from the top)

In this form, the precipitated gold particles are wrapped into cohesive gold foil, creating balls. These range in diameter between 1 and 4 mm. Usually, the ratio between the precipitated powdered material and the cohesive gold wrapping is in the range of 19 to 1.

2. Mat gold (Fig. 1, bottom)

In this form, gold is precipitated mainly through electro-deposition, and it is accumulated in the form of strips or cakes.

Then, they are subjected to a sintering process, in which there will be surface diffusion of the atoms of the particles, creating minimal cohesion between the particles. They can then be transported, cut to specific shapes, and handled during the insertion of the direct gold material into cavity preparations.

The mat gold strips can also be wrapped in cohesive gold foil, creating what is known as mat foil. This facilitates the handling and prevents unnecessary loss of pieces of the material during the insertion procedure.

3. Electralloy (Fig. 1, second from the top)

This is an actual alloy of gold and calcium, with the calcium content in the range of 1%. Alloying induces some improvements in the mechanical properties of the pure gold through slip interference. The alloying process is done before atomization, and the particles are shaped exactly like mat gold. They, too, are subjected to sintering in order to make the specific "cake" or "strip" shapes.

B. Gold foil (Fig. 1, top)

The second class of direct gold material is gold foil. This is the oldest and the most durable direct gold. During manufacture, pure gold ingots are subjected to cold working, thereby creating sheets out of blocks. As the gold is subjected to strain hardening during this process, for further cold working towards the formation of these leaves or sheets, the material should be subjected to proper annealing. This alternating process of cold

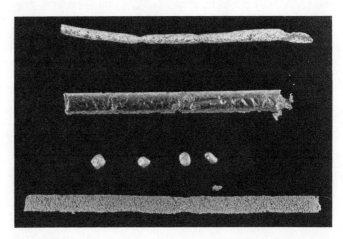

Fig. 26-1. From the top cohesive gold foil, electralloy, powdered gold and mat gold.

working-annealing-cold working continues until the desired thickness of the gold sheet is arrived at. This is usually in the range of 0.001 to 0.007 mm.

Gold foil is supplied in one of four forms:

1. Plain gold foil, which is merely the product of the cold working procedure without any modifications.

2. Corrugated gold foil is manufactured by placing a thin leaf of paper between two sheets of gold foil, after which the whole container accommodating paper leaves and gold foil is ignited. As the paper leaves are burned out, they shrivel, and thereby impart a corrugated shape to the gold foil. It has been proven that corrugated gold foils are more cohesive than the plain ones.

3. Platinum gold foil is an old type of gold foil, which is merely sandwiches of platinum foil between two leaves of gold foil. They are used in stress concentration areas to impart some improved mechanical properties to the gold foil restorations.

4. Laminated gold foil

When a cube of gold ingot is cold worked in order to formulate a sheet, the cubical crystals of gold will be stretched and elongated in a specific direction. If the gold foil of that cube is viewed under a microscope, it appears fibrous, with the fibers parallel to each other in a specific pattern. Mechanically speaking, this type of gold foil material will have directional properties, i.e., it will be resistant to stresses in one direction better than the other. The idea of laminated gold foil is to combine two or three leaves of gold, each from different ingots which have been cold worked in different directions. Although each leaf will be directional in its properties, when combined together, they can be resistant in different directions. Therefore, laminated gold foil is definitely much stronger and much more resistant to stresses than the other forms of direct gold materials.

All different types of direct gold materials can be supplied in a cohesive or a non-cohesive form. The cohesive type of direct gold materials are protected after manufacture by subjecting their surfaces to chlorine or ammonia gases. Although these gases will make the surfaces temporarily non-cohesive, they can be eliminated immediately before inserting the gold into the cavity preparation by the use of heat. It is necessary to treat the gold surfaces with chlorine or ammonia since these gases react with polluting elements to prevent them from permanently contaminating the gold surfaces. They themselves can be eliminated very easily with thermal energy.

For certain procedures, non-cohesive direct gold materials are needed, so manufacturers subject those materials to phosphorous and sulfurous gases, making the surface permanently non-cohesive.

I. Decontaminating and Degassing

The primary reason that direct gold materials are so convenient for building restorations is that they can have complete cohesion of space lattices at room temperature by simply bringing two pieces together and applying pressure to facilitate the cohesion process. It is only necessary to remove any contaminants from the gold surfaces, so that it is possible to create more proximity between the gold pieces. To remove these contaminants, direct gold material should be subjected to a process called degassing or decontamination, which is accomplished simply by applying some thermal energy that can in-

troduce molecular motion in those contaminants, vaporizing them off the surface. Thus the two main objectives of the decontamination process are: (1) to drive impurities off the surface, thus making the surface ready for cohesion, and (2) to keep this surface devoid of any other impurities until complete cohesion occurs during building of the restoration.

Degassing can be accomplished in one of three ways:

A. By an open alcohol flame (Fig. 2)

With this method it is important to use the middle zone of the flame (the high energy reducing zone). Each piece of gold is held in such a zone for three to five seconds before inserting it into the cavity preparation.

B. A mica over a flame

A sheet of mica can be used over any type of flame, and is used somewhat as a heating element. Divide the surface of the mica into several areas to indicate the time the pieces of gold were put on the mica. Maximally, five minutes are allowed for any piece of gold to be heated on the mica.

C. Electric degassing

This is the most controlled and standardized way of decontaminating gold materials. With this instrument, the heated compartment area is made of aluminum. An electric heater controls the time and the temperature. The surface of the heater is divided into small compartments, each accommodating a piece of direct gold. This eliminates the possibility of cohesion of the pieces before they are inserted into the cavity preparation. Maximally, five minutes are allowed for any piece to be kept in the electric decontaminator.

There are certain hazards from overcleaning or overheating of the direct gold materials before their insertion in the cavity preparation. The first hazard is the possibility of recrystallization and grain growth. If this occurs, the mechanical properties of the material will drop substantially. Recrystallization and grain growth are always functions of time and temperature. Therefore, minimal time and temperature to achieve the objectives of decontamination should be used.

The second hazard will be the possible incorporation of impurities from the surrounding atmosphere in the melting or just the very hot surface of gold when it is overheated, or the

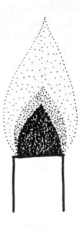

Fig. 26-2

adhesion of those impurities to the gold surface when it is energized by too much heat for too long a time. Precautions should be taken not only to control the time and temperature, but also to avoid degassing the gold in a polluted atmosphere.

The third hazard can occur in those gold materials that are supplied in a sintered form. Overheating during degassing can create an oversintered situation, so that instead of only surface atoms adhering to each other, the whole mass of the particles will adhere to each other. This situation can interfere with the plasticity of the material when it is inserted into the cavity preparation.

The fourth hazard is the complete melting of the surface of the gold. This can make it completely non-cohesive.

The fifth hazard, especially during mass decontamination of direct gold, is that the pieces may tend to adhere before inserting them in the preparation. This is especially likely to happen if they are on mica without being sufficiently spaced from each other, and may lead to larger pieces which are difficult to condense properly.

Insufficient degassing can also create some unfavorable reactions, especially the incomplete removal of the protective gases, thereby making the material only partially cohesive. This will create pitting and porosity within the final restoration.

II. Condensation

A. Objectives for condensation of direct gold materials

The following are the main objectives for the condensation of direct gold material:

1. Wedge initial pieces between dentinal walls, especially at starting points. This is the first and most important step in building a direct gold restoration, for as soon as these pieces are positioned, it is possible to build the restoration over them.

2. Weld the gold pieces together by complete cohesion of their space lattices.

3. Try to minimize the voids in general, and to eliminate them from critical areas like the margins and the surfaces. If complete cohesion of the pieces at every area occurs, there will be no voids. However, gold increments can bridge air entrapments and these may be exposed during finishing or polishing, creating pits on the surface. If such voids occur at the margins, or in the interface between the tooth structure and the gold material, microleakage will increase, followed by a recurrence of decay.

4. Strain hardening of the gold materials which is due to the cold working during condensation. The resulting distortion of space lattices interferes with slip movements and consequently enhances the mechanical properties. In fact, some properties are tripled by this simple act of condensation.

5. Adapt gold materials to the cavity walls and floors. Part of the condensation energy is consumed in bringing the material as close as possible to the cavity walls. This improves frictional retention, decreases microleakage, and reduces recurrence of decay.

6. Elastically deform the dentin of the cavity walls and floors. This objective is facilitated by the elasticity and the high modulus of resilience of vital dentin. As soon as dentin is stressed it will be elastically deformed; yet it will regain its original dimension after varying periods of time, when the direct gold material completely seals the cavity preparation. The return to normal grips the restoration even more, enhancing the frictional retention.

B. Modes of condensation

1. Hand instrument condensation (Fig. 3, A, B, and C)

The condensation energy produced by this method is not always sufficient to fulfill the objectives of condensation. However, it can be used only as a first step in a two-step condensation process, simply to effect the initial confinement of the material within the cavity preparation.

2. Pneumatic condensation (Fig. 4)

This method involves the use of vibrating condensers energized by compressed air. Controlling the air pressure allows adjustments in the frequency and amplitude of the condensation strokes. Although an efficient way, this is not completely controllable.

3. Electronic condensation (Fig. 5)

This is the most efficient and controlled way of condensing direct gold materials. The vibrating condenser heads can have an intensity or amplitude from 2 oz. to 15 lbs. and a frequency of 360 to 3600 cycles/min. The typical apparatus easily permits control of such variables.

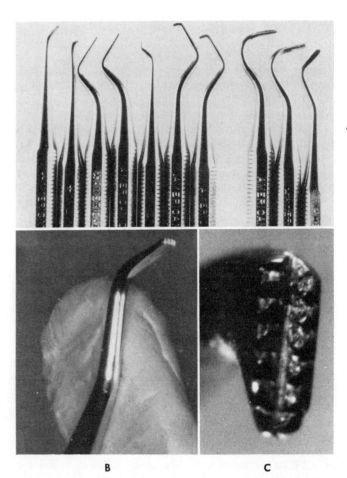

Fig. 26-3. A, Assortment of hand condensers. **B,** Close-up for the shank and nib of a parallelogram hand condenser. **C,** High magnification of the face of the nib of a gold foil condenser.

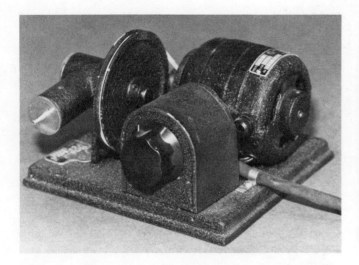

Fig. 26-4

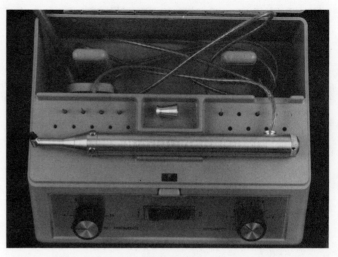

Fig. 26-5

4. Hand condenser and mallet (Figs. 6 and 7)

Although this is the oldest way of condensing direct gold materials, it is still being used. It requires a trained assistant to apply the condensation energy with the mallet. This, in turn, must be in coordination with locating the hand condensers by the operator to the inside of the cavity preparation.

C. Gold condensers

Direct gold condensers have one feature in common: their faces are serrated with pyramidal shaped configurations. (Fig. 3C). This feature will perform three functions:

1. Increase the surface area of the condenser face.

2. Act as swaggers, thus creating lateral forces which will help in fulfilling the objectives of condensation.

3. Establish some triangular indentations in the condensed piece of gold, so that the succeeding increment of gold may be interlocked and immobilized in these indentations.

Condensers for direct gold restorations are provided in different shapes:

a. Round condensers (the bayonet condenser in Fig. 3A) are used mainly to start the direct gold restorations and to establish "ties" in the inner parts of restorations.

b. Parallelogram (Fig. 8) and hatchet condensers (Fig. 9) are used for preliminary condensation and to create the bulk of the restorations.

c. Foot condensers (Fig. 10) are used mainly for cavosurface condensation and surface hardening of the restoration, as well as for bulk build-up.

Condensers for mechanical condensation can be provided for a contrangle or for a straight handpiece. They can be monangled, binangled or bayonet shanked, or even with no angles in their shanks.

D. Principles of condensation

The unique thing about direct gold materials and restorations is that certain principles must be strictly followed to arrive at a successful restoration. Any deviation from such principles leads to immediate failure. These essential condensation principles are as follows:

1. The forces of condensation must be at 45° to cavity walls and floors. In other words, they should bisect line angles (Fig.

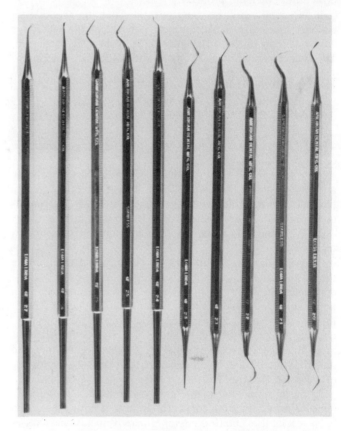

Fig. 26-6. Assortment of hand condensers.

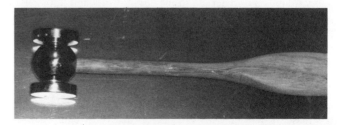

Fig. 26-7. Hand mallet.

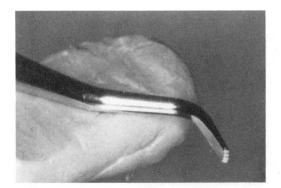

Fig. 26-8

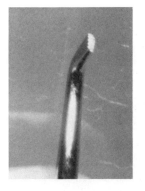

Fig. 26-9

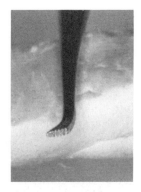

Fig. 26-10

11A) and trisect point angles (Fig. 11B). This leads to the maximum adaptation of gold against walls, floors, line, and point angles, with minimal irritation to the vital pulp-dentin organ.

2. Forces of condensation must be directed at 90° to previously condensed gold. This avoids shear components that can displace or loosen the already condensed pieces of gold. (Fig. 12).

3. Whenever condensing a piece of direct gold, always start at a point on one side and proceed in a straight line to another point on the opposite side, then back to the original side on a different straight line, also starting at and arriving to a specific point. This ensures that the condenser has covered the entire surface of that piece of gold. During these disciplined movements, the condenser should overlap at least ¼ of the previously condensed area. This further assures that each portion of the gold increment has been welded and cold worked and that there are no voids present. This process, called "stepping" ensures the maximal adaptation of the gold to the cavity walls (Fig. 13).

4. Use the minimal thickness of pellet possible, provided that the condensers will not penetrate it. The thinner that the cross-section of each increment is, the easier will be the fulfillment of the objectives of condensation.

5. Energy of condensation

Energy used in condensing direct gold restorations should only be dissipated in fulfilling the objectives of condensation. Additional energy introduced to the field of operation might be consumed in deforming tooth structures or investing tissues of the tooth. Knowing that energy is a product of mass or weight, velocity and time, it is possible to control the amount of energy introduced.

Generally speaking, it is more effective to utilize a lesser amount of energy inside the cavity preparation and to increase energy of condensation gradually as the step-by-step build-up proceeds to the surface. Thus, maximum energy will be used on the surface of the restoration. Condensation energy may be increased by increasing either the frequency or the amplitude of the condensing instrument, and by decreasing the size of the face of the condenser. Remember that condensation energy is inversely proportional to the square of the surface area of the condenser.

The single most important item in the energy dissipation and tissue reaction towards it is the nature of the resistance to that energy. Such resistance is affected by many variables:

a. The more tone that there is in the periodontal ligament,

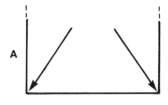

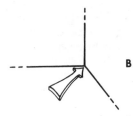

Fig. 26-11

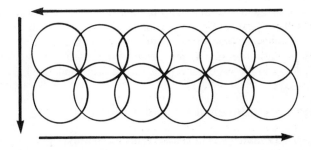

→ Direction of condensing forces
--→ Displacing-loosening shear components

Fig. 26-12

Fig. 26-13

the healthier the periodontium will be, the more resistance there will be to the condensation energy, and the more effective this energy will be in fulfilling the objectives of condensation.

b. The volume of the tooth being condensed against

Logically, the more that the volume of the tooth is, the more will be its ability to absorb energy without deformation and the more will be its ability to resist this energy, allowing fulfillment of the objectives of condensation.

c. The modulus of resilience

The higher that the modulus of resilience of the tooth in which the condensation is occurring is (e.g., vital dentin), the better will be its resistance to deformation.

d. Design factors

Bevelled cavosurface margins, for example, are more resistant to deformation than angular ones. Also, flat floors and walls are more resistant to deforming energy than inclined ones.

e. Operator variables

The operator is the one who decides what type of energy, and at what velocity and amplitude it should be used at different stages of building up the direct gold restoration.

f. Increment size

Minimally sized increments are more effective in realizing the objectives of condensation than larger increments.

g. Technique variables

It helps, especially when using precipitated direct gold materials, to seat the material first, immobilizing it in the cavity preparation, before starting the process of mechanical condensation. This minimizes the loss of gold and helps assure the proper direction of forces against the gold and resisting tissues. Also, during the incremental build-up of the restoration, it is a good idea to periodically check for porosity within the restoration, simply by pressing in with a sharp explorer, and by feeling for any deficiency in the condensation or improper coverage of cavosurface details. It is easier to correct the condensation procedure and to add more increments to fill in these deficiencies, at this time than later.

6. When inserting pieces of direct gold materials, condensation can be either from one periphery of the increment to the other, or, preferably, from the center of the increment to the peripheries. Using the latter method of condensation will minimize bridging trapped air bubbles that will culminate in surface deficiencies in the final restoration.

7. The condensation of precipitated types of direct gold materials should be started by hand. A piece of mat gold (electralloy), coinciding with the shape of the preparation, should be seated in the cavity, or several balls of gold dent necessary to cover the cavity floor or axial wall should be seated rupturing their casing. Then hand condensation is started in the form of a rocking action, preferably from the center to the peripheries, following the same direction of forces and the principles of condensation previously mentioned. When the material is unyielding to the hand condenser, mechanical condensation can proceed.

III. Metallurgical Considerations

A. Metallurgical considerations of cohesive gold foil (Fig. 14)

A cross-section of a properly condensed cohesive gold foil will demonstrate the following features in a metallurgical microscope:

1. The superficial 400 to 600 microns are formed almost completely of solid gold, with no voids. It has been proven that this layer of solid gold is due, mainly, to the act of burnishing.

2. The deepest 200 microns, in contact with a floor, also is composed of solid pure gold with minimal voids. This is due to the resistant nature of the walls or floors against which the gold has been condensed.

3. Serrated portions exist in the bulk of the restoration, with isolated areas of solid gold ranging from 3 to 4 microns in thickness corresponding to the serrated condenser faces. These are areas with no or minimally sized voids.

4. The remainder of the restorations is full of voids, varying in size and number from one location to another.

B. Metallurgical considerations of mat gold restorations (Fig. 15)

In a microscopically viewed cross-section of a mat gold restoration, the following features are apparent. There will be no areas of solid gold, i.e., voids will be spread throughout the restoration, even at the surface. Only strips of solid gold can be found within the restoration, which are actually the gold foil portion of the mat foil. For this reason, mat gold should always be veneered with cohesive gold foil in order to prevent porosity from occurring at the surface.

C. Metallurgical considerations of powdered gold restorations (Fig. 16)

As in mat gold, powdered gold restorations, when viewed microscopically in cross-section, will be full of voids. Only scattered, thin areas of solid gold will be found within the restoration, corresponding to the gold foil encapsulating sheets. Therefore, as with mat gold, it is necessary to veneer powdered gold with cohesive gold foil, in order to establish a solid gold coverage on the surface and at the margins of the restoration.

IV. Mechanical Considerations of Direct Gold Restorations

As can be expected from the metallurgical picture and the mode of condensation of the different types of direct gold

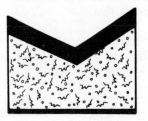 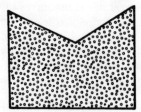

Fig. 26-14 **Fig. 26-15**

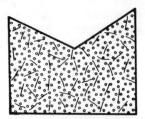

Fig. 26-16

materials, the mechanical properties of each type will differ from the other, especially when measuring the mechanical properties according to their tensile strengths, their knoop hardness numbers, and their density. The following facts summarize the mechanical properties of the different direct gold restorations:

A. Pure cohesive gold foil restorations will be the strongest, the densest, and the hardest of all types of direct gold restorations. This is due to the greater cohesion between the ingredient leaves (foil) in the completed cohesive gold foil restoration as compared to the ingredient particles of the precipitated gold restorations. Cohesive gold foil restorations will have fewer voids, fewer foreign bodies, and a lesser number of component ingredients (that must be joined together) than restorations made of precipitated gold.

B. As previously mentioned, the smaller that the size of the increments during condensation are, the stronger will be the final restoration. This can be explained by the fact that the smaller the increments are, the more will be the available energy required to fulfill the objectives of condensation.

C. To reiterate, the greater that the resistance to condensation is, the more complete will be the fulfillment of the main objective of the condensation, i.e., cohesion, a higher density, producing a harder, stronger restoration.

D. Also, as mentioned previously, the smaller that the size of the condenser is, the better will be the resulting mechanical properties in the restoration. This, of course, is due to the higher energy dissipated by the smaller type condensers.

E. It is practical and effective to combine different materials together in order to take advantage of the best of each. For example, building the bulk of a restoration in the precipitated gold is a feasible, fast process, which will create less trauma to the inner tissues around a cavity preparation. Then veneering that build-up with cohesive gold foil will produce the advantage of a solid gold veneer, with the least number of voids, the greatest mechanical strengths and the most physical resistance. Using this technique, three-fourths to four-fifths of the restoration is built up in precipitated gold, with the remainder being a veneer of cohesive gold foil.

V. General Steps for Insertion of Direct Gold Restoration in a Cavity Preparation

The following can serve as a general outline for the procedure of inserting direct gold materials into a cavity preparation:

A. Three step build-up for the restoration

1. "Tie formation" (Fig. 17)

This involves connecting two opposing point angles or starting points filled with gold with a transverse bar of gold. Such a "tie" forms the foundation for any restoration in direct gold. Of course, its resistance to displacement should be tested before proceeding to the next step.

2. "Banking of walls" (Fig. 18)

This is accomplished by covering each wall from its floor or axial wall to the cavosurface margin with the direct gold material. A wall should be banked in a way that will not obstruct tie formation or banking of other walls in the cavity

preparation. "Banking" should be performed simultaneously on the surrounding walls of the preparation.

3. Shoulder formation (Fig. 19)

Sometimes, to complete a build-up, it is necessary to connect two opposing walls with the direct gold material.

These three steps should completely fill up the cavity preparation, but the build-up should continue until the preparation is overfilled.

B. "Paving" of the restoration

Every area of cavosurface margin portion should be individually covered with excess cohesive gold foil. For this procedure, a "foot" condenser is useful.

C. Surface hardening of the restoration

Utilizing the highest condensation energy in the restorative procedure (i.e., a high frequency and low amplitude), go over the surface of the restoration in all directions, so as to strain harden the surface gold and to fulfill the rest of the condensation objectives at this critical area (surface) of the restoration.

D. Burnishing

As mentioned before, burnishing is the major act in creating a solid gold sheet marginally and on the surface. Burnishing should be done with the proper instruments, moving from gold to tooth surface. Not only will this procedure enhance surface

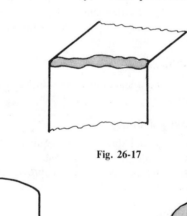

Fig. 26-17

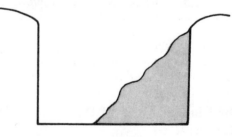

Fig. 26-18

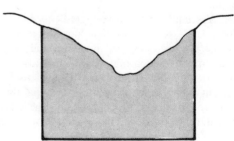

Fig. 26-19

hardening, but it will also adapt the material more to the margins as well as eliminate surface and marginal voids.

E. Margination

Using sharp instruments (e.g., knives and files), moving from the gold surface to the tooth surface, try to eliminate excess in small increments at a time. Do not try to displace or cut a big chunk of the direct gold marginally, as this may displace the whole restoration or cause irreversible damage marginally. This margination process is done until it is possible to visualize the original outline of the cavity preparation. It may be necessary to alternate between burnishing and margination, because margination may expose soft gold or voids. Burnishing can correct these small discrepancies.

F. Burnishing

This process definitely follows margination as a means of closing marginal discrepancies as well as strain hardening the surface.

G. Contouring

In this process, an effort is made to create the proper anatomy of the restoration to coincide with that of the tooth and to be compatible with that of the opposing, contacting, and occluding teeth. It is accomplished using knives, files, or finishing burs. If contouring involves margins, they should be reburnished before final contouring. Further burnishing of non-marginal parts of the restoration may also be needed during the contouring procedure.

H. Additional burnishing

This is done here for the purpose of fulfilling previously mentioned objectives.

I. Finishing and polishing

Minimal finishing and polishing will be required with a properly surface hardened, marginated, and contoured restoration. However, some finishing may be done using precipitated chalk or tin oxide powder on soft bristle brushes or rubber cups.

J. Final burnishing

This is done to ensure closure of marginal voids and other surface discrepancies.

VI. The Biologic Form of Direct Gold Restorations

Question: Are direct gold restorations irritant to the pulp-dentin organ?

Answer: Yes, and the irritating ingredients are:

(1) The energy of condensation, not absorbed by the restorative material, is dissipated into the vital dental tissues creating deformities which may lead to irritation in the pulp-dentin organ. It has been verified that condensation energy forces at right angles to the axial walls or pulpal floors are the most destructive to the pulp-dentin organ. Therefore, the operator should use forces 45° to those walls in an effort to avoid deleterious effects.

(2) The thermal energy in the gold pellet exceeding that necessary for decontamination will also be transmitted to the pulp-dentin organ.

(3) The frictional heat of finishing and polishing.

(4) Galvanic currents, established between cathodic gold and other metallic restorative materials.

(5) Ultrasonic energy resulting from high condensation frequencies can create some (reversible) harm in the pulp-dentin organ.

Question: What is the effect of direct gold restorations at different effective depths?

Answer: With an effective depth of 3-3½ mm., a normal pulp will undergo a healthy reparative reaction. With an effective depth between 1-2 mm, there will be an unhealthy reparative reaction. With an effective depth of less than 1 mm, there will usually be destruction in the pulp-dentin organ. The initial sign is usually cracking in the pulpal or axial wall.

It should be noted that immediately following insertion of a direct gold restoration, the pulp-dentin organ appears to be in a state of disarray. Notable will be the displacement of odontoblasts, areas of internal hemorrhage, and some vesicle formation. However, the pulp will usually return to its preoperative condition (or previously designated reaction) within as little as 24 hours or as long as two weeks. The complete sealing ability of a properly placed restoration enhances the return to normalcy.

Question: What are the protective bases necessary for the pulp-dentin organ?

Answer: With an effective depth of 3 mm or more, no intermediary base protection will be necessary. With an effective depth of 2 mm or more, cavity varnish should be applied on all walls and floors, with the marked exception of the cavo-surface margins.

If the effective depth is between 1-2 mm, a subbase of calcium hydroxide or unmodified ZoE (depending on the condition of the pulp-dentin organ and the location of the preparation) is indicated. This subbase should be covered by varnish, and then a base of zinc phosphate cement. If conditions of the pulp allow calcium hydroxide as the subbase, polycarboxylate cement may be used as the overlying base. Any such circumstance requiring a subbase and/or base must allow all line and point angles of the cavity to be in dentin.

With an effective depth of less than 1 mm, direct gold restorations are contraindicated.

VII. Sealability of Direct Gold Restorations

As mentioned previously, direct gold restorations are the most efficiently sealing permanent restorative materials. Not only does the microleakage space around these restorations have the least dimension of all restorative materials, but the leakage space decreases with time.

It is easy to understand why direct gold materials are so efficient in sealing cavities. The method of condensation creating elastic deformation of the underlying and surrounding dentin, the nobility of the gold materials, the strengths of strained gold materials, especially in very thin cross-sections, and the complete insolubility of the materials in the oral fluids all contribute to this property.

After considering the details concerning the characteristics and principles of manipulating direct gold, one can surmise that direct gold restorations are primarily indicated for

A. Lesions with very limited dimensions and extent.

B. Lesions in which cavity margins can be located on sound enamel surfaces.

C. Lesions in vital teeth, i.e., having a sound pulp-dentin organ, intact supporting periodontium, and the ability to withstand condensation forces.

D. Lesions in which tooth structure left after removal of diseased tissues is bulky enough to create self-resisting walls and pronounced retention modes.

E. Lesions in patients with good oral hygiene, low caries and plaque indices.

F. Lesions with adequate access for detailed preparation and instrumentation.

G. Areas necessary to repair perforations in cast gold alloy restorations.

H. Teeth with no enamel crazing or micro-cracks.

Cavity Preparations for Direct Gold Restorations

Each type of direct gold material requires specific features in the cavity preparation to enable it to be properly inserted and retained.

I. Class I Cavity Preparations for Direct Gold Restorations

A. Simple Class I in molars and pre-molars occlusal surfaces (Fig. 20, A-I)

1. General shape

The outline is similar to Class I cavity preparations for amalgam, but with three modifications:

a. Instead of rounded corners in the triangular and linear fossa areas, these preps have angular corners.

b. The extensions in the facial and lingual grooves in molars will end in a spear-like form, i.e., a pointed termination, rather than rounded.

c. The sweeping curves of the outline form of the cavity preparation compared to those for amalgam are less pronounced. In other words, the whole outline will look more angular than in preparation for amalgam.

2. Location of margins

The facial and lingual margins of these preparations will be on the inclined planes of the corresponding cusps or marginal ridges, so that the width of the cavity will not exceed ⅕ the intercuspal distance. The mesial and distal margins will also be conservatively located on the inclined planes of the corresponding ridge, very close to the adjacent pits.

3. Internal anatomy

The mesio-distal and facio-lingual cross-sections of cavity preparations demonstrate internal features very similar to those found in amalgam Class I, Design 1, with two exceptions:

a. The line and point angles are definite and very angular within dentin substance. Sometimes, at a point angle or at two opposing point angles, it is necessary to prepare starting points, especially if those point angles are not sufficiently sharp or undercut to allow starting a tie of direct gold. The pulpal floor, if it is prepared on two levels due to caries extensions in dentin, has to be made flat using a subbase and strong base material, provided the adjacent line and point angles are in sound vital dentin.

b. The cavosurface margins should be bevelled with a partial

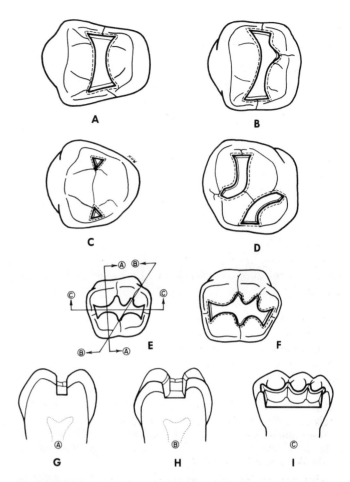

Fig. 26-20. E–I, Class I occlusal preparations for gold foil in all four types of posterior teeth.

enamel bevel. This bevel is at 45° to the direction of the enamel rods and should include at least ¼ of the enamel wall. Its purpose is to protect enamel margins from the condensation energy and to allow coverage of the enamel margins with the durable gold material.

Although the junctions between the dentinal portion of the cavity walls and floors are angular, the junction between the partial bevels on the cavosurface margins should be rounded so as to minimize stresses while condensing gold on the fragile enamel, and also to prevent leaving frail unsupported enamel at these junctions.

B. Compound or complex Class I cavity preparations for direct gold restorations (Fig. 21)

These are Class I cavity preparations with facial and/or lingual extensions. They will have the same general shape, occlusally, as the simple design. The facial and/or lingual extensions will be parallelogram in shape. The location of margins is exactly as in the preparation for amalgam, except the mesio-distal width of the facial and lingual portions of the cavity preparation should be very limited (1 mm, if possible).

The internal anatomy of these cavities will also be similar to the simple design in their occlusal part, and to the amalgam Class I cavity preparation, Design 4, in its facial and lingual parts. However, it is necessary to have starting points at the

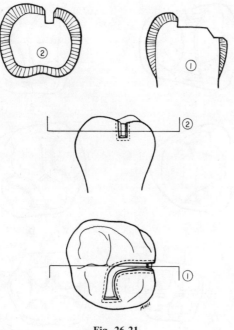

Fig. 26-21

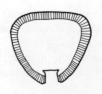
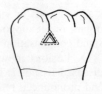

Fig. 26-22

mesial and distal axiogingival corners of the facial and lingual extensions. Again, a partial bevel all around the cavosurface margin is mandatory.

Any further extension of a Class I lesion involving the occlusal and facial surfaces of molars is contraindicated for direct gold materials.

C. Simple Class I cavity preparations on the lingual surface of upper anterior teeth and at the facial and lingual pit areas of upper and lower molars (Fig. 22)

The general shape of this type cavity will be triangular, with the base of the triangle facing gingivally. The location of margins can be anywhere, as the entire area is self-cleansable. Just include the decay and undermined enamel.

The internal anatomy will include a flat axial wall, following the same angulation as the adjacent surface, and surrounding walls in three planes, i.e., an internal, undercut, dentinal plane not including more than ½ of the dentinal walls, a straight second plane formed of enamel and dentin, and a third plane which is the partial bevel. As usual, this involves only ¼ of the enamel wall circumferentially. Whenever these outer plane components join each other, the junction should be rounded. On the contrary, the internal plane components should join each other in an angular fashion.

The previous descriptions for the three types of a cavity preparation for Class I in direct gold materials are basically for cohesive gold foil alone. If one intends to use combinations of direct gold materials, and the bulk of the restoration is going to be in precipitated gold, the line and point angles can be less angular, and starting points will be unnecessary.

Instrumentation for Class I cavity preparation

Instrument utilization is very similar to Class I, Designs 1, 3 and 4 for amalgam, with the exception that one should use smaller burs and hand instruments. For example, use a #168

bur instead of #699 as in case of amalgam, to create smaller preparations. During the final shaping, the angle former may be used more frequently to sharpen internal anatomy. During the preparation finish, a partial enamel bevel should be prepared using the smallest Wedelstaedt chisel in direct cutting strokes, paralleling the preparation margins. Starting points, if required, can be created with a spear bur (see Class V preparations).

II. Class II Cavity Preparations for Direct Gold Restorations

There are three designs for Class II cavity preparations for direct gold materials.

A. The conventional design (Fig. 23)

This is very similar to Class II modern design for amalgam restorations.

1. General shape

The occlusal outline is an exact replica of the simple Class I cavity preparation in molars and premolars, mentioned previously. The isthmus portion will definitely have a reverse S-shaped outline facially and lingually due to the very narrow occlusal preparation in transition to a regular size contact area.

The proximal portion outline will be a one-sided inverted truncated cone. On the upper teeth, truncation will be at the expense of the lingual proximal wall, and on the lower teeth, truncation will be at the expense of the buccal proximal wall. In other words, the inverted truncation is at the expense of the functional cusp side (which is bulkier and more convex).

2. Location of margins

The occlusal portion will have its margins exactly in the same location as the simple Class I on the occlusal surfaces of molars and premolars. However, there is no need for "dovetailing" in locating those margins. The isthmus portion will have its margins located on the inclined planes of the remaining parts of the marginal ridge and the adjacent cusps, so that the width of the cavity will not exceed ⅕ the intercuspal distance.

The margins gingivally will just clear the contact area. There should not be any effort to put the margins subgingivally. Wherever the mere removal of the contact area and the caries cones in enamel and dentin, will put those margins, is the ideal location.

Facial and lingual margins should only include the contact area and the area of near approach. It is not necessary to pass an explorer between the adjacent teeth for clearance, as in the final steps of condensation and in the late stages of finishing and polishing, some separation will occur that will not only facilitate coverage of the proximal margins by direct gold, but also the finishing and polishing at those margins.

If it is necessary to extend the facial margin very far facially

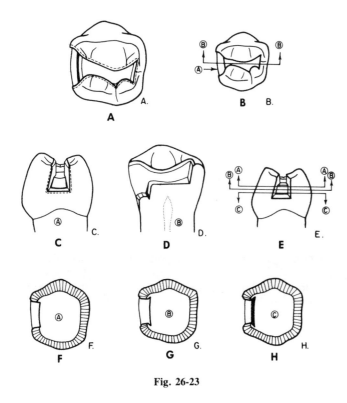

Fig. 26-23

that wall and margin should parallel the facial convexity. This outline will decrease the conspicuousness of the final restoration.

3. Internal anatomy (Fig. 23, C, D, E, F, G, H)

a. A mesio-distal cross-section enables visualization of the proximal, pulpal, axial, and gingival walls and floors. They can be seen to have the same angulation as in Class II, Design 1 for amalgam, with two exceptions:

i. All line angles, with the exception of the axio-pulpal, will be very sharp.

ii. The cavosurface margins are bevelled at almost 45° to the plane of the enamel walls.

b. The facio-lingual cross-section at the gingival one-third indicates that the axial wall will be convex, following the curvature of the proximal surface. The facial and lingual walls may each have four planes: the first one being an inner, dentinal plane making a very sharp and acute angle with the axial wall or with the tangent of the axial wall there; the second plane, or transitional plane, is formed completely of dentin; the third plane is an enamel-dentinal plane following the direction of the enamel rods, facio-proximally and linguo-proximally; the fourth plane is completely in enamel and is a partial bevel, maximally involving ¼ of the enamel wall and at 45° to the enamelo-dentinal wall plane. In extremely narrow preparations the second and third planes may be combined into one, following the direction of the enamel rods (Fig. 23H).

A facio-lingual cross-section in the middle third of the cavity preparation proximally elucidates the same three walls. Each of the facial and lingual walls will have the same planes. The only difference here is that the first (inner dentinal) plane makes a less acute angulation with the axial wall or with its tangent (Fig. 23G).

A facio-lingual cross-section at the level of the pulpal floor

indicates three planes: an inner dentinal plane at right angles to the axial wall or to its tangent; an outer enamel-dentinal plane following the direction of the enamel rods facio- or linguo-proximally, and the third plane or partial bevel, mentioned in the above two sections. Sometimes, in very narrow preparations, the two inner planes will be combined. (Fig. 23F).

A facio-lingual cross-section within the occlusal part of the cavity preparation shows the facial and lingual walls to be in a reverse S-shape, in addition to having a partial bevel on the proximal extent of the cavity walls. (Fig. 23A).

These cross-sections should indicate the existence of a triangular shaped retention area at the expense of the dentinal portion of the facial and lingual walls of the proximal part of the cavity preparation. The base of this triangle is at the gingival floor level and the tip of the triangle is at the pulpal floor level. The retention triangle will open with its widest side to the main part of the proximal cavity preparation. The narrowest side will be internally located. These triangular areas, besides aiding the self-retaining mechanism for direct gold materials proximally, can also act as the starting points for formation of gold ties along the axio-gingival line angle. If the occlusal part of the preparation does not have sharp point angles facilitating the starting of a "tie," starting points can be established with spear burs at two opposing point angles.

The above mentioned design is for cohesive gold foil and is to be modified for a combination of precipitated gold and cohesive gold. One can omit, for instance, the occlusal starting points, and it is possible to make the sharpness of the proximal triangular areas less pronounced.

4. Instrumentation for conventional design

Instrumentation is very similar to that used in preparing a Class II, Design 2 for amalgam. However, smaller dimension instruments are used. Also, the internal anatomy is mainly done with hand instrumentation, especially the line and point angles and the triangular areas. The starting points are done using spear burs and the cavosurface bevels are prepared with a Wedelstaedt chisel, wherever access allows, and with the gingival margin trimmers in many locations.

B. The conservative design

1. General shape (Fig. 24, A and B) of this design is exactly as that of Class II, Design 3 for amalgam restorations.

2. Location of margins (Fig. 24)

This, too, is very similar to that of the same design for amalgam restorations.

3. Internal anatomy (Fig. 24, C and D)

a. *Mesio-distal cross section:*

This section shows a very slanted axial wall, formed of dentin and enamel. The enamel portion is partially bevelled towards the occlusal. The gingival floor is in four planes: an internal, reverse-bevel plane, making an acute angle with the axial wall and formed completely of dentin; a transitional plane, formed completely of dentin and slightly flat; an outer, enamel-dentinal plane following the direction of the enamel rods and, finally, a partial bevel on enamel only, not to include more than ¼ of its extent.

b. *Facio-lingual sections*

In viewing the same four cross-sections as for the conventional design, the first and second sections will be seen as an exact replica of the conventional design. The third cross-

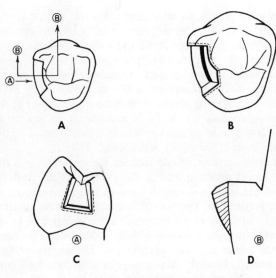

Fig. 26-24

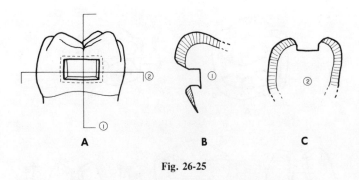

Fig. 26-25

section, just short of the occlusal enamel, shows the termination of the facial and lingual triangular areas. A cross-section occlusal to that will be exactly like that described for the conventional design, except without any occlusal portion. (Fig. 23F)

In other words, the triangular areas, facially and lingually, will extend to just short of the occlusal enamel, leaving a limited thickness of dentin to support the occlusal enamel. The triangular area joins the reverse bevel internally via a rounded junction. The same modifications in cavity preparation can be done to accommodate precipitated type gold, for build-up purposes, as mentioned for the previous design.

4. Instrumentation for conservative design

This is similar to Class II, Design 3 for amalgam, with the same modification in instrumentation, as mentioned with the conventional design Class II for direct gold.

C. The simple design

1. General shape

This is very similar to that for amalgam, except it has a more angular junction between the different margins (Fig. 25).

2. Location of margins

Because the whole surface is self-cleansable, the margins may be placed anywhere on the surface.

3. Internal anatomy (Fig. 25, B and C)

a. An occluso-gingival cross-section (Fig. 25B) will show that the occlusal wall is formed of three planes (assuming that the occlusal margin is located at the occlusal one-third of the involved proximal surface): one plane, in the form of dentin, and at right angle to the axial wall; a second plane inclining occlusal proximally, and formed of enamel and dentin; and a third one in the enamel wall, in the form of a bevel. If the occlusal margin is located at the middle third of the proximal surface, the occlusal walls' two internal planes can be made as one, following the direction of the enamel rods.

The axial wall will be seen in this cross-section to be almost flat. The gingival floor will appear in four planes, because it carries the retention form for such a cavity preparation. The inner plane is formed completely of dentin and is in the form

of a reverse bevel making an acute angle with the axial wall. Next is a transitional plane, formed completely of dentin. The third plane is formed of enamel and dentin and follows the direction of the enamel rods. The final plane is a partial enamel bevel.

b. In a facio-lingual cross-section (Fig. 25C) the axial wall will appear to be flat to only slightly rounded. If the access is very convenient, the facial and lingual walls will have the same anatomy, i.e., each wall will have three planes (assuming that the facial and lingual margins are located in the corresponding third of the involved proximal surface): a dentinal plane at right angle to the axial wall; an outer enamel-dentinal plane following the direction of the enamel rods; and a third plane in the form of a partial enamel bevel. If the facial and lingual margins are in the middle third of the proximal surfaces, the corresponding wall's two internal planes can be combined into one, following the direction of the enamel rods.

On the other hand, if access is not completely convenient, one must choose between a facial or a lingual access. The non-access wall will have the same planes and angulations as in the previous description, but the access side wall will have only two planes: one, enamelo-dentinal in composition, making an obtuse angle with the axial wall, and the second being a partial bevel, enamel only, plane.

Sometimes starting points are prepared at the gingivo-facio-axial and the gingivo-linguo-axial point angles. They will be pyramidal in shape with the base of the pyramid towards the main cavity preparation and with the tip internally located. The direction of those starting points is facio-gingivo-axial and linguo-gingivo-axial, consequently.

The same modifications can be accomplished to make this cavity suitable for precipitated direct gold materials, as described for previous designs; i.e., no starting points and less sharp line and point angles.

4. Instrumentation for simple design

This is the same as Class II, Design 4 for amalgam, with similar modifications as mentioned with the conventional design, Class II cavity preparation to receive direct gold.

III. Class V Cavity Preparations for Direct Gold Restorations

There are four basic designs of Class V cavity preparations, with their modifications.

A. The Ferrier design

1. General shape

The general shape of this cavity preparation is trapezoidal, with the short arm gingivally and the long arm occlusally. This trapezoid shape of cavity preparation has the following advantages:

a. It is the most convenient form for the gingival third cavity preparation, making every corner and margin in the cavity preparation accessible to instrumentation.

b. It will produce the most esthetic shape of a final restoration, as the occlusal margins will be parallel to the occlusal plane. The mesial and distal margins will be partially hidden by the gingiva and paralleling the axial outlines of the facial and lingual surfaces. The gingival margin will be partially covered by the gingiva and paralleling the occlusal plane. This parallelism to anatomical landmarks will make the final restoration less conspicuous.

c. The trapezoidal shape with linear outline will assure prompt paving and margination of the restoration. In other words, one can easily avoid overhangs or overextension with the direct gold materials, as the linear margins have a more predictable location as compared to curved margins.

d. The trapezoidal cavity preparation can facilitate flat walls and planes against which one can condense direct gold safely.

e. The trapezoidal shape cavity preparations are the most conservative for the gingival third lesions.

f. Trapezoidal shape cavity preparations can facilitate the bulkiest retention forms and the most predictably located starting points.

2. Location of margins (Fig. 26)

The location of margins, as designated by Ferrier, is as follows. The gingival margin should be half-way into the gingival crevice. The mesial and distal margins should be partly covered by the gingiva in its ascending path to the interproximal col and partly at, but not involving, the axial angle of the tooth. The occlusal margin is at, but not including, the height of contour. It should be parallel to the gingival margin and both should be parallel to the occlusal plane.

This design can conceivably lead to a massive involvement of tooth structures at the gingival third of the facial and lingual surface. One must assume that whenever the attached gingiva is pronounced and healthy, the fornix is deep and sound, and the tooth is in a very cleansable situation. Therefore, it should be possible to put the margins of a Class V restoration in a more conservative location. This might involve putting the gingival margin supragingivally, or placing the mesial and distal margins away from the axial angles of the tooth towards the center of the facial or lingual surfaces, or the occlusal margin further below the height of contour. Direct gold restorations, with their sealability, can efficiently compensate for such lack of ''preventive extension''

3. Internal anatomy (Fig. 26)

a. In a mesio-distal cross-section, one can visualize a convex axial wall, following the same curvature as the facial or lingual surface.

The mesial and distal walls will appear to be two-planed: one plane is divergent and makes an obtuse angle with the axial wall or its tangent at this location, and it is formed of enamel and dentin; the other plane is in the form of a partial enamel bevel (Fig. 26C).

b. In a gingivo-occlusal cross-section, the gingival wall, assuming it is in the gingival third of the facial or lingual

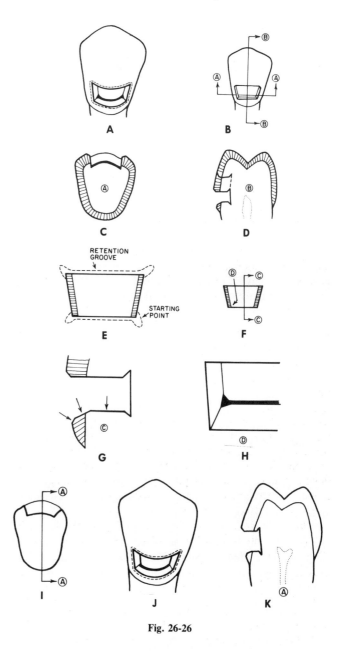

Fig. 26-26

surface, is formed of four planes: an inner dentinal plane (Fig. 26, D and G) resembling a reverse bevel, making an acute angle with the axial wall; a transition plane formed of dentin; a third plane following the direction of the enamel rods, inclining gingivo-facially or lingually; and a final plane in the form of a partial enamel bevel.

If the gingival margin is located on dentin, it will be very difficult to finish gold there because of possibilities of abrading the dentin, gouging the tooth gingivally and subsequent cavitation of the tooth structure there. Therefore, the gingival wall in this instance should be formed of two planes: an internal reverse bevel and an outer flat plane. For those gingival walls made of dentin, special care should be taken not to overfinish the restoration gingivally.

The occlusal wall may have the same four planes (Fig. 26D). The only exception is that the outer planes will be inclining occluso-facially or lingually. If the occlusal margin is located in the middle third of the facial or lingual surface, it will be formed of three planes only: a dentinal reverse bevel internally, an enamelo-dentinal plane following the direction of the enamel rods, and a partial enamel bevel externally (Fig. 26, D and G).

B. Class V cavity preparation with a proximal panhandle extension (Fig. 27)

1. General shape

This cavity consists of two portions; i.e., a facial or a lingual part, whose outline is exactly like the previous design, and a proximal part, parallelogram in shape, as an extension from the facial (or lingual) in the proximal direction.

2. Location of margins

The facial and lingual portions will have their margins in the same location as in the previous design. The proximal portion will have a gingival, occlusal, and facial (or lingual) margin. All margins should be in the gingival embrasure, but they can extend far proximally to the opposite facial or lingual embrasures. In any event, they should be located so as to be accessible for preparation, condensation, finishing, and polishing, with the possible help of some separation.

3. Internal anatomy

The facial or lingual portion will have the same internal anatomy as described for the previous design. The proximal portion will have a flat axial wall. The gingival floor is exactly like the gingival floor of the facial or lingual portion. The occlusal wall is formed only of two planes: a flat internal plane formed of enamel and dentin following the direction of the enamel rods, and a partial enamel bevel plane proximally. There is no internal bevel in the occlusal wall to avoid undermining tooth structure in the contact area (see comparable design for amalgam cavity preparation).

The facial or lingual wall proximally will be formed of two planes: an inner dentino-enamel plane at right angle to the axial wall, following the directions of the enamel rods and a partial enamel bevel plane. The junction between the two axial walls should be perfectly rounded, while other point and line angles should be very angular. The junction between the peripheral partial enamel bevels should be rounded.

C. Class V with uni- or bilateral "moustache" extensions occlusally (Fig. 28)

Sometimes surface defects occlusal to the height of contour are continuous with a gingival third lesion, necessitating their involvement in the Class V cavity preparation and their restorations. So one or two occlusal extensions are added to the basic trapezoidal Class V cavity preparation.

1. General shape

As the name indicates, this design will appear as a unilateral or bilateral "moustache shape" (see comparable design for amalgam cases).

2. Location of margins and internal anatomy

Margins in this design are very similar to those in the first design. However, the additional "extension" portions will have perfectly straight mesial and distal walls ending at a point occlusally. The mesial and distal walls will have the same partial enamel bevel as the rest of the cavity preparation. If it is planned to use only cohesive gold foil, an ideal location for

a starting point, as well as additional retention, is the axial wall of the cavity preparation at the junction of the mesial and distal walls with the occlusal walls of each moustache extension (see comparable design for amalgam cavity preparation).

D. Partial moon (crescent) shape cavity preparation (Fig. 29)

Sometimes, due to the very apical location of the height of contour, or to the gingival inclination of the height of contour, or to the danger of the restoration affecting esthetics, the classical trapezoidal shape will be unacceptable, as it will be involving more than the indicated tooth structures in the cavity preparation. These situations demand a very curved gingival margin in continuation with the mesial and distal margins as if creating part of a circle. The occlusal margin in this modification should follow the height of contour so the general shape will look "semi-lunar."

1. Location of margins

In this modification the mesial, distal, and gingival margins should follow the curvature of the gingivae, and there will be

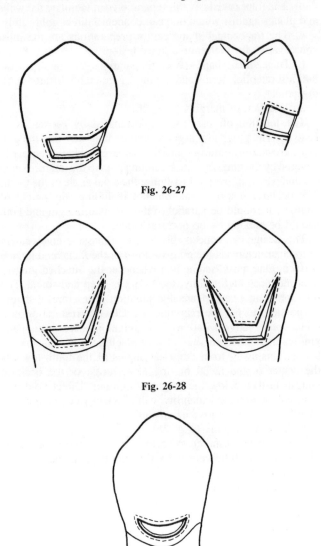

Fig. 26-27

Fig. 26-28

Fig. 26-29

no demarcation between those three margins. The occlusal or incisal margin should follow the curvature of the height of contour, but not include that height of contour. This type of cavity preparation is most frequently indicated in upper and lower cuspids and in upper first premolars. Usually, these preparations will have a very limited inciso- or occluso-gingival width, and if the gingival margins are located subgingivally, almost all of the restoration will be in the gingival sulcus.

2. Internal anatomy

The internal angulation of the walls of this design will be an exact replica of the first design, with the exception that there is no demarcation between the mesial-gingival and distal-gingival walls. However, there is a definite angle between the proximal and the incisal or occlusal walls.

If it is planned to use only cohesive gold foil for any of the previously described cavities, starting points are essential. These starting points should be at two opposing point angles. They should be as deep as 2 mm into dentin, in a direction trisecting those point angles (Fig. 26E). The position of these point angle starting points will determine the direction of the gold ties. For example, if the starting points are at the gingivo-axio-distal and gingivo-axio-mesial point angles, the gold tie proceeds from one point angle to another via the gingivo-axial line angle.

If, on the other hand, it is planned to build the restoration with precipitated gold, the line and point angles need not be as sharp; likewise, starting points are unnecessary (Fig. 26, I, J, and K).

Instrumentation for Class V cavity preparations for direct gold.

This is comparable to that used for amalgam, with the following modifications:

A. It is necessary, usually, to use smaller instruments.

B. A spear bur is created by sharpening the neck of ¼, ½, 33¼, or 33½ bur, much like sharpening a pencil, but making it triangular in cross-section. This is accomplished using a carborundum disc. The reverse bevel dentinal retention form will be primarily prepared with this spear bur by locating it at one involved point angle and dragging it, while revolving, along the line angle to the opposing involved point angle. To primarily prepare the starting points, the spear bur should penetrate the specified point angle, trisecting it with the bur revolving in slow speed. A pointed preparation into the dentin will result.

C. The angle former, or the pointed end of a gingival margin trimmer, can be used to sharpen the reverse bevel and starting points, as well as to connect these retentive starting features with each other and with the rest of the preparation.

IV. Class III Cavity Preparations for Direct Gold Restorations

There are three basic designs for Class III cavity preparations to accommodate direct gold materials. Each is subjected to a number of modifications according to access, esthetics, and remaining tooth structure.

A. The Ferrier design

This design is indicated if, after removal of all the diseased and undermined tooth structure, bulky labial, lingual, and in-

cisal walls remain. This will enable creation of two (three) planed labial and lingual walls and a pronounced boxed incisal retention form within a definite incisal wall. Furthermore, the Ferrier design is indicated if the labial extension of the lesion facilitates minimal extension of the cavity preparation labially. Because of these limitations, this design is more indicated for the distal proximal surfaces of anterior teeth than for the mesial proximal surfaces (less conspicuous). The choice of the Ferrier design is further facilitated if the periodontium and bone support around the tooth are adequate to allow slight separation for access. There is no doubt that preparing this design requires a skillful operator.

1. General shape (Fig. 30)

The Ferrier outline is triangular in shape, involving about two-thirds to one-half of the proximal surface.

2. Location of margins (Fig. 30)

Being a labial and lingual access cavity, the labial and lingual margins should be within the corresponding embrasures. Furthermore, these margins should have certain specifications for esthetic and other reasons:

a. Facially, the margin should be parallel to the calcification lobes.

b. The labial margin should be minimally extended in the labial embrasure, especially for mesial cavity preparations.

c. The labial margin should extend labially enough for the restoration to reflect light toward the adjacent proximal surface.

d. The lingual margin should not encroach on the marginal ridge. In fact, if the marginal ridge must be involved in the cavity preparation, the Ferrier design is contraindicated.

e. The gingival margin should be located ½ to 1 mm apical to the free healthy gingival, following a straight line labio-lingually.

f. The incisal margin will usually be in the contact area. However, if there is a very rounded incisal angle and a fairly pronounced incisal embrasure, this margin may be located within the incisal embrasure.

3. Internal anatomy (Figs. 30D and E)

a. In a labio-lingual cross-section, it can be seen that the axial wall is rounded, but not following the convexity of the proximal surface. The labial and lingual walls will each have

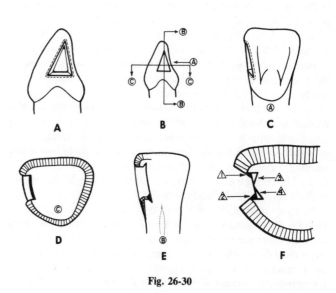

Fig. 26-30

either two or three planes (as in Class II cavity preparation). For example, if there are three planes, they are: an inner dentinal plane at right angle to the tangent of the axial wall; an outer enamel-dentinal plane following the direction of the enamel rods labio-proximally and linguo-proximally; and a peripheral, partial enamel bevel plane.

b. In the inciso-gingival cross-section, the incisal wall appears as in a Class V cavity preparation; i.e., formed of three or four planes. If the incisal margin is at the incisal one-third, there will be an inner dentinal plane, which is part of the boxed incisal retention form; next is a transition, formed completely of dentin; then an outer enamelo-dentinal plane following the direction of enamel rods (inclining inciso-proximally) and, finally, a partial enamel bevel plane. The three-plane arrangement will be as in Class V preparations, when the incisal margin is in the middle third (Fig. 30E). The axial wall will appear ranging from flat to slightly rounded (but less than the convexity of the proximal surface).

In the same cross-section, the gingival wall is formed of four planes: an inner reverse bevelled dentinal plane, a transitional plane, an outer enamel plane following the direction of the enamel rods (inclining gingivo-proximally) and a peripheral partial enamel bevel plane. The incisal retention form is "box-like" in shape, with definite walls directed incisolabio-axially starting at the incisal point angle. It penetrates dentin to a depth of 1.5 mm.

At the gingivo-labio-axial and the gingivo-linguo-axial point angles, there will be pyramidal retention forms with their base facing the cavity and their tip facing the dentin. They are directed gingivo-labio-axially and gingivo-linguo-axially, respectively.

c. All line and point angles should be sharp, with the exception of the junction between the line angles of the cavity preparation proper and those of the retention forms, which should have a rounded junctional relationship. The Ferrier design is mainly for cohesive gold foil, thus these angular line and point angles are essential. Special attention should be paid not to overextend the enamel bevels, especially labially, so as to decrease the conspicuousness of the gold.

4. Modifications for lower incisors

Because the lower incisors are so very delicate, the Ferrier design there should have the following modifications:

a. The labial extent of the cavity should be very limited because of the very wide and accessible labial embrasure.

b. The axial wall should be exceptionally flat because of the minimum convexity of the proximal surface and the relatively pronounced pulp chamber.

c. The lingual wall should be two-planed: one perpendicular enamelo-dentinal plane at 90° to the axial wall, and the other a partial enamel bevel. This prevents leaving undermined enamel resulting from the flatness of the lingual surface and the minimum convexity of the proximal surface.

d. The labial wall may have the same anatomy as the lingual wall, when the labial surface is flat.

5. Instrumentation for Ferrier design

With a ½ round bur, using lateral cutting strokes and axial pressure, remove tooth structure to the proper depth (.02 mm from the DEJ) within the specified outline. Then use the base of an inverted cone bur (33¼) with inciso-gingival strokes, to formulate the lingual wall; with labio-lingual strokes formu-

lating the gingival wall. The side of the same inverted cone bur can be used in inciso-gingival movements to formulate the labial wall. A Wedelstaedt chisel, in direct cutting strokes can be used to cut triangle #1 on the labial wall (Fig. 30F). Next use the linear cutting edge of an angle former in lateral cutting movements to remove triangle #2 on the lingual wall (Fig. 30F). Then, again using the linear cutting edge of an angle former in lateral cutting strokes, cut triangles #3 and 4, from the axial wall (Fig. 30F). A spear bur is used at the linguo-gingivo-axial point angle (directed lingually, gingivally, and axially) in slow revolution to drill almost 1 mm into dentin. Similarly, place the spear bur at the labio-gingivo-axial point angle and repeat the same step (directed labially, gingivally and axially). Finally, use the spear bur put at the incisal point angle (directed labially, incisally and axially) to drill about 1 mm into dentin creating incisal retention. It is now necessary to utilize the cutting edge of the angle former in lateral cutting strokes and, at the expense of the gingival wall along the gingivo-axial line angle, to connect the two gingival point retentions (on a shallower level) "funneling" the junctions between the point retentions and this line angle gingivally.

Also, in the same manner, accentuate the labio-axial and linguo-axial line angle, funneling their junction with the point retentions gingivally and incisally. A bi-bevelled hatchet may be used in direct cutting (shaving) strokes to box up the incisal retention form.

The linear cutting edge of the angle former, using lateral cutting strokes may be used to place the gingival short partial bevel. Then, a Wedelstaedt chisel is used on the labial and lingual cavosurface margins to place the same type of bevel there (Fig. 30).

B. The Loma-Linda design

This design is indicated for a combination of powdered gold build-up with a cohesive gold foil veneer. It is used when access to the lesion is lingual, as dictated by esthetics and the caries extent, or when the lingual marginal ridge is lost or undermined. When there is concern about esthetics, this cavity preparation may have its labial margin in the contact area.

1. General shape (Fig. 31A)

The proximal part of this cavity design will be triangular with rounded corners. The lingual part may have an incisal or gingival "turn" as dictated by access and resistance form (see Class III cavity preparation for amalgam).

2. Location of margins (Fig. 31)

Gingival margins of the Loma-Linda preparation are similar to the Ferrier design. Labial margins, in some situations, may be located in the contact area, making the restoration completely inconspicuous. However, the labial margin will usually have the same locations and specifications as in the Ferrier design. The lingual margin (Fig. 31C) will be located far enough onto the lingual surface to include the marginal ridge and to facilitate access to the internal parts of the cavity preparation.

3. Internal anatomy

a. Viewing an inciso-gingival cross-section (Fig. 31D) the Loma-Linda design appears to have the same anatomy as the incisal gingival section of the Ferrier design, except the line and point angles are more rounded. Also, the incisal internal retention mode appears bulkier than in the Ferrier design.

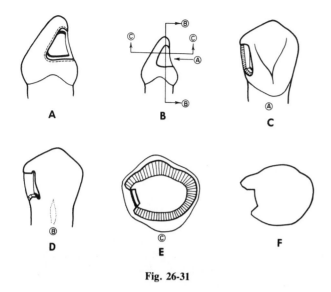

Fig. 26-31

b. In the labio-lingual cross-section (Fig. 31, E and F) if the labial margin is located in the contact area. The labial wall will be formed of two planes: an enamelo-dentinal plane at right angle to the axial wall following the directions of the enamel rods and a partial enamel bevel plane.

If the labial margin is located in the labial embrasure, the labial wall will have the same anatomy as in the Ferrier design. The lingual wall is much shorter than the labial wall. It will have two planes: one following the direction of the enamel rods, and the other being a partial enamel bevel.

c. The point angles gingivally accommodate two cylindrical retention grooves. They will be directed labio-gingivo-axially and linguo-gingivo-axially extending about 1.5-2 mm into the dentin. The incisal retention mode is directed inciso-labio-axial and is cylindrical in form. Whenever the labial margin is located in the contact area, there is no need to put a labio-gingivo-axial retention mode. The line and point angles and the junction between the different retention modes should be bulkier and more rounded than in the Ferrier design.

4. Instrumentation for Loma-Linda design

Using a ½ round bur from a lingual access, remove tooth structure within the contemplated outline at a minimal depth, using axial pressure and lateral dragging. Then, with the base of the 33½ bur, create a labial and a gingival wall from a lingual access using inciso-gingival and labio-lingual strokes respectively. Use the side of the 33½ to create a lingual wall placing the lingual margin on the lingual surface. Create a retention point 1 mm deep with a ¼ round bur directed labially, gingivally and axially at the gingivo-labio-axial point. Similarly, create retention gingivo-linguo-axial point angle by directing the drill gingivally, lingually and axially. Incisally, use the same round bur directed incisally, labially, and axially. With a Loma-Linda hatchet (or the linear cutting edge of an angle former) use inciso-gingival movements to create the different planes for the labial and lingual walls and to round out the axial wall (cut triangles as in Ferrier design).

With the pointed end of the angle former sharpen the gingivo-axial line angle, making it in the form of a groove at the expense of the gingival floor and merging it with the gingival point retentions. Similarly, accentuate the labio-axial and linguo-

axial line angles merging them with the gingival and incisal point retention. Use a bi-bevelled hatchet to box up the incisal retention. Finally, with the linear cutting edge of the angle former in lateral cutting strokes, or with a Weidelstaedt chisel in direct cutting strokes, go over the gingival and incisal margins to be sure that both walls are in two planes, are devoid of frail enamel, and, have a short partial enamel bevel.

C. The Ingraham design

This preparation design is indicated primarily for incipient proximal lesions in anterior teeth where esthetics is the main concern. After removal of diseased and undermined tooth structures, this preparation design will accommodate bulky gingival and incisal walls. Good oral hygiene and low caries and plaque indices are essential indications due to the outline of this design.

1. General shape (Fig. 32)

This preparation is a simple parallelogram in shape.

2. Location of margins

The labial margin of the Ingraham design will be in the contact area, so it is truly invisible labially. The gingival margin just clears the contact area in the gingival embrasure without any predetermined relationship to the gingiva. The incisal margin will be within the contact area. The lingual margin will be on the lingual surface past the marginal ridge, and/or axial angle of the tooth.

3. Internal anatomy

a. Viewing this preparation in an inciso-gingival cross-section (Fig. 32, D, E and F), at the very labial one-third of the cavity (Fig. 32F), the gingival wall will have three planes: an internal dentinal plane, part of a wall accommodating a triangular retention mode, and, inclining apically; an outer enamelo-dentinal plane following the direction of the enamel rods; and a peripheral partial enamel plane bevel. The axial wall will appear to be perfectly flat. The incisal wall will have the same anatomy as the gingival wall, but in the reversed direction.

A similar cross-section at the middle of the cavity preparation (Fig. 32E) will be the same anatomy, except that the internal dentinal planes incisally and gingivally create a less acute angle with the axial wall. Finally, an equivalent cross-section at the very lingual third of the cavity preparation (Fig. 32D) shows each of the incisal and gingival walls having two planes: one flat enamel-dentinal plane at right angle to a flat axial wall and a peripheral partial enamel bevel plane.

In other words, at the expense of each of the incisal and gingival walls there is a triangular area, the base of which is at the very labial end of the cavity preparation and the tip of the triangle is at the lingual one-third of the cavity preparation. The deepest part, then, will be located labially, and it decreases in depth proceeding lingually. Every effort should be made to confine those triangles to the gingival and incisal walls only so that they are not continuous with the proximal surface, as this will negate their retentive affects.

b. Viewing labio-lingual sections (Fig. 32 A and C), the axial wall appears perfectly flat, opening directly to the lingual surface and making a right angle with the labial wall.

The labial wall is formed of three planes: an inner dentinal plane at right angle to axial wall; an outer enamelo-dentinal plane following the direction of the enamel rods; and a marginal partial enamel bevel plane. Lingually, the axial wall will end

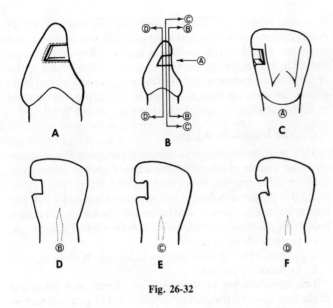

Fig. 26-32

with a partial bevel to protect the enamel on the lingual surface.

4. Instrumentation for Ingraham design

Using a 168 bur from a lingual access, apply axial and labial pressure inciso-gingivally to remove tooth structure within the planned outline. Then use an 8-9 hatchet in direct cutting strokes, to flatten the gingival and incisal walls. Utilize the hatchet in lateral cutting strokes, directed inciso-gingivally, to flatten the labial wall and to place it in the proper angulation.

With a spear bur placed at the inciso-labio-axial point angle, drag it lingually to cut at the expense of the incisal wall. Stop cutting at its middle section. This roughs-in the incisal retention mode. Similarly, place the spear bur in the gingivo-labio-axial point angle, cutting at the expense of the gingival walls to preliminarily establish the gingival retention.

The tip of a suitable size margin trimmer may be used to accentuate the incisal and gingival retention, formulating them into triangular areas. Also use the tip of the gingival margin trimmer to sharpen the labio-axial, the gingivo-axial and the inciso-axial line angles. With the side of the gingival margin trimmer, go over the labial and lingual margins in lateral strokes to be sure that there is no frail enamel rods, and to create the short partial bevel.

Schemes for Inserting Direct Gold into Cavity Preparations

Every design of a cavity preparation to accommodate direct gold materials has a specific step-by-step plan for the gold insertion. These plans are the actual application of the general principles previously mentioned in this chapter.

I. Procedure for Insertion, Finishing, and Polishing of Cohesive Gold Foil in a Simple Class I Cavity Preparation

Begin the restoration by wedging a small piece of gold foil between the three walls surrounding the D.B.P. point angle. Use a rounded hand condenser for this purpose. Hold this segment in place with a gold foil holder using disto-bucco-pulpal pressure. The operator should then pick up a small pellet of cohesive gold foil with a round condenser, pass it in the alcohol flame to clean it, and then insert it in the cavity so that it overlaps part of the originally wedged pellet. These are then cohered together and condensed using disto-pulpal-buccal pressure along the disto-pulpal line angle. With a third segment, the procedure is repeated, always condensing towards the same point angle. This process continues until two-thirds or more of the disto-pulpal line angle is covered with gold. Next, a piece of gold is chosen that will cover the rest of the disto-pulpal line angle. It is cleaned and cohered to the already condensed gold using disto-bucco-pulpal pressure; then the lingual portion is wedged into the disto-lingual pulpal point angle using disto-linguo-pulpal pressure. Condense the uncondensed portion (if any left), using disto-pulpal pressure. This should create a ''tie'' of gold from point angle to point angle. Remove the gold foil holder and test this tie for any looseness. If it is well held in place, proceed with building the restoration.

Bank half of distal and part of the buccal walls with gold using a larger round condenser (the direction of force will be disto-bucco-pulpal); then bank the other half of the distal and part of the lingual walls (the direction of force is disto-linguo-pulpal). At this point, make a tie along the bucco-pulpal line angle which terminates at a spear point angle or at the MBP point angle.

If the tie stops at the mesio-bucco-pulpal point angle, bank the rest of the buccal wall and half of the mesial wall, using mesio-bucco-pulpal forces. If the tie stops at a spear, bank the tied part of the buccal wall in disto-bucco-pulpal direction forces. Then tie the rest of the bucco-pulpal line angle to the mesio-bucco-pulpal point angle and proceed banking the rest of the buccal and a half of the mesial walls using mesio-bucco-pulpally directed forces. Then, make a mesial tie along the rest of the mesio-pulpal line angle. Bank the rest of the mesial and lingual (part of it) walls, using mesio-lingual pulpal condensation forces.

Usually, there will be a concavity at the center of the occlusal surface of gold. It may be filled using a foot condenser, directing forces towards each of the four corners separately. It is possible to rough-in occlusal anatomy in this step.

Pave the margins of the restoration with gold using the foot condenser, being sure that condensation forces bisect the corresponding line angles. Then, surface harden, using the foot condenser at a high frequency, again being sure to use forces which bisect the corresponding line angles.

Burnish from gold to tooth using small ball burnisher, and carve the occlusal anatomy, using a sharp cleoid carver in lateral cutting movements. Burnish again, accentuating grooves and fossae. Now marginate the restoration, using push and pull files. Then burnish once more. After removing the rubber dam and checking the occlusion, remove premature occluding areas using discoid cleoid carvers. Finally, give the restoration a slight shine, using tin oxide with a prophy cup.

To insert direct gold in Class I with lingual or facial extension, the scheme will be similar to that of Class II conventional design, including the use of the matrix. For Class I pit preparations it is similar to what has been described here, but on a smaller section.

II. Procedure for Matricing of Class II Conventional Design to Receive Combination of Powdered Gold and Cohesive Gold Foil

A piece of brass matrix band is cut so that it will cover the tooth surface 2 mm. buccal and lingual to the proximal limit of the preparation and about 3 mm more than the occluso-gingival length of the preparation. This section of matrix is then contoured, festooned, and adapted to the tooth proximally. A wedge (or two) is placed interproximally to adapt the band to the tooth surface apical to the gingival margin of the preparation. Care must be taken to avoid impinging on the gingival cavosurface bevel. A ball burnisher can be used on the inside of the cavity preparation to create the proper convexity in the band, i.e., coinciding with the proximal contour of the tooth. Autopolymerizing acrylic resin is then placed (a small bead at a time with a camel hair brush) over the wedges, filling the buccal and lingual embrasures as well as ½ the occlusal surface of the adjacent tooth.

While the acrylic is hardening, it is necessary to again burnish the band from the inside of the cavity, and to get the band away from the margins (especially the gingival margin) by using a beaver-tail burnisher. (This same technique can be modified to create a matrix for a Class I cavity preparation with lingual or facial extension.)

III. Procedure for Insertion, Finishing, and Polishing of Combination of Powdered Gold and Cohesive Gold Foil in a Class II Conventional Design

Begin the restoration by spearing a ball of goldent with a pointed fine instrument, passing it through the flame (until the created yellow flame is gone) and placing it over one of the proximal retention grooves. Then, process another ball, placing it along the gingivo-axial line angle. Continue this procedure until the whole line angle as well as the opposite proximal retention groove is covered.

With a Loma-Linda condenser, rupture the balls (most of them are ruptured by now) and seat the gold with gentle tapping, rolling motions. Then use the condenser heavily pressing gingivo-bucco-axially in a rocking action, on the powdered gold, making stepping if needed, until the buccal half of the gold is no longer yielding. With the other side of the same condenser repeat this procedure, but directing force gingivo-linguo-axially until the rest of the gold is also no longer yielding. Continue adding and condensing rows of gold balls until reaching the pulpal floor level. There should be a concavity within the gold, facing proximally occlusally. Line the line angles, occlusally, with balls of goldent and condense the same way, with forces directed to bisect the line angles.

It is necessary to remove any powdered gold from the occlusal and proximal margins before beginning to cohere cohesive foil to that already condensed into the preparation. Pick up a piece of cohesive gold foil, clean it in the alcohol flame, cohere it to the already condensed powdered gold at the occlusal bucco-proximal part, condense gingivo-axio-buccally and proceed gingivally until you bank the buccal wall proximally.

Repeat the same procedure starting at the occluso-linguo-proximal corner, banking the lingual wall proximally, using gingivo-axio-lingual forces. Addition of cohesive foil should continue, banking all buccal, proximal, and lingual walls occlusally. Next, pave the margins with gold using the foot condenser, and surface harden all conspicuous gold surface using the same instrument.

Slit the auto-polymerised resin from the occlusal and push the buccal, then the lingual, halves apart with the wedges, then remove the brass matrix band. Pave the buccal and lingual margins, with cohesive gold foil if it is apparent at this stage that they are not properly paved. The remaining steps in the procedure (e.g., burnishing, margination, carving, etc.) should follow the same basic pattern as described for Class I direct gold.

For proximal surfaces burnishing, use a Sparately burnisher, then file the margins occlusally, buccally and lingually, using push and pull files. If you have gross overhang gingivally, use Wilson's knives from the buccal and lingual embrasures to shave them off in small pieces. To marginate the gingival margins use the tip of the Sparately burnisher.

Follow this by burnishing all margins again. Longitudinally cut a sand paper strip (cuttle) to fit the gingival embrasure, tease it through and smooth the proximal gold, gingival to the contact area, in one-direction polishing actions. Then, burnish again. We can use the paper strips used previously and soaked in gold to polish the proximal portion. Upon attaining the appropriate surface finish, remove the dam and check occlusion. Remove prematurities using discoid cleoid. A final shine can be obtained with a tin oxide on a prophy cup.

IV. Procedure for Insertion, Finishing, and Polishing of a Combination of Mat Gold and Cohesive Gold Foil in a Class II Conservative Design

This restoration is started by cutting a piece of mat gold to match the size of the gingival floor of the cavity preparation, passing it in the flame until it becomes brick red in color and then inserting it in the cavity so that it fits the gingival floor with slight excess. A hatchet or a parallelogram condenser is used to seat the gold with light tapping pressure; then, using the same condenser, condense heavily in rocking motions towards the gingivo-bucco-axial, for the buccal half of the gold, then gingivo-linguo-axial for the lingual half of the gold, until the gold is unyielding, and there is a concavity facing proximo-occlusally. After the cavosurface margins are cleansed of any mat gold, the remainder of the restorative procedure follows much the same pattern as previously described for the conventional Class II restorations.

V. Procedure for Insertion, Finishing, and Polishing of a Combination of Mat Gold and Cohesive Gold Foil in a Class V Cavity

Cut a piece of mat gold in the same shape and dimension of the axial wall. Clean it and seat it on the axial wall, using a parallelogram condenser with a tapping action. Heavily condense the mat gold in a stepping and rocking motion, starting from the center towards the corners, with the direction of force trisecting the point angle towards which you are condensing until the gold is not yielding to applied pressure and exhibits a concavity in the center (or the axial wall is not covered at the center). Clear the cavosurface margins from mat gold, using an explorer. Then, pick up a piece of cohesive foil on the tip of a round condenser, clean and cohere it to the mat in the gingivo-distal corner. Then condense it completely in a stepping motion, using forces directed gingivo-disto-axially. Repeat this step several times until you bank half of the gingival and distal walls.

Perform the same procedure to bank the mesial half of the gingival wall and gingival half of the mesial wall, with the forces directed mesio-gingivo-axially. Again, perform the same procedure to bank the occlusal half of the distal wall and the distal half of the occlusal wall with forces directed disto-occluso-axially.

Proceed with the same procedure to bank the occlusal half of the mesial wall and the mesial half of the occlusal wall, with forces directed mesio-occluso-axially. At this point, you should now have a concavity in the center of the restoration with an extremely limited dimension. Fill it with cohesive gold foil in a stepping motion, with forces directed axially. Pave all margins with gold using the foot condenser in forces bisecting the corresponding line angles; then, surface harden the gold using a foot condenser, with high frequency, low intensity malleting. Burnish the gold from the gold to the tooth using the ball burnisher for the occlusal, mesial and distal margins, the beaver tail or Sparately burnisher for the gingival margins.

Contour the restoration using a sand paper disc (cuttle discs) after tapering the head of its screw and coating it with vaseline or petroleum jelly. During this procedure, be sure to keep the disc moving on the gold surface at all times, and be sure it is only lightly touching that surface. Burnish again and marginate the restoration using Stein's knife in lateral cutting strokes while it is partly on the gold and partly on the tooth, and push and pull files in movements from the gold to the tooth surface. Sometimes, we can use the side edges of a Sparately burnisher. This is to be followed by burnishing again.

At this stage you should see the trapezoid outline of the cavity as you originally prepared it. If not, marginate again until we see it. A lustre, if needed, is created with tin oxide and prophy cup. Remove the 212 cervical clamp, inspect the gingiva for any trauma and the tooth surface apical to the gingival margin for any gouging and for any overhang, if present, use a knife or file to shave it. Then burnish the margin again with a sparately burnisher. Apply tincture of iodine or merthiolate to the gingivae. Also, apply a fluoride solution on adjacent enamel.

VI. Procedure for Insertion, Finishing, and Polishing of Cohesive Gold Foil in a Class V Cavity Preparation

Take a piece of gold foil, clean it, then wedge it with a rounded hand condenser in the gingivo-disto-axial starting point. Hold it in place with a gold foil holder. Then, carry a gold pellet with a rounded condenser point in the automatic mallet, clean it, then cohere it to the piece of gold wedged in the starting point, then condense it in a stepping fashion with force directed toward the gingivo-disto-axial point angle. Repeat this several times until the tie covers two-thirds or more of the gingivo-axial line angles. Then, take a piece of gold foil that can cover the rest of the gingivo-axial line angle, cohere

to the already condensed gold, using gingivo-disto-axial pressure. Wedge it in the mesio-gingivo-axial starting point using mesio-gingivo-axial pressure, then condense any uncondensed portion (if left) in stepping motions gingivo-axially. Remove the holder and test the gingival tie with an explorer to see if it is held in place or not. Start cohering gold foil to the already condensed gold, then condence it in a stepping motion at the gingivo-distal corner using forces directed gingivo-disto-axially until you bank the gingival half of the distal wall and the distal half of the gingival wall. Repeat the same on the mesial-gingival corner using forces directed mesio-gingivo-axially until you bank the mesial half of the gingival wall and gingival half of the mesial wall.

Complete the mesial tie by stepping gold on the mesial-axial line angle using mesio-gingivo-axial pressure until you cover two-thirds or more of this line angle. Choose a piece of gold that will cover the rest of the line angle, cohere it to the already condensed gold, and wedge its occlusal end in the mesio-occluso-axial point angle.

Condense toward the mesio-occluso-axial point angle until you bank the occlusal half of the mesial wall and the mesial half of the occlusal wall. Sometimes you need to complete the distal tie, as you did on the mesial, except that the pressure is directed first disto-gingivo-axial, then you wedge toward the disto-occluso-axial point angle.

Bank the distal half of the occlusal wall and occlusal half of the distal wall using pressure directed disto-occluso-axially. You will have a concavity in the center of the restoration; fill it with cohesive gold foil in a stepping motion using forces directed axially. Then proceed with the same steps of paving, contouring, burnishing, finishing, and polishing as described for combinations of mat and cohesive gold foil.

The scheme for inserting direct gold in the other designs of Class V cavity preparation will be with minor modifications to the already mentioned schemes except for preparations with pan-handle extensions where using an S-shaped matrix, as in amalgam, but made of brass instead of stainless steel, is essential prior to insertion of precipitated gold.

VII. Procedure for Insertion, Finishing, and Polishing of Cohesive Gold Foil in Class III Ferrier Design Cavity Preparations

The restoration is begun by condensation of a piece of gold into the linguo-gingivo-axial retention point followed by stepwise condensation along the gingival-axial line angle while holding the original condensed piece in place. After 2/3 or more of the line angle is covered, a final segment is selected to cover the remainder of that line angle. After cohering it to the condensed gold (linguo-gingivo-axially), wedge it gingivo-labio-axially and condense its uncondensed portion (if present) gingivo-axially. You will have a complete gingival tie.

Test the tie retention with an explorer. If in place, bank the gingival wall and the gingival half of the lingual wall, by stepping gold towards the linguo-gingivo-axial corner, using forces in the same direction. After the gingival wall is banked, continue in the same pattern of stepping to shoulder between the lingual and labial walls, with the lingual wall being banked ahead of the labial wall. Any time you arrive at a cavosurface margin, pave the margin with gold, preferably using a foot condenser. *This is the only time it is possible to cover those margins with gold.* Hence forth, they will be inaccessible.

After two-thirds of the cavity is filled, complete the lingual tie (incisal turn) by cohering a piece of gold (that can cover the rest of the linguo-axial line angle) to the already condensed gold, wedging it in the incisal retention form (using inciso-labio-axial forces with a bayonet condenser). Then condense uncondensed portion of the tie using linguo-axial forces. The rest of the lingual wall and all the incisal wall are then banked preferably using the bayonet (round) condenser in inciso-labio-axial forces. Again, whenever you arrive at the margins, pave them with gold.

After banking the incisal wall, continuing in the same direction of stepping, there will be shouldering between a labial and a lingual wall. Continue it until the incisal third of the labial wall is banked. At this stage, a concavity will result in the restoration, facing labio-proximally. This should be filled with gold, using a foot condenser with force directed axially, striving for the proper contour (slight overcontouring) of the restoration. The remainder of the restorative procedure follows much the same pattern as previously described, for the proximal part of Class II restorations.

VIII. Procedure for Matricing for Class III Loma-Linda Cavity Preparation to Receive a Combination of Powdered Gold and Cohesive Gold

To matrice the Loma-Linda cavity, it is necessary to first tailor and place a wedge from the labial, gingival to the gingival margin of the preparation. Then, the softened tip of a stick of gutta-percha is inserted from the lingual into the cavity preparation, until excess appears through the labial. Using a warm carver. the gutta-percha should be contoured and marginated.

Acrylic resin (autopolymerizing) is then applied, using a brush-bead technique, over the labial surface of the operated and contacting teeth, not only filling the embrasure between them, but also covering the incisal edges and the incisal halves of their lingual surfaces. When the acrylic matrix is hardened, the gutta-percha is removed.

IX. Procedure for Insertion, Finishing, and Polishing of Powdered and Cohesive Gold Foil in a Class III Loma-Linda Design Cavity Preparation

Spear a ball of goldent, clean it, and insert it in the cavity over the inciso-labio-axial retention point. Put another cleaned ball along the labio-axial line angle, and so on, until you pave all the labio-axial line angles and cover the labio-gingivo-axial corner. Then, with a Loma-Linda condenser, seat the goldent balls on the walls with gentle tapping. With the same instrument heavily condense the incisal half of the gold inciso-labio-axially and the gingival half gingivo-labio-axially, in rocking stepping motions. Proceed in this fashion seating and condensing goldent balls, one-ball thickness at a time until you fill about three quarters of the cavity in a labio-lingual direction, banking the labial, incisal, and most of the gingival walls, covering the margins whenever you come to them. You will always have a concavity in the gold facing linguo-proximally. Follow this by

inserting a goldent ball or two in the gingivo-linguo-axial retention point and corner. Then condense them using linguo-gingival-axial pressure, filling the retention form and banking the rest of the gingival wall and covering the margin completely.

Fill the rest of the cavity with cohesive gold foil and carefully cover the lingual margin with cohesive foil, using inciso-labio-axial force (for incisal half) and linguo-gingivo-axial force (for the gingival half). Now burnish the gold lingually with a ball burnisher.

Split the matrix at the incisal ridge (chisel or small bur), then remove it together with the wedge. Then, heavily burnish and surface harden the gold labially and lingually using a round burnisher (you may use burnishing burs). Use a sparately burnisher gingivally and incisally. The rest of the procedure is very similar to that used for the proximal part of Class II restorations.

X. Procedure for Insertion, Finishing, and Polishing of Mat and Cohesive Gold Foil in Class III Ingraham Design Cavity Preparation

Cut a piece of mat gold to coincide with the shape and dimension of the labial wall of the cavity preparation. Clean it and apply it on the labial wall. Using a parallelogram or hatchet condenser, seat the gold on the labial wall with light tapping. With the same hand condenser, heavily condense the gold in rocking motions in the incisal half inciso-labio-axially and in the gingival half gingivo-labio-axially, until the gold is unyielding. This creates a continuous labial tie and a concavity in the gold facing linguo-proximally. Clear the labial, incisal, and gingival margins from mat gold. Then, carry a piece of cohesive gold foil on the tip of a round condenser point, clean it, and cohere it to the gold in the inciso-labial corner and condense it in a stepping motion inciso-labio-axially. Repeat this step but cohere the gold pellets to the gold in a gingivo-labial corner, step condensing it gingivo-labio-axially. Repeat these last two steps simultaneously until you bank all the labial wall and most of the incisal and gingival walls. However, whenever you come to a margin, pave it completely with cohesive foil. It is the only time you can get proper access to these margins for condensation. At this stage, you will have a concavity in the gold facing linguo-proximally, so fill it using inciso-axial and gingivo-axial pressure with a foot condenser.

Pave the lingual margin with gold using axio-labial pressure, and the incisal and gingival corners of the restoration using inciso-axial and gingivo-axial pressure. Follow this with surface hardening, burnishing, marginating, finishing, and polishing in the same way as described for the proximal part of Class II restorations.

BIBLIOGRAPHY

Black, G.V.: A work on operative dentistry. Chicago, Medico-Dental Pub. Co., 1917.

Gilmore, et al.: Operative Dentistry. St. Louis, The C.V. Mosby Co., 1977.

Hemphill, W.F.: The use of mat gold. J. Am. Acad. Gold Foil Operators **2**:75, 1959.

Hodson, J.T.: Compaction properties of various gold restorative materials. J. Am. Acad. Gold Foil Op. **12**:52, 1969.

Hodson, J.T.: Microstructure of gold foil and mat gold, Dent. Prog. **2**:55, 1961.

Hodson, J.T., and Stibbs, G.D.: Structural density of compacted gold foil and mat gold. J. Dent. Res. **41**:339, 1962.

Hodson, J.T.: Structure and properties of gold foil and mat gold. J. Dent. Res. **43**:575, 1963.

Hollenback, G.M., and Collard, E.W.: An evaluation of the physical properties of cohesive gold. J. So. Calif. Dent. Assoc. **29**:280, 1961.

Ingraham, R., and Koser, J.: An atlas of gold foil and rubber dam procedures. Seventh ed. Los Angeles, Section on operative dentistry, Univ. of So. Calif. School of Dentistry, 1980.

Iwaku, M., Nagata, N., Hosoda, H., and Fusayama, T.: Edge strength of powdered gold fillings. J. Dent. Res. **45**:1468, 1966.

Koser, J.R., and Ingraham, R.: Mat gold foil with a veneer cohesive foil surface for Class V restorations. J. Am. Dent. Assoc. **52**:714, 1956.

Kramer, W.S., Trandall, T.R., and Diefendorf, W.L.: A comparative study of the physical properties of variously manipulated gold foil materials. J. Am. Acad. Gold Foil Operators **3**:8, 1960.

Lund, M.R., and Baum, L.: Powdered gold as a restorative material. J. Prosth. Dent. **13**:1151, 1963.

Lund, M.R., and Baum, L.: Powdered gold for the Class III restoration. J. So. Calif. Dental Assoc. **33**:262, 1965.

McGee, Inskipp and True: A textbook in operative dentistry. New York, McGraw-Hill Book Co., 1956.

Miller, C.H.: Condensing gold foil. J. Am. Acad. Gold Foil Operators **9**:6, 1966.

Richter, W.A., and Mahler, D.B.: Physical properties vs. clinical performance of pure gold restorations. J. Prosth. Dent. **29**:434, 1973.

Rose, T.K.: On the annealing gold. J. Inst. Metals **10**:150-174, 1913.

Rule, R.W.: Gold foil and platinum centered gold foil: methods of condensation. JADA **24**:1783, 1937.

Shell, J.S., and Hollenback, G.M.: Tensile strength and elongation of pure gold. So. Calif. Dent. Assoc. J. **34**:219, 1966.

Stebner, C.M.: Correlation of physical properties and clinical aspects of gold foil as a restorative material. Dent. Clin. North Am. Nov. 1955, p. 571.

Stronsnider, C.W.: Comparison of specific gravities and hardness of cohesive gold foil malleted with various types of condensors. J. Dent. Res. **24**:61, 1945.

Sturdevant, C., et al.: The art and science of operative dentistry. New York, McGraw-Hill Book Co., 1970.

Taylor, J.B., Stowell, E.C., Murphy, J.F., and Wainwright, W.W.: Microleakage of gold foil fillings. J. Dent. Res. **38**:749, 1959.

Thomas, J.J., Stanley, H.R., and Gilmore, H.W.: Effect of gold foil condensation on human dental pulp. J. Am. Dent. Assn. **78**:788-794, 1969.

Wolcott, R.B., and Vernetti, J.P.: Sintered gold alloy for direct restorations. J. Prosth. Dent. **25**:662, 1971.

Xhonga, F.A.: Direct gold alloys, II. J. Am. Acad. Gold Foil Op. **14**:5, 1971.

Xhonga, F.A.: Direct golds. I. J. Am. Acad. Gold Foil Op. **13**:17, 1970.

CHAPTER 27

Non-carious destruction and disfigurement of teeth

Although decay is the usual cause of tooth destruction necessitating operative procedures, it has been estimated that 25% of tooth destruction does not originate from a caries process. The following are the possible non-caries destructive processes:

 I. Attrition
 II. Abrasion
 III. Erosion
 IV. Localized Non-Hereditary Enamel Hypoplasia
 V. Localized Non-Hereditary Enamel Hypocalcification
 VI. Localized Non-Hereditary Dentin Hypoplasia
 VII. Localized Non-Hereditary Dentin Hypocalcification
 VIII. Discolorations
 IX. Malformation
 X. Amelogenesis imperfecta
 XI. Dentinogenesis imperfecta
 XII. Trauma.

I. Attrition (Fig. 1, A-E)

Attrition may be defined as surface tooth structure loss resulting from direct frictional forces between contacting teeth. Attrition is a continuous, age-dependent process, which is usually physiologic. Any contacting tooth surface is subjected to the attrition process, beginning from the time it erupts in the mouth and makes contact with a reciprocating tooth surface. Attrition affects occluding surfaces and results in flattening of their inclined planes and in facet formation. In severe cases, ''a reverse cusp'' situation might be created in place of the cusp tips and inclined planes. Attrition also affects proximal contact areas, leading to flat, faceted proximal contours, and, in some situations, concave proximal surfaces.

Attrition is accelerated by parafunctional mandibular movements, noticeably bruxism. Although every person has some signs and symptoms of attrition in their dentition, attrition can predispose to or precipitate any of the following:

A. Proximal surface attrition (proximal surface faceting)

This results from surface tooth structure loss and flattening-widening of the proximal contact areas. Because of this process, the surface area proximally, which is susceptible to decay, is increased in dimension. At the same time, cleansability will be hindered due to the decrease in dimensions of the surrounding embrasures. Also, the mesio-distal dimensions of the teeth are decreased, leading to drifting, with the possibility that occluding tooth elements will not be physiologically indicated.

This mesio-distal reduction of teeth dimensions will lead to overall reduction of the dental arch length, with all its sequelae. Finally, due to the above-mentioned situations, the interproximal space will be decreased in dimensions, thereby interfering with the physiology of the interdental papillae. This is coupled with the difficulty of plaque control there, can lead to periodontitis.

B. Occluding surface attrition (occlusal wear)
(Figs. 1A and D, and 2A)

This is the loss, flattening, faceting, and/or reverse cusping of occluding elements. This process can lead to loss of the vertical dimension of the tooth. If the wear is severe, generalized, and accomplished in a relatively short time, there would be no chance for the alveolar bone to erupt occlusally to compensate for the occlusal tooth loss. In this case, the vertical loss might be imparted on the face as a loss of vertical dimension. Both situations will result in overclosure during mandibular functional movements. This situation can strain areas in the stomato-gnathic system not otherwise capable of withstanding these stresses.

On the other hand, if the loss occurs over a long period of time (ten years and more), the alveolar bone can grow occlusally, bringing the teeth to their original occlusal termination. In other words, the vertical dimension loss will be confined to the teeth but not imparted to the face.

Deficient masticatory capabilities of the teeth can also result from occlusal wear. Blunting (flattening) of the cusps will compel the patient to apply more force on the teeth in an attempt to shear food items into swallowable dimensions. These forces can non-elastically strain the muscles, the teeth (leading to more attrition), the periodontium and the joints.

Cheek biting (cotton roll cheeks) is another sequela of occluding surface attrition. With the flattening of cuspal elements through the attrition process, the vertical overlap between the working inclined planes will be lost. This will cause surrounding cheek, lip, or tongue tissues to be fed between the teeth, with a possibility of their being crushed and contused during dynamic tooth contact. Gingival irritation can also occur, due to food impaction and the closeness of the occlusal table to the gingiva.

Decay, as a result of the attrition of the enamel at occluding areas, can occur, because the underlying dentin will be exposed and thereby become more susceptible to decay. This susceptibility is decreased, to some extent, by the high cleansability

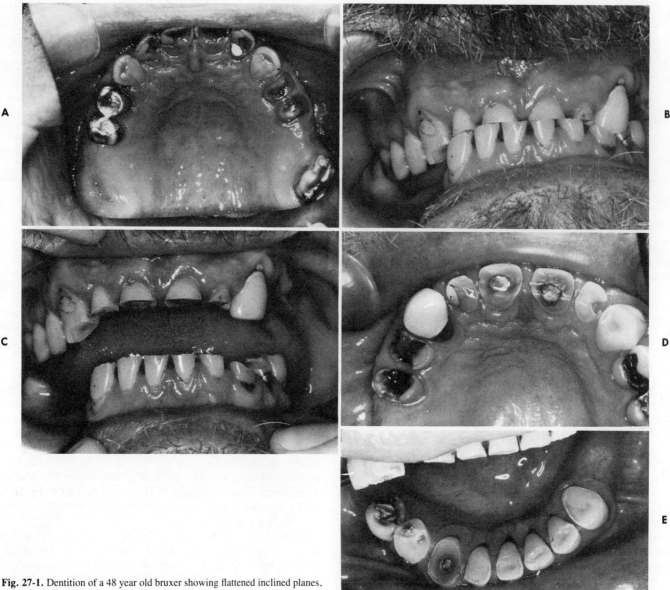

Fig. 27-1. Dentition of a 48 year old bruxer showing flattened inclined planes, reverse cusping, and reverse overlapping. Teeth #8, 9 and 27 are pulpally involved. Tooth #4 is vertically fractured.

of the occluding areas (more frictional movements). However, when the attrition creates "reverse" inclined planes or "reverse" cusps, the decay susceptibility will increase.

Tooth sensitivity is a symptom that can be due to many factors precipitated by the attrition process, e.g., dentin exposure, pulpal and apical strangulation due to excessive nonphysiologic forces, tearing of the periodontal ligaments resulting from the same forces, microcracks (crazings) and stagnation of irritating substrates on the created flat or concave areas of dentin.

Usually, the occluding surface will not undergo symmetrical attrition on both sides of the dental arch, or on opposing arches. As a result, unworn occluding areas will act as interfering (deflecting) points for physiologic mandibular movements (Fig. 2B). TMJ problems can be elicited by one or all of the aforementioned factors, especially the overclosure situation.

This condition will overstretch the joint ligaments. Similarly, stomato-gnathic system musculature problems can be expected as a result of one or more of the aforementioned factors. After severe occluding surface attrition, a predominantly horizontal masticatory movement of the mandible occurs. This type of movement is due to the flat-planed occluding surfaces. To effect some sort of shearing action between opposing teeth, the mandible must be moved farther horizontally, so that the flat-planed teeth can deliver a shearing load on the intervening bolus of food. This horizontal movement can cause extreme strain of the muscles of the stomato-gnathic system.

Treatment Modalities

It should be obvious, from the previous discussion, that attrition can occur in degrees, from involvement of only one

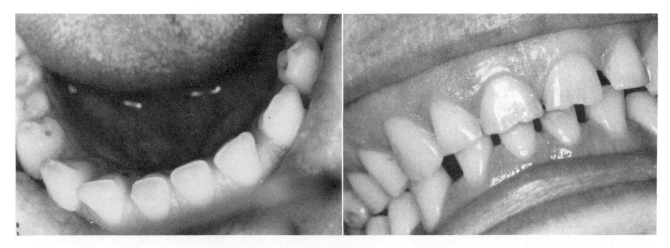

Fig. 27-2

inclined plane to involvement of all occluding surfaces, and from fractional tooth loss to loss of the whole crown portion of the tooth. Sometimes, surface attrition is slower than, and compensated by, intrapulpal deposition of secondary and tertiary dentin. At other times, the attrition is faster than the intrapulpal dentin deposition, leading to direct pulp exposures. In many situations, the pulp-root canal tissues undergo irreversible pathologic changes long before they are perforated (due to cracks and strangulation).

Therefore, treatment must involve several modalities, which should be chosen and initiated in the following sequence:

1. Pulpally involved teeth should be extracted, or undergo endodontic therapy, according to their restorability and future role in the stomato-gnathic system.

2. Parafunctional activities, notably bruxism, should be controlled with the proper discluding-protecting occlusal splints.

3. Myofunctional, TMJ, or any other symptoms in the stomato-gnathic system should be diagnosed and resolved. Sometimes, simply modifying the discluding occlusal splint used in (2) can be the treatment modality resolving both situations.

4. Occlusal equilibration should be performed after all notable symptoms are relieved. Occlusal equilibration might be the only treatment needed, if lost tooth structure is minimal and if remaining structure can be reshaped to effect physiologic, mandibular movements. Occlusal equilibration, by selective grinding of tooth surfaces, should include rounding and smoothing the peripheries of the occlusal tables. Also, one should create adequate overlap between the working inclines. Both features are essential to prevent further cheek biting.

5. During the last three procedures, exposed sensitive dentinal areas should be protected and actual carious lesions should be obliterated. Protection can be accomplished using fluoride solution. The obliteration is achieved by a proper temporary restoration. Also, during the same procedures, the periodontium should be examined and any pathology should be treated.

Fortunately, with extreme loss of clinical crown and vertical dimension, the crown:root ratio becomes very favorable, enhancing the health of the periodontium (except when the sub-

stantial occluding forces are applied horizontally and/or on the completely flattened inclined planes).

6. Restorative modalities can now be initiated. Lost tooth structure due to attrition is at high stress concentration areas. Therefore, only metallic (metallic-based) restorations should be used to replace them. Restorations are only needed in the following situations:

a. Noticeable loss of vertical dimension that has not been compensated for, and that should be regained to effect a physiologic status in the stomato-gnathic system.

b. There is extensive loss of tooth structure in a localized or generalized fashion, necessitating restoring the tooth (teeth) to form and function.

c. Reshaping remaining tooth structures would not, in and of itself, be conducive to occluding inclined planes working in harmony in creating a physiologic mandibular movement.

d. Decay or any other cavitating lesion is superimposed on the attrition reduction of a tooth surface.

e. Worn tooth contour (usually proximally) is not conducive to proper maintenance of the periodontium.

f. A tooth is cracked or endodontically treated.

The most involved restorative modalities are those used to regain lost vertical dimension. They should be accomplished very cautiously and carefully in the following sequence.

Verify and reverify its necessity, i.e., be sure that the alveolar bone did not grow occlusally at the same pace that attrition occurred, because, if the alveolar bone did grow occlusally, bringing the occlusally worn teeth to their customary occlusal location, any building-up restoration could impinge on the freeway space, eliciting and/or aggravating bruxism or other parafunctional habits.

Estimate how much vertical dimension was lost. Arriving at this estimate is a matter of clinical judgment guided by determining the indicated vertical dimension for the patient in the same way it is determined for a full denture construction (from the nasion to the gnathion), and by measuring the vertical dimension, when the patient brings the teeth together. The difference between these two measurements minus the customary measurements for the free-way space (2-3 mm) can give us an estimate of how much we should increase the height of the worn clinical crowns.

Estimate how much additional vertical dimension the stomato-gnathic system can accommodate without untoward effects. It is a well established fact that not all the lost dimension can be tolerated by the stomato-gnathic system, especially if attrition has occurred over a long period (more than 15 years), because there is a certain permanent physiologic accommodation which should not be disturbed. Therefore, if a substantial increase in vertical is planned (more than 2 mm), it is a wise idea to build a temporary restoration or a removable occlusal splint, that can be easily adjusted through subsequent addition or removal of material. Composite (resinous) temporary restorations are most frequently used. They may be retained by etched enamel or extracoronally prepared teeth. With these temporary restorations, establish the minimum increase in vertical at the beginning, periodically adding to it. However, before any addition, the entire stomato-gnathic system should be examined to verify that it is tolerating the previous vertical dimension and is ready for an increase. This process is continued until symptoms of intolerance are observed. At that point, it is necessary to minimally reduce vertical, until these symptoms disappear. The vertical dimension thereby created is the one to which permanent restorations should be built.

The permanent restoration should be done in a cast alloy (cast alloy based) material. A fully adjustable articulator, hinge axis determination, and use of pantographic (stereographic) tracing and facebow records are essential for such cases. These restorations should be cemented only temporarily for an extended period of time, until it is established that no untoward symptomatology will occur.

It should be mentioned here that cases necessitating this treatment modality are rather rare, and all the teeth are usually involved. Patients restored in this way should undergo periodic occlusal equilibration for these restorations after cementation, and they should be warned about possible separation between the teeth as a result of encroaching on the free-way space together with the bruxing nature of these dentitions.

In most situations, no vertical dimension increase is needed. Restorations may still be needed for the other indications, mentioned, and in these cases it is preferable to use cast alloy (cast alloy based) restorations to preserve the remaining tooth structure and to assure the integrity of the supporting tissues.

Because of the short crowns in these cases, it may be necessary to use intraradicular retention means, with or without devitalizing the teeth. Also, extracoronal retention may be the one of choice here to affect the change in the contour and occluding surfaces, in addition to attaining sufficient retention. Splinting of these worn teeth via a cast restoration may be indicated in these situations to increase the resistance-retention forms and also to minimize displacement of teeth after restorations with increased vertical dimension are built.

In cases with a carious lesion or defects superimposed on attrition facets, if the dimension of the lesion is very limited (as usual) and there is sufficient tooth structure around it to accommodate walls, amalgam or direct gold can be used to restore them. If no walls can be created, a cast alloy restoration has to be used. Again, most cases will only need occlusal equilibration and non-restorative protective measures for the exposed dentin.

II. Abrasion (Fig. 3)

Abrasion can be defined as the surface loss of tooth structure resulting from direct friction forces between the teeth and external objects, or from frictional forces between contacting teeth components in the presence of an abrasive medium.

Abrasion is a pathologic process which is usually inseparable from attrition and/or erosion. Although abrasion, like attrition, can stimulate the formation of dentin intrapulpally, causing recession of the pulp and root canal tissues away from the advancing lesion's pulpal limit, sometimes the abrasion rate is faster than the dentin deposition rate. The result is direct or indirect pulpal involvement. Also, many abrasion lesions are close to the gingiva, so plaque control measures can be hindered by abrasion in these areas.

The most predominant abrasion is toothbrush abrasion, occurring cervically, usually to the most facially prominent teeth in the arch (canines and bicuspids). It is usually on the left side for right-handed individuals and vice versa for left-handed people. It progresses very quickly, when the gingiva recedes, exposing root cementum and dentin facially. Tooth brush abrasion's surface extent, depth, and rate of formation is dictated by:

A. The direction of brushing strokes. Horizontal directions are the most detrimental.

B. The size of the abrasive. The larger and more irregular that the abrasive particles are, the more abrasion there will be.

C. The percentage of abrasives in the dentifrice. The higher that the percentage is, the more abrasion there will be.

D. The type of abrasive, e.g., silica abrasives are much more abrading than phosphate and carbonate ones.

E. The diameter of brush bristles. The greater that this diameter is, the more abrasion there will be.

F. The type of bristles. Natural bristles are more abrasive than synthetic (mylar) ones.

G. The forces used in brushing. Of course, the more that force is used, especially in the horizontal direction, the more abrasion there will be.

H. The type of tooth tissues being abraded. The most resistant tissues to abrasion are enamel, especially occlusally. The least resistant is cementum. Dentin, especially cervically, can be very easily abraded.

The clinical signs and symptoms of toothbrush abrasion are very characteristic:

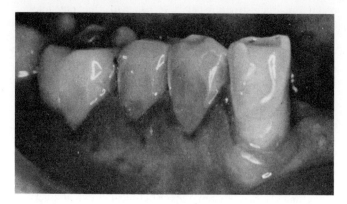

Fig. 27-3

1. The abrasive lesion may be linear in outline, following the path of the brush bristles.

2. The peripheries of the lesion are very angularly demarcated from the adjacent tooth surface.

3. The surface of the lesion is extremely smooth and polished, and it seldom has any plaque accumulation or carious activity in it.

4. The surrounding walls of the abrasive lesion tend to make a V-shape, by meeting at an acute angle axially.

5. Probing or stimulating (hot, cold, or sweets) the lesion can elicit pain.

Knowing the pathogenesis of abrasion, one can understand that toothbrush abrasion is one of many forms of tooth abrasion, e.g., pipe smoking "depression abrasion", which is an abraded depression on the occluding surfaces of teeth at a latero-anterior portion of the arch coinciding with the intraoral location of the pipe stem, results from intrusion and abrasion of the tooth there.

Many other oral habits can create some sort of abrasion, such as chewing tobacco, which can create a generalized occluding surface abrasion. Forcing a toothpick, interdental stimulator, or other solid plaque control modes interproximally can create different forms of proximal abrasion. Certain professional habits, such as cutting sewing thread with incisor teeth, holding and pulling nails with front teeth, or abrasives in the working environment itself, can each create a specific localized or generalized form of abrasion. Pica-syndrome, which is due to the habit of chewing clay (mud), has a specific occlusal abrasion pattern, and other systemic disorders.

There are some iatrogenic tooth abrasions, such as dentures with porcelain teeth opposing natural teeth, or using cast alloys having an extremely higher abrasive resistance than tooth enamel in a restoration opposing natural teeth, or extremely rough occluding surfaces of a restoration enhancing its abrading capability. This latter situation can create abrasion, even if the restorative material is less abrasive resistant than the tooth. Abrasions caused by these iatrogenic factors can be even more destructive if the restoration has occlusal interferences built into it.

Treatment Modalities

After confirming the diagnosis, treatment of abrasion should be pursued in the following sequence:

1. Diagnose the cause of the presented abrasion. There is no use in treating and restoring the teeth if the cause of the abrasion is still in action; otherwise the restoration will be abraded, opposing natural teeth could be abraded, the teeth could move, or the alveolar bone might be resorbed.

2. Knowing the causative factors first correct or replace the iatrogenic dental work. Second try to prevent the patient from practicing the causative habits. If successful in this persuasion, proceed with the restorative treatment as planned (6).

3. If the habit (practice) cannot be broken, restorative treatment can by-pass the effect of the habit. In other words, if it is localized and not interfering with the physiologic function of the stomato-gnathic system, endangering the P-D organ, and—or the periodontium, (e.g., pipe smoking anterolateral

concavities or other localized forms of abrasion) it may be included in the restoration.

The objective of the restoration should be to prevent further destruction of the tooth. Any attempt to restore the tooth to its ideal shape will concentrate intolerable forces (especially abrading ones) on the restoration, with unpredictable and often unfavorable results. If the abrasion is generalized and substantial, the habit (environment) should be discontinued (controlled) by any possible means, because the restorative treatment will involve restoring the teeth to normal configurations in order to establish a functional environment for the stomatognathic system.

4. Abrasive lesions at non-occluding tooth surfaces should be critically evaluated for the need for restoring them. If the lesions are multiple, shallow (not exceeding 0.5 mm in dentin) and wide, there is no need to restore them. If they involve cementum or enamel only, there is no need to restore them.

If a restoration is not indicated for the lesion, the edges of the defect should be eradicated to a smooth, non-demarcating pattern relative to adjacent tooth surface. This is done for esthetic and plaque control reasons. The tooth surface then should be treated with fluoride solution to improve its caries resistance. However, if the lesion is wedge (v)-shaped and exceeds 0.5 mm into dentin, it should be restored.

5. If the involved teeth are extremely sensitive, it is preferable to desensitize exposed dentin before restorative treatment is started. This may take several visits. As in many situations, if the sensitive teeth are restored immediately, they will remain sensitive to thermal changes forever. Desensitization can be accomplished by fluoride solution application (8-30% sodium or stanneous fluorides for 4 to 8 minutes), or ionophoresis using an electrolyte containing fluoride ions (galvanic energy supplied to the tooth in the presence of the electrolyte drives the fluoride ions deep into the dentin).

6. Restorative treatment

If the abrasive lesion involves an anterior tooth or facially conspicuous area of a posterior tooth, at a non-occluding tooth surface, the restoration can be done in one of the direct tooth-colored materials (Fig. 6). In most cases no cavity preparation is needed, if any of the physico-chemically adhering direct tooth-colored materials is used. (Different designs of tooth preparations to suit these situations were described in detail in the chapter on direct tooth-colored restorations.)

Similar lesions which involve a non-conspicuous area in a posterior tooth, should be restored with a metallic restoration. If the cavity preparation to accommodate it will impinge on the pulp and root canal system, the situation can make the tooth sensitive forever or compromise the P-D organ vitality. In this case, one should use one of the physico-chemically adhering direct tooth-colored materials. Although the latter may not be very durable in posterior teeth, their frequent replacement will be a safer treatment modality than encountering the dangers stemming from a cavity preparation and a metallic restoration there. The restorative treatment may then proceed in the same fashion as detailed for treatment of attrition lesions.

III. Erosion (Fig. 4 and 5)

Erosion can be defined as the loss of tooth structure resulting from chemico-mechanical acts in the absence of specific mi-

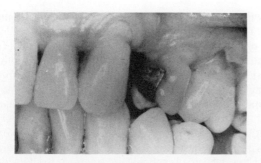

Fig. 27-4

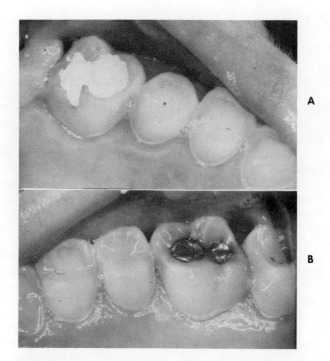

Fig. 27-5. Erosion of the lingual surface of upper premolars and molars as a result of forced regurgitation. (BULIMIA)

croorganisms. Erosion is one of the most predominant oral pathologic changes; in one investigation it was estimated that 18% of the adult population exhibits erosive lesions.

Until now there is no convincing etiology for erosion. It seems that, like decay, it is caused by multiple factors. As expected, many authorities theorize causes and pathogenesis for erosion, but none can explain the process fully. Of these theories the following are most popular:

A. Ingested acid

Ingested acid, with emphasis on citric acid (lemon and citrus fruits), especially if used in large amounts, can participate in or initiate the erosive lesion. Also, other acids, as found in certain beverages and mouth fresheners (deodorizers) can contribute to the erosive process.

B. Salivary citrates

Some authorities have found a correlation between the number and dimensions of erosive lesions and salivary citrates. Others have disproved this correlation.

C. Secreted acids

Acids exist in the gingival crevice, due to the occlusal traumatism (bruxism, interferences, or excessive discluding forces). This acidity of the crevicular fluid has been correlated to both occlusal traumatism and to cervical erosion. Although this acidity cannot be fully responsible for an erosive lesion, it can be a participating factor.

D. Mechanical abrasion

As described in ''Abrasion'', although abrasion cannot explain the characteristic nature of erosive lesions, it can be a contributing factor.

E. Chelating microbial metabolic products

The most prominent product that has been correlated to the erosion processes is pyrophosphate, and although the correlation is not conclusive, it could be one of the contributing factors.

F. Acid fumes

Environmental acid fumes has been statistically correlated to the number of erosive lesions in certain populations.

G. Excessive tensile stresses at the tooth clinical cervix; (Fig. 4.)

Non-elastically deforming tooth contacts, which could be premature or heavy centric, immense working, or balancing, may precipitate intolerable tensile stresses at the tooth cervix, especially facially. The brittle enamel veneer being thin and terminal at this area, could have it's prisms separated from each other, and from underlying dentin. Subsequently it could, be peeled off, or acquire cracks through which acids penetrate and attack. Both lead to the characteristic wedge shape of some erosive lesions.

H. Refused acids

As a result of chronic, frequent regurgitation (forced or nonforced), the stomach's hydrochloric acid can hit the teeth at specific locations, creating a very characteristic type of erosion (lingual surface of the upper teeth, especially molars and premolars (Fig. 5A and B).

I. Salivary flow

The pattern of the salivary flow, as related to intraoral frictional contact between the moving soft tissues and tooth components, is a very interesting and unusual approach to explaining the pathogenesis of erosive lesions.

There have been many attempts to morphologically and therapeutically classify erosive lesions, but none is able to encompass all reported varieties. The erosive lesions are pathognomonic in the following aspects:

1. There is no demarcation between the lesion and the adjacent tooth surface, i.e., an explorer can be passed without any interruption from the lesion to the tooth surface.

2. The lesion surface is glazed.

3. Erosion usually does not affect occluding surfaces, except in very advanced situations, and then only indirectly.

4. The erosion rate is the same for enamel, dentin, and cementum, and, sometimes, for restorative material.

5. The P-D organ reacts by both healthy and unhealthy reparative reactions to the stimulation of the erosive lesion.

6. Adjacent gingiva and periodontium are almost always sound and healthy.

7. Tooth sensitivity to physical, chemical, and mechanical stimuli is always evident and the main complaint of the patient.

8. Carious lesions do not usually occur at tooth surfaces attacked by erosion.

Erosion usually affects people with good oral hygiene. However, it has been reported in patients with a high plaque index. The rate of erosion in active lesions was estimated to be 1 micron per day. Therefore, perforation to the pulp chamber or root canal is very rare with erosive lesions, as the stimulated secondary and tertiary dentin is usually produced at a faster rate than that (1.5-4 micron/day). Erosion affects upper teeth more than lower teeth, especially attacking the facial of cuspids and premolars. The lower anterior teeth facially are a common location for erosion.

Topographically, the extent of teeth involvement with erosive lesions can range from a fine unnoticeable line at the cemento-enamel junction to substantial tooth-substance loss making an hour-glass shape out of a tooth. It should be mentioned that attrition, abrasion, and erosion may work together in creating lesions in teeth, and when all three of these processes are combined, the destruction can be detrimental and rapid.

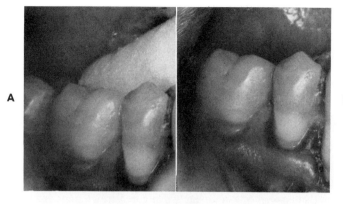

A B

Fig. 27-6

Treatment Modalities

Although the exact cause for erosion is not known, complete analysis of diet, occlusion, habits, chronic vomiting and environmental factors should be performed for patients exhibiting these lesions. Every attempt should be made to correlate the presence of the lesions to possible causes.

After this initial correlation, try to eliminate the causes. The patient should be informed that this *may* not be the cause, but it is the most probable one. He should be told that the treatment to be pursued is mainly symptomatic, and that corrective therapy will, by no means, stop the disease. He should also be told that the process could recur, not only affecting tooth structures, but the restorative material, as well.

Preoperative study models or photographs should be taken and kept for future reference. This is to evaluate the progress of the lesion, if no restoration is the treatment modality, and to see the extent of recurrence, if a restoration is the treatment modality.

There should not be any rush to attempt restorative modalities, except in extremely symptomatic or disfiguring lesions (Fig. 6). It is preferable to observe the rate of the lesion's progress and, according to this observation, choose the most appropriate restorative procedure, or decide if treatment is even indicated at all.

The rest of the treatment is exactly as described for abrasion and attrition, except that, if possible, metallic restorations should be the material of choice if restorations are indicated. Metallic restorations have proven to be more resistant to the erosion process than non-metallic ones. Tooth-colored materials capable of chemico-physical bonding to tooth structure (Fig. 6) can also be used with minimum or no tooth preparation, with the assumption that the restoration may require periodic replacement. The use of these materials is especially indicated when the erosive lesion is extremely deep, badly disfiguring, or when it is expected that the underlying pulp-dentin organ is undergoing advanced degeneration. Again, all

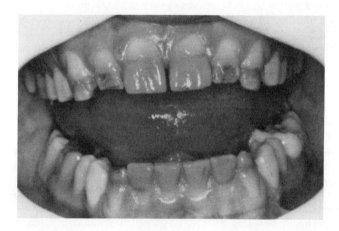

Fig. 27-7

this should be done with the understanding that the lesion might progress around these restorations and even involve them.

IV. Localized Non-Hereditary Enamel Hypoplasia (Fig. 7)

The ameloblasts that are responsible for forming the enamel are very easily injured. During enamel formation, if these cells are irritated, their metabolic product, i.e., the enamel matrix, will not be properly formed, causing certain interruptions and defects. In certain areas, there may be no enamel at all. When the teeth erupt, these defects will be apparent in the crown portion of the tooth (teeth) and this is called localized, non-hereditary enamel hypoplasia. Lesions range from isolated pits to widespread linear defects, depressions, or loss of a segment in the enamel. These defective areas will have different colors from the surrounding enamel, and the discoloration will increase with age, due to their easy stainability from the environment. At some state of the tooth's life, the tooth crown will probably look objectionable.

There are many factors that can injure or destroy the ameloblasts during their formative activities. These include:

A. Systemic disorders

The most prominent of these are exanthemata diseases, nutritional deficiencies (especially vitamins A, C, and D), and hypocalcemia from any cause, or a microbial process as in syphilis.

B. Localized disorders

These include periapical infections of the preceding deciduous tooth (Turner's hypoplasia), traumatic intrusion of the preceding deciduous tooth, etc.

C. Fluorides

Although fluorides arrive to the ameloblasts systemically, they are mentioned here separately because metabolizing fluorides in excessive amounts could poison the ameloblasts and disturb their activities to variable degrees, leading to slightly mottled enamel or a completely disfigured crown in its enamel portion.

The topography of these defects will coincide with the date the disturbance occurred and is very self-indicative.

Treatment Modalities

Since these defects vary in extent and location, there will also be a range of treatment modalities.

If defects are of minimum size (narrow lines or isolated pits or shallow depressions), selective odontotomy can be performed, blending the defects with the remaining tooth surfaces. However, if odontotomy and esthetic reshaping of the tooth enamel cannot produce a pleasing functional effect, it is necessary to resort to direct tooth-colored resinous materials without any mechanical preparations. In other words, only surrounding enamel is conditioned by acids and the resinous material is inserted (see chapter on direct tooth-colored materials). It should be clear that acid etching of fluoride hypoplastic enamel is extremely difficult and non-conducive to efficient retention. Therefore, several applications of conditioning acids should probably be used.

If the defect is at the occluding or contacting area, it is necessary to resort to metallic or cast restorations. However, it should be clear that fluoride hypoplastic enamel is very brittle and chips very easily during tooth preparations and restoration margination. Therefore, every effort should be made to reinforce marginal enamel around these restorations.

If the lesions are discolored and veneering procedures are not planned, vital bleaching can be attempted, but it should be done after selective odontotomy (which will eradicate some discolored areas and may remove the most stained superficial area), and before the acid conditioned enamel-retained restoration. Such vital bleaching can be accomplished in the following way, without the use of any anesthetic:

1. The teeth to be bleached are properly isolated.

2. Adequate prophylaxis is performed for the teeth to be bleached.

3. The teeth are rubbed clean with a cotton pellet containing equal parts of chloroform and ether to dissolve any organic materials that may be present.

4. A mixture of either 5 parts 30% hydrogen peroxide and 1 part ethyl ether carried in a cotton pellet to a full saturation, or sodium perborate and 30% hydrogen peroxide to a pasty form, is prepared.

5. The mixture is applied on the teeth (Fig. 8).

6. A heating element (110-130° F) is applied over the ap-

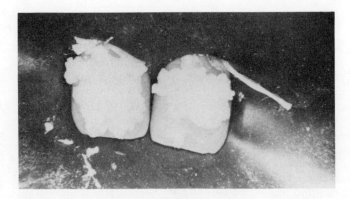

Fig. 27-8

plied mixture for one to three minutes (the patient's report of discomfort should be the time limiting factor, which is why no anesthesia is given).

7. The heating element is reapplied after 1-3 minutes recovery period, being sure the tooth is again covered with the prepared mixture.

The process may take an hour and can be repeated during several visits, until the teeth regain their indicated shade. This procedure may not be successful in all situations. For instance, it is not very effective with greyish and dark brown and sometimes brown discolorations. Also, patients should expect some pulpal sensitivity after each treatment.

If the lesion is completely disfiguring, both in color and in contour, and the involved surface is *not* an occluding one, laminated tooth-colored resinous or ceramic veneers are the treatment of a choice. They can be applied according to the following techniques:

a. Direct technique (Fig. 9, A, B, and C)

i. The veneer (always facial) is premade in different sizes, shades and shapes, but in a thickness not exceeding 0.5 mm. The most appropriate size and shape for the tooth to be veneered is chosen. (Fig. 9A)

ii. The chosen veneer is adjusted by grinding it so that it seats passively on the labial surface of the affected tooth. It should be short of the gingiva, proximal contact area, and incisal edge (Fig. 9B). Although resinous veneers can be applied directly, ceramic types cannot, so the labial surface of the ceramic veneer is covered with a sticky wax, then the veneer is immersed in a 10% solution of hydrofluoric acid, preferably in an ultrasonic bath, for a 15-minute period. This will etch the tooth surface of the veneer for retention.

iii. The tooth is isolated and the enamel is treated and conditioned as described before, to receive enamel retained resinous material.

iv. The bonding resinous material (minimally filled or unfilled type) is flowed on the tooth (see chapter on direct tooth-colored restorations).

v. The veneer is internally lined with the same resinous material and applied on the tooth to its predetermined position.

vi. The veneer should be kept under pressure, until the luting resin is cured (chemically or by light).

vii. Peripheral excesses are removed.

viii. The peripheries are polished and occlusion checked (Fig. 9C).

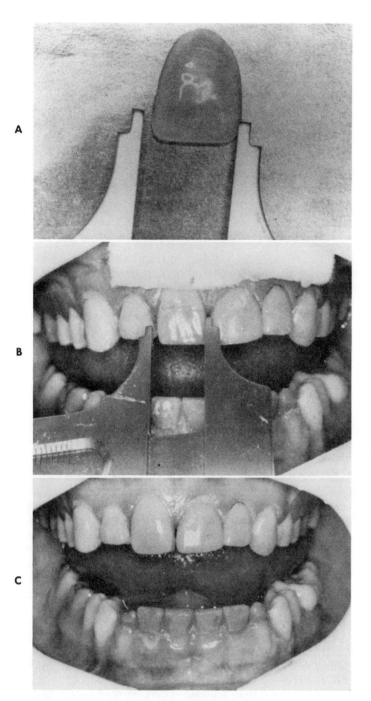

Fig. 27-9

b. Indirect technique

This is a more feasible technique, as the direct technique is extremely time consuming:

i. Prepare study models for the involved arch.

ii. Trim the peripheries of the facial surfaces to be veneered, especially gingivally and proximally.

iii. If using a resinous prefabricated veneer, adjust the veneer to fit passively on the tooth by grinding, additions, or induction heat adaptation (a heated wax spatula brought close to the veneer to soften it, followed by finger pressure). Take

a plaster impression of the labial (facial) surfaces of the involved teeth, either on the study model, after applying a separating medium (soap), or on the teeth surfaces intraorally. The resulting anatomical core will be the holding-adapting mode for the adjusted veneer.

Apply the adjusted veneer on the facial surfaces of the plaster teeth, and apply the plaster core over those veneers. Wrap the entire assembly with a wire to hold it together, and put the assembly in a pressure pan, containing water. Boil the water under pressure for 5-10 minutes, then let it cool, recovering the veneer which will be completely passively adapted to the facial surface.

iv. Veneers can be custom-made from resin or ceramics, following convention techniques of fabricating restorations from either material. The ceramic veneer is then etched internally (as described in the direct technique).

v. The veneer is bonded to the tooth in the same way as we did in the direct technique.

With recent advancements in the material science of composite resins, second through fifth generation types have been developed that can be flowed directly on conditioned enamel and cured in-situ. Certain systems involve the placement, first, of opacifying resins, to mask the labial discolorations.

If veneering is the only way to mask the defect and/or discoloration, but there is no sufficient amount of enamel (form, thickness, distribution, quality, and presence), the laminated veneer will interfere with occlusion (e.g., labial of lower anterior in normal occlusion), the veneering will compromise plaque control measures, or the facial disfigurement is accompanied by tooth structure loss at the contact area, proximal surfaces and/or occluding surfaces, then porcelain fused to metal or cast ceramic full veneering restorations is the modality of choice.

V. Localized Non-Hereditary Enamel Hypocalcification

Just as destruction of the ameloblasts can interfere with the enamel matrix formation, it can also interfere with the mineralization of this matrix, even if it is well formed. This will lead to non-hereditary enamel hypocalcification. The clinical symptoms of enamel hypocalcification will have the same topography as enamel hypoplasia. However, the appearance will be different. Affected areas will not be defective in any way. However, they will appear chalky and soft to indentation, and will be very stainable. Therefore, teeth shades change very fast from chalky to yellow, to brown, dark brown, and/or greyish. If extensive, these lesions predispose to attrition and abrasion. Also, the enamel can be chipped if the lesion involves the entire surface of a tooth.

Treatment Modalities

No attempt should be made for localized odontotomy, etching restorations, or non-veneering types of restorations. If a diagnosis is made early in the tooth's life, while the uncalcified enamel matrix is still intact and the areas are localized, small, and unstained, an attempt at mineralization of the tooth enamel should be made. This procedure can be done using periodic fluoride applications, fluoride ionophoresis, and strict prevention of plaque accumulation in these areas. In many situations mineralization of these decalcified or unmineralized areas could occur to some extent.

Usually, vital bleaching, laminated veneering, composite veneering, and porcelain fused to metal and cast ceramic crowns are the treatments to be used.

VI. Localized Non-Hereditary Dentin Hypoplasia

The odontoblasts are also very specialized cells. Their functions and products (dentin) can be disturbed by environmental irritation, leading to deficient or complete absence of dentin matrix deposition. At this point, the resemblance between the ameloblasts and odontoblasts stops. The ameloblasts are irreplaceable cells, and their disappearance means no enamel in this particular area. However, the odontoblasts are replaceable cells. If they disappear, there will be no dentin temporarily, but dentin deposition will be resumed as soon as other pulp cells start depositing it. In these cases, the defect will be isolated within the dentin substance. The causes for these disturbances are exactly the same as those for localized enamel hypoplasia, and as long as they are covered with the dentin and enamel, there will be no apparent destruction to be diagnosed or treated. However, the situation will be different if these defects are encountered during tooth preparation for a restoration or if the defect is exposed by any other process. In this instance, the defect is part of the preparation or the cavitating lesion that exposed them. Usually, this goes unnoticed, except for sizable defects which change the preparation or the lesion's dimensions. Treatment here could consist of intermediary basing, as it is just an additional dimension to that part of the tooth preparation that is going to be restored.

VII. Localized Non-Hereditary Dentin Hypocalcification

These defects have same causes as hypoplasia. Even though the dentin will be present in substance (no vacancy), it will be softer, more penetrable, and less resilient. The very obvious example of this process is interglobular dentin. Most of the time, the lesion is unnoticed, even when uncovered by a tooth preparation or any other cavitating lesions. The best hedge against problems from the presence of such type of dentin in a tooth preparation is proper intermediary basing (see chapter on intermediary bases and basing).

VIII. Discolorations (Fig. 10)

Although tooth discoloration is not destructive, literally speaking, an unorthodox tooth shade can have a far reaching effect on the affected individual, both socially and psychologically. The dentist is called on frequently to correct this disfigurement.

Discoloration of teeth can be classified from the etiologic aspect as:

A. Extrinsic, a discoloration that is due to surface staining, calculus or any other surface deposits. These can be removed by proper scaling and polishing with the indicated abrasives.

B. Intrinsic, i.e., discoloration which could be created from changes in one or more of the tooth tissues.

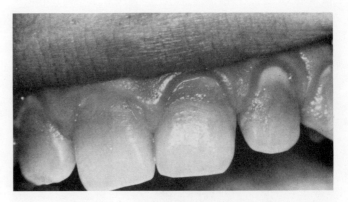

Fig. 27-10

1. Discoloring changes in enamel include hypoplasia and hypocalcification as mentioned before. Very rarely, intrinsic enamel discoloration can be due to externally or internally (systemically) applied agents, due to the extremely low permeability of enamel compared to dentin. Defective enamel from the structural and mineralization aspects can be very permeable and accordingly stainable.

2. Discoloring changes in dentin may result from non-vitality resulting in disintegration of the dentinal tubules' contents, or from pigmentation and staining. The latter can result from external sources, e.g., corrosion products of metallic restorations, medicaments, microbial metabolites, etc. This stainability is facilitated by the dentin permeability, especially if it is hypoplastic, hypocalcified, or dead.

3. Tetracycline discoloration is a sort of permanent staining of the dentin and, to some extent, enamel. It deserves a special mention because of its frequent incidence. Tetracycline administered during the formation of the dentin (enamel) can form complex chelate compounds with both the organic and inorganic components of the dentin (enamel). (The dentin incorporates nine times more tetracycline than enamel.) The created compound is very stable. Such tetracycline staining can occur from the drug crossing the placental barrier and/or being secreted in the milk of the lactating mother. The resulting discoloration ranges from grey brown to dark brown and yellow (Fig. 10).

4. Discoloring changes in the pulp-root canal system can result from pulpal necrosis, in which the disintegration products diffuse through the dentinal tubules from the root canal-pulp chamber system, discoloring the dentin and entire tooth. Such non-vital discoloration will intensify with time due to more disintegration of the products while in the dentinal tubules. This discoloration is usually greyish to dark black. Internal resorption causes a pinkish discoloration at areas where the pulp tissues come close to the tooth surface following resorption of the pulp chamber or root canal walls. Internal hemorrhage, due to excessive instrumentation irritation during cavity preparation, can also cause discoloration from the pulp-root canal system.

Treatment Modalities

1. Discoloration due to extrinsic causes can be resolved as mentioned before.

2. Intrinsic discoloration in enamel and dentin can be treated in the same way localized non-hereditary enamel hypoplasia and hypocalcification is treated.

3. Intrinsic discoloration due to discoloring changes in the pulp-root canal system should be treated as follows. If tooth non-vitality is the cause, endodontic therapy should be instituted. After successful treatment, proceed with the following sequence of treatment:

a. Non-vital bleaching

Evacuate the pulp chamber and root canal portion of the clinical crown from any root canal treatment medicaments or fillings; then, irrigate the evacuated area with a mixture of chloroform and ethyl-ether. Prepare mixtures as in vital bleaching (five parts 30% hydrogen peroxide and one part ethyl-ether in a cotton pellet or a paste of sodium perborate in 30% hydrogen peroxide), and place the mixture into the evacuated pulp-root canal and apply heat inside (110-130° F). In this case, it is possible to maintain the heat longer to obtain better results than with vital bleaching (no pulp tissues to be concerned with). The process can be repeated several times to obtain satisfactory results. The inner part of the evacuated area, especially facially, should be filled with a very white shade of silicate cement, and the rest of the area can be restored with another indicated restoration.

b. If non-vital bleaching does not end with pleasing results, it may be necessary to resort to laminated veneer or porcelain fused to metal or cast ceramic veneering restorations as described before.

If internal resorption is the cause for the discoloration, initiate endodontic therapy, and after successful completion of the endodontic treatment, clean out the concavity(ies) in the pulp chamber walls created by the internal resorption and fill it with a suitable tooth-colored material, possibly silicate cement, and proceed with the regular restorative procedures.

If internal hemorrhage has caused the discoloration, the tooth should be covered with ZOE or a ZOE cemented temporary for a while. This will facilitate the resolution of the hemorrhage. If discoloration does not disappear in time, if darkening occurs, or if confronted with degenerative pulpal symptoms, endodontic therapy may be necessitated.

IX. Malformation

Malformation can be either in micro- or macroforms, and is usually of hereditary origin. The most common type of malformation is one or two teeth (usually upper lateral) that are noticeably smaller in size than surrounding ones, with pointed incisal edges (peg teeth). Malformation should be differentiated from the illusion that can occur when there is a substantial discrepancy between tooth size and jaw size. This situation might give the impression of too large or too small teeth. Nevertheless, this should not be corrected by restorative procedures, but rather with orthodontic treatment.

Treatment Modalities

1. If the affected tooth is properly aligned in the arch and has intact enamel and is not subjected to extensive occluding forces (is not a discluding tooth), conditioning of the enamel and building the tooth up with a direct tooth-colored resinous material will be the treatment of choice, at least for a temporary period of time.

2. If the affected tooth is malaligned, repositioning should be performed before any restorative treatment (see chapter on restoration of badly broken down teeth).

3. If the affected tooth does not have sufficient quality enamel to retain a restoration similar to that described in (1) or if the tooth (after a restoration) can be subjected to excessive occluding forces, it is preferable to select porcelain fused to metal or cast ceramic veneering restorations as the treatment modality.

X. Amelogenesis Imperfecta (Fig. 11)

These lesions result from genetically determined abnormalities in the formative stage of enamel unassociated with evidence of biochemical or systemic diseases. They can be autosomal dominant traits (hypocalcification, hereditary generalized and localized hypoplasia), or they can be X-linked trait (hypomaturation) or a recessive trait (pigmented hypomaturation). The abnormality could be in the matrix formation leading to hypoplasia or it could be in the mineralization leading to hypomineralization.

These lesions usually affect one type of dentition, and only the enamel. There is a variety of these imperfecta diseases and attempts have been made to classify them. Although every type of class has certain clinical features, generally speaking, the classes of hypoplasia imperfecta affect several teeth (may be the entire dentition) with the following symptoms:

A. Thin enamel

B. Open contact

C. Small teeth, with short roots, very limited pulp chambers and root canal dimensions

D. Delay in eruption

E. Sometimes the enamel is glassy (prismless)

F. There may be some discoloration, usually yellow

G. The enamel could look wrinkled

H. All signs of severe occlusal wear

In the same aspect, the class of hypomineralization imperfectas have the following general clinical features (Fig. 11):

1. The enamel is usually stained (yellow or black). It may be chalky at early stages of life.

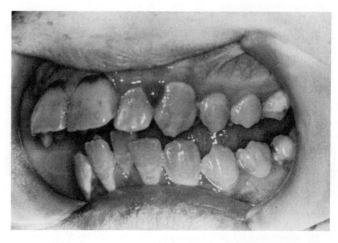

Fig. 27-11

2. The enamel chips easily.

3. The enamel can be very soft in consistency (cheesy).

4. Although teeth will have normal forms when they erupt, they have dull surfaces readily stainable by age. The stains become darker with time.

5. The enamel is worn away very easily in life with all signs and symptoms of severe attrition (may be to the gum line).

Treatment Modalities

Early diagnosis is the key to a relatively successful treatment. Only two modalities can be used in most cases.

1. Selective odontotomy esthetically reshaping the teeth. This is a repeated procedure that is needed throughout the lifetime of the tooth because of the frequent changes in shape (attrition).

2. Full veneering includes procedures with metallic, metallic based, or cast ceramic restorations. At no time should these restorations oppose a natural tooth, i.e., occluding teeth should be restored at the same time with the same materials.

In extensive conditions, lengthy, comprehensive periodic evaluation should be practiced before trying any restorative work on these patients, as the teeth are easily chipped. This situation can happen during a tooth preparation or during service. If enamel imperfectas are not associated with dentin imperfecta, the restorative prognosis can be favorable. In any event, conservative non-restorative treatment should be tried first, before resorting to restorative procedures.

XI. Dentinogenesis Imperfecta
(Fig. 12, A and B)

These are also genetically dictated classes of diseases, affecting the formation and/or maturation of the dentin matrix in the absence of any obvious systemic or biochemical changes. Again, several attempts have been made to classify them according to the trait, although most of them are autosomal dominant. There are other classifications according to their extent and clinical features, and others according to the association with osteogenesis imperfecta. At any rate, there are at least eight types (classes) of these imperfectas reported in the literature.

Generally speaking, the one most frequently reported is the hereditary opalescent dentin. It may have some features of the other types also. A summary of these features are:

A. The color may be from grey, brown, yellow-brown to violet.

B. Most of them exhibit a translucent hue.

C. The enamel, although intact, is easily chipped because of the defective dentino-enamel junction.

D. The crowns are overcontoured.

E. The roots are short and slender.

F. There are signs and symptoms of extensive attrition.

G. The dentin is devoid of tubules.

H. The dentin contains a lot of interglobular dentin.

J. The decay process, if initiated, will spread laterally.

J. Root canal and pulp chamber space is obliterated.

K. Dentin hardness and resilience is almost half that of normal dentin.

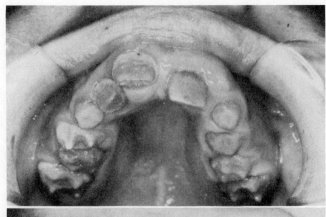

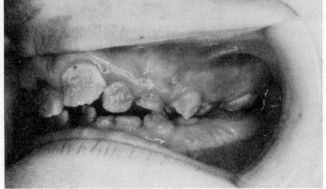

Fig. 27-12

Treatment Modalities

Any possible success for treatment depends upon early diagnosis and care. Only two possible treatment modalities can be used here, namely, selective odontotomy and permanent full veneering. There should not be any false security in preparing these teeth, because of the absence of the pulp chamber and root canals, as these teeth are very susceptible to fracture, especially by instrumentation forces. There should not be any attempt to use intracoronal or intraradicular retention modes. Therefore, the only retention possible is an extracoronal reinforcing-protecting veneering restoration. Splinting between these teeth is one way to avoid root fracture, which, unfortunately, should be expected by both the patient and the dentist.

XII. Trauma

Separation and/or loss of tooth structure as a result of trauma frequently occurs necessitating dental treatment. Trauma that leads to these mishaps can be from substantial impact forces (exceeding the fracture limit of involved tooth structure), as from a fall, a blow, or sudden biting on a hard unyielding substance (Fig. 13 and 14). Trauma can also result from long standing repetitive cyclic loading forces that are less than the breaking point of tooth structure, but definitely more than their endurance limits. Trauma resulting from such cyclic loading occurs over a long period of time, and can also result in periodontal break-down, in addition to tooth fracture or cracking (Fig. 15). Such cyclic, non-physiologic loading always results from occlusal interferences, especially the balancing type.

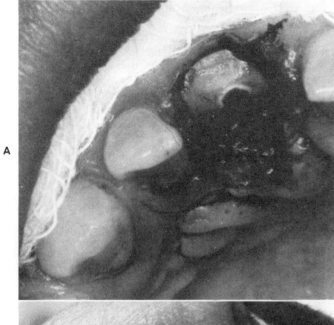

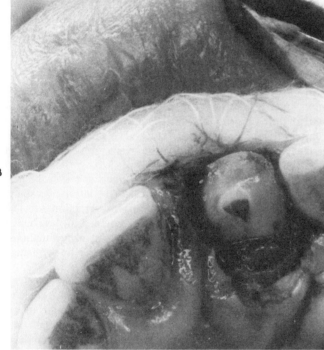

Fig. 27-13

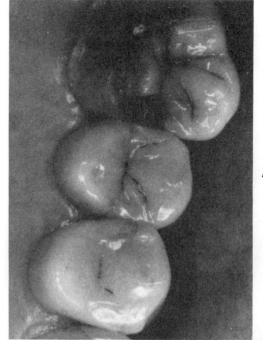

Fig. 27-14

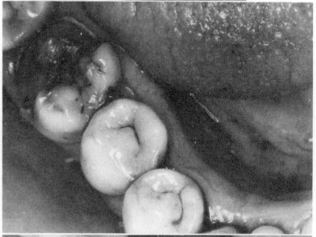

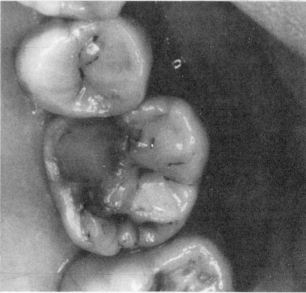

According to Ellis, injuries to natural teeth can be classified into eight classes:

Class 1: Simple fracture of the tooth crown, involving little or no dentin

Class 2: Extensive fracture of the tooth crown, involving considerable dentin but no pulp (Fig. 14)

Class 3: Extensive fracture of the crown, involving considerable dentin and exposing the pulp

Class 4: A traumatized tooth which becomes non-vital with or without loss of crown structures

Class 5: Tooth lost as a result of trauma

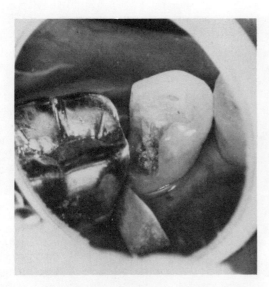

Fig. 27-15

Class 6: Fracture of the tooth root, with or without loss of crown structure (Fig. 13)

Class 7: Displacement (dislocation) of a tooth (teeth), without fracture of crown or root

Class 8: Fracture of the crown en masse, with the broken crown pieces retrievable

Ellis' classification is an excellent therapeutic classification. However, it only encompasses the tooth defects originating from high magnitude forceful impacts, although cyclically applied low magnitude forces can produce similar effects as described under any of the eight Ellis' classes. The effects take place in stages, i.e., incremental types of tooth fracture. Frequently, at one of these stages a failure will occur, which can be the same as one of the failures described in Ellis' classes. There will be clinical symptoms indicating these incomplete fractures, cracks or incomplete cyclic dislocations of the involved teeth. Therapeutically, each of these incomplete traumatic situations deserves a class of its own. Therefore, two classes are added: Class 9—incomplete fracture of the tooth or cracked tooth; and Class 10—cyclic incomplete dislocation of the tooth.

Understandably, there can be combinations of any of the 10 classes.

Treatment Modalities

There are three therapeutic bases for the treatment of traumatized teeth:

1. Accurate and detailed diagnostic data should be collected, as described in the chapter on restoration of badly broken down teeth. In addition, data on the status of the root condition and development is necessary. Any injury to oral and paraoral tissues should be recorded and taken into consideration during the therapy.

2. The patient should be aware of the fact that vitality of the tooth at the time of the examination does not mean that the tooth will be vital by the end of the treatment or later in life, as the traumatic energy may start a degenerative process in the P-D organ that can lead to immediate pulp necrosis or a very delayed, slowly progressing (sometimes over ten years) one.

3. Sometimes, due to the incomplete tooth development and/or the extent of tooth involvement, or early stages of passive tooth eruption when the accidental tooth defect occurred, the tooth will need two sets of restorative modalities. The first one is a provisional restoration until the tooth completes its development, its passive eruption is stabilized, or endodontic therapy is successfully completed. The second one is a permanent restoration.

The following is a scheme of the suggested treatment for each class:

Class 1

1. Smoothing the edges and peripheries of the defect is sufficient in most cases.

2. Esthetic reshaping of the involved area and similar areas on symmetrical teeth may be necessary.

3. If the defect involves a relatively large surface area of an anterior tooth not correctable by either (1) or (2), surrounding enamel can be conditioned, and the area restored in a resinous direct tooth-colored material. The area can be filled directly with ASPA, after proper tooth treatment, provided the restoration will not be occluding (see chapter on direct tooth-colored restorations). If it is a posterior tooth, a metallic restoration should be used (see chapter on restoration of badly broken-down teeth).

Class 2

In most cases, two sets of restorations are indicated. The provisional restorations can be Class IV, Design 3 or 4 for anterior teeth, according to the location and extent of the defect. For posterior teeth, it can be an amalgam restoration, according to the principles mentioned in the chapter on restoration of badly broken down teeth.

The permanent restoration is usually indicated after the provisional one fulfills its objectives (i.e., after confirming a sound pulp-dentin organ, or completion of passive eruption, etc.). It should be selected and designed as mentioned in the chapter on restorations of badly broken down teeth. In many situations, the provisional restorations can actually serve as the permanent ones.

Class 3

For these cases, the pulp and root canal therapy should be initiated immediately. In most cases, for the purpose of esthetics, space maintenance, and facilitating successful pulp and root canal therapy, the tooth crown should be built up. In these latter situations proceed according to the following sequence:

A. Make initial pulp therapy, e.g., pulp extirpation, pulpotomy, or in some cases direct pulp capping (if indicated, see Chapter 14). In extirpation and pulpotomy situations, leave a dry cotton pellet in the pulp chamber or its entry site, or inject an elastomeric impression material into the pulp chamber and let it set.

B. Build up the tooth crown with a provisional treatment restoration. This can be a pin-retained restoration, or etched-enamel retained direct tooth-colored restoration, etc. In general, follow the principles of building a badly broken down tooth.

C. For further endodontic therapy steps make an access cavity preparation through the hardened treatment restoration (done in step B) to the pulp chamber. (The residual dry cotton pellet or elastomeric ''plug'' will guide, indicate and confirm the entry to the pulp chamber.)

D. Proceed with the indicated endodontic therapy. When it is successfully completed, proceed with step E.

E. The created access cavity preparation through the restoration, together with the involved pulp chamber, and sometimes a part of the root canal(s), should be obliterated with the same material used to build up the crown, with or without premade posts in the root canal(s). The choice of a post should be according to the rules mentioned in the chapter on pin- and post-retained restorations. In this way, the provisional treatment restoration is converted to a foundation for a cast or cast alloy based reinforcing-protecting type of a restoration.

F. After successful direct pulp capping or endodontic therapy with the subsequent foundation, proceed with restoring the tooth as mentioned in the chapter on principles of restorations of badly broken down teeth.

Class 4

Proceed according to the following sequence:

A. If the tooth crown is intact, immediately initiate endodontic therapy.

B. If the tooth crown is fractured, proceed as in Class 3.

C. If the tooth crown is discolored, especially in conspicuous teeth, and a veneering permanent restoration is not planned, use non-vital bleaching or laminated veneering procedures, as mentioned early in this chapter. The latter procedure(s) can only be done after successful endodontic treatment.

D. If the tooth is discolored beyond any possible bleaching, laminated veneering is contraindicated (and esthetics is a great concern) and/or it has a provisional treatment restoration (from B), the tooth should be veneered with cast alloy-based or cast ceramic restoration.

Class 5

Accidental tooth loss or fracture beyond any restorative capability should be replaced with a prosthesis. If the loss occurred early in life, where fixed permanent prosthesis is contraindicated, a provisional fixed bridge can be used. The pontic tooth can be a plastic denture tooth that should be chosen and adjusted to occupy the space and function of the lost tooth. To facilitate attachment of the plastic tooth to the adjacent abutment teeth, it should accommodate two steel rods (0.050''). The steel rods are joined to the artificial tooth through light or chemically cured resin in prepared cavities in the tooth, embedding the steel rods. Concurrently, the steel rods should fit in similar cavities at each of the adjacent natural teeth. The cavity in the natural tooth should be undercut and enamel conditioned. The protruding rods from the artificial tooth will be embedded in the composite resin that will fill these cavities in the abutment teeth, thus creating a provisional bridge. An electrochemically etched, non-noble alloy based bridge, to be retained by conditioned enamel through a luting composite resin, might also be used as a provisional prosthesis. In this case, the pontic can be a porcelain fused to the metal base. When conditions allow, a permanent fixed cast (cast alloy based) bridge should replace the provisional bridge.

Class 6

Root fractures can be classified therapeutically as cervically horizontal, midradicularly horizontal, apically horizontal, and vertical.

A. Cervically horizontal (slightly oblique) (Fig. 13) fractures are always accompanied by a complete loss of the crown or crown looseness, necessitating its removal. The treatment procedure here is endodontic therapy, preferably a one-visit procedure. Then, the remaining tooth structure is handled the same way as a badly broken down tooth, with subgingival-infrabony location of the margins of the defects. As mentioned later (chapter on badly broken down teeth), any indicated periodontal surgery, intensional extrusion, etc. (to bring the gingival margin of the defect occlusal to the attaching epithelium) should be accomplished before proceeding with the regular restoration of badly broken down, endodontically treated tooth.

B. Midradicularly horizontal (slightly oblique)

1. If tooth vitality is assured, immobilization, using one of the procedures mentioned in the chapter on restorations of badly broken down teeth, is the only treatment required, until signs of repair are evident (splinting could be permanent as healing takes several years).

2. If tooth vitality is doubtful or the tooth became non-vital, endodontic treatment should be instituted and successfully completed. Then a splinting, reinforcing stainless steel (chrome cobalt) rod should be cemented, joining the two root fragements together. The tooth should be permanently splinted to adjacent teeth.

C. Apically horizontal (or slightly oblique root fracture)

If the tooth vitality is assured, it should be left without any interferences. However, if the tooth becomes non-vital or its vitality is doubtful, endodontic therapy should be instituted and the apical root fragment is surgically removed. Attempts to join and splint the apical fragment to the main root, especially when surgery is not feasible, can interfere with the apical seal of the root canal.

D. Vertical root fracture

It is extremely difficult to diagnose this type of fracture. Only through symptoms of isolated periodontal pocketing next to the fracture line, tooth non-vitality, loosened retrograde filling, or especially by reflecting a muco-gingival flap exposing a fracture line can diagnosis be accomplished. Vertical root fracture is usually caused by overcondensation during root canal filling, overly energetic insertion of root canal posts, or impact trauma. Vertical fracture of the root has a very unfavorable prognosis as it always propagates quickly to the tooth crown, thereby connecting the peridontium and pulp root canal tissues with the infected oral environment. There will be no way to seal this created avenue. Almost always, the root affected by this type of fracture should be eradicated. This means extraction of a single rooted tooth and hemisectioning or partial amputation of multirooted teeth. In a few situations, where the fracture line is confined to a segment of a tooth and does not cross to the opposite side of the root, a cavity preparation which would cause the fracture line to be obliterated with amalgam might be the solution of choice. In even fewer situations, the loosened segment of the fractured root is removed, leaving the rest after rounding its edges, which may be without root canals.

Class 7

In this class, after proper reduction of the tooth and/or replacing it in its socket (if it is a reimplantation, root canal debridement and obliteration should be done prior to the reduction), the tooth (teeth) should be splinted to adjacent ones, using one of the different methods described in the chapter on restorations of badly broken down teeth.

Class 8

Cases falling under this class are usually reported immediately after the tooth fracture, so the pulp is vital, even if it is exposed. In these cases, if the separated crown portion is retrieved and intact, the following should be done:

A. Clean the retrieved tooth piece and keep in a sterile saline solution.

B. If the pulp is involved, initiate and complete endodontic therapy, preferably in a one-visit procedure.

C. The enamel surface at the fracture line of the remaining tooth and the intact broken portion should be conditioned and primed.

D. If the tooth is endodontically treated, the pulp chamber should be filled with composite resin. In both [endodontically and none-endodontically treated teeth] situations, the two pieces are brought together, and kept under pressure until the primer and the composite resin set.

E. The enamel surrounding the junctional line between the two fragments is conditioned and primed as usual, and composite resin is flowed there to further join the two fragments.

This type of restorative treatment modality should be considered a provisional restoration, especially if the involved tooth is one that is laterally loaded during functional mandibular movements. Eventually, the tooth will be treated as in Class 3 or 6 (cervical root fracture). However, for an immediate esthetic restoration, this is an excellent treatment modality.

Class 9

It is a very well documented fact that there are as many, if not more, incomplete tooth fractures as there are complete fractures. The latter can be an immediate incident as a result of impact forces (discussed before) or the last and most confirmed symptoms of a long standing incomplete fracture. It seems that more and more of this type of tooth destruction is being seen, which is due both to more awareness of the possibility of their occurrence and to better diagnostic tools.

There are many possible reasons for the high incidence of cracked teeth in modern dentitions, e.g., more people keep their teeth in older age, with accompanying and more possible steep cusps, highly calcifying intermediary bases, use of high speed equipment in tooth preparation, use of pins or posts in retaining restorations, etc.

There are numerous factors that encourage such incremental cracking of teeth. These include:

A. Premature occluding contacts, especially in lateral mandibular excursions. Balancing contacts are the most predisposing.

B. Very wide and deep intracoronal restorations (especially MOD restorations).

C. Disclusion mechanism including posterior teeth, especially without any canine components.

D. Forced-in retention modes of a restoration, e.g., pins, cements, etc.

E. Vibrating rotary instruments, especially high speed ones.

F. Posterior teeth cusp inclines and groove dimensions not compatible with the progressive and immediate side shifts of the mandibular movements.

G. Habits (see attrition and abrasion).

H. Severe thermal cycling in the oral environment.

I. Non-vitality of tooth structures (totally and locally).

J. Hypermineralization or dehydration of tooth structures.

K. Sharp deep surface fissures or grooves, extremely sharp line and point angles of a preparation in a tooth, and any internal or external sharp details that may act as shear lines for a crack culminating in a fracture.

L. Loose intracoronal restorations. This situation will magnify the shear stresses within the tooth.

The diagnosis of a cracked tooth is one of the most perplexing of all dental diseases. Usually the patient will show one or more of the following signs and symptoms. Frequently, the chief symptom is pain, indicating combinations of pulpitis and periodontitis at different levels, depending on the degree of periodontal and pulpal involvement with the crack. The same stimuli provoking these types of pain can be used here for diagnosis (thermal, osmotic pressure changes, etc.). Usually, the tooth looks intact, without any restoration or with an apparently sound restoration. The patients almost always show evidence of good plaque control. The patient will frequently complain that the pain is elicited while chewing, since posterior teeth are more frequently involved than anterior ones. The frequency of occurrence in posterior teeth is in the following order: second lower molars, first lower molars, and maxillary premolars. The rest of the posterior teeth are seldom affected.

Upon applying pressure on segments of the tooth, one at a time, one application can start the painful episode. Such pressure can be applied by wood sticks, mirror handles, inlay seaters, amalgam pluggers or asking the patient to bite on a rubber wheel.

If the tooth contains an amalgam restoration, the corrosion products of the amalgam might stain the crack. The stained crack can be apparent from the tooth surface or seen only after removing the amalgam. Also, transillumination, using fiber optic or incandescent light, can show the crack when the light is brought close to it. Furthermore, some coloring dyes can show up the crack by staining the accumulated plaque within it. Examples of these dyes are methylene blue or mercurochrome, etc.

In many situations the crack is apparent to the unaided eye without staining or transillumination, but usually accompanied with enamel crazing. So, whenever enamel crazing is discovered, further examination of the enamel and dentin should be done to verify or negate the presence of a crack.

Any of the possible predisposing factors should be explored, for a radiograph can show an apparently completely sound tooth. However, infrequently, a crack might appear in it, if it is sizable enough and in the plane shown by the radiograph.

Periodontal break-down can be evident at the site of the crack (connected or disconnected pocket). This is due to the detachment of the periodontal membrane ligaments from the tooth at the site of the crack. In many situations, this could be the first sign of a crack. An orally apparent crack can be explored using a sharp explorer pressing it pulpally, as this might elicit the pain episode. Relieving the tooth from occluding with opposing tooth (teeth), especially in lateral excursion could stop the pain for a time, until the tooth supererupts to occlude again with its opposing partner. Banding the tooth with a cemented orthodontic or copper band can also stop the pain episode.

Treatment Modalities

After thorough examination, if a cracked tooth is suspected to be the cause of the patient's symptoms, the following provisional treatment should be done.

1. Relieve the tooth from eccentric occluding contacts. In some severe cases, it should also be released from centric ones.

2. Cement a circumferential band around the tooth (orthodontic or copper band).

In many situations the pain is completely alleviated by the two above mentioned treatment modalities.

3. If the signs of pulpitis (or pulpal degeneration) persist after (1) and (2), proceed with endodontic therapy. While in the pulp chamber and root canal system, look for any continuity of the crack with the root canal walls or subpulpal floor, because if the latter situations are verified, the tooth should be extracted or undergo hemisectioning or amputation. If there is no crack continuity to these anatomical landmarks, complete endodontic treatment.

4. If the tooth contains an intracoronal restoration or a carious lesion, it should be removed and a temporary ZOE restoration should be inserted and kept there for at least two weeks (with the band on). Sometimes the temporary is mixed with a staining dye to verify the extent and propagation of the crack.

5. Any periodontal defect caused by the crack should be explored and corrected. If the crack involves the clinical root, the periodontal correction should be in such a way as to prevent the crack in these areas from being continuous with the oral environment (clinical crown). Otherwise the tooth should be extracted or the root amputated or hemisected.

The permanent restoration should be done only after:

a. Cracked tooth, occurrence, and extent are verified.

b. Endodontic therapy, if indicated, is successfully completed.

c. The pulp-dentin organ and the periodontium have recovered from the degeneration caused by the presence of the crack.

The permanent restoration will be in the form of a reinforcing-protecting type of cast or cast based restoration, usually accompanied by a foundation, so as to minimize the necessity for intracanal preparation for the reinforcing final restoration.

Class 10

To adequately treat this cyclic incomplete dislocation, the extent and cause of periodontal break-down should be detected. From this, indicated periodontal therapy should be instituted, which usually includes occlusal equilibration. After eradicating the causes for the periodontal break-down, sometimes the tooth needs to be immobilized, at least for a while, to enhance and assure periodontal healing (Fig. 16). The immobilization is done after reducing the tooth to its physiologic position (can be easily attained here), and in one of the several splinting modes mentioned in a chapter on the restoration of badly broken down teeth.

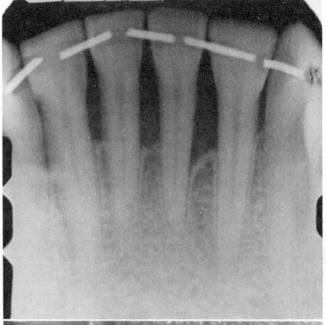

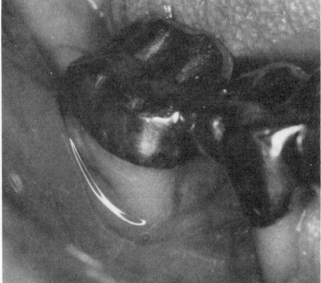

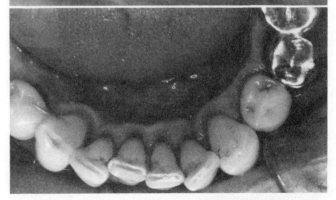

Fig. 27-16. A, Provisional splinting of lower incisors, affected by Class 10 trauma, to adjacent cuspids. **B,** Permanent splint to hemisectioned tooth #30. **C,** Provisional splint to tooth #28 with tooth #27.

BIBLIOGRAPHY

Abbey, L.M., and Lombard, J.A.: The etiological factors and clinical implications of pica: report of case. J. Am. Dent. Assoc. **87**(4):885-887, 1973.

Ainamo, J.: Relationship between occlusal wear of the teeth and periodontal health. Scand. J. Dent. Res. **80**(6):505-509, 1972.

Bakdash, M.B.: Anomalous destruction caused by the use of toothpicks. Oral Surg. **46**(1):167-168, 1978.

Bales, D.J.: Pain and the cracked tooth. J. Indiana Dental Assoc. **54**:15, 1975.

Bates, J.F., Stafford, G.D., and Harrison, A.: Masticatory function—a review of the literature. 1. The form of the masticatory cycle. J. Oral Rehabil. **2**(3):281-301, 1975.

Bergstrom, J., and Lavstedt, S.: An epidemiologic approach to toothbrushing and dental abrasion. Community Dent. Oral Epidemiol. **7**(1):57-64, 1979.

Berry, D.C., and Poole, D.F.: Attrition: possible mechanisms of compensation. J. Oral Rehabil. **3**(3):201-206, 1976.

Blattner, R.J., Heys, F., and Robinson, H.B.: Osteogenesis imperfecta and odontogenesis imperfecta. J. Dent. Res. **21**:325, 1942.

Bodecker, C.F.: Enamel hypoplasia. J. Dent. Res. **20**:447, 1941.

Bow, P.: Dentinogenesis imperfecta—a method of semipermanent restoration. J. Dent. Assoc. S. Afr. **33**(6):293-300, 1978.

Brodie, A.G., and Sognnaes, R.F.: Erosionlike denture markings possibly related to hyperactivity of oral soft tissues. J. Am. Dent. Assn. **88**(5): 1012-1017, 1974.

Brown, K.E.: Reconstruction considerations for severe dental attrition. J. Prosth. Dent. **44**(4):384-388, 1980.

Brucker, M.: Studies on the incidence and cause of dental defects in children II. Hypoplasia. J. Dent. Res. **22**:115, 1943.

Bruggen Cate, H.J. ten.: Dental erosion in industry. Br. J. Ind. Med. **25**(4):249-266, 1968.

Bull, A.W., and Bradley, D.J.: Erosion and the problem of control. Aust. Dent. J. **14**(5):293-294, 1969.

Cameron, C.E.: Cracked tooth syndrome. J. Am. Dent. Assn. **68**:405, 1964.

Cameron, C.E.: Cracked tooth syndrome: Additional findings. J. Am. Dent. Assn. **93**:971, 1976.

Charbeneau, G.T., Bozell, R.R., 3d.: Clinical evaluation of a glass ionomer cement for restoration of cervical erosion. JADA **98**(6):936-939, 1979.

Christen, A.G.: Candy breath mints, acidic beverages, and traumatic brushing—suspected factors in tooth erosion and abrasion: case report. Tex. Dent. J. **94**(5):10-12, 1976.

Dahl, B.L., Krogstad, O., and Karlsen, K.: An alternative treatment in cases with advanced localized attrition. J. Oral Rehabil. **2**(3):209-214, 1975.

Darling, A.I.: Some observations on amelogenesis imperfecta and calcification of the dental enamel. Proc. R. Soc. Med. **49**:759, 1956.

Davis, W.B.: A comparison of dentine abrasion data generated by radiotracer and surface profilometer methods. J. Oral Rehabil. **6**(2):177-181, 1979.

Davis, W.B., and Winter, P.J.: The effect of abrasion on enamel and dentine and exposure to dietary acid. Br. Dent. J. **148**(11-12):253-256, 1980.

Downs, W.G.: Studies in the causes of dental anomalies. J. Dent. Res. **8**:367, 1928.

Eccles, J.D., and Jenkins, W.G.: Dental erosion and diet. J. Dent. **2**(4):153-159, 1974.

Eccles, J.D.: Dental erosion of nonindustrial origin. A clinical survey and classification. J. Prosth. Dent. **42**(6):649-653, 1979.

Eccles, J.D.: The treatment of dental erosion. J. Dent. **6**(3):217-221, 1978.

Ellis, R.G., and Davey, R.W.: The classification and treatment of injuries to teeth of children. 5th ed. Year Book Medical Pub., Inc., 1970.

Elzay, R.P., and Robinson, C.T.: Dentinal dysplasia. Oral Surg. **23**:338, 1967.

Fishman, L.S.: Dental and skeletal relationships to attritional occlusion. Angle Orthod. **46**(1):51-63, 1976.

Fuks, A., Anaise, J., Westreich, V., and Gedalia, I.: Effect of fluoride supplementation of a citrus beverage on the erosion rate of molars of hamsters. J. Dent. Res. **52**(5):1149, 1973.

Fuller, J.L., and Johnson, W.W.: Citric acid consumption and the human dentition. J. Am. Dent. Assn. **95**(1):80-84, 1977.

Gabrovsek, J.: New thesis on the development of erosion and dental caries. J. Dent. Res. **49**(5):1020-1024, 1970.

Gibbard, P.D.: The management of children and adolescents suffering from amelogenesis imperfecta and dentinogenesis imperfecta. Int. J. Orthod. **12**(4):15-25, 1975.

Gwinnett, A.J., and Jendresen, M.D.: Micromorphologic features of cervical erosion after acid conditioning and its relation with composite resin. J. Dent. Res. **57**(4):543-549, 1978.

Harte, D.B., and Manly, R.S.: Four variables affecting magnitude of dentifrice abrasiveness. J. Dent. Res. **55**(3):322-327, 1976.

Hiatt, W.H.: Incomplete crown-root fracture in pulpal-periodontal disease. J. Periodontol. **44**:369, 1973.

Hodge, H., Finn, S.B., Lose, G.B., Gachet, F.S., and Bassett, S.H.: Hereditary opalescent dentin. II. General and oral clinical studies. J. Am. Dent. Assn. **26**:1663, 1939.

Hodge, H.C., Finn, S.B., Robinson, H.B., Manly, R.S., Manly, M.L., Van Huysen, G., and Bale, W.F.: Hereditary opalescent dentin. III. Histological, chemical and physical studies. J. Dent. Res. **19**:521, 1940.

Hollinger, J.O., and Moore, E.M., Jr.: Hard tissue loss at the cemento-enamel junction: a clinical study. J. N.J. Dent. Assoc. **50**(4):27-31, 1979.

Hurst, P.S., Lacey, L.H., and Crisp, A.H.: Teeth, vomiting and diet: a study of the dental characteristics of seventeen anorexia nervosa patients. Postgrad. Med. J. **53**(620):298-305, 1977.

Larsen, M.J.: Dissolution of enamel. Scand. J. Dent. Res. **81**(7):518-522, 1973.

Lawrence, L.G.: Cervical glass ionomer restorations: a clinical study. Dent. J. **45**(2):58-59, 63, 1979.

Levine, R.S.: Fruit juice erosion—an increasing danger? J. Dent. **21**(2):85-88, 1973.

Low, T.: The treatment of hypersensitive cervical abrasion cavities using ASPA cement. J. Oral Rehabil. **8**(1):81-89, 1981.

McKay, F.S., and Black, G.V.: An investigation of mottled teeth. Dent. Cosmos **58**:477, 627, 781, 894, 1916.

McLachlan, W.: Tooth damage from use of citrus fruits. Br. Dent. J. **131**(9):385, 1971.

Meister, F., Jr., Braun, R.J., and Gerstein, H.: Endodontic involvement resulting from dental abrasion or erosion. J. Am. Dent. Assn. **101**(4):651-653, 1980.

Mendis, B.R., and Darling, A.I.: Distribution with age and attrition or peritubular dentin the crowns of human teeth. Arch. Oral Biol. **24**(2):131-139, 1979.

Mendis, B.R., and Darling, A.I.: A scanning electron microscope and microradiographic study of closure of human coronal dentinal tubules related to occlusal attrition and caries. Arch. Oral Biol. **24**(10-11):725-733, 1979.

Patterson, S., and El-Kafrawy, A.H.: Tooth discoloration and cosmetic bleaching. Current therapy in dentistry. Vol. 6, 1977, St. Louis, C.V. Mosby Co., p. 504.

Radentz, W.H., Barnes, G.P., and Cutright, D.E.: A survey of factors possibly associated with cervical abrasion of tooth surfaces. J. Periodontol. **47**(3):148-154, 1976.

Renson, C.E.: Attrition, abrasion, erosion and the temporomandibular joint. Dent. Update Nov.-Dec. 75; **2**(6):283-288.

Reynolds, J.M.: Occlusal wear facets. J. Prosth. Dent. **24**(4):367-372, 1970.

Rowe, A.H.: A palliative treatment for severe enamel erosion. Br. Dent. J. **133**(10):435-436, 1972.

Ryan, A.S.: A preliminary scanning electron microscope examination of wear striation direction of primate teeth. J. Dent. Res. **58**(1):525-530, 1979.

Sarnat, B.G., and Schour, I.: Enamel hypoplasia (chronologic enamel aplasia) in relation to systemic disease: a chronologic, morphologic and etiologic classification. J. Am. Dent. Assoc. **28**:1989, 1941; **29**:67, 1942.

Schafer, Hine and Levy.: Textbook of oral pathology. Philadelphia, Saunders, 1974.

Shear, M.: Hereditary hypocalcification of enamel. J. Dent. Assn. S. Afr., **9**:262, 1954.

Shelling, D.H., and Anderson, G.M.: Relation of rickets and vitamin D to the incidence of dental caries, enamel hypoplasia and malocclusion in children. J. Am. Dent. Assoc. **23**:840, 1936.

Skogedal, O., Silness, J., Tangerud, T., Laegreid, O., and Gilhuus-Moe, O.: Pilot study on dental erosion in a Norwegian electrolytic zinc factory. Community Dent. Oral Epidemiol. **5**(5):248-251, 1977.

Snyder, D.E.: The cracked tooth syndrome and fractured posterior cusp. J. Oral Surg. **41**:698, 1976.

Sognnaes, R.F.: Periodontal significance of intraoral frictional abrasion. Periodont. Abstr. **25**(3):112-121, 1977.

Sognnaes, R.F., and Ducasse.: An extreme case of vestibular denture wear. J. Calif. Dent. Assoc. **5**(8):54-56, 1977.

Sognnaes, R.F., Wolcott, R.B., and Xhonga, F.A.: Dental erosion. I. Erosionlike patterns occurring in association with other dental conditions. J. Am. Dent. Assn. **84**(3):571-576, 1972.

Spanauf, A.J.: Erosion arising from a nutritional factor with concomitant bruxism. A clinical case report. Aust. Dent. J. **18**(4):233-234, 1973.

Spanko, J.E.: The eminent canine. J. Prosth. Dent. **34**(1):48-52, 1975.

Standlee, J.P., Caputo, A.A., and Collard, E.W.: Dental defects caused by some twist drills and retentive pins. J. Prosth. Dent. **24**:185, 1970.

Stern, N., and Brayer, L.: Collapse of the occlusion-aetiology, symptomatology and treatment. J. Oral Rehabil. **2**(1):1-19, 1975.

Sylvestri, A.R.: The undiagnosed split-root syndrome. J. Am. Dent. Assn. **92**:980, 1976.

Toda, Y., Shirato, M., Tohnai, K., Fujii, H., Tesato, S., Takehana, S., and Ito, A.: A scanning electron microscopic study of dentinal tubules in dead tracts. J. Nihon Univ. Sch. Dent. **22**(1):1-9, 1980.

Toller, P.A.: A clinical report on six cases of amelogenesis imperfecta. Oral Surg., **12**:325, 1959.

Tronstad, L.: Scanning electron microscopy of attrited dentinal surfaces and subajacent dentin in human teeth. Scand. J. Dent. Res. **81**(2):112-122, 1973.

Tronstad, L., and Langeland, K.: Histochemical observations on human dentin exposed by attrition. Scand. J. Dent. Res. **79**(3):151-159, 1971.

Via, W.F., Jr.: Enamel defects induced by trauma during tooth formation. Oral Surg. **25**:49, 1968.

Volpe, A.R., Mooney, R., Zumbrunnen, C., Stahl, D., and Goldman, H.M.: A long term clinical study evaluating the effect of two dentifrices on oral tissues. J. Periodontol. **46**(2):113-118, 1975.

Weinmann, J.P., Svoboda, J.F., and Woods, R.W.: Hereditary disturbances of enamel formation and calcification. J. Am. Dent. Assn. **32**:397, 1945.

White, D.K., Hayes, R.C., and Benjamin, R.N.: Loss of tooth structure associated with chronic regurgitation and vomiting. J.A.D.A. **97**(5):833-835, 1978.

Wictorin, L.: Effect of toothbrushing on acrylic resin veneering material. II. Abrasive effect of selected dentifrices and toothbrushes. Acta Odontol. Scand. **30**(3):383-395, 1972.

Wolpoff, M.H.: Interstitial wear. Am. J. Phys. Anthropol. **34**(2):205-227, March 1971.

Xhonga, F.A.: Bruxism and its effect on the teeth. J. Oral Rehabil. **4**(1):65-76, 1977.

Xhonga, F.A., and Sognnaes, R.F.: Dental erosion: progress of erosion measured clinically after various fluoride applications. JADA **87**(6):1223-1228, 1973.

CHAPTER 28

Principles for restoration of badly broken down teeth

The emphasis in this chapter will be on the general principles guiding the operator in designing restorations for teeth whose mutilation or disease exceeds the restorative capacity of any previously described designs and modalities. In order to restore a tooth permanently when confronted with such extensive tooth destruction, the systemized, disciplined approach described herein is essential to the success of the procedure.

Posterior Teeth

An operator may have a mental image of a restorative design, material, and technique when examining a badly broken down tooth; however, four basic steps should be taken before finalizing that design and executing it (Fig. 1). They are:

I. Evaluate the P-D organ and the periodontium of the tooth to be restored, preferably before the patient is anesthetized.

II. Remove all undermined enamel. There is no place for such enamel in all permanently restored posterior teeth.

II. Clean all surrounding walls from dentin that is diseased or is otherwise a liability to the mechanical stability of the contemplated restorations.

IV. Treat the pulpal and axial walls with intermediary bases, as previously described in chapters 13 and 14.

Evaluation of Remaining Tooth Structures (Fig. 2)

At this point, the operator must make a mental note of the dimension and nature of the remaining tooth structures mechanically, biologically, and cariogenically (Fig. 3). This is vitally important if the final restoration is to be built up in the most acceptable fashion; i.e., sacrificing the least amount of dental tissues, time and expense, using the most indicated material and technique, and creating the least irritation to dental tissues. To obtain this information, the operator should engage in the following procedure.

I. Recollection of the Stress Pattern in Posterior Teeth and Correlating It to the Remaining Tooth Structure and Conditions

This correlation should emphasize four things. First, is the locations of the tooth in the arch and the opposing items should be noted. Remembering that stresses are maximum at second

premolar and first molar teeth, design features to counteract such stresses should be maximized in restorations for these particular teeth. Remember, too, that stresses are more induced and better resisted in upper than in lower teeth. On the other hand, functional stresses are least in teeth opposing a bridge pontic, a denture, an inclined tooth (if the occluding cusp is not a plunger one) or a space.

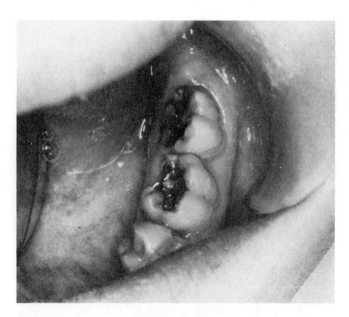

Fig. 28-1

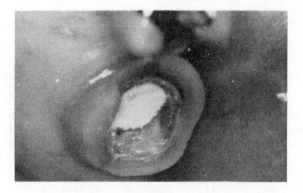

Fig. 28-2

435

Secondly, if the remaining tooth structures contain stress concentration areas (Fig. 4), (e.g., marginal ridges, crossing ridges, cusps, a junction between clinical crown and clinical root, and/or axial angle of the tooth, etc.), the restoration should be designed in a way that will not induce additional stresses at these areas. Every effort should be made to keep these critical areas of the tooth undisturbed by the restorative process. Any weakening or loss of these parts will necessitate drastic design changes.

Third, the functional, non-functional (orbiting), or over-functional cuspal elements should be noted by examining the involved teeth during static and functional mandibular movements. The operator can then recognize the nature of the stresses that can be expected in the remaining tooth structures, especially the occluding ones. From this information (Figs. 2 and 3) a decision can be made about the ability of these parts of the tooth to withstand stresses without failure. If they cannot, these intolerant portions of the tooth should be replaced or protected by appropriate restoration design changes.

The fourth emphasis is that if the remaining tooth structures contain naturally weak areas; e.g., thin dentin bridge, exposed subpulpal floor, nearby bifurcation, cementum, etc., they should be recognized and every effort should be made not to involve them in the mechanical problems of the future restoration, or in the stress pattern of the restored tooth.

II. Diagnosis and Recognition of the Vital Capability of the Tooth or the Part of the Tooth Being Restored

Since non-vitality usually implies hypermineralization and/or dehydration of the tooth dentin, such a decrease in dentin fluids is recognized mechanically by a drop in ultimate strength, an increase in brittleness, and a decrease in modulus of resilience of dentin. This should be differentially diagnosed according to the following criteria.

A. If the tooth is totally non-vital; i.e., endodontically treated, the operator should first confirm all signs and symptoms of successful endodontic therapy as revealed by:

1. An apical seal with complete obliteration of the root canals without under- or overfilling.

2. A lack of radiographically recognizable apical radiolucency, or evidence of a present one being reduced in dimension.

3. A lack of pain during percussion on the tooth.

4. A lack of pain from pressure at the periapex from either the facial or the lingual sulcus.

5. A lack of fistula.

The operator must then recognize the technique used in the root canal treatment including the materials used to obliterate the root canal system. The post-endodontic use of the pulp chamber or root canal system in the retention form of a restoration necessitates different procedures for each technique or material used.

The most important criterion to note is the dimension of the pulp chamber relative to the dimension of the future restoration. Also to be evaluated are the number of the opposing walls in the pulp chamber and their occlusal inclinations and surface dimensions. The closer that the ratio of these dimensions is (i.e., pulp chamber size relative to restoration size) and the more opposing walls with generous surface dimensions there

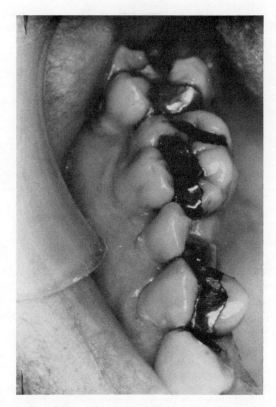

Fig. 28-3

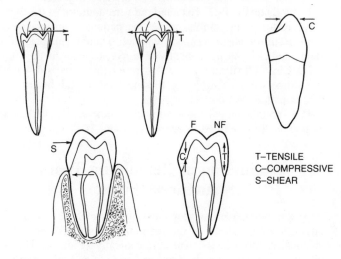

T—TENSILE
C—COMPRESSIVE
S—SHEAR

Fig. 28-4

are, the greater will be the possibility of using the pulp chamber as a principal retention form for the future restoration.

Furthermore, the more root canals there are, the greater will be the possibility of using some of them to accommodate auxillary, anti-rotation, and reciprocal means of retention. Such canals are easier to incorporate into the restorative design when their shapes are more regular and they are more readily accessible from their pulpal orifices. Of course, the larger that the diameter of the root canal is, the better will be its chances of accommodating a restorative material as a retentive extension from the restorations.

The second most important criterion to diagnose and evaluate with regard to a non-vital tooth is the bulk of the remaining tooth structure surrounding the opening of the root canal. As mentioned before, this is an area of maximum stresses. If, indeed, the root canals are to be used as retention modes, the more bulk that they have at this location, the safer will be the use of these root canals as retention modes.

B. If only parts of the tooth are non-vital (e.g., dead-tract areas), they, too, should be recognized so the operator can avoid locating retention modes there. This will eliminate the possibility of cracking or fracture failure. If anatomically possible, non-vital areas should be prepared such that they are surrounded by flat floors and ledges.

C. If parts of the tooth are only partially vital (e.g., calcific barrier, sclerosed dentin, and tertiary dentin), they, too, should be recognized as areas unacceptable for housing retention modes. If it is absolutely unavoidable to locate retention modes there, the least stressing modes should be prepared and used. However, they must be augmented with more retaining reciprocal and adjacent retention modes. Such augmenting modes should involve fully vital tooth dentin in addition to the partially vital areas.

In reality, non-vital and partially vital dentin in an otherwise vital tooth is usually located far inside the cavity (tooth) preparation close to the pulp and root canal system where retention modes are contraindicated anyway.

III. Cariogenic Evaluation of Remaining Tooth Structures

This should proceed according to the principles mentioned in the descriptions of outline form. This will help decide which areas of the remaining tooth structure are to be involved in the tooth preparation.

IV. Correlative Three-Dimensional Evaluation

The operator should carefully study the radiographs as well as make a physical examination of the tooth to have a good idea about the dimension and nature of remaining enamel and dentin and their relation to invested pulp chamber and root canal system. This evaluation will also assist the operator in correlating the pulp system to the surface configuration of the crown and root surfaces, the investing periodontal tissues, and the surrounding musculature.

V. Possibilities, Locations, and Dimensions of Resisting Flat Planes

It is necessary to always be on the lookout for the possibility of creating flat planes in the remaining tooth structure at right angles to the direction of the occlusal loading, without compromising the tooth biologically (Fig. 5). This is the most effective resistance form in a tooth preparation for any restorative material. To be maximally resistant, flat planes should have bulky tooth structure apical to them, as this will dilute and properly resist induced stresses. This is why the ideal location for these planes is in the tooth structure peripheral to the pulp chamber and root canal system, where the tooth structure apical to these flat planes can extend as far as the root tip or at least the closest furcation. Also, the closer these planes

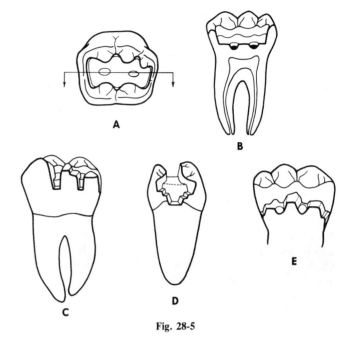

Fig. 28-5

are to the occlusal surfaces, the greater will be their bulk. The more surface area of these flat planes that there is, and the closer they are to the applied forces, the more efficient will be their resisting capability. However, any dimension or location for these planes is acceptable. They should be part of the tooth preparation as their effect is cumulative. These flat planes can be in one or more of the following forms:

A. Pulpal floor (Fig. 5, A and B)

Although it is always at the regular depth (0.5 mm from the DEJ), forming part of the peripheries of the tooth preparation, it can and should be prepared at different levels. This design feature will be advantageous from the standpoints of both retention and tooth structure conservation.

B. Gingival floors (Fig. 5, C and D)

These always form one or more of the lateral peripheries of a tooth preparation, taking full advantage of the tooth structure bulk apical to their location. They, too, can and should be formed of different levels in three dimensions (proximo-axially, bucco-lingually, and gingivo-occlusally).

Both pulpal and gingival floors should ideally be entirely flat. However, this is a situation that is anatomically not feasible in most cases of badly broken down teeth. The next logical choice, then, is a peripherally flat circumference, or at least flat in two opposite areas, leaving the rest of the floor in whatever shape it was left in by the destruction (Fig. 5, A and B).

C. Tables (Fig. 5C)

These flat planes are to be located in areas of reduced (or completely lost) cusps, axial angles, marginal ridges, or crossing ridges. Again, they may be formed in different levels.

D. Ledges and shelves (Fig. 5E)

These are flat planes prepared in bulky lateral surrounding walls, usually reciprocating with one or more flat planes to achieve stability and proper resistance. They are always indicated where one of the previously mentioned flat planes is either not opposed to another flat plane, or cannot otherwise be prepared.

VI. Crazing

The presence of craze line continuous with the peripheries of the destruction or the contemplated preparation margins (Fig. 48) can be the precursor for partial or complete fracture of the tooth. This is the reason why they should be diagnosed and properly evaluated before any restorative attempts.

Although there is no age limitation for the incidence of these crazings (microcracking), they are usually found in older people, where the tooth has been hypermineralized and dehydrated. In many instances they are found in teeth that have been either subjected to previous restorative procedures, or endodontically treated, or subjected to trauma. If such microcracks are suspected but not seen, it may be necessary to use a special dye applied on the doubtful area with small cotton pellets (e.g., red or blue dyes, mercurochrome, tincture of iodine, and fluorescent dyes).

If the presence of microcracks is confirmed, the operator must evaluate their nature and effect by first looking for any signs and symptoms of a cracked-tooth syndrome (incomplete tooth fracture), e.g., history of pain simulating that of combined pulpitis and periodontitis. It may be possible to elicit pain by trying to separate part of the tooth with applied pressure using a mirror handle, orange wood stick, or inlay seater. Pain on percussion or commencement of pain by pressing the tip of a sharp explorer into one of the discovered cracks (see section on trauma in a chapter on non-carious destruction of teeth) are quite diagnostic.

If cracked-tooth syndrome is confirmed, further evaluation of the cracks is unnecessary, for the treatment will involve them all without any discrimination. However, if it is not confirmed, then simply counting the number of microcracks adjacent to the (contemplated) preparation margins facilitates restorative design decisions. If the cracks are numerous (more than 5-6), the treatment will be the same as for cracked-tooth syndrome, but if there are only a few (less than 5-6/area) in contact with the preparation margin, investigate their extent and involvement to see if they are confined to enamel, involve underlying dentin, or penetrate to the pulp tissues and periodontium.

VII. Surface Deformities

If surface defects or decalcifications are present, adjacent to either the peripheries of the destruction or to the anticipated margins of the preparation, the need to involve these defects in the tooth preparation or restore them separately should be decided. The decision to involve them will depend on their size, the possibility of self-retention of a restoration in a separate preparation for them, and the possibility of the preparation being extended to involve them without drastic modifications and involvement of sound tooth structures.

VIII. Proximal Drifting of Tooth Due to its Own Tissue Loss

A loss in mesio-distal dimension of the dental arch to an extent that the arch will no longer accommodate the broken

down tooth restored to its natural dimensions, contour, and contact-occluding interrelationship (Fig. 6, A and B), necessitates one of two treatment modifications.

First, the possibility of restoring the tooth to a reduced dimension should be explored; e.g., making a bicuspid out of a tricuspid premolar. Before making such a decision, the operator should be confident that the newly anticipated contouring, contacting, and occluding tooth components will be physiologic and non-interfering with the biologic and cariogenic soundness of the surrounding tooth structures. Although it is not a recommended procedure, restoring teeth to reduced di-

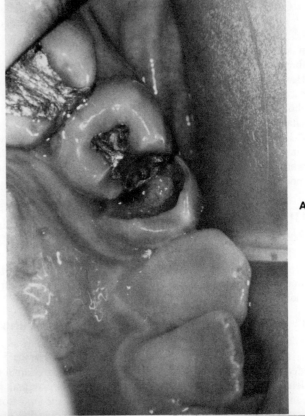

A

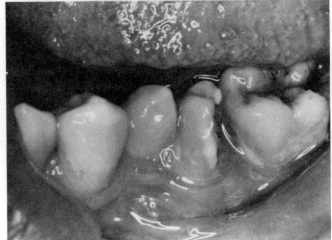

B

Fig. 28-6

mensions can be done for teeth with a doubtful prognosis and/ or for teeth that have drifted minimally. On the other extreme, such a procedure can be used on extensively drifted teeth that are beyond repositioning.

ecHowever, trying to restore a tooth in such a situation can be a futile experience. The proper axial contour and adequate contact areas, as well as the indicated occluding surface components, will seldom be achieved without moving the tooth (teeth) back to their normally indicated positions, thereby regaining the mesio-distal dimension of the dental arch. This is the *second* and most sound *alternative,* i.e. regain the lost space. If this is contemplated, the operator should evaluate:

A. The distance the tooth must travel to arrive at its original location.

B. The number of teeth and their roots to be moved (especially the overall root surface area).

C. The amount of interceptal bone between the teeth (roots).

There are innumerable ways to achieve such tooth movement. If the tooth in question is the only one to be moved and/ or the drifting distance is slight (up to 2 mm), and it has the proper amount of interceptal bone, then wood wedges, over-contoured temporary restorations, or separating wires can be used (as mentioned in the chapter on contact and contour) to effect the necessary relocation. However, if space loss involves more than the tooth and/or it is a sizable distance, but with sufficient interceptal bone intervening (more than 2 mm), orthodontic tooth movement could be undertaken, using a variety of appliance designs, to move the tooth (teeth) according to the diagnostic criteria you have just collected. E.g., decide on the most acceptable direction of movement, solidify the segment of the arch opposite to that direction by brackets and arch wire (labial and/or lingual arches). Then cut a coil spring 2-3 mm longer than the dimension you need to regain. Place the arch wire through it and force it to stay between the brackets of the teeth to be moved and the closest tooth of the anchor segment. Periodic activation of the coil spring is needed (Fig. 6C). Removable appliances can be used with retractors, anchored to the base of the appliance.

If the drifting results in root-to-root contact or if it is beyond orthodontic therapy, the tooth in question should be removed if it is single-rooted. If it is multirooted, it may be hemisectioned, leaving intact the bony supported segment to be restored to a reduced dimension.

REGAINING LOST MESIO-DISTAL DIMENSION

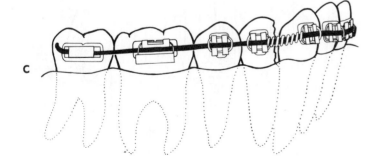

c

IX. Gingival Margin Location Relative to the Periodontium Components (Fig. 7)

The gingival peripheries of the destruction should be recorded, and the gingival margins of the contemplated restoration should be decided upon (see chapter on single tooth restoration and the periodontium). If the gingival limit of the destruction is located supra-gingivally, even with the free gingiva, or within the gingival crevice, and the adjacent periodontium has adequate width of attached gingiva and fornex depth, no change in the periodontium is needed to maintain the periodontium. Regular procedures (as mentioned in the chapter on single tooth restoration and periodontium) should be followed. If the gingiva covering the apical end of the tooth destruction is hyperplastic, a gingivectomy (usually using electrosurge) may be performed, in order to expose the apical limits of the defect.

If the gingival limitation of the destruction is apical to the bottom of the gingival crevice, but still suprabony, the width of the attached gingiva (for facial and lingual defects) and the occluso-apical thickness of the interdental papillae (for proximal defects) should be evaluated relative to the attaching (den-to-gingival) epithelium and the apical limit of the defect. If sufficient width of the attached gingiva or thickness of the interdental papillae is verified, the apical limit of the defect can be exposed by gingivectomy procedures without changing the artchitectural contour of the surrounding periodontium. However, if gingivectomy procedures would unfavorably affect the peridontium, a full thickness muco-gingival flap should be reflected, so that the entire periodontal apparatus may be repositioned and reattached apical to the gingival limit of the defect.

When the apical limitation of the destruction is infrabony, yet there can be sufficient bone support for the tooth after the bone occlusal to the apical limit of the defect is removed,

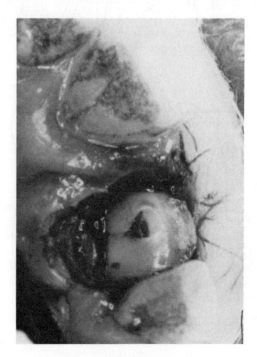

Fig. 28-7

together with enough bone to create a 2-3 mm attaching epithelial zone with sound tooth surface apical to the apical limit of the destruction, a full thickness muco-gingival flap is again utilized, exposing the indicated site and amount of bone to be removed by osteoectomy. Again the reflected flap is re-attached apical to the gingival limit of the defect.

If the apical end of the defect is infrabony, but osteoectomy and apical repositioning of the investing periodontal apparatus component cannot be performed due to insufficient supporting bone or fear of exposing important anatomy, etc., *intentional extrusion* of the tooth may be attempted in order to expose the apical end of the destruction supragingivally, facilitating restoration of the tooth. There are several methods for accomplishing this:

If the tooth is endodontically treated, wire hooks can be temporarily cemented within the root canals, so that each hook protrudes from the tooth occlusally. The tooth is moved occlusally using a rubber elastic attached on one side to the hook(s) and on the other side to any anchoring device, maintaining the pulling forces parallel to the long axis of the tooth being extruded. The anchoring device can be either a heavy

wire crossing over the tooth and attached to occlusal (incisal) surfaces of adjacent teeth (Fig. 8A), or a hawley appliance, or brackets attached to the adjacent teeth, or brackets attached to opposing teeth (Fig. 8B).

If the involved tooth is vital, facial or lingual brackets (with or without bands) should be attached close to the gingival line of the tooth. The adjacent teeth (at least one on each side) should each have a bracket, but located more incisally (occlusally) on the facial or lingual surfaces. Elastic bands are hooked to the brackets in a way to be located apical to the bracket of the tooth to be extruded (Fig. 8C).

If the tooth is vital, but does not have enough facial or lingual surfaces to accommodate a bracket, cemented or threaded pins with hooks may be inserted in the deepest portions apically. The anchorage can be any of those previously mentioned. Elastic bands are hooked to both the anchorage device and the hooked pins in the tooth to be extruded (Fig. 8D).

In all situations the occlusal (incisal) surfaces should be periodically adjusted to make room for sufficient extrusion, until the apical termination of the destruction appears supragingivally. Also, the anchorage should be planned, so that the movement will occur to the affected tooth, not to the anchoring ones. The extruded teeth should be evaluated as any periodontally affected and treated teeth. As the surface topography

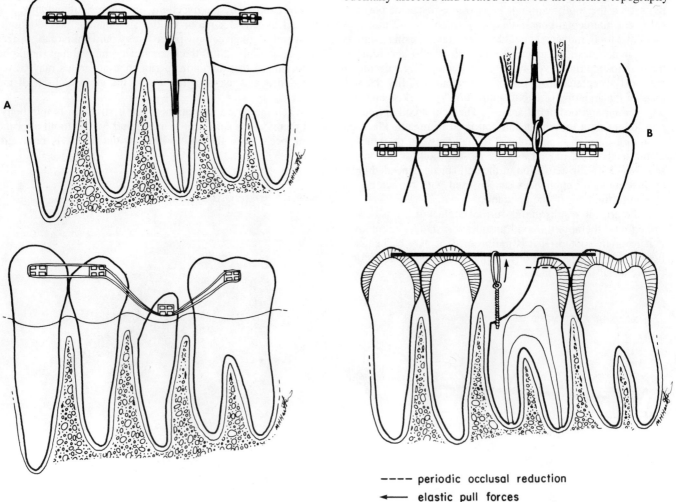

---- periodic occlusal reduction
◄— elastic pull forces

Fig. 28-8

of the new clinical crown and the stress pattern in the tooth and the involved periodontium will be similar.

In any of the previously mentioned situations, if the depth of the facial or lingual vestibule is not physiologically deep enough, i.e., partially or totally depriving the peridontium of its attached gingiva, restoring defects at these areas will be doomed to failure from periodontal and/or cariogenic breakdown. Sulcular deepening may be performed to obtain the indicated fornex depth and attached gingiva dimension.

X. Badly Broken Down Teeth Whose Periodontium Has Been Affected and Treated

When restoring badly broken down teeth that have undergone periodontal therapy, the operator can expect to confront one of several problems in the remaining tooth structures.

First, he may encounter the exposure of unusual anatomy, due either to the healing recession of the gingiva or as a result of the disease process. These unusual anatomies for a crown surface can be in the form of concavities (Fig. 9), flat surfaces, deep grooves, and/or flutes. Each will necessitate modifications in the usual features of the preparation if they approximate the area of destruction.

Second, a furcation exposure (Fig. 10), ranging from a simple exposure of the occlusal flutes to the furca proper to through-through connection between two opposite furcations, will necessitate special design features, if involved in the area of destruction.

Third, because of bone loss, there may be a biologically negative crown to root ratio (Fig. 11), challenging the resistance of the tooth and the contemplated restoration.

Fourth, because of the taper of the root, if a proximal lesion is present, the tooth preparation will have a very thin dentin bridge axially, endangering the status of the P-D organ (Fig. 12).

Fifth, for the same reasons just mentioned, the gingival floor for a proximal preparation in the root portion will be very narrow, minimizing its resistance-retention capabilities (Fig. 12).

Sixth, because of the root taper and presence of surface concavities there, preparing the tooth for a cast restoration can be nearly impossible, or, at the very least, involve a consid-

erable amount of tooth structures occlusal to the root portion in an attempt to remove undercuts in the preparation.

Seventh, periodontally treated teeth may have been affected by primary or secondary traumatism which may still be present at this stage of therapy. Any traumatism or its symptoms should be corrected by the restorative procedure or intercepted prior to the restoration, with the indicated occlusal equilibration.

Eighth, periodontally affected and treated teeth will have multiple facets at the contact area and/or occlusal surfaces, which may accompany mesio-distal and occluso-apical loss of tooth structure. These facets should be involved in a tooth preparation if any margin comes close to them. They may complicate reproduction of contact and contour in the final restoration.

Ninth, because of uneven bone loss accompanied by gingival recession, two opposing axial portions of a destruction and preparation may not have symmetrical lengths in their axial walls. Consequently, the locations of the gingival floors (margins) at the opposite axial surfaces will be uneven (Fig. 12). This situation may create imbalance in the resistance and retention form, necessitating modifications to increase the length of the short side of the restoration; e.g., gingival pin.

Tenth, a missing adjacent tooth (teeth) is a usual occurrence with dentitions affected by periodontal diseases. This situation leads to numerous modifications in the restorative design, e.g., use of the involved teeth as an abutment for a prosthesis. Also, loss of teeth can lead to tilting, rotation, extrusion, or drifting of teeth with the predictable sequelae necessitating modifications in the restorative design.

Eleventh, the supereruption of teeth (Fig. 13), although not always a result of periodontal problems, usually occurs as a

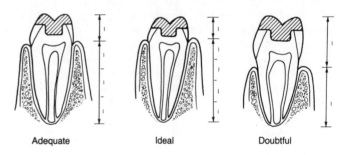

Adequate Ideal Doubtful

Fig. 28-11

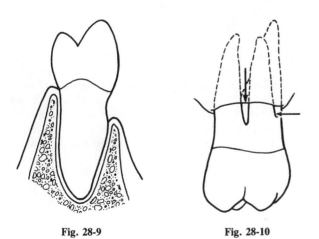

Fig. 28-9   **Fig. 28-10**

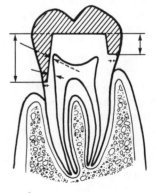

Fig. 28-12

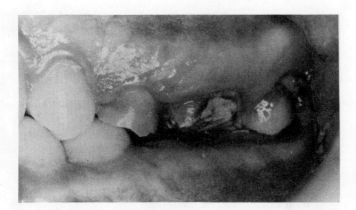

Fig. 28-13

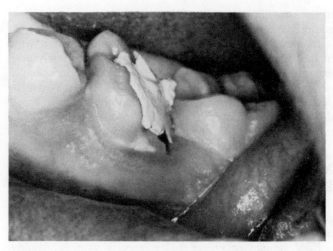

Fig. 28-14

result of the loss of opposing tooth (teeth). Supereruption can complicate presented problems by:

A. Necessitating the reduction of the involved tooth occlusally.

B. Requiring replacement of opposing missing teeth to prevent further extrusion.

C. Exposing an extruded tooth furcation and root surfaces.

D. Causing changes in the location and the nature of the contact areas.

E. Creating a biologically negative crown root ratio.

F. Causing the usual resistance, retention, and P-D organ problems associated with elongated clinical crowns.

Twelfth, the periodontium will require more than the usual care, as plaque control is made more difficult by exposure of the root surface anatomy.

Thirteenth, tipping of cusps or an entire tooth as a result of the loss of the mesio-distal dimension (Fig. 14), missing or loose-movement of adjacent teeth, can change occluding and contacting characteristics of the tooth, putting it at a disadvantage from the resistance point of view. Therefore, teeth should be moved back to their physiologic position and/or interfering cuspal elements should be selectively ground before restoring them.

Fourteenth, loose teeth can not only complicate instrumentation, but may also necessitate future splinting, possibly in the contemplated restoration.

Fifteenth is the possibility of *hemisectioning* or root amputation of a periodontally affected multirooted tooth. Hemisectioning is a procedure by which a segment of a multi-rooted tooth, which is confirmed unrestorable or periodontally affected beyond repair, is removed, leaving a sound restorable part of the tooth. It may be indicated for multi-rooted teeth, in situations of severe bone loss (less than ¼ normal bone support is left) that is confined to less than all the roots; when severe root decay is confined to less than all the roots of the tooth; and when proximal drifting of the multi-rooted tooth with complete loss of the interceptal bone results in root-to-root contact between adjacent teeth. It is also indicated for teeth with very subgingivally (infrabony) located decay restricted to ½ or less of the tooth, wherein surgical or extrusion exposure of the apical limit of the decay is not feasible.

Hemisectioning can be done in the following sequential steps:

1. Root canal therapy must be performed first.

2. With a long-shanked cylindrical round-ended diamond stone or carbide bur separate the indicated root(s) from the intact part of the tooth through the corresponding furcation (Fig. 15). As much as possible, trim the tooth structure lip formed by removal of the furcation there.

3. Extract the unwanted separated root(s).

4. One may need to make a flap opening to the area to do some osseous contouring, root planning for the kept root(s), and curettage. Close the operation area, using sutures and a periodontal pack.

5. The remaining tooth portion may need a temporary restoration and provisional splinting until periodontal healing is completed.

When it comes to restoring the remaining parts of the hemisectioned tooth (around 3-4 months after, for complete epithelialization of the periodontium), certain evaluations will dictate the restorative design.

If the remaining tooth portion is in the form of a bicuspid (lower molars missing one root or upper molars missing two roots) or a narrow elongated molar (upper molars missing lingual root), or a triangular table (upper molars missing mesio-buccal or disto-buccal roots), the final restoration must be in that same shape. Moreover, the occlusal configuration should be related to the underlying bone support and root structures, as areas of the newly created clinical crown to be stressed in the restorative design should be well supported by the underlying resisting root bone complex.

The location and type of the sectioning lip must be noted, as the gingival margin of the restoration should cover it. Usually, after the hemisection, the remaining tooth portions will need a foundation prior to a final restoration. As the hemisected tooth is usually to be used as an abutment, at least to replace the missed portion of the tooth, it should be evaluated as any abutment tooth.

Sixteenth, dimensions of newly created embrasures is at its maximum. A situation that may be necessary for proper plaque control but may be predisposing to further periodontitis if not restored or maintained properly.

Seventeenth, the possibility of *bicuspidization* should be

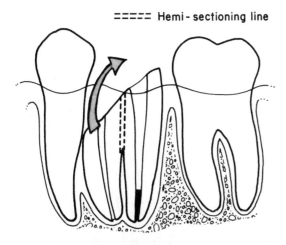

===== Hemi-sectioning line

Fig. 28-15

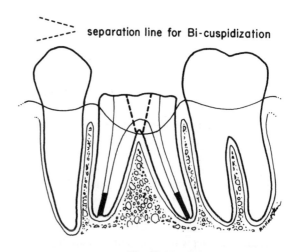

- - - - - separation line for Bi-cuspidization

Fig. 28-16

evaluated as a viable procedure by which, for example, a double-rooted molar tooth is sectioned in the middle to create two bicuspids. The procedure is indicated for:

a. Teeth with deep uncleansable exposed furcation(s).

b. Unresolved horizontal pockets in the mesio-distal direction or facio-lingual direction, accompanying a furca involvement.

c. Apical furcation decay.

d. Divergent roots with sufficient intraradicular bone to be the future interceptal bone of the created bicuspids.

If the space between the two sections of the tooth is not enough to allow for adequate axial contour, contacts, and embrasures for future restorations, look for the possibility of orthodontic separation of the bicuspidized molar segments. This will necessitate:

i. A space between the separated teeth parts and adjacent teeth with sufficient interceptal bone there.

ii. Favorable root(s) inclination and anatomy as related to its (their) movability by orthodontic means.

iii. The availability of anchorage sites.

From this, the type of orthodontic appliance, the amount of forces and their direction, and time to accomplish the desired separation for proper contact and contour of the formed bicuspids are decided.

The bicuspidization procedure can be done in the following steps:

A. Root canal therapy for the indicated tooth is performed.

B. With a long-shanked, round-ended (nose-ended) cylindrical diamond stone or carbide bur cross the tooth at its indicated furcation, involving the lesion if present there and removing the sectioning tooth structure lip(s) (Fig. 16).

C. A provisional temporary restoration splinting the two separated segments of the tooth is constructed and cemented in place.

D. Flap operation for the involved area may be needed to eradicate the remaining part of the pockets. In addition, there may be some osseous contouring, root planning, and curettage, followed by suture and periodontal packs.

E. After removal of sutures and packs, the periodontium is left to heal and epithelialize with the temporary provisional splinting restoration in place.

F. If orthodontic separation is indicated, the two bicuspids are banded and separated by springy devices or dragged toward banded adjacent teeth with elastic bands.

After healing and creation of sufficient space the two created bicuspids are evaluated as any periodontally affected and treated tooth with emphasis on:

1. The type of embrasures to be created between them and between each one and the adjacent tooth, as they should be conforming to the newly created periodontium and attachments.

2. The type of occlusion (statically and functionally) on the created bicuspids and accordingly the possible stress pattern, so the restoration design will be conforming and resisting.

Restorations for periodontally treated teeth can be done only if:

a. The periodontium did heal as symptomatized by:

i. The free gingivae stopped receding. They are firm and properly cuffing the tooth.

ii. Attached gingivae are intact and pronounced.

iii. No measurable pocket and no gingival bleeding.

iv. No indication of further bone loss.

v. No indication of occlusal traumatism.

vi. Oral hygiene and plaque accumulation is well under control.

b. The periodontium is in the process of proper healing.

c. The restoration(s) is (are) needed to facilitate and/or promote the healing of the periodontium.

Mechanical Evaluation of Lost Tooth Structure Preparatory to Designing the Retention-Resistance Features of the Tooth Preparations

During this portion of the pre-operative evaluation, the operator must envision the restoration replacing lost tooth structures being subjected to functional loading, and then try to plan the best tooth preparation to both retain this restoration and make it resistant to these loads. Certain criteria must be considered here.

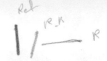

I. The Dimension and Nature of the Destruction Relative to that of the Tooth

Occluso-apical destruction presents more retention than resistance problems, as the restoration build-up in a longitudinal direction definitely encounters displacing forces. Bucco-lingual and mesio-distal destructions pose both resistance and retention problems. This is because, in addition to the loss of tooth structure, decreasing the substance for housing retention modes, a large surface area of the restoration will be subjected to displacing loads, while remaining thinned tooth substance will be less resistant to the direct loading.

The loss of the stress concentration area of a tooth poses a major resistance problem necessitating certain restorative design features. Naturally, the area should house "self-resistance" features for the replacing part of the restoration. These include bulk, slanting wall angulations toward the fulcrum, flat floors, and proper fulcrum features for the center of the restoration.

In addition, the restoration should be designed in the stress concentration area so as not to encounter additional stresses from retaining *other* parts of the restoration, or stemming from additional forces directly applied there. Finally, special retention features should be added to the stress concentration area in the form of nearby "immobilizing modes". These serve to decrease micromovement of the restoration thereby sparing this part of the restoration any additional stresses resulting from such movements.

II. Partial or Complete Loss of a Cusp

After removing all undermined enamel, a cusp should be evaluated in the following sequence:

A. Is it functional or non-functional? (This is an arbitrary nomenclature, as each type is stressed in a different way and pattern.) Generally, replacing a non-functional cusp poses more resistance-retention problems than replacing a functional cusp. As mentioned before, the stresses in the non-functional cusps are more displacing and destructive than on the functional cusp.

B. What are the types (working or balancing) of cuspal inclined planes involved in the destruction? Generally, the nature of loading on the working incline is much more than on the balancing incline.

C. What is the width of the destruction (loss) relative to the intercuspal distance? This is the most important measurement. (It should be measured in the bucco-lingual directions in all posterior teeth and in the bucco-lingual and mesio-distal directions in posterior teeth having more than one cusp facially and/or lingually [Fig. 17].) As mentioned before, at conventional depths (1.5-2 mm), the loss of width can be detrimental to the resistance form of the remaining portion of the cusps if it exceeds ⅓ to ½ the intercuspal distance. This situation is aggravated in a deeper preparation. It is in these cases that protective resisting measures should be introduced into the restorative design. Usually, horizontal structural loss is deviated toward one cusp more than the other (Fig. 18). This situation should be noted, as only the cusp toward which the destruction is deviated may need additional design changes.

D. The bucco-lingual partial loss of a cusp from the occlusal direction can create both resistance and retention problems that need to be solved in the restorative design. This is due to the increased exposure of the restoration to loading and to less cusp bulk remaining for self-resistance.

E. The mesio-distal partial loss of a cusp, if not accompanied by bucco-lingual loss, can only pose resistance problems. These stem from exposing part or all of the restorations' mesial and/or distal inclined cuspal planes to direct loading.

F. The occluso-apical partial loss of a cusp usually creates retention problem with slight resistance problem. This type of loss actually decreases the resistance problems in the remaining

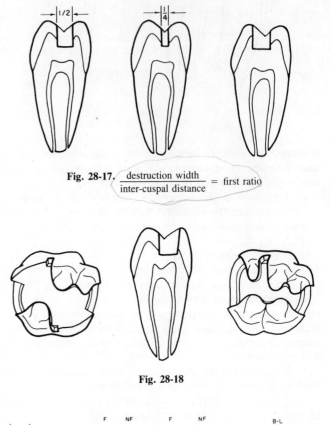

Fig. 28-17. $\dfrac{\text{destruction width}}{\text{inter-cuspal distance}}$ = first ratio

Fig. 28-18

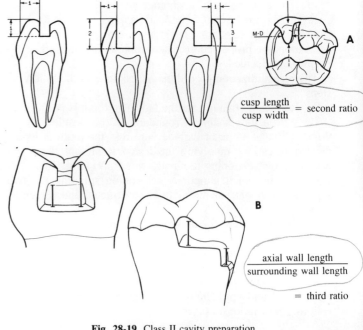

$\dfrac{\text{cusp length}}{\text{cusp width}}$ = second ratio

$\dfrac{\text{axial wall length}}{\text{surrounding wall length}}$

= third ratio

Fig. 28-19. Class II cavity preparation

cuspal tooth structures due to the indirect loading of the remaining cuspal elements.

G. The length of the remaining part of the cusp relative to its width, is the second most important measurement (Fig. 19A). The ideal ratio for this measurement is one or less. Usually, if the ratio exceeds two, cuspal protections and reinforcing measures should be incorporated in the restorative design, especially when using restorative materials stronger than the tooth structure.

H. In restorations involving two or more surfaces, the occluso-gingival length of the axial wall relative to that of the surrounding walls, should be in a ratio of 1:2 or more (Fig. 19B). Anything less will seriously compromise retention and resistance.

I. The complete loss of a cusp (Fig. 20) imposes major retention and resistance problems for the restoration. The resulting restorative design should include all features required in replacing a stress concentration area.

J. Cusp loss (partial or complete), complicated by loss(es) of other stress concentration areas or parts of areas (Fig. 20) should be recognized and recorded. In this situation, the operator's clinical judgement, experience, and imagination should lead to the following objectives:

1. Retention-resistance modes at different areas of the preparation not counteracting or neutralizing each other

2. If possible, immobilizing retention modes next to a lost stress concentration area, reciprocating with a retention mode for the same means of immobilization in another lost stress concentration area, e.g., two opposing proximal grooves next to two opposing lost cusps

3. If anatomically possible, two or more lost stress concentration areas having the same principal, auxillary, and/or reciprocal means of retention, e.g., an external box between two lost facial cusps in a molar

4. Preparing retention-resistance modes for one area so as not to impinge on the self-resistant bulk of another involved or uninvolved area (see chapter on Class II)

5. If the final restoration involves two or more stress concentration areas, retention modes for one stress concentration area should not immobilize the restoration there more than the retention modes for another stress concentration area and the vice versa should also be observed, as the part with less immobilization will have its micromovement extremely exaggerated, even if its modes are quite sufficient for its own potential movement. Overimmobilization for one area can direct stresses to the closest stress concentration area in the restoration.

III. Partial or Complete Loss of a Marginal or Crossing Ridge (Fig. 21)

As these ridges are the belting elements between the buccal and lingual cusps, they should be observed from several aspects:

The *width* of the partial loss, relative to the intercuspal distance, is the most important measurement for these anatomical landmarks. It is closely associated with the same measurement in cusp loss, and should be compared prior to planning a restorative design. The closer that the ratios are, the greater will be the chances of having the same treatment. However, the farther apart that the ratios are, the more will be the necessity for *different* design features for the cusps than for the ridges. Generally speaking, the more that the horizontal loss of the ridge is, especially at a depth more than 2 mm, the more the resistance and retention problems for the previously ridge held cuspal elements will be. In any event, whatever the crossing destruction width for these ridges, the reinforcing-and-protecting measures should be part of the same measures applied to adjacent connected cuspal elements.

Bucco-lingual deviation of the partial ridge loss, toward functional or non-functional cuspal elements (i.e., leaving more bulk of the ridge toward the opposite side), is an important observation to make in order to correlate with the adjacent cusp's width to length ratio. The cuspal width dimension, in the form of a ridge, is more of a positive sign for self-resistance than the same dimension in a non-ridge area. This is because of the tooth structure thickening in such an area.

Thinned ridges in the mesial and/or distal direction (crossing

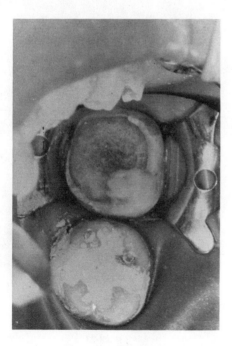

Fig. 28-20

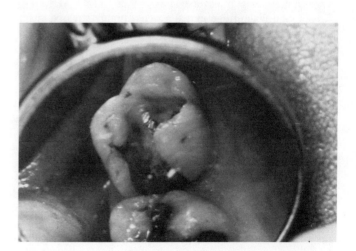

Fig. 28-21

and proximal marginal ridges) and in the facial and/or lingual direction (facial and lingual marginal ridge) is a situation most often observed in occlusally attacked ridges. Generally speaking, intact and even thickness of ridges are important to maintain in any dimensions, as there is a drastic drop in the self-resistance of adjacent cuspal elements when they are lost, Also, the amount of thinning in three directions is very influential in shaping the self-resistance of the ridge as well as the combined cuspal elements. Because of all of these factors, the following criteria should help decide how to handle thinned ridges:

A. If the thinned parts of the marginal ridges are not involved in occluding contact during centric and functional relations, any thickness as low as 0.5 mm is adequate, provided the cavity depth at that point does not exceed 2 mm, and the adjacent axial surface is intact.

B. If the thinned part of a marginal ridge comes in contact with opposing cuspal elements during centric or excursive relations, it should have at least 1.5-2 thickness at its thinnest cross-section which is always at its occlusal or pulpal ends. If it is thinner than that, it should be crossed.

C. In cases of oblique and transverse ridges, even if they are in static or dynamic occlusal contact, do not cross them unless they are as thin as 0.2 mm, provided the cavity depth at that point does not exceed 2 mm.

D. If the conditions mentioned above are not satisfied, and if it is necessary to cross the ridge, the crossing should be confined to the thinnest portion only, if this places the created cavity margins in self-cleansable areas. Otherwise, it is necessary to include more of the ridge to satisfy these basic principles.

E. The crossing depth should be confined to the minimum thickness of the restorative material that can be self-resistant (e.g., 1.5 mm in amalgam and 0.5 mm for cast alloy). Furthermore, the ridge thickness or length: width ratio of 1 should be achieved without consideration to the depth of the rest of the preparation. This latter feature may be used provided it will locate the gingival margin of the preparation (in case of proximal marginal ridges) at a self-cleansable area and will not interfere with the retention features of the final restoration.

F. If anatomically feasible, in place of a partially or totally crossed ridge, leave an elevation of tooth structure (struss) connecting separated cusps and remaining segments of the ridge to help resist transverse stresses (see Class I, Design 4). This is vital if the ridge joined a weak, highly stressed cuspal element with a stronger, bulkier one.

G. Complete loss of the ridge is usually accompanied by critical intercuspal dimensions of the destruction as well as a high cusp length-to-width ratio. It necessitates reinforcing-protective features previously described.

H. Ridge loss (partial or complete), complicated by loss of other stress concentration areas, requires the operator to follow the same criteria as for the partial or complete loss of a cusp.

IV. Partial or Complete Loss of Axial Angle(s)

This creates major resistance problems for the contemplated restoration and remaining tooth structures. This is not only because the axial angles are the place for the most concentrated and deleterious stresses, but also it is fairly difficult to immobilize the restoration there without involving adjacent tooth

parts externally. This situation may complicate the stress situation more. It (they) should be examined and evaluated in the following order (Figs. 20, 22, and 23).

A. Is the involved axial angle at the functional or non-functional side? Since more mechanical problems can be expected on the non-functional side axial angles than the functional side ones, more stress concentration features should be introduced in the preparation design on the non-functional side.

B. What is the location of loss relative to the rest of the axial angle? (This includes terminal partial loss or midway partial loss.) Terminal loss(es) (Fig. 23), especially at the oc-

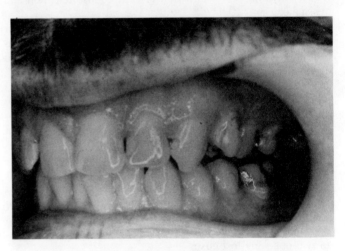

Fig. 28-22

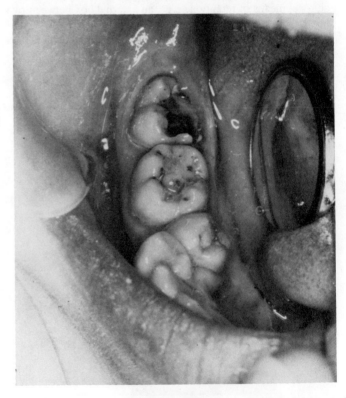

Fig. 28-23

clusal end, are more detrimental than midway loss(es) (Fig. 22). This is because a restoration replacing an occlusally lost axial angle will definitely be a part of an occluding cuspal element, with substantial direct loading at this critical area. Also, a restoration replacing an apically lost axial angle will be subjected to maximum shear loads, both on the functional and non-functional side. These loads, if not completely displacing the restoration, at least challenge the resistance form at that location. In addition, terminally located axial angle portions of a restoration, especially occlusally, are more difficult to retain than midway portions. This is because in the occluso-gingival direction they have tooth structure on one side only (occlusally or gingivally).

C. What is the dimension of the loss?

1. A loss in the occluso-apical direction is the most detrimental in terms of resistance form. The more that the involvement is in this direction, the less will be the resistance of the future restoration, necessitating more drastic tooth design changes to protect more of the stress concentration area.

2. Loss in a pulpal direction is biologically and anatomically the most detrimental. From these aspects it can be hazardous if it is close to the pulp chamber (mesio-buccal), the tooth is multi-rooted, it is accompanied by substantial occluso-apical loss, and/or the adjacent pulp chamber or root canals are large.

3. Loss in the horizontal direction is the least detrimental, as most of the involvement of the axial angles includes the entire axial angle in this direction.

4. Complete loss of the axial angle (Fig. 24) sometimes occurs. If the tooth preparation is to end occlusally at that location, i.e., with the occlusal termination of the clinical root, it is always accompanied by partial or complete loss of adjacent cusp; it should be handled in the same way in terms of design changes.

V. Cavity Preparation Depth, Pulpally, Axially and Gingivally

This should be observed not only because of the biological importance (pulp-dentin and periodontium organs), but also because of its influence on the number and locations of different levels for the pulpal floor, axial walls, and gingival floors. In addition, depth is very critical in deciding on the desirability of protecting/reinforcing features for the adjacent cusps or ridges, as well as the design of such features.

VI. The Junction Between the Clinical Crown and the Clinical Root

In evaluating this area, the operator should observe the following in relation to the future restoration and the restored tooth (Fig. 25):

A. Is the crown-root junction partially involved in the parameters of the destruction, or is this involvement necessitated for biologic and cariogenic reasons? If this is the case, one can expect resistance problems in both the restoration and remaining tooth structure there, necessitating the previously described restorative design features of a stress concentration area. The stress situation there will be aggravated by decrease of bulk in the remaining tooth structure in one or more of the three possible directions at the area of involvement. The most detrimental loss is axially (toward the pulp chamber and root canals), thinning the tooth structure in the direction of maximum shear stresses, which are the most lethal to the tooth substances mechanically.

B. If the parameters of the future restoration do not involve the true junction, how far from that junction will the closest margin of the restoration be?

C. When confronted with partial involvement of the clinical root-clinical crown junction, where are any nearby areas in the remaining tooth structure in which to locate immobilizing modes?

D. If the tooth preparation comes close to this junction, retention modes for the future restoration should not be inserted there.

E. In case of three dimensional complete loss of the crown-root junction (i.e., the occlusal periphery of the remaining tooth structures are levelled with the gingival margins), any retention modes should be placed inside the root substance and a newly created junction between a clinical crown, almost completely formed of restorative material, and a clinical root, almost completely formed of tooth structure, should be reinforced by a

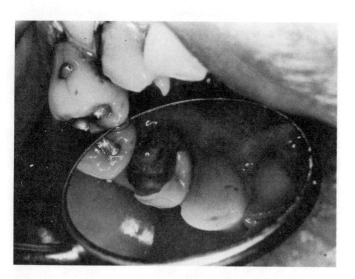

Fig. 28-24

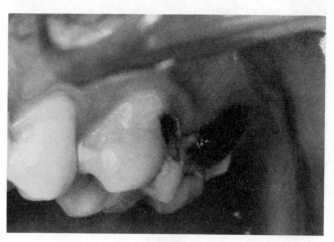

Fig. 28-25

material stronger than those forming the clinical crown and root.

VII. Occlusal Abnormalities That Change the Relative Position, Functionality, and Stress Pattern of Cuspal Elements

Such an evaluation should attempt to elucidate any localized abnormalities (Fig. 26), e.g., crossbite, tooth rotation, tilting, extrusion, intrusion, or version. It should be determined at this point if the tooth is going to be correctly repositioned by orthodontic treatment, in which case a provisional restoration must be placed and the final restorative design delayed until after successful orthodontic therapy.

However, if orthodontic treatment will not be undertaken, occluding restoration parts in both static and dynamic relationships should enter into the restorative design. The direction of tooth inclination or version should also be diagnosed and recorded, because the tooth preparation design and instrumentation will need to be modified according to these inclinations.

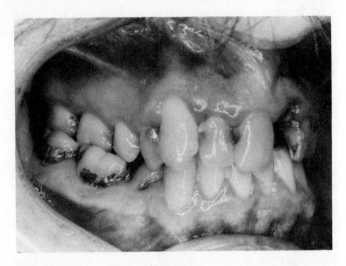

Fig. 28-26

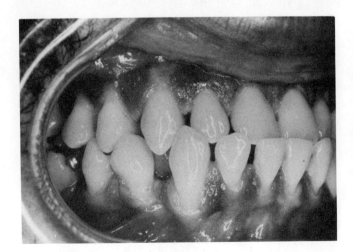

Fig. 28-27

Similarly, the direction of tooth rotation should be recognized and the clinical surfaces should be correlated to the anatomical ones. Through this correlation, too, the design and instrumentation for the restoration will be modified. In addition, the amount (percentage) of intrusion or extrusion should be recorded. If normal crown substances are placed subgingivally, or normal root anatomy areas located supragingivally, they should be recorded, because they will influence the restorative design. Finally, the entire stomatic-gnatho system should be examined by occlusal analysis in an effort to discover any abnormalities (e.g., interferences) that must be corrected prior to and via the restorative design and execution. This is done to assure that the restoration will not be detrimentally loaded in this unideal position.

Next, generalized occlusal abnormalities (Fig. 27) should be diagnosed and the possibility of orthodontic therapy should be explored. If such therapy is not feasible, the situation could be handled as with localized problems, although with less than adequate results. If they are minor localized occlusal abnormalities that can be corrected by restorations, e.g., edge-to-edge occluding teeth, minor crossbite, rotated teeth or misplaced teeth, etc., all efforts should be made to predict the stress pattern in the remaining tooth structure and future restoration that will make the normal occluding contact with opposing teeth.

VIII. The Possibility that the Tooth Will Be Used as an Abutment for a Prosthesis
(Fig. 28)

For example, if the restored tooth is to be one of the retainers for a fixed bridge or a removable partial denture, the restoration must be designed with a dual purpose.

In both situations, the additional stresses as well as their type, magnitude, direction, and concentrations in the restoration and remaining tooth structures, should be predicted with adequate safety margins. This is not difficult if the operator knows the type and direction of displacing forces on the prosthesis, and correlates them to the remaining tooth structure and the intended restorations.

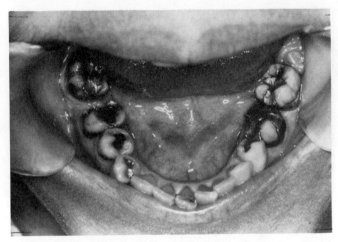

Fig. 28-28

IX. Determining Whether or Not the Tooth Will Be Splinted to Another Tooth as a Part of Overall Treatment, and, if so, if the Tooth is a "Splint*er*" or a "Splint*ee*"

The "Splint*er*" restoration and remaining tooth structures can accommodate more stresses than the "splint*ee*", which must partially depend on the "splint*er*" tooth for resistance and retention forms. If the splinted teeth are part of a prosthesis attachment or retainer, the "splint*er*" will invite even more stresses in addition to these already mentioned. Of course, it is not only the amount of lost tooth structure that decides whether the tooth be a "splint*er*" or a "splint*ee*", but it is also the amount of bone support around the tooth.

The amount, direction and concentration of stresses in the remaining tooth structure and replacing restoration of the splinter can be calculated with safety margins by combining the possible stresses in the splint*ee* and the prosthesis (if it is to be used) and add them to that of the splint*er* under normal loading situations. But initially one should recognize which tooth is the splint*er* and which one is a splint*ee* and plan our restorative design accordingly.

X. Relative Length of the Restored Clinical Crown to the Clinical Root

Normally, this ratio should be 1:3. The less that the ratio is, the stronger will be the resistance form of the entire tooth to the loading stresses. The resilience of the periodontal membrane and supporting bone is responsible for absorbing and dissipating most of the mechanical energy applied on the tooth. When these investing tissues are decreased in dimension, resulting in an increased crown:root ratio, much of the applied forces must be resisted by the tooth structures themselves. The stress is further exaggerated by increased surface area of tooth exposed to loading in an offset crown:root ratio. Therefore, when the contemplated restoration and/or the remaining crown structure will create a crown:root ratio more than 1:3, the restorative design should be modified to reduce the increased stresses. This may be accomplished, for example, by reducing dimensions of occluding surfaces, decreasing the steepness of inclined planes, rounding the occlusal terminations of cuspal elements, and minimally involving cuspal elements in excursive and disclusive mechanisms.

XI. Unusual Strength and Power in the Bite of the Patient and any Habits that Might Introduce Different and/or Additional Types of Magnitude and Directions of Stresses

These include bruxism, pipe smoking, tobacco chewing, ice chewing, etc. Once recognized and observed, they should be analyzed, recording the affected occluding cuspal elements, approximate magnitude, type and direction of expected stresses on the contemplated restoration. All of this will fa-

cilitate any design modifications which the situation might necessitate.

XII. Tilting of the Destructed Tooth

Such tilting may be due to original eruption pattern; or non-bodily drifting caused by, missing adjacent teeth, proximal tooth structure loss, or periodontal disease. When confronted with a broken down and tilted tooth, one should consider the ideal treatment, i.e., orthodontic uprighting. Several factors influence the decision to upright a tooth, including the amount and direction of tilt, the amount and condition of investing bone to be involved in the orthodontic movement, the root surface area of the tilted tooth and the changes in occluding cuspal elements and contacting tooth components which would result from uprighting; or any vertical or closing tendencies as indicated by the Y-axis, gonial angle, and mandibular angle. If the decision is made to upright the tooth, there are several techniques available to effect such movement, ranging from the same-arch anchor devices to opposing arch ones. The resulting conditions substantially simplify the restorations for such a tooth. An example of this technique is:

A. A removable appliance (modified Hawley) is constructed so that it will be retained by the rest of the teeth and contains an incisal inclined plane to release occlusion not to interfere with uprighting. Retracting springs, anchored to the appliance are attached to the tooth surface toward which the tilting occurred and activated in the reverse direction. The spring should be activated periodically.

B. A fixed appliance in the form of solidifying-tying together a good segment of teeth anterior or posterior to the tilted tooth, e.g., teeth ## 27, 28, 29, and 30, to act as an achorage to upright a tilted tooth, tooth # 31, (Fig. 29). All teeth are connected with an arch wire (sequential from 0.016 to 0.018 × 0.025"). In addition, there is an uprighting device, e.g., a Helix looped wire with a loop at the tilted tooth and free arm to be attached to the anchoring teeth' arch wire. The Helix loop is activated to place intrusion forces on the anchoring teeth and rotating extruding forces on the tilted tooth (Fig. 29). In both procedures periodic occlusal adjustments and frequent disclusion of teeth are needed to allow the uprighting movement.

On the other hand, if the decision is made to restore the tilted tooth as is, the operator must evaluate a different set of problems. For example, how the restorative design will deal with other than normal occluding surfaces, especially with some cuspal elements overloaded while others are not loaded at all. The restorative design might have to deal with exposed root anatomy and possibly a furcation on the side of the tooth opposite the tilt. Furthermore, when instrumenting tilted teeth, the operator must make a conscientious effort to avoid over-

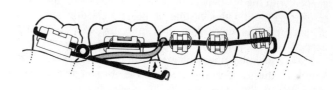

Fig. 28-29. Uprighting of tilted tooth #31.

cutting on one side and undercutting on the other (tilted) side. Similarly, when preparing internal retention modes, there is a very real danger of perforating either to the surface or the pulp.

At any rate, in evaluating these teeth for a restoration, one should look for the degree of tilting relative to the long axis of the tooth, using a radiograph. One should also explore if the loading in the tilted part is tolerated by investing periodontium, will further tilting occur, if the same type of loading is reproduced in the restoration, or will no further tilting happen due to opposing tooth contact preventing it. Finally consider the possibility of adequately preparing these teeth for restoration without the above mentioned hazards.

Planning the Restorative Design

Most of the restorative modalities have been described in detail elsewhere in this text. For restoration of badly broken down teeth, these modalities should be used intelligently where they are most indicated. These applications should be done with whatever modifications are necessary in order to achieve their goals successfully. During this part of the chapter an attempt will be made to describe in detail the treatment modifications and specific procedures required for certain exemplary cases. As of today, amalgams, casts or combinations of both are the only permanent restorative materials for posterior teeth. So, with this in mind, following are principles to be followed in the restorative design.

I. Management of Total or Partial Cuspal Loss

As mentioned before, the ideal length:width ratio of a totally self-resistant cusp is one or less. Therefore, when using amalgam, a material which depends on its resistance and retention form on remaining tooth structures,

A. If the average cusp length:width ratio is 2 or more on the functional side, the non-orbiting cusp should be capped or replaced completely with amalgam.

B. If the average ratio is 3 or more on the non-functional side, the orbiting cusps should be capped or replaced completely with amalgam.

In case of cast restorations, which are dependent on tooth structure only in their retention form.

C. If the cusp length:width ratio is more than 1 on the functional side, the cusp should be capped or replaced in cast material.

D. If the ratio is more than 2 on the non-functional side, the cusp should be capped or replaced in cast material.

E. Ideally, the width of a preparation should not exceed one-fourth to one-third the intercuspal distance, when restoring a tooth with amalgam, if the horizontal width of the preparation exceeds one-half the intercuspal distance, the cusp should be capped with the restorative material. On the other hand, when restoring a tooth with a casting, if the cavity width:intercuspal distance ratio is more than one:three, the cusps should be capped as well as be reinforced or protected in some way.

F. The ideal length of the axial wall is half (or more) of the length of the surrounding cavity walls. In restorations using amalgam, if the axial wall length is less than one-third the length of surrounding walls, capping of cusps is indicated. In cases involving cast restorations, if the axial wall length is less than one-half the length of surrounding walls, reinforcing or protecting those surrounding walls by capping cusps is indicated.

The specific design features for capping or replacing cusps with amalgam were described in detail under Class II, Design 6 cavity preparations. However, in addition to the features mentioned therein, a stress concentration area design feature should be added, as described earlier in this chapter.

The design features for capping, shoeing, or replacing cusps by castings were described in the chapter on design of tooth preparations for cast restorations. Further design features which should be added include:

1. Stress concentration area design features as described earlier in this chapter.

2. Facial or lingual "skirting" of shortened or badly thinned cusps, instead of counterbevels.

3. Expanded use of reverse secondary flares to tie preparation components together.

4. Extended, exaggerated bevels to reinforce minimally involved cusps.

II. Management of Total or Partial Loss of Axial Angles

When axial angles are to be involved, the maximum details of stress concentration area design features, as previously described, should be incorporated. In addition, there should not be any acute-angled marginal tooth structure at this area. Rather, margins should be right-angled, if using amalgam, and obtuse-angled, if using a casting. Also, the restorative material, if completely replacing the axial angle, should have its maximum bulk at that location, as compared to the other parts of the restoration. If a casting is the restorative mode, the axial angle could be protected or reinforced using skirts, reverse secondary flares, or collar extensions. Under no circumstances should retention features be placed at the site of a lost axial angle. Immobilization can be accomplished with retention features placed at other nearby locations.

III. Management of Partial or Complete Loss of Marginal and Crossing Ridges

Both amalgams and cast materials can either partially or totally replace marginal and crossing ridges. However, only casting can protect or reinforce these areas. Preparations for replacement can be as any of the previously described designs of a tooth preparation. Preparations for protection or reinforcement might take the form of extended bevels, overangulated bevels, counterbevels and sometimes skirts.

IV. Management of Partial or Complete Loss of the Crown-Root Junction

Using either amalgam alloys or cast materials, crown-root junctional areas can be replaced. Naturally, amalgam requires greater bulk than a cast material in this area. When using either material, do not put retention modes at the crown-root junction. Cast restorations can reinforce or protect thinned cross-sections of the area through the Ferrule effect, described in the chapter dealing with the restoration of root canal treated teeth. Cross linking retention modes are valuable in this area.

V. Management of Enamel Crazing (Microcracking)

If it is confirmed that a tooth demonstrates the signs and symptoms of cracked tooth syndrome, and/or if cracks are numerous and have an unlimited extent, care should be taken not to involve them in the tooth preparation. The tooth in these cases will need an amalgam foundation, then restoration with a reinforcing or protecting type of cast restoration, such as an onlay or full veneer casting, to splint together the separated portions of the tooth.

If cracks penetrate deep into dentin or to the pulp-root canal system and/or the periodontium, they should not be involved in the tooth preparation, as the tooth will need a restorative design as mentioned above. This may be done after endodontic therapy if the P-D organ has been affected beyond its reparative capabilities. If cracks are limited in number and penetrate enamel only, with no traces in dentin, enamelectomy may be performed and the reduced areas to be involved in the final cavity preparation.

If cracks are limited in number, and only part of the enamel is involved, enameloplasty can be tried until the cracks are eradicated. Then the thickness and nature of the remaining enamel should be evaluated relative to the future restoration. If this enamel is of sufficient dimension and maintains the capacity to support marginal tooth structure, it should be left untouched. Otherwise the area should be included in the final cavity preparation.

A. Stress receiving and stress inducing components of the tooth structure-restoration complex should be kept away from recognized involved weak areas of the tooth

Examples of this are: avoid putting tables and flat gingival floors over or near the furcation, don't use a subpulpal floor as a load receiving area, avoid putting retention modes in thinned dentin bridges or dentin around the furcation, and avoid directly loading thinned dentin bridges, etc.

B. Preparation margins should be located so that they do not contact opposing teeth during masticatory cycles

In such large restorations, there is great possibility of bending thinned cavity walls away from the restoration as in Fig. 30A and of moving the restoration away from the cavity walls as in Fig. 30B.

C. Junctions between different parts of the preparation must be rounded

This is especially true in junctions acting as fulcra, for reasons mentioned before.

D. Isthmus areas in the future restoration should be recognized, and an effort should be made to prevent failure there

This is carried out by increasing restorative material bulk and by bringing the fulcrum close to the area of anticipated maximum stresses, as described before.

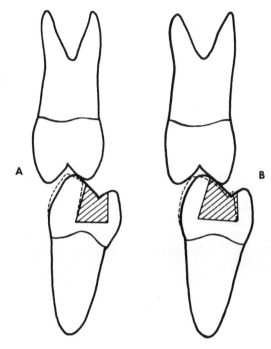

Fig. 28-30

E. Surface decalcifications or defects

If these are adjacent to the destruction (Figs. 26 and 28) to be involved in the preparation, they can be handled by either a boxed extension (for amalgam or casting), a grooved extension (for amalgam and casting), or secondary flares, reverse secondary flares, skirts, and elongated overangulated bevels (for cast restorations).

VI. Tilted Teeth

As previously discussed, the ideal treatment for tilted teeth is orthodontic uprighting, followed immediately by restoration. However, if orthodontic therapy is not feasible and/or if tilting is slight, the tooth is stable, and the surrounding periodontium can withstand loading, the tooth can be restored right away. However, certain modifications in the restorative designs will be warranted.

First, it will be necessary to allow maximum loading stresses to be applied away from the direction of inclination. This is possible by changing the tooth's occluding anatomy in the restoration in a way which creates maximum functional contact away from the inclination. However, this may necessitate additional reciprocal retention at the side toward which the tooth is tilted.

Second, the occluding surfaces should be built in such a way that the applied functional forces on the restoration will not predispose to further tilting. Both of these modifications should be executed without creating any centric or excursive interferences for physiological mandibular movements, or predisposing the investing periodontium to any breakdown.

Finally, it is important to visualize the tooth structure in three dimensions in its tilted position so as to avoid undercutting, overcutting, or perforations during tooth preparation.

VII. Crosslinkage Using Cemented Pins or Posts (Fig. 31)

Such additional retentive and resisting modes are indicated for four specific restorative situations:

A. Cases in which the occlusal one-third to one-half of a cusp have sufficient bulk to withstand stresses, but it is locally discontinued at its apical base by lateral spreading of the decay (Fig. 31A)

B. Cases in which there is an extensive cervical lesion (Class V) continuous with a Class II lesion (Fig. 31B)

C. Cases in which it is necessary to reinforce the junction between the anatomical crown with the anatomical root (Fig. 31C)

D. Teeth with incomplete fractures which make it necessary to join the partially separated segments together (Fig. 31D)

The technique for the first two indications is as follows:

1. The distance between the contemplated locations for the two opposing pin channels is measured, and a piece of wire 3-4 mm longer than the measured distance is cut and adjusted.

2. Pin channels are prepared. One should be deeper than the other (usually the root pin channel is the deeper one).

3. A pin should be tried and adjusted so that when it is seated to the full depth of the deeper channel, it does not penetrate the shallower one.

4. Cement is mixed and flowed into the pin channels. Also, the pin ends are soaked with cement. The pin is inserted into the deep channel, and aligned with the orifice of the shallower one. Then it is inserted into the shallow pin channel only to a depth that will not disengage it from the deeper channel. The procedure for indication (C) may be any cemented post technique as described in the chapter on pin- and post-retained restorations. The procedure for (D) is similar to that for (A) and (B), but it is in the horizontal direction. For indications A, B and D, cemented pins obliquely located and crossing each other could be used (Fig. 31A and D).

VIII. Retention Features

Different retentive modes have been mentioned and described in detail throughout this text, usually in conjunction with specified tooth preparation designs. In restoring badly broken down teeth any of these means may be used without the necessity of including the entire preparation design features that were described within. In addition, these basic retention features should follow certain rules of usage:

A. Always recognize and analyze the displacing forces on the anticipated restoration, observing and recording the origin, termination, and fulcrum of its movements. As practically as possible, locate the retention modes at one and preferably at both ends of the moving part away from the fulcrum.

B. The retention modes should fit the restorative technique and materials, e.g., counterbevels should not be used with amalgam alloys restorations.

C. Retention modes should not introduce intolerable stresses in the remaining sound tooth structures, e.g., threaded pins in root canal treated teeth.

D. Locking retentive modes should have sufficient tooth structure bulk in the area of the tooth that will receive stress as a result of this locking activity.

E. Retention modes should have sufficient tooth structure bulk, peripheral to them to be self-resistant.

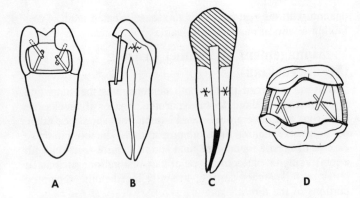

Fig. 28-31. A, Two vertically oblique reciprocating pins crossing each other. **B,** one vertical continuous pin. **C,** root canal post. **D,** obliquely horizontal pins crossing each other.

F. No single retention mode should work alone; rather, it should be augmented by auxillary and reciprocal means. This is to minimize failure and to decrease stress concentrations in both tooth structure and the restorative material.

G. A replacement of stress concentration areas should have a nearby retentive mode.

H. Retentive modes should be comparable in their locking capability to the magnitude of the displacing forces, and these locking components should be in the opposite direction to that of the displacing forces.

I. There should be complete compatibility, reciprocity, and synchronization between the retention and resistance forms of the tooth structure-restoration complex. If not contradicting and interfering with the resistance form, every segment of the preparation should have its own retention modes, if possible. This is to minimize interdependency of one part of the restoration on the other for retention, so that minimal stresses will be induced at junctional areas of the restoration.

J. Retention means should not compromise the biologic integrity of the involved tooth structures and surrounding oral tissues.

IX. Resistance Features

The only limitation to resistance form features is the clinician's imagination. Many of these design features have been mentioned throughout this text. As with retention form, although certain resistance modes have been described in conjunction with other designs, it is not necessary to use the other features of these designs when using its resistance modes.

In using the resistance features previously described, the following rules of usage should be observed:

A. As practically as possible, the resistance features in the remaining tooth structures should not be at the expense of the resistance features of the restorative material, and vice versa.

B. "Bulk" is the most efficient, practical, and most easily accommodated resistance feature.

C. Creating planes at right angles to anticipated loads is the second most effective resistance form. Of course, the greater that the dimensions of these planes are, the more will be the resistance. Also, the resistance effect of several planes is cumulative.

D. Junctional areas should be studied carefully and retention interdependency of the joined segments there should be evaluated. If such an interdependency is obvious, all possible resistance features should be placed there.

E. Resistance forms of the restoration and remaining tooth structures should be synchronized with occlusion in both its static and its dynamic form.

F. Details of the resistance features should be designed for both the restoration and remaining tooth structures, always minimizing shear stresses as much as possible.

G. Non-vital tooth structures (partially or totally) are the least resistant to stresses, especially in thin cross-sections. This is the reason why design features should include reinforcing and protecting aspects by a more resistant restorative material than the tooth structures, e.g., capping, skirt, collars, etc. For ideal resistance form, weakened tooth structures should be replaced or reinforced (Fig. 32) with a stronger restorative material. This is a condition that necessitates certain design features in the remaining tooth structure to fully utilize the reinforcing capabilities of these restorative materials (e.g., surface extensions, caps, shoes).

H. One resistance feature in a tooth preparation should not aggravate stress patterns in other areas of the preparation or the restoration.

J. As mentioned in the discussion of retention features, resistance features should be in complete cooperation with retention features without each nullifying the other's capabilities.

J. Resistance features should not interfere with the biologic integrity of the involved and surrounding tissues.

K. Resistant items in a preparation should direct forces along the most advantageous angulation for the tooth roots, investing bone, and periodontal ligament; i.e., along the long axis of the tooth.

L. Flat planes, at right angles to applied forces, will receive all the applied forces and react accordingly. If it is thought that the resisting status of the flat plane cannot withstand applied forces without failure, the effect of these forces can be reduced by inclining the plane. Stress reduction is proportional to the amount of the inclination. The inclination should preferably be directed to a more resisting item in the preparation.

X. Restorative Design Features for Endodontically Treated Teeth

After verifying the success of root canal therapy and collecting the necessary data the restorative design may be planned with the following considerations:

A. If marginal and crossing ridges are intact, amalgam restoration in a Class I, Design 8 can be the final restoration.

B. If one or more of the marginal ridges or crossing ridges are involved in the cavity preparation of an endodontically treated tooth, amalgam must act as a foundation for a reinforcing type of cast restoration.

C. If the pulp chamber has 2 mm and more dimensions in three directions, has dimensions amounting to one-fifth the amount of lost tooth structure, has at least two intact opposing walls, and one or more of its roots is sizable enough to accommodate amalgam to a depth of 4 mm, use Class I or II, Design 8 cavity preparation for an amalgam restoration or foundation.

D. Use posts and pins, as described in detail in the chapter

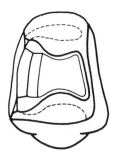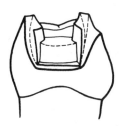

Tooth Preparation for Reinforcing-Protecting Restoration

Fig. 28-32

on pin- and post-retained restorations, if conditions mentioned in "C" are not fulfilled.

E. Any badly broken-down, endodontically-treated tooth (with one or more marginal ridges or crossing ridges lost) should have a foundation (substructure), usually in amalgam, under its restoration (superstructure) which is usually made of a cast material. This design is necessary to avoid further intraradicular instrumentation if this type of restoration should fail. Removing previous intraradicular retention modes usually invites root fracture (Fig. 38).

The amalgam foundation under a casting is also necessary to eliminate undercuts for the cast restoration tooth preparation without the necessity of sacrificing massive amounts of sound tooth structures. Furthermore, less micromovements of the restorations inside the root canals and pulp chamber occur if the restorative procedure is done in two parts, rather than one. This is because the inner portion (foundation) will be indirectly loaded, especially if the peripheral segments of the cast restoration are in contact with tooth structures. This arrangement also predisposes to less stresses in the pulp chamber and root canal walls, with a lowered possibility of fracture there.

More simplication and standardization of the restorative technique is accomplished if done in two segments, rather than one. Less intraradicular instrumentation with less residual stresses and always less tooth structure involvement is assured when using a two-piece restoration rather than a one-piece.

Amalgam is the ideal plastically inserted material for a foundation because of the following advantages:

1. Amalgam has minimum porosity if it is properly condensed.

2. Due to the inherent properties of the material and the incremental insertion procedure, accompanied by the condensation energy, amalgam will have the maximum adaptability to retention modes, tooth preparation surfaces, and details. As a result, the foundation will exhibit adequate strength and minimum leakage, a characteristic that improves with age (especially in the presence of a casting alloy covering a restoration).

3. Of all plastically inserted materials, the strength of amalgam is the most comparable to that of the wrought metal retentive modes and the restorative cast material.

4. Modern amalgam can be prepared for the superstructure reduction as soon as fifteen minutes after insertion.

5. Amalgam can be seen radiographically, facilitating future diagnostic procedures.

6. Amalgam can be completely dried from moisture, thereby

allowing adequate retention and setting of the luting cement for the covering casting.

7. Amalgam has a contrasting color from tooth structures. This characteristic can facilitate finishing and subsequent marginal removal of amalgam at barely accessible and visible areas gingivally.

The use of presently available composite resins as a foundation for a cast restoration superstructure should be restricted for several reasons. First of all, there is the difficulty of finishing and completely removing composite from margins subgingivally. This is a necessary step to allow the cast restoration superstructure to be the most peripheral material. This same drawback becomes worse, if the composite is not radiopaque. The high porosity of composite is an inherent characteristic (Fig. 33). Unfortunately, the bulk pack way of inserting it enhances this problem leading to extensive leakage problems, in addition to lowering its strength. The characteristic water sorption of composite resins, combined with this porosity, will lead to retainment of moisture despite attempts to dry it. This moisture content will prevent adhesion of any luting cement to the composite, or inhibit proper setting of the cement resulting in a possible cementation failure.

In addition to bodily and interfacial leakage between their components, composite resins show poor adaptability to retention modes and cavity details. This may lead to future leakage, with possible marginal break-down.

F. The Ferrule Feature

As mentioned in a chapter on pin- and post-retained restorations, the ferrule effect is the most important resistance feature in a restoration for an endodontically treated tooth. Utilizing this feature, the cast restoration should encompass the tooth circumferentially, bringing its components together to efficiently resist splitting and to assure maximum reinforcement for the remaining tooth structure (Fig. 34). To do this the cast restoration should involve sound tooth structure at least 2 mm apical to the gingival periphery of the foundation. This may take the form of a skirt, collar, counterbevel, veneer or exaggerated bevels.

XI. Restorative Design Features for Badly Broken Down, Periodontally Treated Teeth

Restoration of badly broken down periodontally treated teeth, especially those previously suffering from advanced periodontitis, or intentionally extruded, pose quite a challenge to the clinician.

The following are the areas in the restorative design that should be emphasized for previously periodontally affected but treated teeth:

A. Tooth preparation

Tooth preparation should emphasize the following features:
1. Try to put gingival margins supragingivally (Fig. 35).
2. When preparing for cast restorations, the bevels, especially the gingival bevels, should be exaggerated in extent and angulation in order to involve adjacent wear facets and root surface defects or root surface anatomical anomalies.
3. The preparation for a cast restoration should incorporate a variety of skirts, secondary flares, and reverse secondary flares to eradicate peripheral marginal undercuts created by the taper of any exposed root portion of the tooth.

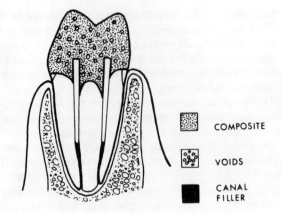

COMPOSITE

VOIDS

CANAL FILLER

Fig. 28-33

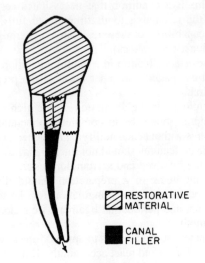

RESTORATIVE MATERIAL

CANAL FILLER

Fig. 28-34

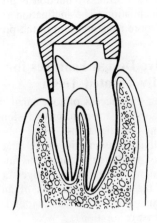

Fig. 28-35

4. Avoid placing any margin in the furcation. Maximally the margin may be at the very occlusal limit of its occlusal flutes. To involve the furcation will create a restored tooth with a doubtful cariogenic and periodontal prognosis. When confronted with margins that will end in the furcation proper, due to the extent of destruction, it is necessary to think of other

restorative modalities, e.g., hemisectioning or bicuspidization, as alternatives.

5. For all types of restorations, the preparation walls and floors in place of a flat, concave or fluted root surface areas should follow the same configuration as the replaced root surface. This is to avoid involving or encroaching on the root canal system, to create an even thickness of the restorative material, and to facilitate a definite surface termination at the margins.

6. A tooth preparation for a cast restoration that involves root surface concavities or flutes, besides having its walls (axial surfaces) replace these anatomies with the same configuration (concave or fluted), should have the established imitating configuration of these walls (axial surfaces) over the entire surface occluso-gingivally. This is necessary to assure absence of undercuts in the path of the preparation, and to facilitate a definite marginal termination gingivally.

7. For amalgam restorations the gingival floor will almost always be one-planed axio-proximally (facially or lingually).

8. For amalgam restorations proximally there are a number of indications for Class II, Designs 4 and 5.

9. The gingival floor margins and finishing lines that come close to a furcation should follow the apico-occlusal curvature of the furcation in the horizontal direction (Fig. 36).

10. Gingival floor or finishing lines immediately occlusal to a furcation should have an apical inclination (divergence) so as to dissipate and eliminate forces accumulation.

11. Gingival floors immediately occlusal to a furcation should be accompanied by mesial and distal (facial and lingual) flat ledges or gingival floors away from the furcation (Fig. 36). These flat-planed areas should have an inclination which is at right angles to the occluding forces (long axis of the tooth), so that no forces will concentrate stresses in the furcation tooth structures.

12. To facilitate plaque control in fluted areas of the root or inlets to the furcation, a simple widening of the flutes without restoration can be done. If the flute is to be produced in the restoration, but on a wider scale than originally present, the preparation wall (axial surfaces) at the fluted areas should have the same curvature and flare as the contemplated restoration, and not as the original flute.

B. Proximal contact and axial contour of the restoration

The final restoration for periodontally treated teeth, espe-

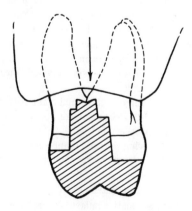

Fig. 28-36

cially those previously involved in an advanced periodontitis situation, should have certain modifications in their axial contour.

Occluso-apically, the contour should be less pronounced than usually found in teeth not previously affected with periodontitis. This is more applicable to the facial and lingual axial contour than to the proximal ones, and it should not interfere with the contour of the unrestored areas of the tooth. This configuration will improve the plaque control around the periodontium.

The surface configuration of the root anatomy, whether it is a concavity, flatness, or flute, if involved in the preparation, it should be reproduced with the same configuration in the final restoration. Furcation flutes, if reproduced in the final restoration, should involve the entire surface apico-occlusally to assure proper plaque control at the critical furcation area. Restorations involving part of the cemento-enamel junction, but away from the furcation, should have a flat surface area occlusal to the CEJ in a horizontal direction to assure the integrity of the area.

The horizontal axial contour of the restoration should follow the same contour as the replaced tooth surface to assure the biologic integrity of the adjacent periodontium. As mentioned before, replacing the tooth contour in these directions is more biologically important than replacing it in occluso-apical directions. Contact areas, too, should be in the most physiologic location, replacing any created facets there with the proper convex configuration.

C. Occluding surfaces and control of occlusal forces

After periodontal therapy, there usually are ungained bone losses compromising the ability of involved teeth to comply with physiologic occlusal loading. To add to the problem, many of the proprioceptive nerve endings within the periodontium are lost reducing the ability of the neuro-muscular mechanisms to recognize overloading on the invested tooth and to react accordingly. If this is the case with the tooth (teeth) being restored, certain modifications in restorative design must be considered.

If the restoration is to replace all occluding surfaces, the width of the occlusal table should be reduced, minimizing the amount of forces to be received by the tooth. The heights and inclinations of cuspal elements should also be reduced, to minimize lateral forces on the tooth.

If it is practically possible, the crown:root ratio should be decreased to improve the root resistance features of the tooth (e.g., in extruded teeth). This resistance is also enhanced by controlling parafunctional habits through occlusal splints, removal of interferences, and by building the restoration without excursive or centric interferences. Finally, if it is proven that the tooth (teeth) with this presented bone support cannot stand anticipated occlusal loading without failure, splinting should be considered in the restorative design.

XII. Splinting

Teeth splinting should be designed so that bone support of the splinted teeth is shared. Sometimes even the resistance and retention capability of the splinted teeth is shared. It is always advantageous to include a corner tooth with a long root in the splinting assembly and the splint should be designed so that the stronger tooth will receive the applied forces before the weaker. This will assure the weaker tooth is being indirectly loaded. The decision to splint can be controversial, and there are many factors involved:

1. If tooth mobility exceeds three to four degrees, endangering the integrity of the periodontal ligament and attaching bone and placing the tooth in a traumatic location, splinting should be considered.

2. If the tooth is required to play a major mechanical role in the dentition, e.g., if it is going to be an abutment for a fixed prosthesis or partial denture, and it has lost more than ⅓ of its bone support, it should be splinted to a stronger tooth. The same thing should be done if the tooth is going to be included in a disclusion mechanism of the mandible, etc. Usually, splinting should be considered in any overloading situation where the teeth have less than one-half to one-third of the maximum bone support remaining.

3. As part of periodontal therapy, if the tooth is to be immobilized to assure periodontal healing, it should be splinted.

4. A tooth may be splinted to improve resistance and retention form.

5. A tooth may be splinted to prevent further movement after orthodontic and/or periodontic therapy.

6. Several teeth may be splinted in order to create a restorative splint with a greater or lesser number (or dimensions) of teeth for functional or cosmetic reasons.

The number of teeth to be splinted will be decided upon by the number of teeth that need additional support (splintee) and, most importantly, the nature of needed bone support. This can be arrived at by determining the amount, location and type of supporting bone for the teeth (tooth) that need splinting (splintee). Accordingly, one can obtain the same information about

the lost bone. From this calculated data one can locate the needed nature of the bone support in adjacent teeth (splinters). For example, two splintees may need one splinter or one splintee may need two splinters, depending on the availability of the type, location and extent of the indicated supporting bone in the splinter.

Whether the splintee tooth should be between two splinters or peripheral to them is decided upon by the availability of splinter tooth. The first arrangement can be ideal but it cannot be fulfilled in every case, depending on the factors previously mentioned.

The type and amount of resistance and retention features in the splinter and splintee should be designed so that the splinter will have most of the share of locking and resisting. This may affect the number of teeth to be involved as certain number of splinters may not take care of the resistance-retention needs of the splintee(s).

The splint should be designed to immobilize the splinted teeth in the three possible directions. Adequate plaque control and readily accomplished maintenance should be assured in the choice and in designing of the splint. A choice between different types of splinting modalities can be arrived at after describing the available types and their indications.

Types of Teeth Splints

A. Provisional splints (Fig. 37)

1. Removable types
a. Occlusal splints, usually used for occlusal therapy, may have an attached facial arch wire to support the tooth (teeth) in the labio-lingual direction. The splint itself will immobilize

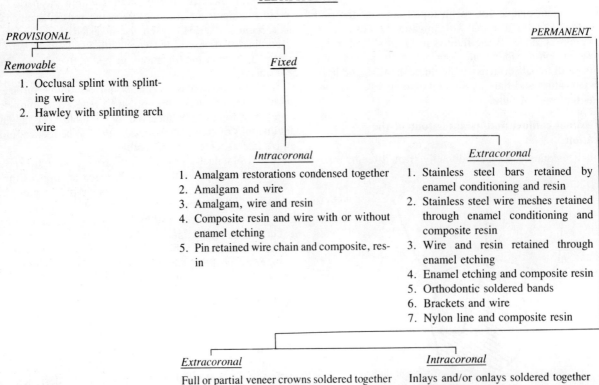

TEETH SPLINTS

PROVISIONAL — PERMANENT

Removable
1. Occlusal splint with splinting wire
2. Hawley with splinting arch wire

Fixed

Intracoronal
1. Amalgam restorations condensed together
2. Amalgam and wire
3. Amalgam, wire and resin
4. Composite resin and wire with or without enamel etching
5. Pin retained wire chain and composite, resin

Extracoronal
1. Stainless steel bars retained by enamel conditioning and resin
2. Stainless steel wire meshes retained through enamel conditioning and composite resin
3. Wire and resin retained through enamel etching
4. Enamel etching and composite resin
5. Orthodontic soldered bands
6. Brackets and wire
7. Nylon line and composite resin

Extracoronal
Full or partial veneer crowns soldered together

Intracoronal
Inlays and/or onlays soldered together

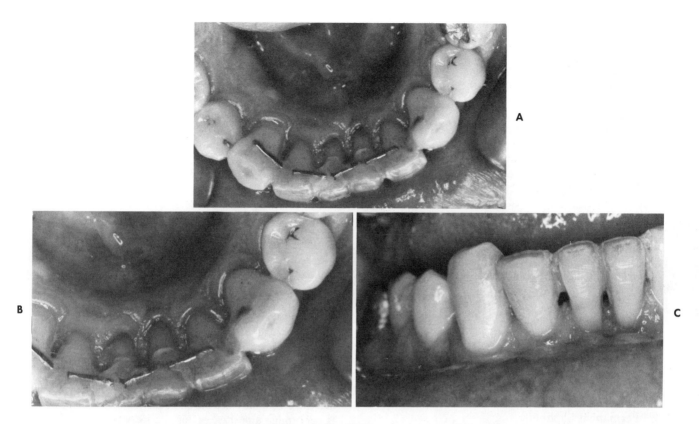

Fig. 28-37

the tooth in the mesial, distal, and occluso-apical direction. It is ideal if the splint is needed in conjunction with occlusal therapy. The main disadvantage of this removable splint is that its action is not continuous, except when the patient is wearing it.

b. The Hawley appliance with splinting facial arch wire is a regular Hawley appliance with a similar facial arch wire as in the occlusal splint. It produces the same action as the occlusal splint, with a possibility of more disengagement of the upper from the lower teeth during the immobilization period.

2. Fixed types

a. Intracoronal

i. MOD amalgam restorations condensed together in the involved teeth, making a one piece amalgam

Prior to condensation, all involved teeth are matriced and wedged at the same time. Then sufficient length and width of the intervening band material is cut (scissors or burs), so as to create bulky junctions between restorations. The remaining band material interproximally, together with the wedges and the matrixed gingival margin of the preparation, should not be disturbed in order to assure the creation of a physiologic gingival embrasure with adequate marginal adaptability. After condensation, the splinting amalgam should be carved to confirm adequate embrasures, especially gingivally.

ii. Amalgam and stainless steel wires

This intracoronal splint is similar to the confluent MOD amalgams, but after partially condensing the amalgam restoration over part of the proximal portion and covering part of the pulpal floor, stainless steel wires, in the diameter of 0.050″ or more, are laid mesio-distally across the preparations occlusal

to the condensed amalgam. More amalgam is then condensed over the wires.

iii. Amalgam-wire and resin intracoronal splints

These are usually indicated if amalgam restorations are already present or separate MOD amalgam restorations are to be built for the individual teeth. A fissure bur is used to cut a mesio-distal groove in the amalgam restoration, not involving all the contact areas. Then, with a 33¼ or ¼ bur, cut facial and lingual undercut retention in the created groove on the entire occlusal amalgam, mesio-distally. A wire is laid into the created groove and covered with composite resin.

iv. Another similar intracoronal splint involves placement of composite resin and wires in cut grooves, with or without acid etching (Fig. 37).

These grooves are cut at the mesial and distal aspects of a tooth, preferably away from occluding areas. The grooves should not cross the whole tooth mesio-distally (3-4 mm horizontal involvement is adequate), and they should be at least 2 mm deep with their lateral walls undercut. If enamel is available, it should be conditioned as mentioned before. Pieces of 0.050″ diameter wire are cut to fit these grooves connecting between the indicated teeth. Composite resin is mixed and some is introduced into the grooves, but not to fill them completely. Then the pieces of wire are inserted. Additional composite is then added to cover the wire and completely fill the grooves. The composite is then finished and polished in the usual way.

v. Fitting a wire chain within a continuous groove on the lingual surfaces of adjacent teeth

The chain may be stretched and stabilized using threaded pins to hold it against underlying dentin. The anchored chains are then covered with composite resin to complete groove obliteration.

These five techniques provide very stable splints, but they require regular adjustment, finishing, and polishing. In addition, plaque control is fairly difficult there, so it should be continuously emphasized to the patient.

b. Extracoronal

i. Many of the extracoronal provisional splints are very similar in that they involve acid etching of either facial or lingual enamel of adjacent teeth and imbedding either stainless steel bars (rectangular in cross-section), stainless steel wire mesh, or round stainless steel wire (.050″ in diameter), within composite resin bonded to the etched enamel. In fact, on anterior teeth with minimal displacing occlusal loading, composite alone, bonded to facial or lingual enamel, may suffice as a provisional splint.

ii. Orthodontic bands, properly fixed to involved teeth, may be soldered together and then cemented to serve as a provisional splint.

iii. Orthodontic brackets may be bonded to acid etched enamel with composite resin. Attaching an orthodontic wire to the brackets, either with elastics or with ligature wires, creates a provisional splint holding the involved teeth together.

iv. Finally, nylon line, which is similar to, but thicker and more rigid than fishing line, may be imbedded in composite resin that is bonded to acid-etched enamel facially or lingually.

B. "Permanent" splints

1. Extracoronal

"Permanent," extracoronal splints take the form of full or partial veneer crowns soldered together, or cast together.

2. Intracoronal

"Permanent" intracoronal splints take the form of inlays or onlays soldered or cast together.

Both types of permanent splints can have horizontal threaded or cemented pins to improve their attachment to the involved tooth. The joints between any splinting castings should be deviated occlusally. This facilitates a larger gingival embrasure for better plaque control. Between visits during the construction of a permanent splint, temporary or provisional restorations should be splinted together to assure tooth immobility during the cast fabrication.

The choice between these numerous types of splints is a matter of clinical evaluation and judgement. However, the following guidelines may be applied in the process of this evaluation:

a. If the involved teeth are intact and splinting is to be only temporary (e.g., a matter of months), in order to create the proper stability of the weaker teeth, the removable types of splints are most indicated.

b. Of course, provisional types of splints should be considered before the permanent ones if at all possible. This will facilitate evaluation of results and a decision about the validity of the entire idea of splinting for the particular situation. This is an especially valuable technique because splinting sometimes aggravates the periodontal situation more by complicating plaque control measures and by depriving the clinician from one of the most important diagnostic tools, i.e., tooth mobility.

c. Intracoronal provisional splints are the most stable of all provisional splints. They do not interfere with occlusion or normal architecture and maintenance of the oral and paraoral tissues. Furthermore, they can be used for several years.

d. Intracoronal provisional splints do require tooth structure removal (cavity preparation), which is, of course, a permanent change. This is the reason why they are the most indicated splints when there is already a restoration or lesion in the involved areas.

e. Extracoronal provisional splints are reversible, i.e., they do not necessitate any loss of tooth structure. However, they may interfere with normal activities of the cheek, lip and tongue and, to some extent, plaque removal and maintenance measures.

f. Intracoronal provisional splints can be the most inconspicuous splints, especially if formed out of composite resin.

g. The permanent intracoronal types of splints are the least irritating to the periodontium.

h. All permanent types of splints are the final restorations that the splinted teeth should have, if splinting is to be part of the restorative treatment plan for the life of these teeth.

i. Teeth splinted with provisional fixed splints should be evaluated after varying periods of time (one year or more), physically and radiographically, to ascertain the involved teeth's support and stability. If, after this evaluation, the involved teeth prove to be self-supporting, the splints should be removed and the teeth restored individually. If, however, support does not improve, permanent splints should be constructed and cemented, provided the clinician is convinced that splinting is performing a positive action, periodontally.

j. Usually, provisional removable splints are all that is needed. However, if after the designated time (e.g., four months) the objectives of splinting are not fulfilled, or if the individual teeth migrate back after not using the splint for a while, a fixed provisional splint should be built for the indicated teeth before a decision is made to permanently splint.

XIII. Foundations Versus Restorations

In many situations of badly broken down teeth, the tooth needs a foundation made either of amalgam or sometimes even composite resin. Following that, a permanent restoration is made of a cast material. The tooth preparation for an amalgam foundation is exactly the same as its preparation for an amalgam restoration. However, the tooth preparation for a final cast restoration of the tooth with a foundation is a little different from the tooth with no foundation. These differences will be elucidated later.

Indications for a Foundation (Build-Up) Prior to a Reinforcing-Protecting Cast Restoration

A foundation, or build-up may be indicated in one or more of the following situations:

1. Root canal treated teeth with one or more of their marginal or crossing ridges involved

2. In a tooth with all non-functional and/or half or more of the functional cusps to be replaced

3. A tooth to be used as an abutment for a fixed prosthesis or partial denture with one or more of its cusps completely lost

4. A second premolar or first molar (or any tooth with an

above average loading situation) with MOD or more involvement, including crossing ridges, with a width averaging ⅔ and more of the intercuspal distance

5. A tooth with the occlusal half (or more) of one of the axial angles of the non-functional side and/or the occlusal half (or more) of both axial angles on the functional side are lost, together with the adjacent cusps

6. A tooth with a deep axial cervical lesion facially and/or lingually, involving more than two of its axial angles and ⅔ or more of its occluso-apical dimension

7. If 60% or more of the tooth structure is lost and has to be replaced

8. For teeth that have some of their forming components cross-linked together with pins

9. For cracked teeth, teeth showing signs and symptoms of cracked-tooth syndrome, or teeth with multiple unlimited crazing (microcracks), to avoid further cracking or thinning of remaining tooth structures due to instrumentation, the tooth is built up in the most conservative preparation with an amalgam foundation. Then a cast restoration is used to cover (reinforce) and bind together the separated tooth segments, usually in an extracoronal fashion.

10. Amalgam foundations for the badly broken down tooth can function as a provisional restoration for very young patients, in dentitions with uncontrollable caries, or other situations when cast restorations are contraindicated. The foundation will serve as a provisional restoration until a more appropriate age and cariogenically controlled conditions occur. Then a cast restoration may be indicated.

11. For short or shortened teeth, in which it is biologically and mechanically safe to lengthen them with à foundation build-up prior to a cast restoration

12. In tilted teeth, when orthodontic uprighting is not feasible, crown portion uprighting can be done through foundations made of a cast alloy or amalgam, involving the whole crown. A cast restoration can be used over them, which, most of the time, is part of a fixed prosthesis, going in the insertion path direction of that prosthesis.

In all of these situations, build-ups are advisable for the following reasons:

a. Teeth with such destruction unavoidably accommodate multiple undercuts in the path of a preparation for cast restoration. Trying to eliminate these undercuts can lead to unnecessary loss of vitally needed sound tooth structures in such an already weakened tooth. Building the tooth up with an amalgam foundation can safely obliterate such undercuts, while preserving sound tooth structure.

b. Foundation material will occupy some of the space created by the lost tooth structure, thereby minimizing the amount of casting material (especially expensive noble metals) for the covering restoration.

c. Amalgam, or any foundation material, will be in direct contact with the weakened tooth structure to be covered with the cast restoration. When this composite structure (tooth + foundation + restoration) is loaded during function, weakened tooth structures will be stressed the least, as forces will be indirectly delivered to them through the amalgam or any other foundation material used.

d. In badly broken down teeth indicated for cast restorations, with deep involvement axially and pulpally, amalgam as a foundation material will seal the avenues to the pulp chamber and root canal system. This is facilitated by its good adaptability, minimal leakage, and improved sealability with age, especially in the presence of a cast alloy over it. These advantages cannot be exhibited by a cast restoration alone.

e. In deep cavity preparations indicated for cast restorations, amalgam as a foundation external to the proper intermediary basing (subbase plus base or varnish), can incorporate two or more insulating media to different environmental shocks. This includes the cementing media of the cast restoration, as well as the amalgam itself, as an insulating medium.

f. Using amalgam (or any other material) to build-up lost cusps or axial angles of a tooth will establish ideal reciprocal retention forms for a cast restoration covering them.

g. With amalgam (or any other material) as a build-up material, axial surfaces and other components of a tooth will work as auxillary retention forms for the covering cast restoration.

Both situations mentioned in (f) and (g) are not realized if the tooth is to be restored directly by a cast restoration alone.

h. In situations when the bucco-lingual width of an occlusal involvement of a tooth to be restored in cast restoration exceeded ¾-⅘ the intercuspal distance, the remaining cuspal elements are so thin that directly capping the cusps with cast restorations will be impossible without completely losing them together with the axial length of the preparation. This, in turn, will decrease the resistance and the retention forms. Building the tooth in amalgam first will facilitate keeping all or part of these cusps. Where the lost part is replaced in amalgam, the tooth preparation for the casting is not deprived of its needed axial length and its vitally required cuspal tooth structures.

i. In deep, wide, cervical lesions involving multiple axial angles, amalgam foundations can minimize axial depth for the cast preparation, eliminate distorting axial cavities and minimize trauma to the very close pulp tissues.

j. By building-up badly broken down teeth to a fairly regularly shaped tooth with an amalgam foundation, the tooth preparation design for a cast restoration and its execution can be greatly simplified, with little modification from the norm. This saves money, time and effort, in addition to assuring more possibilities of success.

k. If marginal failure occurs to the final cast restoration in the future, the foundation might still be intact, so deep re-entry to the cavity preparation may not be necessary, minimizing irritation (Fig. 38).

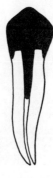

Fig. 28-38. Marginal failure for this cast restoration will necessitate further intracanalicular instrumentation which could be detrimental for the entire tooth.

l. In restoring some extensively destroyed teeth, pins and other prepared or premade retention modes may be necessary. Incorporating them in an amalgam foundation to be covered by a pinless (postless) cast restoration is more feasible and practical than involving those premade retention modes in the cast restoration. This is because a cast restoration without pre-made retention modes is much easier to fabricate. Also, these pinless (postless) cast restorations are, mechanically, better tolerated by the tooth than pin-containing (post containing) cast restorations without a foundation.

XIV. Design Features of a Tooth Built-Up in an Amalgam Foundation (or Any Other Material) Prior to a Protecting/Reinforcing Cast Restoration

In addition to the different features for preparations, for cast restorations already described in detail, the following should also be fulfilled:

No intracoronal preparation should be performed into an amalgam foundation, i.e., if the amalgam foundation involves the entire occlusal surface or part of it, preparing it for a casting restoration should be in the form of surface occlusal reduction, like preparations for full veneer restorations (Fig. 39). *Do not prepare external boxes, internal boxes, or grooves in the amalgam foundation*. Any of these can create thin amalgam walls, reducing the bulk of amalgam and subjecting it to stress concentration beyond its tolerance (Fig. 40).

The margins for the cast restoration should be located on sound tooth structure, 2 mm or more apical to the gingival margin of the foundation (Fig. 41). This will facilitate adequate finishing lines or other types of termination for the cast restorations. Furthermore, it will assure minimal ion and electron transfer back and forth between the amalgam and the cast alloy. Such galvanic current is of some clinical significance. The resulting corrosion and accelerated deterioration of underlying amalgam could leave vacancies in the immediate area (e.g. open margins), resulting in increased microleakage. Locating the casting margins on sound tooth will also allow the resto-

ration's lateral resistance and retention modes to directly involve this strong, unattacked part of the tooth structure. This, in turn, results in a maximum ferrule effect. Furthermore, locating casting margins on sound tooth structure imposes only one interface marginally, as opposed to two or more interfaces.

In addition to having a direct contact with tooth structures marginally, it is preferable for the cast restoration to have two pairs of opposing flat planes in tooth structure at right angle to occluding forces and the long axis of the tooth (Fig. 42). These can be in the form of ledges, floors, tables, or combinations of these. Besides giving the advantages mentioned previously, flat planes can make most of the occluding forces delivered directly to the intact, strong, better part of the underlying tooth structure. This minimizes loading on the foundation. At least 1.5 mm amalgam thickness should be left under the cast material, especially over tables (Fig. 43) and pins (Fig. 41), to provide self-resistance.

Under no circumstances should the amalgam foundation accommodate boxes, grooves, or any other intracoronal retention modes for the cast restoration (Fig. 40). As a result of preparing the two pairs of flat opposing planes mentioned above, intracoronal lateral walls in amalgam may be produced as a by-product. In this case, the internal and external peripheries of these walls should be extremely rounded (Fig. 42).

An amalgam foundation should never be used as a location for a premade retention mode, e.g., pins. It should be re-emphasized that the *only* retention the foundation should supply is reciprocal and auxillary retention through its surface area and lateral frictional locking as a whole.

In preparing finishing lines or flat planes in tooth structure beyond an amalgam foundation, clear the margin of amalgam (composite) creating a ledge (underhang). Then extend the preparation axially (for flat plane), or apically (for bevels or finishing lines, etc.)

From all of these design features it should be evident that the use of a foundation preceding a cast restoration must be planned ahead. The decision to build-up a foundation should not be made after restoring the tooth, when the need for a reinforcing/protecting restorative modality is recognized.

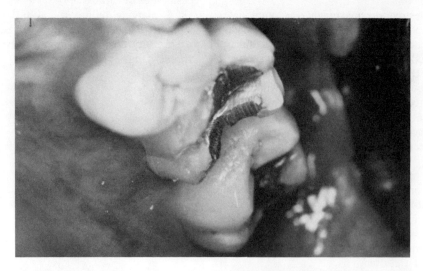

Fig. 28-39. Preparing a tooth for an onlay restoration, the occlusal reduction of the amalgam foundation is similar to that for full veneer crown.

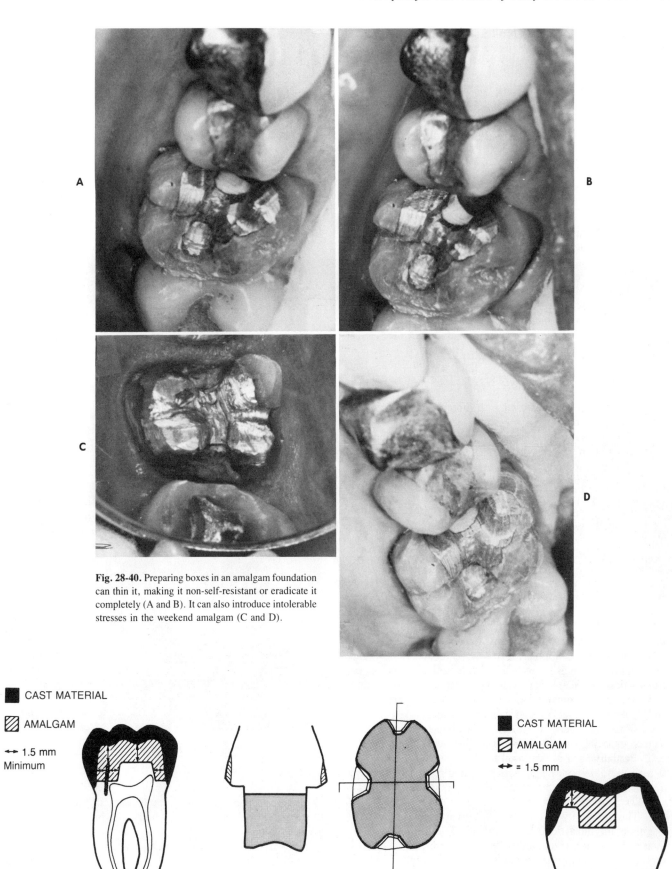

Fig. 28-40. Preparing boxes in an amalgam foundation can thin it, making it non-self-resistant or eradicate it completely (A and B). It can also introduce intolerable stresses in the weekend amalgam (C and D).

■ CAST MATERIAL

▨ AMALGAM

↔ 1.5 mm
Minimum

Fig. 28-41

Fig. 28-42

■ CAST MATERIAL

▨ AMALGAM

↔ = 1.5 mm

Fig. 28-43

Anterior Teeth

In restoring badly broken down anterior teeth (Figs. 44 and 45) many of the same design features mentioned for posterior teeth will be utilized. In anterior teeth, restorations should be done using tooth-colored materials, with the exception of three situations in which metallic, non-tooth-colored materials may be used. These situations are *the distal of the cuspids, foundations for reinforcing cast restorations,* or as *a substructure for a porcelain superstructure.*

The following are the suggested sequences in which badly broken down anterior teeth are evaluated, prepared and restored:

A. First, evaluate the status of the P-D organ and the attaching periodontium, as mentioned before.

B. Second, clear surrounding walls of irreparably attacked and unwanted enamel and dentin and apply the appropriate intermediary base.

C. Mechanically evaluate remaining tooth structure.

Because of the limited tooth volume in anterior teeth, their peculiar loading situation (anterior determinant of mandibular movement), esthetic requirements, etc., thorough mechanical evaluation of the remaining tooth structure as well as the contemplated restoration is essential. This evaluation should take into consideration one of the following three restorative possibilities:

I. Can the tooth be restored with direct tooth colored materials or amalgam?

II. Can the tooth be restored directly with a cast or cast-based restoration? What type?

III. Must the tooth be first built up with a foundation before being restored with a reinforcing/protecting cast or cast-based restoration?

Of the above-mentioned choices, of course, the one affording maximum restorative benefit with the least amount of tooth involvement should be the restorative plan. All of these decisions should be made after comprehensive evaluation of the loading situation (both static and dynamic), together with recalling probable stress patterns in anterior teeth (see Chapter 10). All of this must be correlated not only to the remaining tooth components, but also to the areas to be replaced.

The correlative evaluation of anticipated stress patterns should emphasize certain salient features:

a. Stress concentration areas of anterior teeth include lingual marginal ridges, incisal angles and ridges, axial angles, lingual concavities, cervical areas, and the distal surface of canines

b. Transverse and vertical components of force during static and dynamic contacts of upper and lower teeth

c. Weakened areas, e.g., undermined enamel and incisal angles, especially when destruction approaches these areas

d. Partially vital or non-vital tooth or parts of a tooth

e. Types, points of application, and direction of possible displacing forces on the contemplated restoration (Figs. 46 and 47)

f. The possibility of creating a gingival floor

This is the most important resistance feature in a proximo-incisal restoration (foundation) for an anterior tooth. It is essential to pre-operatively evaluate: whether the gingival floor will consist of enamel and dentin, or just dentin; its proximity to the area of application of forces; the amount of dentinal bulk

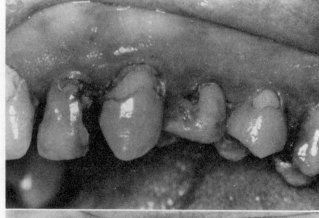

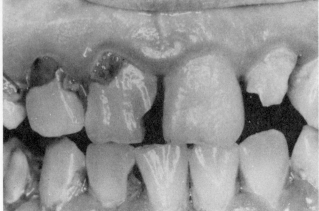

Fig. 28-44

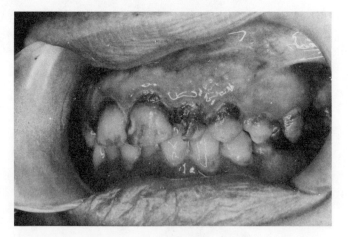

Fig. 28-45

available for retention modes; the location of the floor relative to surrounding anatomy; and, finally, the location of the gingival floor relative to the C.E.J.

g. Overlapping of teeth, which sometimes aggravates stress situations, and other times prevents any loading whatsoever

In addition, overlapping changes the carogenic susceptibility of involved surfaces.

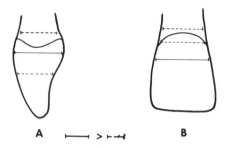

Gingival Floor at ⊢——⊣ Is More Advantageous Mechanically
Than at ⊢—⊣ Position

Fig. 28-46

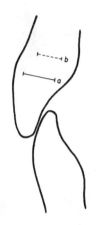

Gingival Floor at Position *a* Is More
Preferable Than at Position *b*

Fig. 28-47

h. Cracks and crazing, which are managed exactly as in posterior teeth (Fig. 48)

i. Tooth thickness labio-lingually at the incisal ridge and angle

The higher this measurement, the greater the resistance capability of the entire tooth.

j. The dimensions of destruction relative to the dimensions of remaining tooth structure

The higher that this rating is, the more favorable becomes the third restorative option, i.e., a foundation to be covered with a casting or a casting based restoration.

D. Esthetic concerns

Before restoring any anterior tooth, it should be evaluated esthetically for design features with the best cosmetic results. Any surface discoloration beyond the major defect should be examined to see its extent and to determine if bleaching is feasible, or if it is necessary to include in the tooth preparation. In many circumstances, a complete veneering with a cast-moldable ceramic or cast based porcelain crown is indicated.

Usually, the esthetic concern for the upper teeth is greater than for the lower. In addition, cosmetic problems are more obvious and demanding on the mesial aspects of these teeth than the distal. Of course, labial destruction is more disfiguring cosmetically than at any other location on the tooth.

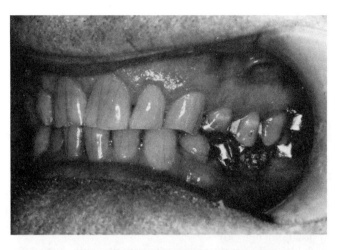

Fig. 28-48

Lip lines, during both speaking and singing, define the conspicuous areas of the teeth. In fact, their location can definitely affect the location of margins. An open-mouth smile should be observed, as well, to ascertain the number of teeth displayed and the predicted conspicuousness of a restoration.

The possibility of improving esthetics by extending, over-contouring, or otherwise changing the configuration of the tooth should be considered and enter into the overall plan of treatment. This should also include esthetic reshaping of adjacent teeth, to be undertaken prior to or after restorative treatment. The possibility of making the upper incisor ridge line parallel to the top of the lower lip to improve esthetics should also be considered. All of these esthetic considerations must, of course, not compromise the phonetic, anatomic, or anti-cariogenic necessities of the tissues involved.

E. Phonetic considerations

It is a well established fact that speech impairment can result from some loss of anterior tooth structure. The degree of impairment should be identified and corrective restorative measures undertaken, specifically using the following:

1. Evaluate "F" sounds, during pronunciation of which the incisal edges of the upper incisors touch the vermillion border of the lower lip.

2. Evaluate "V" sounds, during pronunciation of which the incisal edges of the upper incisors touch the inner side of the lower lip, just within the vermillion border.

3. Evaluate "S" sounds, during pronunciation of which the incisal edges of the lower anteriors come into the closest possible proximity of the lingual surfaces of the upper anteriors that is short of actual contact.

Phonetics, likewise, should not compromise esthetic, anatomic, or anti-cariogenic requirements of the involved teeth.

Planning the Restorative Treatment Design

At this stage the amount and nature of remaining tooth structure can be positively recognized and/or predicted, and the operator should have adequate data to choose between the three possible routes for restoring the tooth (teeth) in question.

I. Build the Tooth Up with a Foundation Form (Substructure) to be Covered with a Reinforcing/Protecting Restoration (Superstructure) (Fig. 49)

Usually, a ceramic or porcelain fused to cast veneer restoration is the superstructure of choice. It is indicated in the following situations:

1. A root canal treated tooth, if any proximal surface is involved

2. Loss of the two incisal angles together with more than half the proximal surfaces of the tooth

3. Loss of more than 50% of the tooth structure (Fig. 50)

4. Loss of more than one axial angle to a depth more than the anticipated axial reduction for the reinforcing/protecting restoration (Fig. 50)

5. A cracked tooth or one with multiple, unlimited crazing in its enamel, and/or with defects at axial depths deeper than the axial reduction for the veneering crown

6. A shortened tooth due to the nature of the destruction or to the removal of undermined undesirable tooth structures

7. A tooth to be used as an abutment for a fixed prosthesis or partial denture and whose defect involves one or more of the stress concentration areas to a depth more than the usual reduction for the moldable ceramic or cast based porcelain restorations

8. Multiple defects (Class III, IV, and V) in the same tooth (Fig. 50), having depths more than the axial reduction of a veneer crown and having a lot of undercuts

9. Remaining tooth structure accommodating multiple undercuts, the elimination of which could be detrimental to self-resistance of the remaining tooth structures

As previously pointed out for posterior teeth, foundations are the ideal solution to obliterate them.

10. Similar indications as for posterior teeth, especially for the distal of the cuspid

Anterior foundations, too, are preferably made in amalgam, but sometimes in composite resins and rarely in cast alloy. Despite the material, they should have internal dentinal retention forms (refer to the chapter on pin- and post-retained restorations and the chapter on cast restorations). Enamel etching (conditioning) should not be used as a primary means of retention here.

The choice of amalgam as a foundation is the most preferable for the same reasons mentioned for posterior teeth. The foundation design features, too, are very similar to those mentioned for posterior teeth.

II. Reinforcing/Protecting Restoration Without a Foundation or Build-Up

A moldable ceramic casting or porcelain fused to cast crown is, again, the treatment of choice. It is indicated in the following situations:

1. In all situations mentioned for Choice I, where the depth of the defect does not exceed the regular axial reduction depth for the contemplated cast or cast based porcelain restoration

2. Remaining tooth structure with the necessary axial length to retain the reinforcing-protecting restoration

3. In all situations mentioned for Choice I where the defects

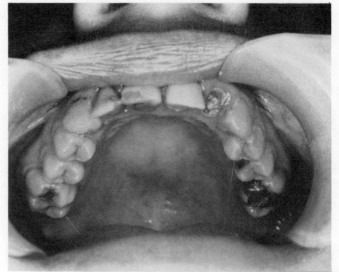

A

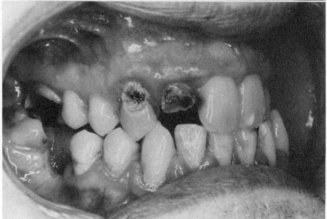

B

Fig. 28-49

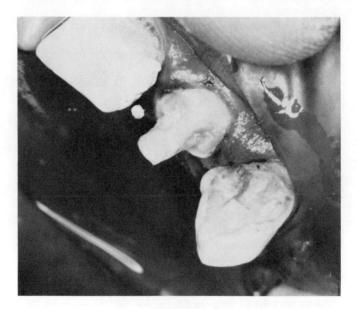

Fig. 28-50

do not create multiple undercuts that cannot be eradicated by the preparation for the protecting-reinforcing cast or cast based porcelain restorations

4. In situations where permanent discoloration in tooth structures is beyond the resolving limit of conservative restorative modalities, i.e., direct tooth color restorations with or without acid conditioning, or bleaching, or laminated veneering, etc. Complete veneering tooth-colored restorations will be the only indicated restorative modality.

5. Both labial and lingual walls are completely lost bilaterally, plus the incisal angles and the remaining tooth structures have insufficient enamel to be conditioned for proper retention

6. Lost tooth structure replacement in direct tooth-colored material can only be retained with auxillary means of retention

7. Distal of a cuspid destruction indicated to be restored in cast material

III. Restoration with Direct Tooth-Colored Materials

It is indicated for situations not necessitating aforementioned choices I and II.

The following should be done:

1. Recognize the access direction. This decision is dictated by esthetics (lingual) and the extent of the destruction (either labial or lingual), as mentioned before.

2. Recognize the nature of the remaining enamel. As enamel can be used for retention in some direct tooth-colored material restorations, its absence will dictate other types of retention. If enamel is present, its thickness, configuration, and undermined nature should be noted, especially around the defects. The existence of hypoplasia and/or hypocalcification must be evaluated. If permanently and conspicuously discolored enamel is to be eliminated, the operator must weight the removal of such discoloration against the possibility of loss of retentive ability (see Chapter 10).

3. The operator must strive to create a gingival floor in keeping with the specifications previously mentioned (see chapter on direct tooth-colored materials). The gingival floor must be prepared as pronounced, surfacewise, as possible, and at a right angle to the long axis of the tooth, if possible (Figs. 46 and 47). It may be prepared at different levels with different segments, if the destruction will not allow only one level. The gingival floor must be placed as close to the loading location as possible. It should contain the most locking retention means as possible, as it will be in a location to best resist displacing forces. If the adjacent gingival enamel is amenable to etching, the operator should create hollow-ground bevels to provide more surface area for etching.

4. An effort to keep the incisal angle should be made. The loss of this angle will drastically complicate the mechanical problems of the restoration. Maintaining the viability of the angle is possible if the operator can at least keep part of it, refrain from putting incisal retention if the incisal margin is close, and does not make any angulation in the incisal wall that may undermine the incisal angle or accentuate the incisoaxial angle if it comes close to the incisal angle.

5. If possible, the operator should create a labial and/or lingual wall, a vitally important criterion for the retention and resistance of the restoration (if it is intracoronal) as well as for the remaining tooth structure. The possibility of these walls should be evaluated according to the following criteria:

a. Could the preparation have *both* labial and lingual walls or only one? If it can only have one, will it be at the occluding or non-occluding side? Of course, two walls are preferable to one. But if only one is possible, it is preferable to have it on the occluding side rather than on the non-occluding side. In both preferred situations, it will be possible to have occluding forces indirectly delivered to the restoration. Accordingly, the presence of these walls dramatically improves the resistance and retention forms.

b. Can the wall(s) be one- or two-planed? Of course, two planes with one of them at a right (acute) angle to the axial wall are more resisting and retaining than one plane diverging proximally. A one-planed wall at a right (acute) angle to the axial wall will be the most advantageous, but it may be impossible to prepare because of anatomic and cariogenic limitations.

c. The more that the anticipated axio-proximal dimensions of the walls are, the better will be the resisting and retaining capability of these walls.

d. The more that the anticipated inciso-gingival dimensions of the walls are, the better will be their retaining capabilities.

e. An increased percentage of undermined enamel in the wall will increase retention form, but will concurrently reduce the resistance capability of the replacement–tooth structure complex.

f. The larger that the angle at which the labial and lingual walls meet incisally is, the better will be the resistance form of the restoration (foundation). This is because they will accommodate bulkier material there. In addition, there will be a greater possibility of accommodating a bulky incisal retention form within this angle.

g. The more right or acute-angled that the junction is between the labial and lingual walls with the axial wall, the more will be the retention form.

h. As the area of the anterior tooth just incisal to the cemento-enamel junction is the bulkiest portion of this tooth, if the labial and lingual walls involve part of this bulky area, they can accommodate a sizable retention form.

i. Similarly, the amount of dentin the labial and lingual walls contain affects the size of retention grooves that can be placed in each without undermining any enamel.

j. If it is necessary to create better labial and lingual walls, extend the gingival floor apically, involving sound tooth structures to accommodate at least short labial and lingual walls. Every surrounding wall in any dimension will add to the resistance-retention of the restoration-tooth structure complex. Furthermore, their effect is cumulative.

k. The labial and lingual walls should create rounded line and point angles with the axial walls.

6. Prepare and condition the enamel circumferential to the destruction (preparation) in the way described in a chapter on direct tooth-colored restorations.

7. With the exception of enamel etching, these items can be applied when preparing the tooth for a foundation prior to the reinforcing protecting restorations.

8. The rest of the principles are as described for posterior

teeth, and are in the chapters on direct tooth-colored restorations.

BIBLIOGRAPHY

Amsterdam, M., and Rossman, S.K.: Technique of hemisection of multirooted teeth, Alpha Omegan **53:**4-15, 1960.

Baum et al.: Operative Dentistry. Phildadelphia, Saunders, 1981.

Black, G.V., and Black, A.P.: A work on operative dentistry. Vol. I and II, 6th ed. Chicago, Medico-Dental Pub., 1924.

Charbenear et al.: Principles and practice of operative dentistry. Philadelphia, Lea and Febiger, 1980.

Gilmore, H.W., et al.: Operative Dentistry. 3d ed. St. Louis, The C.V. Mosby Co., 1977.

Ingber, J.S.: Forced eruption. Part I: A method of treating isolated one and two wall infrabony osseous defects. Rationale and case report. J. Periodont. **45:**199, 1974.

Ingber, J.S.: Forced eruption: Part II: A method of treating nonrestorable teeth, periodontal and restorative considerations. J. Periodont. **47:**203, 1976.

McGhee, W.H., True, H., and Inskipp, F.E.: A textbook of operative dentistry. New York, McGraw-Hill, 1956.

Palomo, F., and Kopczyk, R.A.: Rationale and methods for crown lengthening. J. Am. Dent. Assn. **96:**257, 1978.

Penny, R.E., and Kraal, J.H.: Crown-to-root ratio: Its significance in restorative dentistry. J. Prosth. Dent. **42:**34, 1979.

Rosen, H.: Operative procedures on mutilated endodontically treated teeth. J. Prosth. Dent. **11:**973-986, 1961.

Rosen, H., and Gitnick, P.J.: Integrating restorative procedures into the treatment of periodontal disease. J. Prosth. Dent. **14:**343-354, 1964.

Index